Rockwell Model 3
Slide Rule Memory
Electronic Calculator

Audiological Assessment

Edited by
Darrell E. Rose, Ph.D.
Mayo Clinic
Rochester, Minnesota

PRENTICE-HALL, INC., ENGLEWOOD CLIFFS, NEW JERSEY

PRENTICE-HALL INTERNATIONAL, INC., London
PRENTICE-HALL OF AUSTRALIA, PTY. LTD., Sydney
PRENTICE-HALL OF CANADA, LTD., Toronto
PRENTICE-HALL OF INDIA PRIVATE LIMITED, New Delhi
PRENTICE-HALL OF JAPAN, INC., Tokyo

13-050807-1

Library of Congress Catalog Card Number: 71-123408

Printed in the United States of America

Current printing (last number):

10 9 8 7 6

Contributors

Jerome G. Alpiner, Ph.D.
University of Denver
Denver, Colorado

Kenneth W. Berger, Ph.D.
Kent State University
Kent, Ohio

William T. Brandy, Ph.D.
West Virginia University
Morgantown, West Virginia

D. Thane R. Cody, Ph.D.,M.D.
Mayo Clinic
Rochester, Minnesota

Samuel G. Fletcher, Ph.D.
Alabama Medical Center
Birmingham, Alabama

Noel D. Matkin, Ph.D.
Northwestern University
Evanston, Illinois

Geary A. McCandless, Ph.D.
University of Utah
Salt Lake City, Utah

Eugene D. Mindel, Ph.D.,M.D.
Michael Reese Hospital and Medical Center
Chicago, Illinois

Joseph P. Millin, Ph.D.
Kent State University
Kent, Ohio

Wayne O. Olsen, Ph.D.
Northwestern University
Chicago, Illinois

Lloyd L. Price, Ph.D.
Florida State University
Tallahassee, Florida

Paul A. Rittmanic, Ph.D.
Department of Mental Health
Dixon, Illinois

David C. Shepherd, Ph.D.
Syracuse University
Syracuse, New York

Gerald A. Studebaker, Ph.D.
University of Oklahoma School of Medicine
Oklahoma City, Oklahoma

Jack Tompkins, Ph.D.
Texas State Technical Institute
Waco, Texas

McCay Vernon, Ph.D.
West Maryland University
Westminster, Maryland

Jack A. Willeford, Ph.D.
Colorado State University
Fort Collins, Colorado

Preface

As the field of audiology has grown into a full-fledged profession, the amount of information necessary for the student to have at hand has become prohibitive in its original form. Although there are a number of excellent texts relative to audiology, there is not a wide coverage of the methods used in audiological assessment. This book delineates what the authors feel are some of the most important concepts in audiology, with particular emphasis on the administration of specific tests and the analysis of test results.

The editor wishes to point out to the new student that none of the material presented is meant to be a definitive answer to the problems resulting from hearing loss, but is instead intended to lead to a better comprehension of the field of audiology. The book is designed to be more of a guide to an understanding of the functions of tests rather than an all-inclusive coverage of the field or a "how to do it" cookbook on testing techniques.

It will become obvious to the reader that only a mild attempt has been made to have the chapters conform to any set organizational scheme. The authors, in many cases, have not attempted to hide their biases on specific topics. But with the exception of the chapter by Vernon and Mindel (*Psycho-*

logical and Psychiatric Aspects of Profound Hearing Loss), no strict philosophies are evidenced, although underlying each chapter are strong, if unstated, philosophies.

Prior to publication, this chapter by Vernon and Mindel created some controversy; however, whether or not you are in favor of the manual method of educating the deaf, this chapter will prove interesting. It was only after working for two years with *deaf* adults that the editor gained an appreciation of the magnitude of the social and educational problems facing individuals who are educationally deaf. Based upon this experience and upon a thorough study of the chapter by Vernon and Mindel, the editor finds it difficult to disagree with their philosophy, however controversial it may seem.

In at least one instance, a bibliography of materials not completely covered in the chapter is presented. Although there is by necessity some overlapping in the chapter, rather complete, independent bibliographies are presented for each chapter. As is the case with any book, all aspects of the field have been impossible to cover, and additional literature is presently available to the reader.

DARRELL E. ROSE
Rochester, Minnesota

Contents

5 Public School Hearing Conservation 133

Jerome G. Alpiner, Ph.D.

6 Pure-Tone Audiometry 167

Lloyd L. Price, Ph.D.

1

Sound Generation and Transmission

Jack Tompkins, Ph.D.

Everyone has a certain intuitive knowledge about sound generation and propagation. For example, we are aware of the fact that sound is generated by vibrating objects. We learn at an early age how to create sounds by beating a drum and by plucking or striking a tightly stretched wire. We can often feel the vibration associated with the sound.

Further, we are aware that sound can travel from some point, as from a stage, and will reach, in time, the distant points of a large auditorium. We have all probably had the unhappy experience of not being quite able to hear a speaker if we have been seated in the back rows of such a large auditorium. So, we are made aware that sound intensity diminishes the farther it travels from the source. In addition, we are conscious of the fact that sound requires a perceptible amount of time to travel even moderate distances. We can summarize this knowledge of sound in the following formalized statements of fact:

1. Sound is generated by vibratory motion.
2. Sound can be transmitted through a medium which delays it and attenuates its intensity.
3. Sound can be received at a point distant from its origin.

Further investigation of sound generation and transmission is merely a process of examining the physical nature of these underlying facts. Taking them in turn, let us first examine vibratory motion.

Vibratory Motion

To understand and be capable of analytically describing vibration, we should understand a concept called SIMPLE HARMONIC MOTION. It is descriptively named. Harmonic means repetitive or cyclical and, as far as motion in physical systems is concerned, it is the simplest to describe. In fact, it is a fundamental unit into which more complex motions are reduced for purposes of analysis.

One useful illustration of simple harmonic motion is that of a weight suspended by a spring attached to a rigid overhead support. Such a system is illustrated in Figure 1.1A. At rest, the weight assumes a quiescent or zero position and remains motionless. If it is pulled downward and then released, it will start to bob up and down along a vertical line. In theory, this system can be considered to have no frictional losses, so that it will continue this up-down vibratory motion forever or until stopped by some external force. This system forms what is called a SIMPLE HARMONIC OSCILLATOR.

This vibrating system is a form of oscillation, and the number of up-down cycles the weight experiences in one second is termed the FREQUENCY OF OSCILLATION. The time required for one cycle is called the period of oscillation, or simply the PERIOD. For example, if the weight makes 100 complete up-down cycles in one second, it is said to oscillate at a frequency of 100 cycles per second. A frequency of one cycle per second is called a HERTZ; so, more properly, the frequency of oscillation would be said to be 100 Hertz (abbreviated Hz). Correspondingly, the period of oscillation is $\frac{1}{100}$ second. This relation between frequency and period may be expressed in a mathematical equation as

$$f = \frac{1}{T} \tag{1}$$

where f = frequency in Hertz

T = period of oscillation in seconds

This oscillating spring-mass system can be analyzed by imagining a pencil being attached to the mass and positioned to mark on a strip of paper, as shown in Figure 1.1B. If the system is set into oscillation and the strip of paper moved laterally to the direction of motion of the mass, a time graph of the mass motion will be produced. Such a graph would look like the one shown in Figure 1.1B. Now the exact repetitive form of the motion is evident.

Next, compare this graph to that of the simple trigonometric sine function. This is done by selecting some angles and finding the corresponding sine of the angle in any trigonometric function table. We would then be graphing the equation

$$y = \sin \Theta \tag{2}$$

where Θ = selected angles in degrees

When this is done, the graph of equation (2), as shown in Figure 1.1C, will be seen to have exactly the same form as that of the mass displacement in the simple harmonic oscillator. So, we may use equation (2) to describe mathematically the motion of the simple harmonic oscillator with one

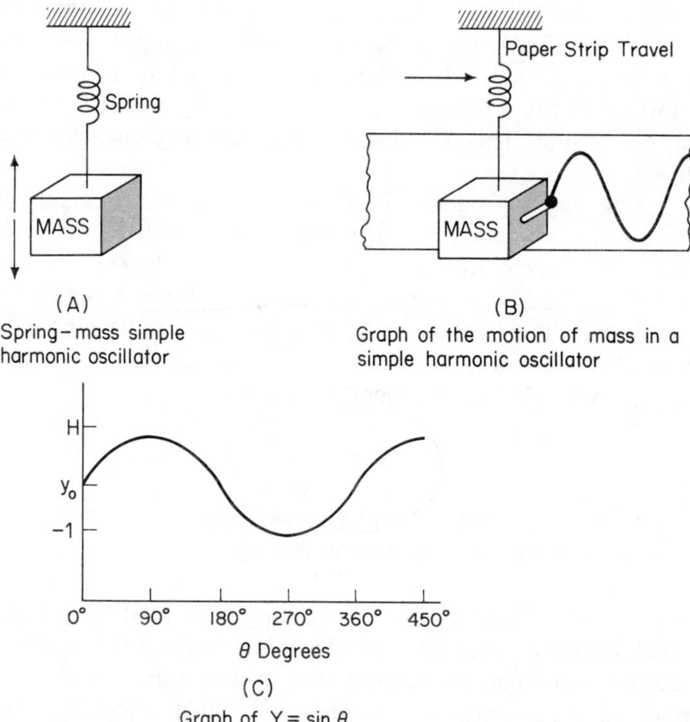

FIGURE 1.1 (A) Illustration of how a mass suspended by a spring will bob up and down to make a simple harmonic oscillator. (B) An imaginary graph of the motion of the mass made by attaching a pencil in such a fashion as to let it mark on a strip of paper moving laterally. (C) Graph of equation $y = \sin \Theta$, showing it is the same form as the graph in (B).

minor change, because the values of sine Θ range only between $+1$ and -1. Since there is no theoretical limit to the maximum excursion our weight may experience in the harmonic oscillator, we must multiply the sine function by the maximum displacement. If we designate this maximum as Y_{max}, then our equation is

$$y = Y_{max} \sin \Theta \tag{3}$$

where y = displacement at any instant
Y_{max} = maximum displacement

One major use of having an equation for the harmonic oscillator is to provide a way of describing the displacement at any instant in time. Yet time is not a factor in equation (3); so we must relate the angle Θ to time. This can be done in the following way.

Notice the sine function repeats every 360° and correspondingly, the graph of mass displacement repeats every cycle. By comparison we can say each cycle of motion is the equivalent of 360° of angular rotation. Thus, in our previous example where the frequency was 100 Hz (100 cycles per second) we could say it had the equivalence of 100 times 360° or 36,000° of rotation per second. This is called an equivalent angular velocity (degrees per second).

Expressing angular velocity in degrees per second is acceptable, but it is more commonly expressed in radians per second. Since there are 2π radians in 360°, there would be 200π radians in 36,000°; therefore, an angular velocity of 36,000° per second equals 100 times 2π or 200π radians per second. Note this is obtained by multiplying 2π radians in 360° by the frequency of oscillation of 100 Hz.

We may express this in a general equation by

$$\omega = 2\pi f \tag{4}$$

where ω = angular velocity in radians per second
f = frequency of oscillation in Hertz

The preceding illustrates how a vibrating or oscillating system can be considered to have an equivalent angular velocity. Since it has an equivalent angular velocity (radians per second), then in some time period t, it can also be considered to have rotated through an equivalent angle of Θ radians as shown by

$$\text{angle} = \frac{\text{radians}}{\text{seconds}} \times \text{seconds} = \text{radians}$$

or

$$\text{angle} = \text{angular velocity} \times \text{time}$$

from which we write by substituting mathematical symbols for these quantities

$$\Theta = \omega t \tag{5}$$

where t = elapsed time in seconds
ω = angular velocity in radians per second

Now if we substitute relation (5) for Θ in equation (3), we have the desired formula from which we can calculate the mass displacement at any time. This is the mathematical description of the simple harmonic oscillator

$$y = Y_{\text{max}} \sin \omega t \tag{6}$$

or alternatively by using (4),

$$y = Y_{\text{max}} \sin 2\pi ft \tag{6a}$$

Such a system as described could produce a sound that would be perceived by a listener to have a certain loudness and pitch. The loudness of the sound, again as perceived by a listener, is proportional to the maximum amplitude of the displacement of the weight, and the pitch is determined by the frequency of oscillation.

Another system similar to that of the suspended mass is shown in Figure 1.2A. This is a rather stiff steel bar fastened rigidly at one end. If the free end is struck, it will vibrate and may produce an audible tone. The mass of the bar would be equivalent to the mass of the previous system and the stiffness of the bar would be represented by the spring in the previous system. So, our original spring-mass system will serve as an

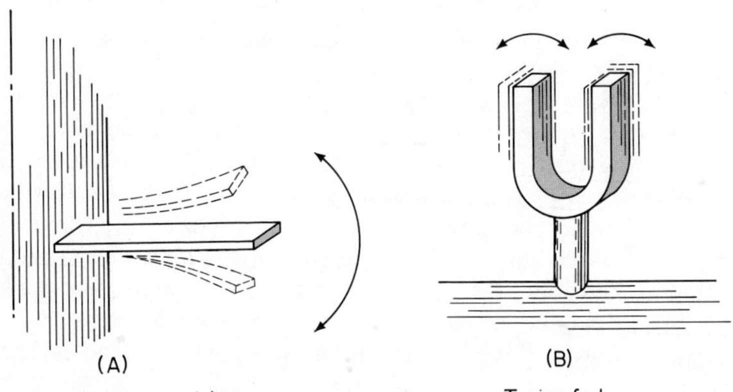

FIGURE 1.2 Two examples of simple harmonic oscillators: (A) A simple steel bar held rigidly at one end and set into vibration is another example of a simple harmonic oscillator. (B) Two steel bars joined at the base to make a tuning fork is a slightly more complex example of a simple harmonic oscillator.

analogy for the vibrating bar. The motion of the tip of the bar is, to a good approximation, simple harmonic motion. The displacement of the tip can be computed by using either equation (6) or (6a).

When two bars are joined at the base, a tuning fork is made as in Figure 1.2B. If struck, it would produce a sound at its characteristic or natural resonant frequency. Though this is a more complex mechanical arrangement, our original system would still be a valid analogy. Thus, the mathematical and physical processes just described can be applied to a number of simple vibrating sound-producing systems, which testifies to its fundamental importance.

Wave Propagation

Next we should explore the nature of propagated sound. Instead of attaching a pencil to the oscillating spring-mass system of Figure 1.1A, assume a light rope of some considerable length is attached in its place. Again, start the system to oscillating and observe what happens to the rope.

If we could "freeze" the rope motion by taking a still picture, we would see that along its length it has the same shape as our original sine-wave graph. However, if we took a rapid sequence of still pictures, we would see that this sine-wave shape appears to be moving away from the point of attachment to the mass. The crest of any wave appears farther down the rope with each successive photograph. This is illustrated in Figure 1.3.

If we had a clearly marked spot on the rope, we would also observe from our series of photographs that this spot would move only in the vertical direction that is transverse to the direction of the apparent motion of the wave down the length of the rope. For this reason, it is called TRANSVERSE WAVE MOTION.

There would be a certain distance between points occupying the same relative position in successive waves—for example, the distance between two successive crests. This distance is called the WAVELENGTH and is usually represented by the greek letter λ. One wave is generated with each cycle of oscillation. Then the time required to produce one wavelength is the period of oscillation. Stated differently, in a length of time equal to the period of oscillation, the wave appears to move down the rope a distance of one wavelength. In one second there are f cycles of oscillation, so in one second, a wave would appear to move down the rope f times the wavelength. The wave is then said to be propagated at a velocity of $f\lambda$ units per second. This is illustrated by the following dimension equation:

$$\text{velocity} = (\text{wavelength}) \times \text{frequency}$$

$$\text{velocity} = \frac{\text{meters}}{\text{cycle}} \times \frac{\text{cycles}}{\text{second}} = \text{meters per sec}$$

If we substitute mathematical symbols for these quantities, we have the following equation for the velocity of propagation:

$$v = f\lambda \tag{7}$$

where v = velocity of propagation
f = frequency in Hz
λ = wavelength

Next we should extend our equation of simple harmonic motion to describe the displacement of any point along the length of rope as a function of time. As the equation now stands, it describes only the displacement of the point of attachment of the rope to the mass. At any instant in time as we move away from this point of attachment, the rope has varying

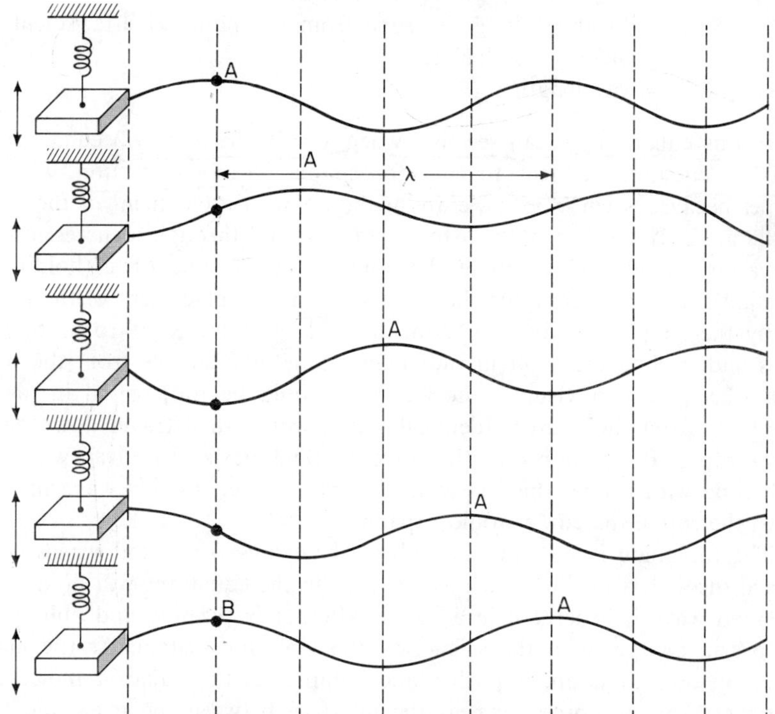

FIGURE 1.3 Apparent wave motion generated by attaching a piece of string to the mass of a simple harmonic oscillator. The crest of any arbitrary wave such as point A appears to move to the right as the mass bobs up and down. As the crest A moves away, a succeeding crest B appears at the left and also moves toward the right. Any marked point such as the heavy dot only moves up and down as transverse to the direction of wave motion.

amounts of displacement according to its sine-wave shape we observed in our imaginary photographs. An equation that describes both the frequency and motion of points along the length of the rope is called the EQUATION OF A WAVE. The following is one mathematical formulation of this equation:

$$y = Y_{max} \sin\left(2\pi ft - \frac{2\pi x}{\lambda}\right) \tag{8}$$

or

$$= Y_{max} \sin 2\pi\left(ft - \frac{x}{\lambda}\right) \tag{8a}$$

where y = displacement of a point on the rope
Y_{max} = maximum or peak displacement
f = frequency of oscillation in Hertz
x = distance along the rope from the point of attachment at which y is calculated
λ = wavelength

In this equation we can see that when $x = 0$, the term x/λ equals zero and the equation reduces to that for simple harmonic motion. This is proper because when $x = 0$, we are at the point of attachment of the rope to the mass. If we then allow x to increase from 0 through a succession of increasing values and compute the corresponding value of y (holding t constant), we would compute the exact sine-wave displacement of the rope.

By the simple expedient of attaching a large number of ropes to the mass and leading them off in radial directions, like spokes from the hub of a wheel, we can visualize how a wave could be propagated in many directions from the source. Identical waves would then travel down each of the ropes. If we connected the corresponding crests of a given wave on each rope with a line, this line would form a circle. As this wave moved down the ropes, the circle would expand.

The foregoing is not an exact physical analogy for sound waves conducted through a medium such as air, though the equations will hold true. A sound wave is generated in a gas by alternately pushing and pulling at the gas in contact with the surface of the vibrating system. As the mass moves in one direction, it pushes and compresses the adjacent molecules thus increasing the pressure near the interface between the mass and the gaseous medium. Then, as the mass moves in the opposite direction in its vibratory cycle, it pulls some gas molecules with it and decreases the pressure. With each cycle of oscillation, the gas molecules are alternately compressed then rarefied, which creates in the surrounding space alternate zones of increased and decreased pressures, respectively. These zones of pressure differences give rise to what is called a PRESSURE GRADIENT. The alternate zones of high and low pressure are radiated outward in a fashion similar to that of the wave traveling down the rope with one difference. The sound wave is propagated because the gas molecules move in a line in the same direction as the pressure gradients. So, the medium moves in the same direction as the wave travels whereas in the former case, the medium (rope) moved transverse to the direction of wave motion. Sound-wave propagation through a gas is an example of longitudinal wave motion.

If, at some instant in time, we could examine the air pressure along a radial line leading from a vibratory system and graph it as a function of distance from the source, we would see that the pressure is of sine-wave form. Also, these sine waves of pressure would appear to move away from the source. Therefore, our mathematical expression for the equation of a wave can be applied to the pressure-wave form.

Returning to the rope example, if the tension in the rope is increased (by stretching the rope tighter), the wavelength would also increase. Then, according to equation (7), the velocity of propagation would increase, which it would in fact do. By experiment, it can be verified that the velocity of propagation in such a system can be computed by

$$\text{velocity} = \sqrt{\frac{\text{tension}}{\text{mass per unit length}}} \tag{9}$$

where typically,[1]

velocity = meters per second (or centimeters per second)
tension = Newtons (or dynes)
mass = kilograms (or grams)

The corresponding relation by which the velocity of propagation in a gas may be computed is similar but somewhat more complex. It is

$$\text{velocity} = \sqrt{\frac{\gamma \times \text{pressure}}{\text{density}}} \tag{10}$$

where typically

velocity = meters per second
pressure = Newtons per square meter
γ = constant volume specific heat (1.4 for air)

The similarities between (9) and (10) should be noted. The rope tension plays the same role as gas pressure, mass per unit length is the counterpart of density (which is mass per unit volume). Further account must be made for other properties of gases and this is done by inserting γ, the constant volume specific heat of the gas. The value for γ may be found in various tables of physical constants for a given gas. Typical values of sound velocity in several gaseous media are given in Table 1.1.

[1] In this and other equations it is only necessary to be consistent in units. British Gravitational, MKS, or CGS units may be used.

Table 1.1 VELOCITY OF SOUND IN GASEOUS MEDIA AT 0°C AND ONE ATMOSPHERE PRESSURE

Media	*Velocity*
Air	331.5 meters per second
Carbon Dioxide	258.0 meters per second
Helium	970.0 meters per second
Nitrogen	337.0 meters per second
Oxygen	317.0 meters per second

The velocity of propagation is also dependent upon the temperature of the gas. If the velocity of propagation of sound is known at any temperature, t_1, the velocity at any other temperature t_2, can be obtained from the following relation,

$$\frac{V_1}{V_2} = \sqrt{\frac{t_1^0 + 273}{t_2^0 + 273}} \tag{11}$$

where

V_1 = velocity of sound at t_1^0C

V_2 = velocity of sound at t_2^0C

Sound propagated through air does not travel in one line like the wave down a rope; instead, it radiates uniformly in all directions.

If we observe and follow the crest of a sound wave, we would notice that it is spherical in shape. Any given pressure crest appears to expand outward into a larger and larger sphere. Following each crest by one wavelength would be another crest.

There is a fixed amount of sound energy imparted to the air with each cycle of oscillation. All this energy is originally contained in a very small spherical shell immediately adjacent to the sound producer. Then it begins to expand and move outward. Assume the sound power in this small shell is F watts, and the radius of the shell is r_1. Then the area of the spherical wavecrest is found (as the area of any sphere) by

$$A_1 = 4\pi r_1^2$$

The power per unit area is the power, F watts, divided by this area. This power per unit area is the sound intensity at a distance r_1 cm from the sound source. This is expressed in the following formula:

$$I_1 = \frac{F}{4\pi r_1^2} \tag{12}$$

where

I_1 = the sound intensity in watts per square centimeter at a distance r_1 centimeters from the source

F = the sound power in watts

r_1 = the radius of sphere in centimeters

As the sound wavecrest moves uniformly outward, it must cover a larger and larger area (much like the surface of an expanding balloon). Finally at some distance r_2, it covers an area

$$A_2 = 4\pi r_2^2$$

and now the power per unit area (intensity of the sound at a distance of r_2 cm) is

$$I_2 = \frac{F}{4\pi r_2^2}$$

and the ratio of intensities at the two different distances r_1 and r_2 cm from the source becomes

$$\frac{I_1}{I_2} = \frac{\dfrac{F}{4\pi r_1^2}}{\dfrac{F}{4\pi r_2^2}} = \frac{r_2^2}{r_1^2}$$

from which

$$I_2 = I_1 \frac{r_1^2}{r_2^2} \tag{13}$$

The fact that sound intensity diminishes as the square of the distance from the source is the reason it is said to follow an INVERSE SQUARE LAW.

For equation (12) to have full meaning, it is necessary to know the relationship between the pressure waves, which are the true physical substance of a sound wave, and the corresponding intensity.

First, it should be understood that the pressure waves of sound cause molecules of gas to acquire a velocity. Because of this, energy is being propagated with the sound wave and this energy is manifested in the velocity of the gas molecules. From basic physics it is known that work equals the product of force times distance, and power is the time rate of doing work. Thus,

$$\text{work} = \text{force} \times \text{distance}$$

and

$$\text{power} = \frac{\text{force} \times \text{distance}}{\text{time}}$$

Since distance divided by time is velocity, we may further state that

$$\text{power} = \text{force} \times \text{velocity}$$

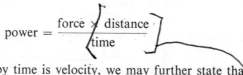

In a sound wave the force is due to pressure differences (pressure gradients) between adjacent zones in the radiated wave, and the velocity of the gas molecules is also proportional to the pressure and physical properties of the gas. Averaging over one wave, it can be shown that the sound intensity is

$$I = \frac{P^2}{2\rho v} \tag{14}$$

where

P = pressure in dynes per square centimeter
ρ = density of gas (1.22×10^{-3} gram per cubic centimeter for air)
v = velocity of propagation of wave centimeters per second
I = sound intensity in watts per square centimeter

An important fact to be observed is that the sound intensity is proportional to the square of the pressure amplitude, because both force and velocity are dependent upon the pressure. Thus, a fourfold increase in intensity requires a twofold increase in the pressure amplitude. Near the threshold of hearing, the pressure is 0.0002 dyne/cm^2, which produces a sound intensity of 10^{-16} watts/cm^2.

When comparing intensities of two different sounds, it is often convenient to use in place of a simple ratio, a unit which is equal to ten times the logarithm of the ratio. This is the DECIBEL. Accordingly,

$$IL = 10 \log \frac{I_1}{I_2} \tag{15}$$

where

IL = intensity level in decibels
I_1 = intensity of a given sound in watts per square centimeter
I_2 = intensity of a reference sound (commonly taken as 10^{-16} watts per square centimeter for threshold of hearing)

Typical intensity levels are given in Table 1.2.

TABLE 1.2 SOUND INTENSITIES

Sound	*IL*
Threshold of hearing	0 dB
Whisper	+20 dB
Conversation	+60 dB
Painful Sensation	+120 dB

Quite commonly we desire to express the ratios in terms of sound pressure instead of in intensities. Accordingly, since the intensity, as we see from equation (14), is proportional to the pressure squared, the ratio becomes

$$PL = 10 \log \frac{P_1^2}{P_2^2} \tag{16}$$

$$= 20 \log \frac{P_1}{P_2} \tag{16a}$$

where

PL = pressure level in decibels
P_1 = pressure of given sound in dynes per square centimeter
P_2 = pressure of reference sound (commonly taken as 0.0002 dyne per square centimeter as the threshold of hearing)

Loudness should not be confused with intensity level. While they are related, they are not the same. LOUDNESS is a purely subjective interpretation of a sound wave and is a psychophysiological phenomenon. If a sound intensity is multiplied by a factor of 100, it will not be interpreted to be 100 times as loud. Instead, it is more nearly proportional to the logarithm of the intensity ratios.

Another unit, the PHON, has been devised to make quantitative measurements of the loudness or auditory sensation of a given sound.

The loudness of sound is determined in the following way. The intensity of a reference tone is adjusted until it sounds equally as loud as the sound being measured. The amount, in decibels, by which the intensity of the reference tone is increased over its specific threshold-of-hearing value, is the loudness level in Phons. The reference note used is a 1,000 Hertz pure tone and the reference pressure and intensity are 0.0002 dyne per cm^2 and 10^{-16} watts per cm^2 respectively.

At the reference frequency, the Phon and the decibels are equal. However, since the threshold of hearing actually varies with the frequency, at other frequencies the Phons and decibels will not be equivalent. For example, a sound loudness of 40 Phons at 1,000 Hz requires 40-dB sound pressure level above threshold. To produce the same 40 Phons of loudness at 100 Hz, approximately a 53-dB sound pressure level is required.

Receiving sound waves involves having some object or system that can respond to the radiated pressure waves. There are many devices which can perform this function. A thin metal diaphragm suspended in the sound-conducting medium will respond to pressure differences as the sound wave passes by. Higher pressure on one side bends the diaphragm, deflecting the center toward the lower pressure on the opposite side.

If this diaphragm is attached to an appropriate electrical signal generator, the sound wave that causes the diaphragm to be deflected could be converted into an analogous electrical signal. We then have a microphone. This is an example of what is broadly termed a TRANSDUCER. The sound pressure waves are said to be transduced to corresponding electrical signals.

The human ear is also a transducer. It converts the sound pressure waves into a complex series of electrical nerve impulses that are in turn transmitted to appropriate areas of the brain.

It is assumed that the reader is primarily interested in audiology and that he either has acquired, or is in the process of acquiring, an understanding of the human hearing mechanism in considerable depth. Further discussion along this line will not be included here. (See "Anatomy and Physiology of the Auditory System," by Samuel G. Fletcher.)

Appendix

DECIBEL NOTATION

The concept of expressing measurements in terms of decibels was originally conceived and defined in terms of electric power. The decibel is fundamentally defined as

$$\mathrm{dB} = 10 \log \frac{p_1}{p_2} \tag{1}$$

dB = decibels of power gain or loss

p_1 = power in watts

p_2 = power in watts

In electrical circuits power is expressible in terms of voltage and current by

$$p = \frac{E^2}{R} \tag{2a}$$

$$p = I^2 R \tag{2b}$$

where

E = voltage across resistance R

I = current flow through resistance R

R = resistance in ohms

By substituting (2a) in equation (1), we can obtain

$$\mathrm{dB} = 10 \log \frac{E_1^2/R_1}{E_2^2/R_2} \tag{3}$$

where

E_1 = voltage across resistance R_1

E_2 = voltage across resistance R_2

Equation (3) may be reduced to

$$\mathrm{dB} = 10 \log \left(\frac{E_1^2}{E_2^2}\right)\left(\frac{R_2}{R_1}\right)$$

$$= 10 \log \frac{E_1^2}{E_2^2} + 10 \log \frac{R_2}{R_1}$$

$$\mathrm{dB} = 20 \log \frac{E_1}{E_2} + 10 \log \frac{R_2}{R_1} \tag{4a}$$

Now if $R_1 = R_2$, the last term becomes 10 log 1, which is zero, so we are left with

$$dB = 20 \log \frac{E_1}{E_2} \tag{4b}$$

which is the commonly used decibel expression for voltage gain or loss.

Similarly if we substituted (2b) into (1) we would obtain

$$dB = 20 \log \frac{I_1}{I_2} + 10 \log \frac{R_1}{R_2} \tag{5a}$$

and if again $R_1 = R_2$, the second term is zero, and we are left with

$$dB = 20 \log \frac{I_1}{I_2} \tag{5b}$$

However, if the resistances are unequal, then we must retain the second term in both of these equations.

In applying this fundamental unit to sound intensities, we must consider the following: Sound intensity is

$$I_1 = \frac{F_1}{4\pi r_1^2}$$

from which

$$F_1 = 4\pi r_1^2 I_1 \tag{6}$$

where

F_1 = sound power in watts
I_1 = intensity of sound at a distance r_1 centimeters from source in watts per square centimeter

In decibel notation we can write

$$dB = 10 \log \frac{F_1}{F_2} \tag{7}$$

where

F_1 = one sound power in watts
F_2 = second sound power in watts

Substituting (6) in (7), we have

$$dB = 10 \log \frac{4\pi r_1^2 I_1}{4\pi r_2^2 I_2}$$

or

$$dB = 10 \log \frac{I_1}{I_2} + 20 \log \frac{r_1}{r_2} \tag{8}$$

Again, if the two intensities are measured at the same distance from the source, then $r_1 = r_2$, so the second term is zero and may be omitted. If this is not true, it must be taken into account.

In dealing with pressure in decibel notation we start with

$$I_1 = \frac{p_1^2}{2\rho_1 v_1} \tag{9}$$

where

I_1 = sound intensity in watts per square centimeter
p_1 = sound pressure in dynes per square centimeter
ρ_1 = gas density
v_1 = velocity of propagation in centimeters per second

Using (9) in (8) we have

$$\text{dB} = 10 \log \frac{\dfrac{p_1^2}{2\rho_1 v_1}}{\dfrac{p_2^2}{2\rho_2 v_2}} + 20 \log \frac{r_1}{r_2}$$

This reduces to

$$\text{dB} = 10 \log \frac{p_1^2}{p_2^2}\left(\frac{\rho_2 v_2}{\rho_1 v_1}\right) + 20 \log \frac{r_1}{r_2}$$

which may be further reduced to

$$\text{dB} = 20 \log \frac{P_1}{P_2} + 10 \log \frac{\rho_2 v_2}{\rho_1 v_1} + 20 \log \frac{r_1}{r_2} \tag{10}$$

If the two sound pressures P_1 and P_2 are measured in the same medium under the same ambient conditions, then ρ_1 equals ρ_2, and v_1 equals v_2, whereupon the second term is 0 and may be omitted. If these conditions are not met, then it should be retained. Similarly, if the two pressures are measured at the same distance from the source, then r_1 equals r_2 and this term drops out; we are left with a commonly used form for decibel of pressure gain or loss:

$$\text{dB} = 20 \log \frac{P_1}{P_2} \tag{11}$$

On some occasions the second and third terms of equation (10) have been omitted and equation (11) has been used inappropriately. We should always be on guard against improper decibel calculations since this obviously leads to errors and ambiguities.

Another common error is to simply apply the decibel calculation to any two quantities that are vaguely (if at all) related to power. Obviously we can take twenty times the logarithm of the ratio of any two arbitrary quantities. However, this would be a misapplication of the unit in the strict sense.

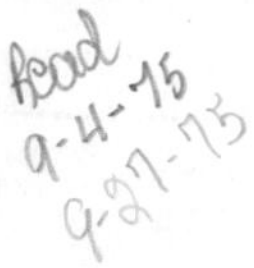

2

Anatomy and Physiology of the Auditory System

Samuel G. Fletcher, Ph.D.

The audiologist who seeks to describe and measure responses to auditory stimuli must be deeply interested in the biological characteristics of the auditory system. The ear, which is the primary structure of auditory behavior, is a masterpiece of biological engineering. The structural and functional efficiency and economy of this complex organ buried within the hardest bone of the body continues to challenge the most sophisticated investigations. Occupying a space of only about one and one-half inches, the ear is capable of focusing sound energy, transmitting it with essentially no loss of energy through a series of variable channels, and transforming it into a code of nerve impulses which can be interpreted by the brain. Naturally within the limits of a single chapter of a book, one can hope only to present a framework upon which a reader may attempt to apprehend and apply anatomical and physiological information concerning the ear that has been and is still rapidly accumulating.

The chapter is arranged in the order that sound follows as it enters and passes through the auditory channels to its eventual arrival in the brain. At the end of each of the first three major divisions of the auditory system, a short discussion of embryonic development is given. This kind of information is increasingly useful in understanding problems in audition that have their origin in congenital disturbances.

The auditory system is most easily visualized as a coarticulation of four components which differ from almost their first moment of formation (Figure 2.1). These are: (1) the EXTERNAL EAR, which receives and conducts sound and reflects the direction of the vibratory field; (2) the MIDDLE EAR, which transmits and amplifies the vibrations; (3) the INNER EAR, which analyzes the sound waves, transduces the vibrations to electrochemical energy, and initiates nerve signals and, finally, (4) the SENSORY PATHWAYS, which relay the nerve signals to the brain and other processing centers where the final assessment of the acoustical incident is made, and from whence instructions are fed to other parts of the body and back to the ear itself.

The External Ear

The outer portion of the ear is the AURICLE or PINNA, which is in the form of a shell attached to the side of the head at about a 30° angle (Figure 2.2). It consists of an external fold, the HELIX, which circles the auricle superiorly and posteriorly and continues forward to the TRAGUS projecting over the canal.

A small thickening or nodule called DARWIN'S TUBERCLE is frequently found along the upper ridge of the helix. Sometimes this is rather prominent and, instead of facing forward, may protrude to the side or even behind, as it does in the ear of the macaque monkey. When the tip points upward, it is known as a "satyr-tip."

The ANTIHELIX is also a concentric ridge. It lies parallel to the helix and encircles posteriorly the deepest depression called the CONCHA or shell. The concha lies in the center of the auricle. At its upper portion the antihelix divides into two limbs, the UPPER and LOWER CRURA, which enclose a small depression called the TRIANGULAR FOSSA. The furrow-like depression between the helix and antihelix is called the SCAPHOID FOSSA because it is shaped like the keel of a boat. The inferior extremity of the auricle is the LOBULE which lacks cartilaginous support.

The auricle is attached to the skull by three muscles, vestigial in man but which give animals extremely good precision in auditory orientation. This attachment is further strengthened by anterior and posterior ligaments.

The auricle funnels into the EXTERNAL AUDITORY MEATUS or ear canal. Enclosed in the meatus and the first recesses of the auricle is about 4 cc of air. The outer third of this 25 mm canal has a cartilaginous skeleton, while the skeleton of the inner third is bony. Its diameter shows individual variation from 4 to 10 mm. The diameter gradually decreases to reach its narrowest dimension at an isthmus not far from where it terminates blindly at the TYMPANIC MEMBRANE or eardrum.

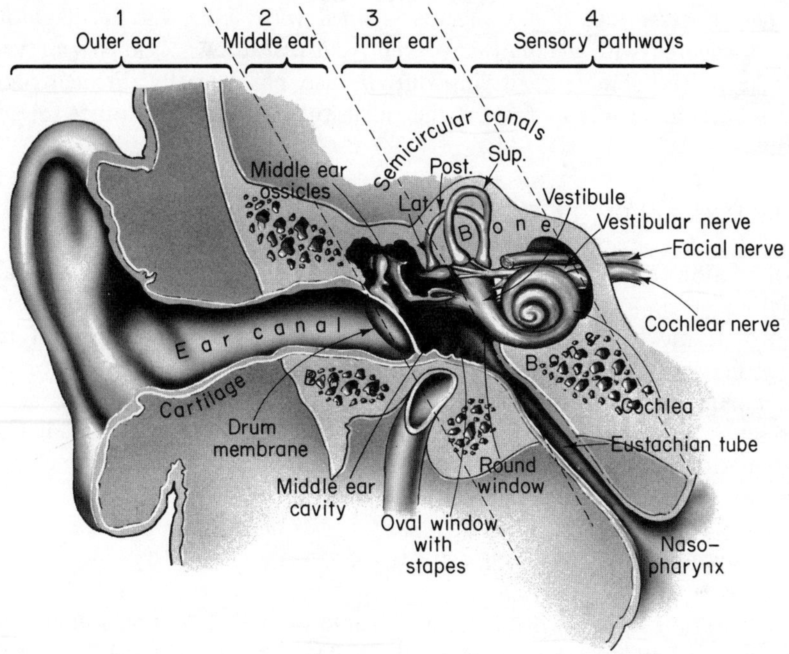

FIGURE 2.1 The human ear

Source: Zemlin, Willard R. "The Ear." *Speech and Hearing Science: Anatomy and Physiology*. Englewood Cliffs, New Jersey: Prentice-Hall, Inc., 1968, (*From* three unpublished drawings of the Anatomy of the Human Ear by Max Brodel.)

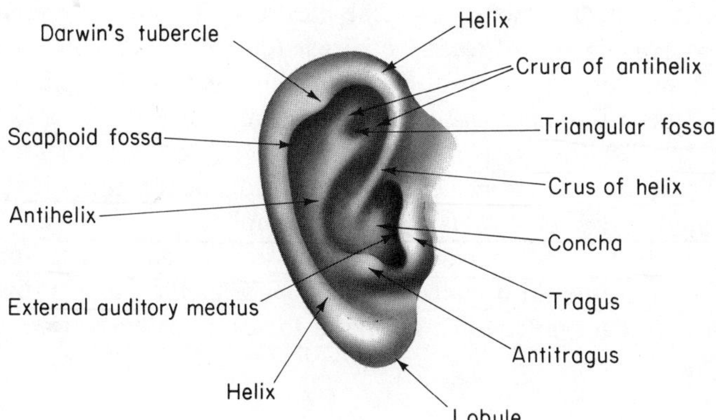

FIGURE 2.2 The auricle (pinna).

Source: Zemlin, Willard R. "The Ear." *Speech and Hearing Science: Anatomy and Physiology*. Englewood Cliffs, New Jersey: Prentice-Hall, Inc., 1968.

The inner surface of the meatus is lined with skin. The cartilaginous part is covered with glands that secrete yellowish-brown CERUMEN or wax that keeps the skin from drying out. It also has laterally directed hairs and sebaceous glands to prevent the intrusion of insects and other foreign bodies.

INNERVATION OF THE EXTERNAL EAR

Sensation is provided to the superior and posterior surface of the earcanal and the superior two-thirds of the eardrum by the auriculo-temporal branch of the trigeminal nerve (V). The nervus aricularis branch of the vagus nerve (X) serves sensation to the anterior and inferior surfaces of the earcanal and to the inferior one-third of the eardrum. The vagus nerve also serves sensation in the pharynx and larynx. For this reason, stimulation or irritation in the earcanal may arouse the cough reflex as though the pharynx or larynx were stimulated.

EMBRYOLOGY OF THE EXTERNAL EAR

The auricle develops from six embryonic mounds or hillocks that arise from the second branchial or hyoid arch. These are seen first in the sixth-week embryo and are well formed by the third month of fetal life. No external auditory meatus is present at first, however. With the sole exception of the tragus, all parts of the auricle develop from these hillocks. The tragus comes from the first arch. Because of this difference in embryonic origin, the point at which the tragus and other structures meet is the site of occasional preauricular fistulas.

During the second month of fetal life, a solid core of epithelium is formed and extends inward from the auricle toward the shallow middle ear, which is beginning to be formed as an extension of the pharynx. The thickened disk at the inner end of this epithelial core is destined to become the outer layer of the tympanic membrane. During the sixth month, the rather delicate epithelial core begins to break down. By the middle of the seventh month, this process is typically complete and an open canal is present. It may be seen that developmental arrest could cause absence of the auricle before the third fetal month, absence of the earcanal before the sixth month, or later in fetal life, atresia of the canal with a normal auricle.

The Middle Ear

The middle ear consists essentially of a group of air cavities containing the OSSICLES—the MALLEUS, INCUS, and STAPES—and their muscles. The tympanic membrane separates the earcanal from a cavity on the other side known as the TYMPANIC CAVITY or TYMPANUM. Recently it has been shown that with the exception of the tympanic membrane and part of the posterior wall and roof of the tympanum, the entire tympanic cavity and the EUSTACHIAN TUBE which connects the middle ear with the pharynx, is ciliated and lined with mucous glands (38). These cilia are arranged so that their sweeping motion can carry mucous and other debris from the cavity through the eustachian tube to the nasopharynx.

THE TYMPANIC MEMBRANE

The TYMPANIC MEMBRANE is a thin, transparent, elastic membrane which on inspection has the appearance of a smooth, glistening, pinkish, pearl curtain slanted inward at the deepest point of the external auditory meatus. The membrane is tightly stretched on a bony frame. In its upper section is a less tense area called the PARS FLACCIDA or SHRAPNEL'S MEMBRANE. This area is bounded anteriorly and posteriorly by thickened borders called the MALLEOLAR FOLDS. The remainder of the membrane is termed the PARS TENSA. The lateral surface of the tympanic membrane is concave. The deepest part of the concavity, the UMBO, corresponds with the flattened tip of the handle (manubrium) of the malleus, which is imbedded in the membrane.

Although it has a thickness of only one-tenth mm, the tympanic membrane is composed of three layers: An outer cutaneous layer of skin, an intermediate layer of connective tissue fibers, and an inner mucous layer which is for the most part a single layer of cells continuous with the mucous membrane lining the tympanic cavity. The middle layer is most important because it provides resiliency to the membrane. This layer has an outer sheet of thin, straight radial fibers stretched like spokes in a wheel between the umbo and the fibrous ANNULAR SULCUS, which attaches the membrane to the tympanic element of the temporal bone. The inner sheet consists of circular fibers especially prevalent around the periphery and in a strip between the periphery and the umbo.

OSSICLES OF THE MIDDLE EAR

As noted, the tympanic membrane is attached to the most external of the interarticulated middle-ear ossicles. Consequently, movements of the ossicles reflect those of the membrane itself. The length of the malleus is about 8 mm, three of which form the CAPUT or head, one the COLLUM or neck, and four the MANUBRIUM or handle. The axis of the head forms an angle of 140° with the axis of the handle (*see* Figure 2.3).

The head of the MALLEUS rests in an upper compartment of the tympanic cavity called the EPITYMPANIC RECESS. Above the malleus is the TEGMEN or roof of the cavity. The head of the malleus is attached to the tegmen by a thin ligament, the SUPERIOR MALLEOLAR LIGAMENT. A lateral and an anterior ligament also attaches the malleus to surrounding bone to provide fixed-point stability.

The INCUS articulates with the malleus at the INCUDOMALLEOLAR JOINT. Shaped something like a premolar tooth with very divergent roots, it has a

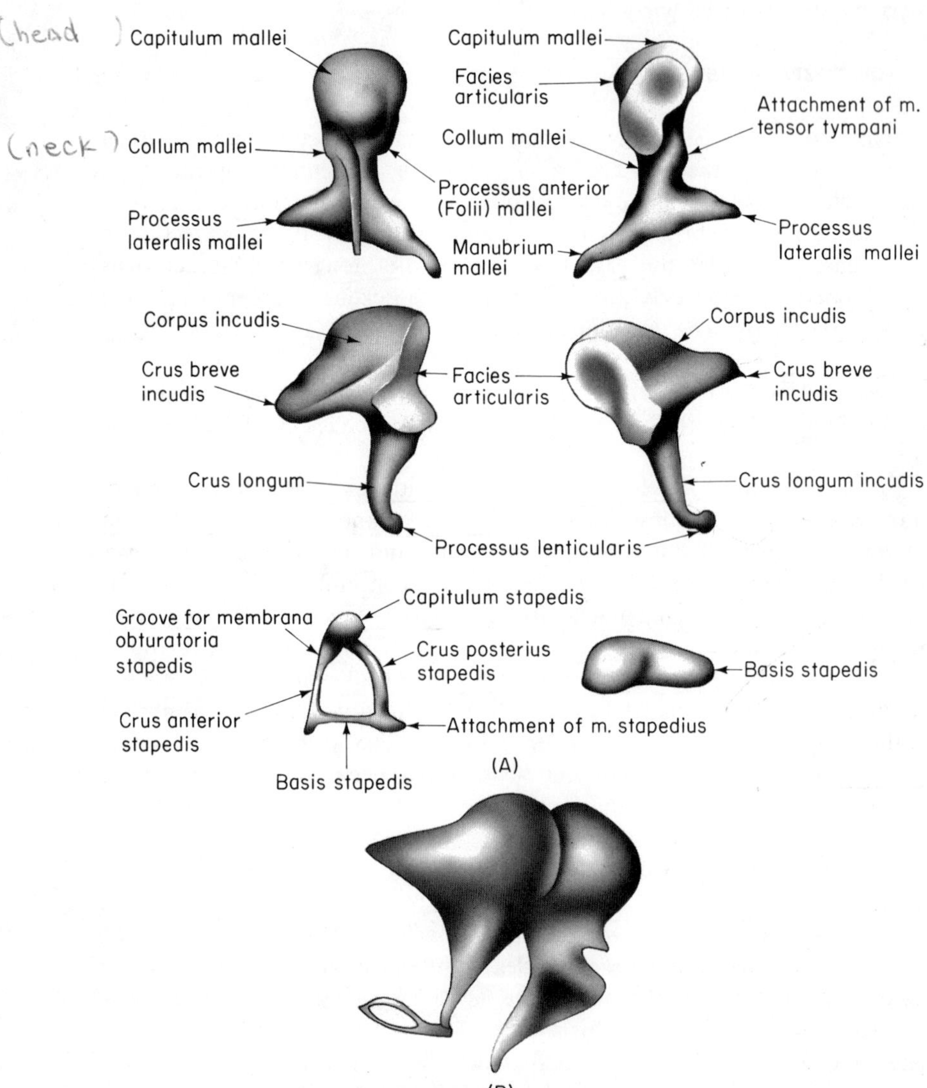

FIGURE 2.3 (A) The ossicles (according to Woërdeman). (B) Articulated ossicles of the left ear.

Source: Woërdeman, H. *Atlas d'Anatomie Humaine.* P.O.F., Paris, 1956. *Courtesy of Dr. Willard R. Zemlin.*

thickened upper end with two slender processes or crura arising from it—a long one and a short one. The short process is directed almost horizontally toward the posterior end of the epitympanic recess, where it is fastened by ligaments to the wall. The long process of the incus extends downward and medially to a place posterior to and nearly parallel with the handle of the malleus. On its lower extremity, which is bent medially, is a minute spherical bone, the LENTICULARIS, for articulation with the head of the stapes. The lenticular process is the smallest bone in the body.

The STAPES consists of a head, a slightly constricted neck, and two crura that diverge around the OBTURATOR FOREMEN and attach to a footplate. The footplate is framed in the oval window (FENESTRA OVALE) of the vestibule of the inner ear which it seals hermetically by means of the ANNULAR LIGAMENT.

The ossicular joints are unique from other joints in the body in that they do not have overlying muscles to sustain their articular contact. Rather, they depend entirely on an elastic capsular component to keep the cartilaginous synovial joint surfaces in contact (17).

MUSCLES OF THE MIDDLE EAR

Movements of the ossicles may be modified by two muscles: the TENSOR TYMPANI and the STAPEDIUS. The latter is the smallest muscle in the body. The tensor tympani is lodged in a compartment immediately above the eustachian tube on the anterior part of the tympanic cavity. It is separated from the eustachian tube by a bony and fibrous partition.

The tensor tympani muscle originates from the upper part of the eustachian tube and the inside surface of its own canal. The muscle then tapers into a small round tendon that turns at a right angle as it leaves its canal, passes laterally across the tympanic cavity, and attaches to the upper end of the malleolar handle. Contraction of this muscle pulls the handle medially and thereby reduces sensitivity to loud sounds. The muscle is supplied by a motor branch from the trigeminal cranial nerve (V).

The stapedius muscle is completely encased in a small pyramid of bone jutting out on the back wall of the tympanic cavity. A delicate tendon of the stapedius enters the tympanum through a tiny aperture on the summit of the pyramid and is attached to the posterior surface of the neck of the stapes. Contraction of this muscle inhibits the rocking motion of the stapes in the oval window and also reduces sensitivity of the ear to sound pressures (19). The muscle is supplied by a branch of the facial nerve (VII).

The combined attenuation from the tensor tympani and stapedial muscle to loud sound is about 20 dB (31). The muscles have a latency of about 20 msec between the onset of sound and the movement of the ossicles to which they are attached. Therefore, they are less effective in protecting the ear against sudden loud noises such as a gunshot than they are to sustained sound. These latencies diminish with increasing sound intensity. Fisch and Schulthess (10) found that stapedial latencies were reduced to as little as 10 msec to sound above 100 dB in intensity.

Liden et al. (25) recently generated data that suggested that stapedial contraction favors "passage of high frequencies by reducing the transmission of the low frequencies to the cochlea." This high-pass filter effect was originally postulated by Stevens and Davis (45). Simmons (41) suggests that by this mechanism the listener can actually tune his ear to reduce specific physiologic noise.

THE EUSTACHIAN TUBE AND OTHER STRUCTURES

Mention has been made of the EUSTACHIAN OR AUDITORY TUBE. This tube is 30 to 40 mm long and extends between the tympanum and the pharynx. The lateral third of the tube, that part near the tympanic cavity, has walls that are supported by bony tissue.

At its most narrow section it measures only 1 to 2 mm in diameter. The remainder of its wall, 24 to 25 mm, is supported by cartilage. The part supported by cartilage is typically closed except during certain physiological activities such as swallowing or yawning.

Dilation of the auditory tube to equalize pressure on each side of the tympanic cavity is accomplished by contraction of the DILATOR TUBAE division of the TENSOR VELI PALATINI MUSCLE with some assistance from the LEVATOR VELI PALATINI MUSCLE.

As the eustachian tube opens into the pharynx, its orifice on the upper lateral wall is encircled by the TORUS TUBARIUS CARTILAGE. In the human adult the tube has an upward angulation which facilitates drainage. In the infant this upward angulation has not yet matured, thus drainage of the middle ear is more difficult (15).

Several other structures of the middle ear are worthy of mention without elucidation. These are the MASTOID ANTRUM and the MASTOID AIR CELLS, which communicate posteriorly from the epitympanic recess; the FACIAL NERVE, which is embedded in the posterior wall of the tympanum; the ITER CHORDAE NERVE (Chorda Tympani), which crosses from the canal of the seventh nerve through the tympanic cavity to join the fifth cranial nerve and serve taste sensation in the tongue; and the ROUND WINDOW (fenestra rotunda) or secondary tympanum on the medial wall.

EMBRYONIC DEVELOPMENT OF THE MIDDLE EAR

The embryonic primordia of the middle-ear cavity is an outpouching of the pharynx (foregut) which extends toward the body wall between the first and second branchial arches in the third week of development. The flattened end of this pouch forms a primitive tympanic cavity.

During the second month, the ossicles begin to take shape but are still enveloped in connective tissue above and lateral to the developing middle-ear cavity. By the fourth month the ossicles are formed but it is not until the seventh month that they are enclosed within the cavity. The malleus and incus are derived from Meckel's cartilage (which also provides the mandible) in the first branchial arch. This accounts for associated developmental disturbances involving both the mandible and the ossicles such as in the Treacher-Collins syndrome. The stapes arises later from the second arch and is not fully formed until after the fourth month. Elliott and Elliott (6) note that the one constant in congenital anomaly of the auditory ossicles is "at least a remnant of the malleus handle."

Pneumatization of the tympanic cavity is not completed until after the seventh month. Pneumatization of the tympanic antrum and of the mastoid bone itself is not begun until after the fifth month and is apparently not completed after childhood, or even as late as puberty.

The Inner Ear

The oval and round windows of the middle ear open into the elements of the inner ear (Figure 2.4). Because of its complicated channels and passages, the inner ear is also called the LABYRINTH. In actuality the labyrinth consists of two sets of cavities. One is the OSSEOUS LABYRINTH which is a series of bony canals within the petrous part of the temporal bone. The other is the MEMBRANOUS LABYRINTH which consists of a series of communicating sacs and ducts suspended within the osseous labyrinth and is filled with a fluid called ENDOLYMPH. The space in the osseous labyrinth not occupied by the membranous labyrinth is filled with a fluid called PERILYMPH. The membranous labyrinth does not float freely in the perilymph. Rather, it is attached to the osseous walls by numerous threads of connective tissue.

DIVISIONS OF THE INNER EAR

Two main divisions of the labyrinth are distinguishable posteriorly and anteriorly: a 3 by 5 mm cavity, the bony VESTIBULE; and a very narrow membranous canal, the DUCTUS REUNIENS, communicating between them.

The posterior division of the labyrinth, seat of the organs that sense movements of the head and orientation of the body in space, is made up of the SEMICIRCULAR CANALS, the UTRICULUS, and the SACCULUS. The five openings of the three canals (two of the canals fuse at one extremity) enter into the utriculus. Near their entrance they present enlarged extremities, the AMPULLAE, in which the sensory termination of the vestibular nerve, the AMPULLAE CUPULA, is found.

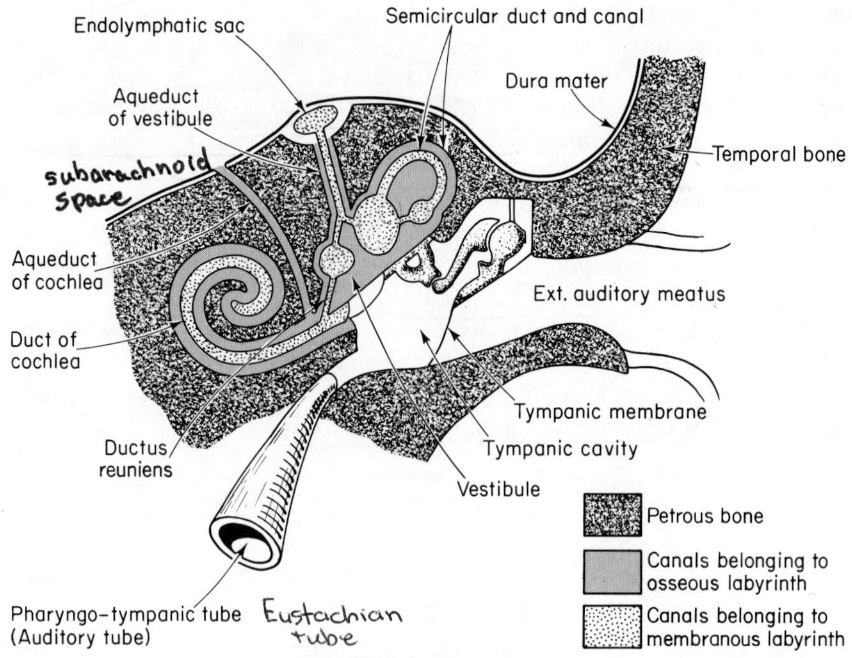

FIGURE 2.4 A general scheme of the ear.

Source: J.C.B. Grant. *An Atlas of Anatomy*. 4th ed. Baltimore: The Williams and Wilkins Company, 1956.

The utriculus is connected to the sacculus by the utriculo-saccular endolymphatic duct which is in turn connected to the cochlear endolymphatic duct by the ductus reuniens. Thus, the vestibular divisions of the labyrinth form part of the total volume of fluid to which sound is delivered. In some cases of abnormality they must be taken into consideration. They need not be considered further here, however, with the mechanism of hearing.

The anterior division of the labyrinth is coiled like a snail shell and for this reason is called the cochlea. The auditory function is delegated to this organ.

The Cochlea

As shown in Figure 2.5, the cochlea has a central bony pedestal called the MODIOLUS which acts as an inner wall for the coiled tube which wraps about 2 and 3/4 turns around it. Projecting from and spiraling around the modiolus is a thin shelf of bone, the SPIRAL LAMINA. From this shelf a tough membrane, the BASILAR MEMBRANE, stretches across the tube and attaches to the outer wall at the SPIRAL LIGAMENT. This separates the tube

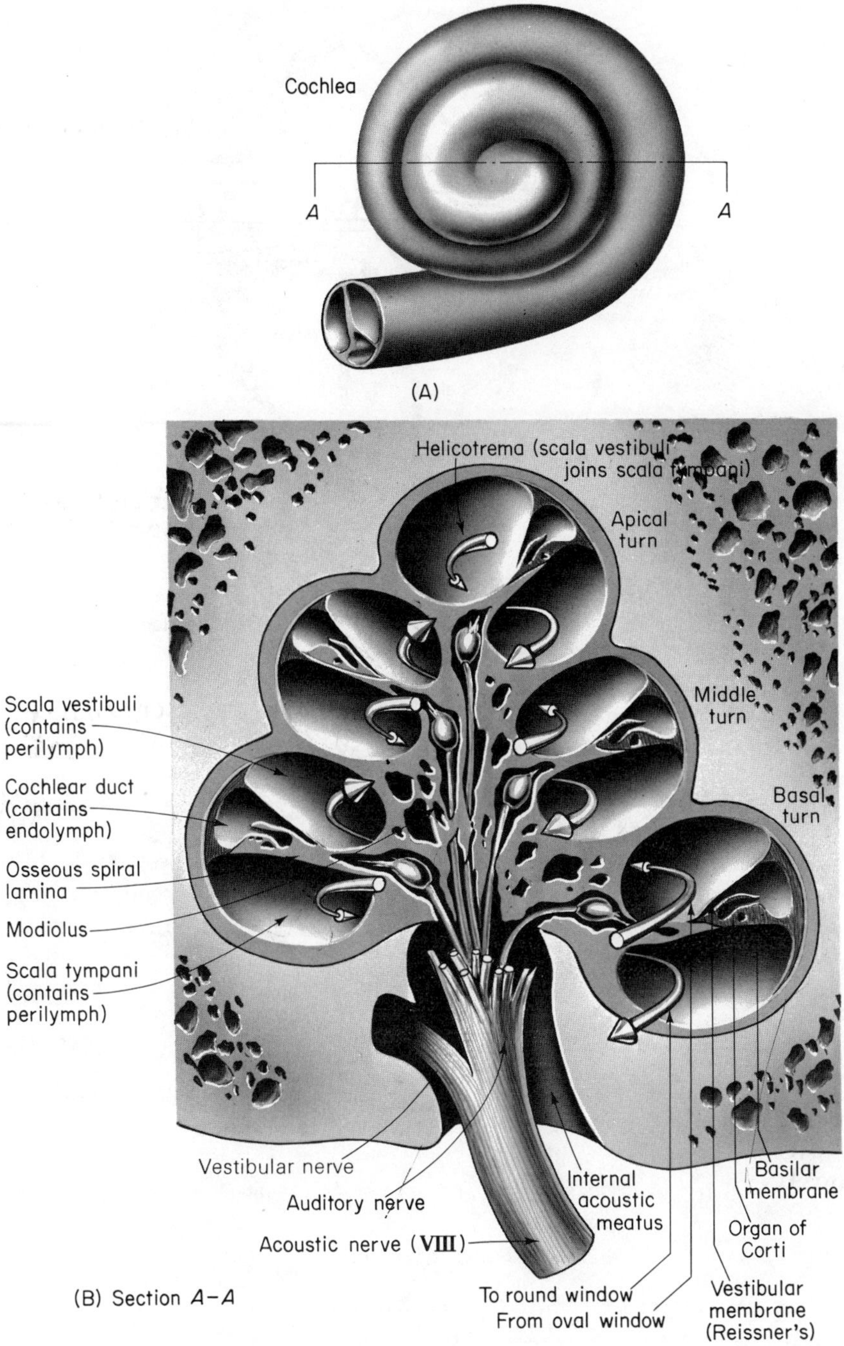

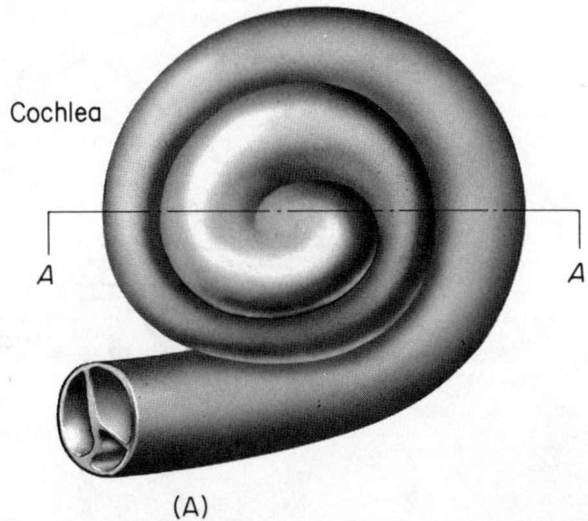

(A)

Helicotrema (scala vestibuli joins scala tympani)
Apical turn
Middle turn
Basal turn
Scala vestibuli (contains perilymph)
Cochlear duct (contains endolymph)
Osseous spiral lamina
Modiolus
Scala tympani (contains perilymph)
Vestibular nerve
Auditory nerve
Acoustic nerve (VIII)
Internal acoustic meatus
Basilar membrane
Organ of Corti
To round window
From oval window
Vestibular membrane (Reissner's)

(B) Section $A-A$

FIGURE 2.5 (A) Cochlea. (B) Cross-section of cochlea.

Source: Ciba Clinical Symposium, 1962.
Science: Anatomy and Physiology. Englewood Cliffs, New Jersey: Prentice-Hall, Inc., 1968.

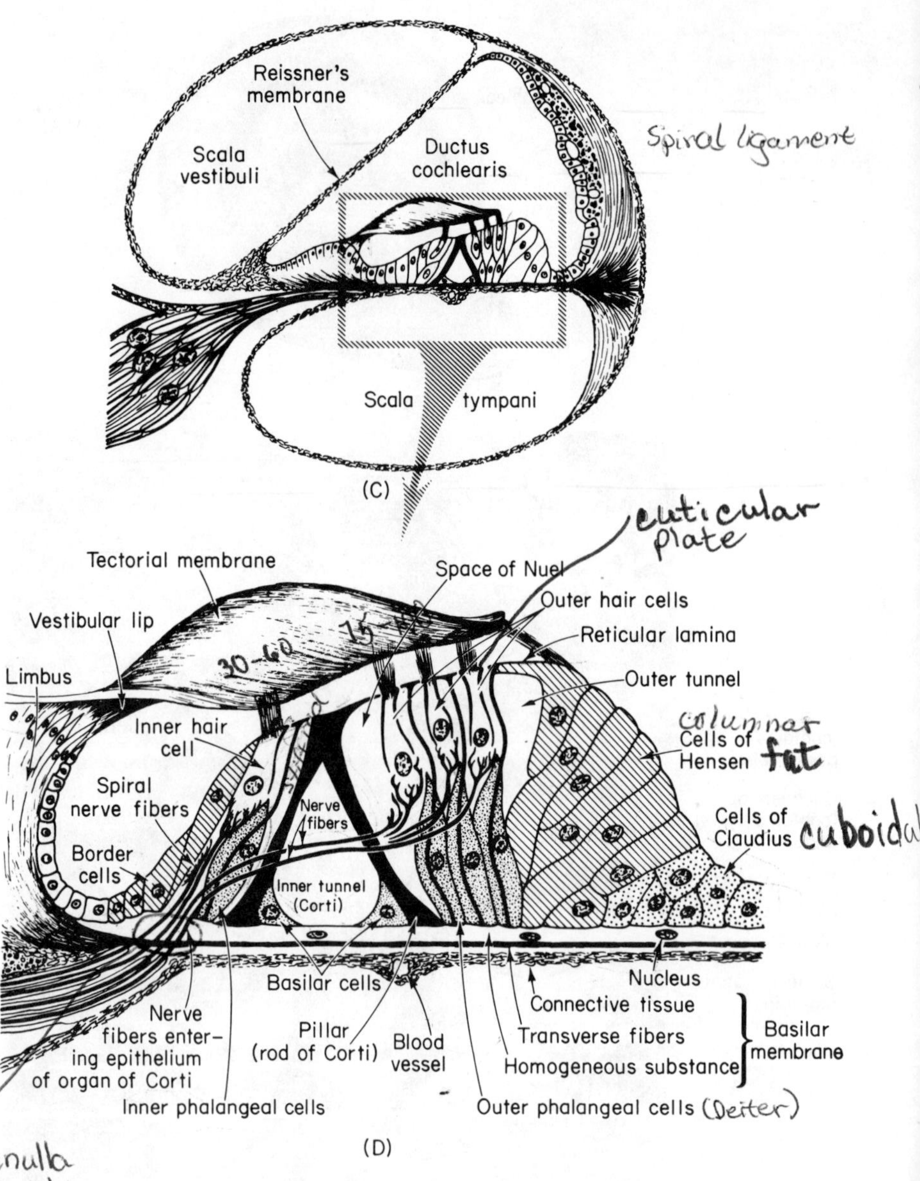

FIGURE 2.5 (C) Enlargement of part of a cross-section or cochlea. (D) Organ of Corti.

Source: See FIGURE 2.5 (A) and (B).

into two passages for its full length except for a small opening at the apex, known as the HELICOTREMA. In this free space at the summit the two passages join. The upper canal of the cochlea, the SCALA VESTIBULI, begins in the vestibule near the oval window and ends at the helicotrema. The lower canal, the SCALA TYMPANI, begins at the helicotrema and ends at the round window which is covered by a thin membrane separating this passage from the tympanic cavity.

Near the round window is the COCHLEAR AQUEDUCT. This is a small 6 to 7 mm straight channel which connects the scala tympani with the fluid-filled subarachnoid space surrounding the brain. It may function as a regulating mechanism whereby pressures between the inner ear and the subarachnoid space could be equalized. Its small diameter of 0.09 to 0.1 mm would restrict such activity to a very slow rate, however (2, 37).

A second duct, the VESTIBULAR AQUEDUCT, serves to balance pressure in the endolymphatic system. This duct exits from the sacculus and passes through the petrous pyramid. Upon emerging, it dilates to form the blind ENDOLYMPHATIC SAC in the posterior cranial fossa under cover of the dura mater. Thus, a direct exchange with the cerebro-spinal fluid is not possible. Rather, the endolymphatic sac could release pressure in the endolymphatic system only by expanding like a balloon as it accepted additional fluid. Again, its small dimension would restrict this function to a very slow rate.

The cochlea measures only about 5 mm from base to summit and has a breadth of about 8 mm across the base. The spiral tube is about 35 mm long. The basilar membrane within the spiral tube is about 32 mm long and tapers in width from 1/2 mm at the apex to 1/20 mm at the basal turn. It is made up of about 24,000 individual fibers (strings) arranged in parallel and at right angles to the length of the membrane.

Extending diagonally from the spiral lamina to the outer wall of the cochlea is REISSNER'S MEMBRANE. It is the thinnest membrane in the cochlea with a thickness of just one or two somewhat flattened cells. Reisner's membrane extends along the whole passage of the cochlea to join the basilar membrane at the helicotrema and form a completely sealed sac called the COCHLEAR DUCT or SCALA MEDIA. It is the endolymph-filled, membranous

Endolymph	*Perilymph*
High potassium content	Low potassium content
Low sodium content	Relatively high sodium content
Low protein content	High protein content as compared with endolymph or cerebrospinal fluid
High positive electric potential	Negative electric potential compared with endolymph
Variable mucopolysaccharids in different species of animals	Variable mucopolysaccharids according to species

scala media of the cochlea that communicates with the sacculus via the ductus reuniens. The other two passages, the scala vestibuli and scala tympani, contain perilymph. The outer wall of the scala media is covered by the STRIA VASCULARIS (i.e., vascular strip), which has a dense layer of capillaries and specialized cells believed to secrete the endolymph (3, 23). The chemical contrast between the two fluids is shown in the table on page 29 (adapted from Ormerod, 33).

THE ORGAN OF CORTI

The sensory organ which transforms sound waves into neural impulses is on the vestibular surface of the basilar membrane in the scala media. The cells and structures that belong to this organ are called collectively the ORGAN OF CORTI.

The organ of Corti has two kinds of elements. One element is purely supportive and provides the framework of the structure. The other consists of hair cells, which are the specific sensory structures with nerve fibers. These are embedded in the supportive elements. The cells of the organ of Corti are nurtured by the endolymph and perhaps by cortilymph (see below) and therefore are freed from blood vessels, which could introduce additional noise into the endolymphatic channel.

The most central part of the supporting network of elements in the organ of Corti are the INNER and OUTER RODS (pillars) OF CORTI, which form a triangular tunnel with part of the basilar membrane between them. These are thick, stiff bodies which broaden out at their base. They divide the organ into inner and outer portions. On the inner side of the tunnel of Corti is a single row of hair cells, the INNER HAIR CELLS, supported by a row of INNER PHALANGEAL CELLS, or "finger-like" cells, and other smaller supporting cells of Held. On the outward side of the tunnel rods are three and sometimes four rows of smaller OUTER HAIR CELLS which are supported by phalangeal cells of Deiters and have prominent intracellular spaces between them.

Engström (7) has called attention to the difference in the fluids in the tunnel of Corti and in the intercellular spaces around the outer hair cells. He emphasized that although the general ionic content of this fluid is similar to perilymph, considerably more macromolecular elements, possibly protein, were present. Spoendlin (44) speculated that these elements were nutritional in nature for the base part of the external hair cells. With this uniqueness in mind, Engström suggested that the fluid contained in the tunnel of Corti be termed CORTILYMPH. Thus, each outer hair cell is in direct contact with two different fluids. The endolymph bathes the top of the cell and the cortilymph bathes the major part of the cell from the intercellular spaces. Each of these fluids is rich in potential nutrients.

The upper edges of the phalangeal cells supporting both the inner and outer hair cells contact each other to form a compact network. This network of cells is called the RETICULAR MEMBRANE. The cilia or hairs penetrate the reticular membrane and are imbedded in the gelatinous TECTORIAL MEMBRANE (18) which winds in spiral fashion along the whole length of the organ of Corti.

Extending outward from the outer hair cells and their phalangeal supportive cells (CELLS OF DEITERS) are the CELLS OF HENSEN, which are large supporting cells with fat globules. They are an integral part of the organ of Corti and form a series almost equal in width to the rest of the organ. They are of unequal height and are built closely to the cells of Deiters. A line of cube-shaped CELLS OF CLAUDIUS completes the lining of the vestibular surface of the basilar membrane to the spiral ligament.

About 3,500 cells of approximately 12 μ in diameter are contained in the inner row of hair cells and about 20,000 cells of approximately 8 μ in diameter are in the outer row. The inner hair cells are shaped like a jug with a wide base. Where they come in contact with neighboring cells, well-marked intercellular spaces are present. They are inclined in the same direction as the inner rods and have from thirty to sixty hairs on their surface which are 3 μ to 4 μ in length and 0.32 μ in diameter.

When sound waves pass through Reissner's membrane and impinge upon the tectorial membrane, distortional forces develop on the hair cells giving rise to a cochlear response called COCHLEAR MICROPHONICS. This response is found to be a faithful reproduction of the waveform of the stimulus up to moderate intensities of sound stimulation. At the present time the microphonics are generally believed to arise in the hair-bearing end of the hair cells as the result of an ionic current flow through the cells (23). The precise way in which the mechanical motion of the sound wave is registered at different points along the cochlea and exactly how the hair cells are stimulated are still matters of considerable conjecture (3, 29, 30, 47).

The outer cells are cylindrical in shape with a round base. They lie with their bases in special hollows formed by the cells of Deiters and incline parallel to the outer rods. The number of hairs on the hair cells varies around seventy-five but may reach as many as 100. The auditory hairs are more conspicuous on the outer hair cells than on the inner, but are only about 0.15 μ in diameter. Davis (5) found that the outer cells are more easily damaged by sound than the inner cells. Many investigators have shown them more sensitive to drugs.

Iurato (22) summarized the biological zones of the hair cells as follows: (*see* Figure 2.6).

> The apical zone, composed of the cuticle and the auditory hairs, is the device that receives the mechanical impulses generated by the hairs touching the tectorial membrane.... The underlying part, called the intermediate zone, well supplied with endoplasmic organoids, is the zone supplying the necessary energy to convert and amplify the mechanical stimulus. The perinuclear zone appears to handle conduction, while at the levels of the recepto-neural junction the impulse passes to the nerve fibers.

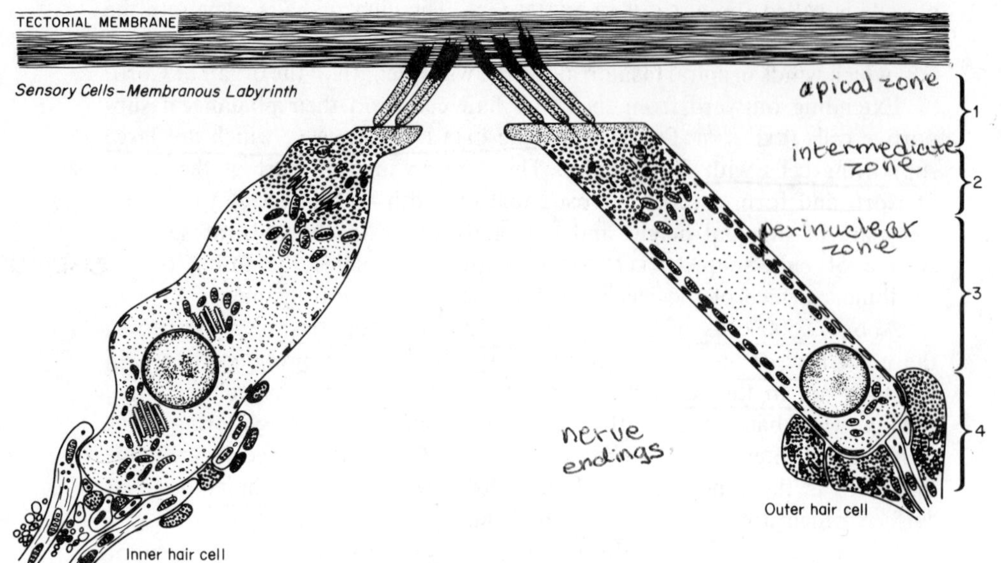

FIGURE 2.6 Diagram of the basic observations on the submicroscopic structure of the sensory cells of Corti's organ. From top to bottom: (1) apical zone, (2) intermediate zone, (3) perinuclear zone, and (4) nerve endings.

Source: Iurato, M.D., Salvatore. "The sensory cells of the membranous labyrinth," *Archives of Otolaryngology*, **75**: 312–28, 1962. By permission of the Journal of the American Medical Association.

Embryonic Development of the Inner Ear (34)

The primordium of the membranous labyrinth is the first part of the ear to appear in the embryo. This is first indicated in the third week of development when a vaguely marked thickening of the ectoderm is found on either side of the primitive brain in the area subsequently to become the medulla. By the end of the third week this AUDITORY PLACODE has taken shape as a sharply differentiated plate. The placode invaginates to form the AUDITORY PIT during the fourth week. As the pit deepens, its opening at the surface is closed and an epithelial space, now known as the AUDITORY VESICLE, is formed.

In the ensuing days the auditory vesicle enlarges and changes from spheroidal to an elongate oval shape with a more expanded dorsal portion. This dorsal portion will develop into the vestibular part of the membranous labyrinth while the more slender anterior part will become the cochlea.

By the end of the sixth week of development, conspicuous phalanges push out from the vestibular portion of the main vesicle. As they do so, their central portions become thin and finally undergo resorption so that the original semilunate flanges become converted into looplike ducts to form the semicircular canals.

While the semicircular canals take shape, the main vestibular portion of the vesicle becomes subdivided by a progressively deepening constriction into a more dorsal utricular and a more ventral saccular portion. The semicircular canals then open off the utriculus. Near one of the two points of communication with the utriculus, each canal forms a local enlargement known as an AMPULLA, within which develops the sensory area, the CRISTA. Specialized areas called MACULAE develop later in the sacculus and utriculus.

The cochlear part of the membranous labyrinth elongates rapidly in the sixth week and develops a sharp bend in its distal end. During the seventh and eighth weeks, elongation continues at an accelerated rate and the initial bend develops into the 2 and 3/4 spirals of the cochlea duct. As the cochlear duct is thus elongated, its original broad connection with the vestibular portion of the membranous labyrinth becomes narrowed to the slender ductus reuniens.

The cochlear division of the eighth nerve follows the cochlear duct as it grows in length, and its fibers fan out all along the duct. A bandlike ganglion, the SPIRAL GANGLION, is formed adjacent to the cochlear duct.

By the close of the third month the membranous labyrinth has achieved almost its adult configuration. During this time the mesenchyme surrounding the membranous labyrinth has become increasingly concentrated to form a cartilaginous shell with delicate strands of connective tissue developed to suspend the membranous labyrinth.

The first primordium of the organ of Corti becomes apparent in the third month of development as a localized thickening of the epithelium on the floor of the cochlear duct. The process of differentiation begins in the basal part and spreads gradually to the apex. McGrady and his coworkers (28) found that differentiation of the basal parts of the cochlea coincides with the onset of its function. For instance, in one species of opossum, sound frequencies from 500 to 6,000 Hz were perceived in the lower turn from the second to the fifty-ninth day of fetal life in the pouch. Only after the fifty-ninth day, when the middle and upper turns were developed, did the fetus respond to sound frequencies from 300 to 10,000 Hz, and on the sixtieth day from 200 to 20,000 Hz.

From the third to the fifth month, the entire cochlear duct undergoes considerable expansion. The tectorial membrane, formed over the epithelial thickening, becomes more extensive; and the developing organ of Corti beneath it begins to show marked specialization with the formation of the hair cells. During the sixth month, some resorption occurs within the organ of Corti itself to form the tunnel of Corti, which will later be supported by the developing supporting elements designated as the rods. The tunnel of Corti seems to develop later than the fluid spaces around the outer and inner hair cells (9, p. 33). The inner ear has practically its adult size at birth.

The Sensory Pathways

The route of the acoustic signal through the mechanical pathways to its sensory conversion in the middle ear will be summarized first in our discussion of the sensory pathways. We will then consider the central neurological relays that enable the message to reach the brain and other processing centers for interpretation and reaction of the acoustic stimulus.

The process of audition begins when longitudinal sound waves, transmitted through air, are funneled by the auricle into the external auditory meatus and collide with the tympanic membrane at the end of this blind tunnel. The tympanic membrane moves in response to this compression-rarefaction collision. Energy thus collected by the tympanic membrane is transferred to the ossicular chain system of the middle ear, which amplifies the pressure by a lever and an "hydraulic press" type of action. The movement of the stapes in the oval window of the labyrinth vestibule transmits the sound waves to the fluid of the scala vestibuli. A high degree of impedance-matching by the ossicular chain between the air and fluid phase enables this transfer of sound energy without significant loss.

The acoustic vibrations now continue in the perilymphatic fluid and through Reissner's membrane to the endolymphatic fluid. From thence the vibrations are impressed upon the tectorial membrane in such a fashion that the hair processes in the organ of Corti undergo a distortional force between the tectorial membrane and the basilar membrane. This force is the stimulus that triggers hair cell activity which, in turn, generates nerve impulses. By some manner not presently agreed upon, high tones are registered near the base of the cochlea and low tones at the apex. Energy travels around the helicotrema as well as through the basilar membrane to be absorbed by the round window.

Sound may also reach the inner ear by other routes although the above route is the most important. Two such routes are: (1) directly across the middle ear to the round window membrane by air waves instead of through the ossicles, and (2) by transmission of sound to the inner ear through the bony structures of the skull. Inherent in both of these alternative routes of sound transmission is a great loss in acoustical energy necessary to activate the inner ear. Therefore, under normal conditions these routes do not usually contribute to audition.

COCHLEAR NERVES

Auditory nerve impulses per se in the sensory pathway begin at the inner and outer hair cells, which differ from each other morphologically and also have a different pattern of innervation.

The nerve fibers to the cochlear hair cells pierce the basilar membrane at the habenula perforata. As they exit from the spiral lamina and pierce the basilar membrane, they lose their myelin sheaths that have served to insulate them from each other. From there to their terminations on the hair cells, they course as naked nerve fibers, entirely unsheathed (42). Some of the fibers take a short, radial course primarily to the inner hair cells. These are, therefore, called RADIAL FIBERS. Many of the fibers terminate just beneath the hair cell, while others ascend the sides and may achieve considerable length before terminating (43). Each inner cell is associated with one or two such radial fibers. Galambos (11) noted that this nerve-to-cell arrangement would afford a clear basis for an hypothesis of a one-to-one relation between place on the basilar membrane and place in the central nervous system to extract the frequency of a sound signal.

Fibers destined for the external hair cells traverse the tunnel of Corti and for the most part spiral along the organ of Corti for 2 or 3 mm before terminating at the hair cells. These are therefore called SPIRAL FIBERS. They tend also to supply many different hair cells by numerous branches before ending. The nerve endings to the external hair cells are in contact only with the base of the cell. Galambos (11) suggested that this nerve-to-cell arrangement could afford the basis for a "diffuse relationship" interpretation of sound frequency analysis.

A third type of nerve fiber is also present in the cochlea. This is a fiber with nerve endings containing numerous vesicles. Under the electron microscope these endings appear "much granulated" compared with the knoblike endings of the other nerves. On the basis of similarity between these "much granulated" nerve endings and motor nerve endings in other parts of the body, Engström (8) postulated that these were EFFERENT FIBERS whereas the others were afferent. Ishii et al. (20) found biochemical evidence that "all plexises within the organ of Corti contain fibers [that have]... both efferent and afferent components." These finer efferent fibers wind among the other two and are in extensive synaptic contact with the dendrites from both outer and inner hair cells (21, 32). They belong to the descending auditory tract, which likely inhibits activity of the cochlear nerves. Galambos found reduced sound activity following electrical stimulation of the cochlear nerve in the cat and suggested that this was the result of such efferent inhibition.

The afferent nerve fibers, which are bipolar neurons, leave the hair cells of the cochlea, pass by their cell bodies in the SPIRAL GANGLION of Corti, and join other such axons in the modiolus to form the COCHLEAR NERVE.

ACOUSTIC NERVE

As the cochlear nerve leaves the auditory capsule in the petrous bone, it is joined by the VESTIBULAR NERVE from the sensory organs in the semicircular canals, the sacculus and the utriculus. The two nerve bundles together are thereafter referred to as the ACOUSTIC NERVE (VIII). The acoustic nerve joins the facial nerve (VII) and they pass through the internal auditory meatus in the petrous pyramid of the temporal bone.

The bundle of fibers from the cochlea retains its frequency representation as it passes through the acoustic nerve (25). That is, the fibers in the middle of the high-frequency range run straight through the nerve as the axis. The other fibers are twisted spirally around these in ropelike fashion. Those from the apex of the cochlea spiral one way and the ones from the base in the opposite direction. This arrangement is likely a reflection of the twisting which occurred in the embryonic cochlea as it was coiled into its final spiral form.

The auditory nerve has been called a "bottle neck" of auditory sensation because all of the afferent and efferent impulses to and from the brain must pass through this single bundle of approximately 30,000 nerve fibers. The nerves are not scattered anatomically like those serving cutaneous or proprioceptive sensation. Thus, the auditory nerve is liable to total disruption or impairment. On the other hand, the possible efficiency of this arrangement for direct stimulation has been recognized in recent attempts to circumvent a nonfunctioning cochlea (40).

VENTRAL AND DORSAL COCHLEAR NUCLEI

When the acoustic nerve emerges from the internal auditory meatus, it enters the medulla; and the cochlear and vestibular divisions are again separated. The cochlear nerve synapse at the ventral and dorsal cochlear nuclei (Figure 2.7). This is one of the main switching centers in the auditory system. Lorente de No (26) has differentiated thirteen different subdivisions of the cochlear nucleus on the basis of the differences in the way the cells are arranged and the way incoming fibers terminate upon them.

All afferent fibers from the cochlea enter the medulla, divide into ascending and descending collaterals, and make synapses in each of these thirteen distinct subdivisions of the cochlear nucleus complex (11). Thus, each fiber terminates upon a great many cells. Again the frequency characteristics of the cochlea are maintained. Fibers from the apex of the cochlea, where low tones are registered, separate at the side and inferior margin of the nucleus, while those from the base, projecting the high tones, bifurcate in the midposterior margin of the nucleus. The conclusion is that in some, if not all of its thirteen subdivisions, the geographical (spatial) arrangement for frequency that was established in the cochlea is repeated in this first central nucleus of the auditory system. In other words, "the cochlea is 'unrolled' at the cochlea nucleus, not just once, but repeatedly" (11). Furthermore, frequencies that are not near the "best frequency" for the particular auditory area are inhibited or suppressed (15). Similar frequency projections are retained in higher nuclei and on the brain itself where the

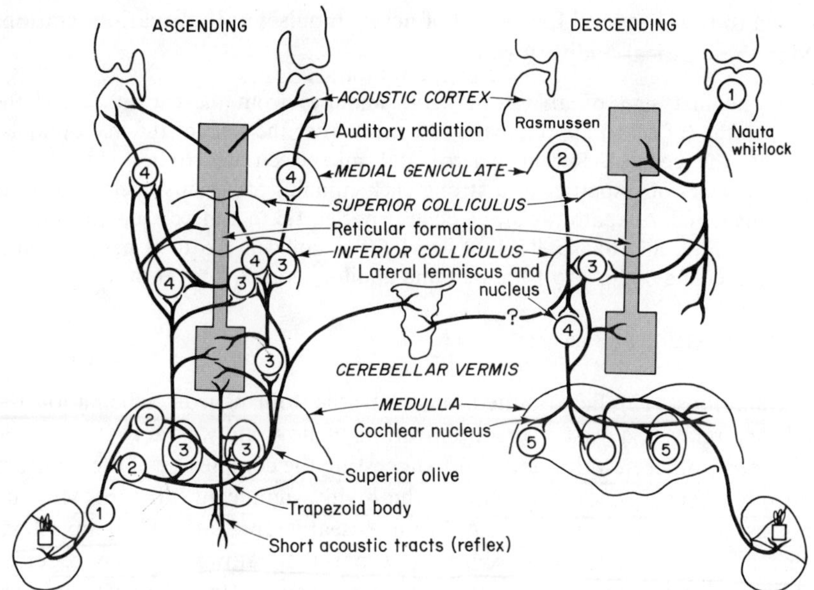

FIGURE 2.7 Diagram of the auditory pathways showing ascending and descending connections.

Source: Galambos, R. "Mechanisms in Audition," *Laryngoscope*, 68:393, 1958.

high tones terminate deep within the auditory cortex, while the low tones end in the outer folds near the surface.

From the dorsal and ventral cochlear nuclei, complex interconnections establish several paths to the cortex and to other important relay centers in subcortical areas as shown in Figure 2.7.

HIGHER RELAY CENTERS

Classical studies of the auditory tracts have emphasized a four-neuron path (35, pp. 24–7). The first neuron runs from the cochlea to the synapse at the dorsal and ventral cochlea nuclei. The second-order neuron was supposed to travel from these nuclei to synapse in the superior olive, the accessory superior olive, the nucleus of the trapezoid body, and the nucleus of the inferior colliculus. The third-order neuron then passed by way of the lateral lemniscus to synapse at the medial geniculate body and, finally, the fourth-order neuron traversed the auditory radiations to the superior temporal gyrus of the cerebral cortex. The anatomical features of each of these major relay stations are discussed in detail in Galambos' excellent review (11).

Tasaki (46) summarized some interesting data from a variety of studies related to time required for arrival of nerve impulses at these various stations along the classical auditory route:

> The first sign of arrival of nerve impulses from the ear appears in the cortex (of a cat) approximately 10 m sec after the start of the microphonics in the cochlea. Recent macro- and microelectrode studies indicate the latencies of responses to a strong click stimulus at various nuclei along the main auditory pathway are: Cochlear nuclei, 1.5 to 2 m sec ; superior olivary complex, approximately 4 m sec; inferior colliculus, 6 to 9 m sec ; medial geniculate body, 7 to 10 m sec ; and auditory cortex, 8 to 12 m sec.

ALTERNATE RELAY ROUTES

Galambos (12) has pointed out that the four-neuron schema of the auditory relay is a vast oversimplification of now known facts.

Among other new developments suggesting the complexity of the auditory and other sensory-motor systems is the highly significant work of Magoun and his coworkers at the UCLA Brain Research Institute. Their investigations have revealed the presence of a parallel pathway in the reticular formation of the brain. Incoming fibers moving up the classical auditory pathway send off shoots into these and other more medial regions of the brain including the cerebellum. Gernandt and Ades (14) were able to demonstrate the existence of "a diffusely projecting spinal system" which seemed to link descending tracts in the spinal cord with reticular formation connections to elicit reflex-type responses to sound stimulation.

Various synaptic relays through the alternate routes allow messages to be delivered to the cortex and other neural centers. Magoun (27, p. 188) notes that "in its ascending and descending relations with the cerebral cortex, the reticular system is intimately bound up with, and contributes to most categories of higher nervous activity... in most of the central integrative processes of the brain." Animal studies have been performed wherein the classical auditory avenues have been sectioned leaving only the alternate lines intact. Such animals are highly disabled in auditory activities for the first few weeks after such an operation. After several months they seem to be able to regain the ability to perform well in auditory situations (12).

DESCENDING AUDITORY TRACTS

The descending auditory tracts illustrated in Figure 2.7 have received less attention than the ascending tracts. In 1946 Rasmussen (36) first clearly identified and described an efferent bundle which consisted of nerves originating in the superior olive region of the medulla. The fibers from one side of the medulla in this bundle were traced to the opposite side of the medulla and thence peripherally to a spiral bundle next to the ganglion cells of the cochlea. In 1953 he traced these fibers to the organ of Corti and concluded that they terminated on the hair cells. A variety of studies since that time have confirmed the presence of this efferent system and have also suggested additional routes at essentially all levels of potential auditory interaction (20, 24). Additional clarification of the efferent systems may be expected.

From the welter of details in the discussion of the anatomy and physiology of the auditory system, certain main facts or principles of organization emerge. The central fact is the old but clearly confirmed observation that a remarkable orderliness exists at all levels of the auditory system. The system is so delicately arranged and balanced that almost infinitesimally small forces in the acoustic signal can be faithfully transported, recorded, and relayed to higher centers with remarkable integrity. This relay system incorporates mechanical, hydraulic, and electrical transducers and amplifiers which seem to operate so efficiently that a tremendous amount of information is transmitted to the brain, while relatively little additional noise is injected into the transmission channel.

The ear also has a built-in system to protect its biological integrity from unwanted or undesirable stimuli. This system extends from the noise-reducing muscles of the middle ear, through the inhibitory efferent nerve endings on the hair cells of the cochlea, and apparently in inhibitory endings throughout all of the major relay centers of the brain.

Many gaps remain in our knowledge of the auditory system. Some of the information cited is based on experiments on animals far removed from man and therefore is open to question in its application to man. This is especially so concerning studies of nervous pathways. Nevertheless a meaningful body of information is available upon which new knowledge of the basic structure and function of the auditory system, as well as new approaches to audiological evaluations, may be built.

We can only conclude that the ear does indeed represent truly a masterpiece of engineering that will challenge and excite us as scientists and clinicians for many years to come.

Bibliography

1. Anson, B. J., J. A. Donaldson, R. L. Warpeka, and T. R. Winch. "A critical appraisal of the anatomy of the perilymphatic system in man." *Transactions of the American Otological, Rhinological, and Laryngological Society*, **71**:488–509, 1964.
2. Bekesy, G. von. "Pressure and shearing forces as stimuli of labyrinthine epithelium." *Archives of Otolaryngology*, **84**:122–30, 1966.
3. Buch, N. H., and M. B. Jorgensen. "Eustachian tube and middle ear Embryology and Pathology." *Archives of Otolaryngology*, **79**:472–80, 1964.

4. Citron, L. D. Exley, and C. S. Hallpike. "Formation, circulation, and chemical properties of labyrinthine fluids." *British Medical Journal*, **12**:101–4, 1956.
5. Davis, H. "Biophysics and physiology of the inner ear." *Physiological Review*, **37**:1–49, 1957.
6. Elliott, G. B., and K. S. Elliott. "Some pathological, radiological, and clinical implications of the precocious development of the human ear." *Laryngoscope*, **74**:1160–71, 1964.
7. Engström, H. "The cortilymph, the third lymph of the inner ear." *Acta Morphologica Neerlando-Scandinavia*, **3**:195, 1960.
8. Engström, H. "On the double innervation of the sensory epithelia of the inner ear." *Acta Oto-Laryngologica*, **49**:109–18, 1958.
9. Engström, H., H. W. Ades, and J. E. Hawkins, Jr. "Cellular pattern, nerve structures, and fluid spaces of the organ of Corti." *Contributions to Sensory Physiology*, Vol. 1: New York: Academic Press, 1965.
10. Fisch, U., and G. U. Schulthess. "Electromyographic studies on the human stapedial muscle." *Acta Oto-Laryngologica*, **56**:287–97, 1963.
11. Galambos, R. "Neural mechanisms of audition." *Physiological Reviews*, **34**:497–528, 1954.
12. Galambos, R. "Neuroanatomy and physiology of the auditory system: Short Course." 42nd Annual Convention, *American Speech and Hearing Association*, 1966.
13. Galambos, R. "Suppression of auditory nerve activity by stimulation of efferent fibers to the cochlea." *Journal of Neurophysiology*, **19**:424–37, 1956.
14. Gernandt, B. E., and H. W. Ades. "Spinal motor responses to acoustic stimulation." *Experimental Neurology*, **10**:52–66, 1964.
15. Graves, G. O., and L. F. Edwards. "The eustachian tube: A review of its descriptive, microscopic, topographic, and clinical anatomy." *Archives of Otolaryngology*, **39**:359–97, 1944.
16. Greenwood, D. D., and N. Maruyama. "Excitatory and inhibitory responses areas of auditory neurons in the cochlear nucleus." *Journal of Neurophysiology*, **28**:863–92, 1965.
17. Harty, M. "The joints of the middle ear." *Zeitschrift für Mikroskopisch-Anatomishe Forschung*, **71**:24–31, 1964.
18. Hilding, A. C. "Studies on the otic labyrinth. 1. On the origin and insertion of the tectorial membrane." *Annals of Otology, Rhinology and Laryngology*, **61**:354–70, 1952.
19. Hilding, D. A. "The protective value of the stapedius reflex: An experimental study." *Transactions of the American Academy of Ophthalmology and Otolaryngology*, **65**:297–307, 1961.
20. Ishii, T., Y. Murakami, and J. Balogh, Jr. "Acelycholinesterase activity in the efferent nerve fibers of the human inner ear." *Annals of Otology, Rhinology and Laryngology*, **76**:69–82, 1967.
21. Iurato, S. "Efferent fibers to the sensory cells of Corti's organ." *Experimental Cell Research*, **27**:162–64, 1962.
22. Iurato, S. "The sensory cells of the membranous labyrinth." *Archives of Otolaryngology*, **75**:312–28, 1962.
23. Katsuki, Y., K. Yanagisawa, and J. Kanzaki. "Tetrathulammonium and Tetradotoxin: Effects on cochlear potentials." *Science*, **151**:1544–45, 1966.

24. Kiang, N. Y. S., R. R. Pfeiffer, W. B. Warr, and A. S. N. Backus. "Stimulus coding in the cochlear nucleus." *Transaction of the American Otological Society*, **53**:35–58, 1965.
25. Liden, G., B. Nordlund, and J. D. Hawkins, Jr. "Significance of the stapedius reflex for the understanding of speech." *Acta Oto-Laryngologica*, Supplement, **188**:275–79, 1964.
26. Lorente de No, R. "Anatomy of the eighth nerve. The central projection of the nerve endings of the internal ear." *Laryngoscope*, **43**:1–38, 1933.
27. Magoun, H. W. *The Waking Brain.* Springfield: Charles C. Thomas, Publisher, 1963.
28. McGrady, Jr., E. "The embryology of the opossum." *American Anatomical Memoir* 16. Philadelphia: Wistar Institute of Anatomy and Biology, 1938.
29. Mygind, S. H. "Functional mechanism of the labyrinthine epithelium." *Archives of Otolaryngology*, (I) **82**:452–561, 1965; (II) **82**:587–90, 1965; (III) **83**:3–9, 1966.
30. Naftalin, L. "Some new proposals regarding acoustic transmission and transduction." *Cold Spring Harbor Symposia on Quantitative Biology*, **30**:169–80, 1965.
31. Neergaard, E. B., H. C. Anderson, C. C. Hansen, and O. Jepsen. "Experimental studies on sound transmission in the human ear. III: Influence of the stapedius and tensor tympanic muscles." *Acta Oto-Laryngologica, Supplement*, **188**:280–86, 1954.
32. Nomura, Y., and I. Kirikae. "Innervation of the human cochlea." *Annals of Otology, Rhinology and Laryngology*, **76**:57–68, 1967.
33. Ormerod, F. C. "The metabolism of the cochlear and vestibular end-organs." *Journal of Laryngology and Otology*, **75**:562–73, 1961.
34. Patten, B. M. *Human Embryology.* New York: The Blakiston Company, 1953.
35. Rasmussen, A. T. *The Principal Nervous Pathways.* New York: The Macmillan Company, 1935.
36. Rasmussen, G. L. "The olivary peduncle and other fiber projections of the superior olivary complex." *Journal of Comparative Neurology*, **84**:141–219, 1946.
37. Ritter, F. N., and M. Lawrence. "A histological and experimental study of cochlea aqueduct pathway in the adult human." *Laryngoscope*, **75**:1224–33, 1965.
38. Sade, J. "Middle ear mucosa." *Archives of Otolaryngology*, **84**:137–43, 1966.
39. Scheer, A. A. "Correction of congenital middle ear deformities." *Archives of Otolaryngology*, **85**:269–77, 1967.
40. Simmons, F. B., C. J. Mongeon, W. R. Lewis, and D. A. Huntington. "Electrical stimulation of acoustical nerve and inferior colliculus." *Archives of Otolaryngology*, **70**:558–67, 1964.
41. Simmons, F. B. "Perceptual theories of middle ear function." *Annals of Otology, Rhinology, and Laryngology*, **73**:724–39, 1964.
42. Smith, C. A., and E. W. Dempsey. "Electron microscopy of the organ of Corti." *American Journal of Anatomy*, **100**:337–68, 1957.
43. Smith, C. A. "Innervation patterns of the cochlea: The internal hair cell." *Annals of Otology, Rhinology, and Laryngology*, **70**:504–27, 1961.

44. Spoendlin, W. H. "Ultrastructural features of the organ of Corti." *Transactions of the American Otological Society*, **50**:61–82, 1962.
45. Stevens, S. S. and H. Davis, *Hearing*. New York: John Wiley and Sons, 1938.
46. Tasaki, I. "Hearing." *Annual Review of Physiology*, **19**:417–38, 1957.
47. Vinnikov, J. A. and L. K. Titova. "Cytophysiology and Cytochemistry of the organ of Corti: A cytochemical theory of hearing." *International Review of Cytophysiology*, **14**:157–91, 1963.

neoplasm - n; a new growth of tissue serving no physiologic function : TUMOR

collagen - n.: an insoluble fibrous protein that occurs in vertebrates as the chief constituent of connective tissue fibrils + in bones & yields gelatin + glue on prolonged heating (w) H_2O.

dyscrasias - n. an abnormal condition of the body.

3

Otologic Assessment and Treatment

D. Thane R. Cody, Ph.D., M.D.
Mayo Clinic
Rochester, Minnesota

The History

In the assessment of hearing impairment, one should remember that disorders of the audiovestibular system may be the first manifestation of neoplasm of the nasopharynx, multiple sclerosis, collagen diseases, disorders of the reticulo-endothelial system, blood dyscrasias, or cerebrovascular arteriosclerosis. Making a diagnosis of conductive hearing impairment or sensori-neural hearing loss and ignoring the fact that this complaint is only one manifestation of a serious and perhaps life-threatening disorder can be a tragic error. In assessing hearing impairment, therefore, the examiner, in addition to obtaining a history of past, present, and familial otologic complaints, must also be prepared to obtain a careful history of complaints referable to other systems. Naturally, it is not the responsibility of the audiologist or otologist to obtain a complete general medical history on all patients with hearing impairment. The first few minutes spent talking with the patient or his relatives will help to determine the direction the inquiry should take and how detailed the history must be. In addition to hearing impairment, other symptoms of disorders of the ear are tinnitus, vertigo, aural pain, aural discharge (otorrhea), aural sensation of fullness theatened -

or pressure, increased aural sensitivity to sound (recruitment and hyperacusis), and distortion in pitch (diplacusis). Any one or more of these symptoms may coexist with loss of hearing.

HEARING IMPAIRMENT

The age of the patient at the time of examination and the age at onset of impairment of hearing help the examiner in determining what historic facts he must try to obtain. For instance, if a two-year-old child is suspected of being hard-of-hearing and has not developed any speech, emphasis is going to be placed on a prenatal, natal, neonatal, and familial history. If the child has recently been examined by a pediatrician, has no obvious congenital malformations, and appears to be mentally bright, then a careful inquiry into the health of the mother during pregnancy may elucidate the cause of the problem. A history of rubella, particularly during the first trimester of pregnancy, would explain a bilateral severe sensori-neural hearing impairment in the child. A history of theatened abortion, which could have resulted in anoxia to the fetus, could possibly be responsible for hearing impairment. A history of the mother having multiple abortions prior to a successful pregnancy with the patient would lead to the suspicion that the mother was infected with syphilis and would make mandatory the serologic testing of both parents and child. If the father is Rh positive and the mother Rh negative, erythroblastosis fetalis would be suspected as a possible cause of the hearing impairment. Such a history would be particularly incriminating if there were several older siblings and the patient was jaundiced at, or shortly after, birth. Difficulties in delivery and problems in resuscitation of the baby at birth, which could have resulted in anoxia, may have been the etiologic factor.

If the child was premature, and particularly if it was born during the 1950's, a thorough history of whether or not the child received prophylactic antibiotics after birth and the type of antibiotic given are extremely important factors. It is well documented that severe sensori-neural hearing impairment developed in many premature infants who received dihydrostreptomycin during the 1950's. Usually dihydrostreptomycin was administered in combination with penicillin. The elucidation of a history of a severe illness, such as meningitis, during the neonatal period may provide the clue to the cause of a severe hearing loss. Obviously, in assessing the auditory problem of a two-year-old child, inquiry into the occurrence of congenital hearing impairment in parents, siblings, grandparents, uncles, aunts, and cousins also can be helpful to the examiner.

In a sixty-year-old patient who has noticed a gradual onset of difficulty in hearing, it will be apparent that the emphasis in the history will be quite different from that of the two-year-old child. A detailed history of the prenatal and neonatal periods would be unnecessary, but a family history of hearing impairment might be of value and the patient should be queried. If hearing impairment has developed in other members of the family during adult life, the examiner would suspect the possibility of presbycusis or otosclerosis. In addition, a history of excessive exposure to noise may be of aid in determining the etiology of a hearing disorder in a sixty-year-old patient.

The examining physician should determine whether the hearing loss is unilateral or bilateral and, if it is bilateral, whether or not the impairment occurred simultaneously in both ears. It is important to establish whether or not the patient thinks that he hears better with one ear than with the other, because oftentimes, even though the pure-tone audiometric threshold, the speech reception threshold, and the speech discrimination scores are identical in each ear, the patient still says that he hears better with one ear than with the other. All surgical procedures for restoring conductive hearing loss have a small but significant risk that the hearing will be made worse. Because of the possibility of this complication, when surgical treatment is indicated, it is mandatory to operate on the ear that objectively has the poorest hearing, and when audiometric results show the hearing impairment is the same bilaterally, it is prudent to operate on the ear that the patient subjectively thinks is worst.

The speed with which hearing impairment develops can vary from a few seconds to many years. The sudden onset of severe or complete unilateral or bilateral hearing impairment in a patient in his teens or twenties during or shortly after an infection of the upper respiratory tract would make the examiner highly suspicious of viral labyrinthitis. This would be particularly likely if the patient had the symptoms and signs of mumps and the virus had been cultured. On the other hand, if a sixty-five-year-old patient who has not had a recent infection of the upper respiratory tract and who is known to have hypertensive heart disease awakens one morning with complete unilateral deafness, the etiologic factor would most likely be a vascular accident in the inner ear.

Hearing impairment may develop rapidly over weeks or months. An example of this is the bilateral sensori-neural hearing impairment that not uncommonly occurs in patients a few weeks or months after they have received dihydrostreptomycin or neomycin. In a situation in which the hearing loss first appears four months after use of the antibiotic has been discontinued and rapidly progresses to complete deafness, the patient may not relate the hearing impairment to intake of the drug. It is the examiner's job to ferret out this important information.

Hearing impairment also may develop over many years. It is not always easy to elicit a history of gradual development of hearing loss, and the physician must be cognizant of this problem. A patient may have been aware only of a hearing impairment for several months, because during that period the air-conduction threshold in both ears had reached, or dropped below, the 40-dB level. The slow development of hearing impairment hid the fact from the patient until the problem became critical. The same difficulty may exist with gradually developing unilateral hearing impairment. After the hearing loss has become severe, the patient may suddenly notice that he cannot hear with the affected ear, although he has been quite unaware of the insidious development of impairment. Careful questioning will often reveal that the patient's relatives and friends had suggested for years that he should have his hearing checked, for they had become aware of the problem long before the patient had, or at least before he was willing to concede that he had hearing loss.

Fluctuation in auditory acuity may be associated with disorders of both the middle ear and the inner ear. Fluctuation with an overall tendency to progressive deterioration in hearing ability is characteristic of Meniere's disease, latent labyrinthitis associated with congenital syphilis long after the infection has been adequately treated, and Cogan's syndrome (nonsyphilitic interstitial keratitis associated with audio-vestibular symptoms). In many instances it is difficult to be certain, on the basis of the history, whether periodic changes in auditory acuity have occurred. The patient may be a poor observer or the hearing impairment may be so severe that it is impossible for him to recognize rather minor fluctuations. In these situations the only way in which the presence of fluctuation can be established is by obtaining serial audiograms. Even when there is a definite history of exacerbations and remissions in the hearing impairment, it is ideal to document this by repeated audiometric testing.

The patient's ability to function in a noisy environment can help in the differential diagnosis of the type and etiology of hearing impairment. The patient who has bilateral conductive hearing loss due to otosclerosis often will remark that he hears conversation better while driving in a car with the windows open. The reason for this is simply that his hearing loss masks out some of the excess ambient noise, while a person in the same car with normal hearing finds it more difficult to hear when the windows are open and tends to speak louder. On the other extreme are the patients who have a high-tone sensori-neural hearing loss, such as frequently occurs in presbycusis. These patients may first become aware of a hearing problem because of difficulty in understanding conversation at a cocktail party or large meeting.

Strangely enough, the patient who comes for assessment of hearing impairment may have worn a hearing aid with benefit for ten years, but he may leave the aid at home on the day of the examination and may not mention the fact that he has used one. It is important, both from the point of view of diagnosis and for future rehabilitative measures, to ascertain whether or not the patient has tried a hearing aid. If a hearing aid has been used, it is necessary to determine the type; whether it was worn in the ear (air-conduction) or behind it (bone-conduction); whether binaural hearing aids were used and, if so, the benefit derived from their use; and how much of the time the patient actually used a hearing aid. The patient also may be reluctant to mention previous operations on the ear and the historian must inquire specifically about such treatment. The information that the patient underwent fenestration, stapes mobilization, or stapedectomy on one ear for hearing impairment with resultant improvement in hearing quickly establishes otosclerosis as the probable cause of the hearing loss in the other ear.

TINNITUS

An annoying noise, often described as ringing, hissing, humming, buzzing, roaring, cricket-like chirping, or a seashell sound, may be heard by the patient in the ear with impaired hearing. This complaint is called TINNITUS and may occur with any type and degree of hearing loss. Tinnitus may be intermittent or constant and may vary in intensity. Oftentimes the tinnitus accompanying hearing impairment is the patient's chief complaint. The degree of annoyance may be related to the intensity, the patient's emotional stability, or both. Although the noise heard by the patient is usually nonpulsatile, occasionally it may pulsate in rhythm with the heart beat and in such instances is often described as a "swishing" or "thumping" sound. Pulsatile tinnitus not uncommonly occurs when there is a conductive hearing loss due to fluid in the middle ear, such as in acute or chronic suppurative otitis media and secretory otitis media.

VERTIGO

Dizziness may be another associated symptom of hearing impairment and to the patient this term can mean many things. It is up to the examiner, and frequently this can be extremely difficult, to determine exactly what the patient does mean by this complaint. True VERTIGO is the term used for any hallucination of movement, no matter what its character, and frequently it occurs as the result of lesions of the inner ear involving both the auditory and vestibular systems, such as in Meniere's disease. Lesions confined to the vestibular components of the inner ear may be the cause, as well as lesions in the brain stem, particularly those of a vascular nature, and, rarely, lesions of the temporal lobe of the cerebrum. It is important to acquire as accurate a description of the vertigo as possible including the duration of attacks, the frequency of attacks, precipitating factors, and the association of the vertiginous episodes with nausea, vomiting, excess perspiration, and diarrhea. Severe attacks of objective rotatory vertigo are associated with ataxia; however, severe unsteadiness may develop as the result of an inner-ear disorder without rotatory vertigo. As a matter of fact, it is the rule rather than the exception for patients to experience severe unsteadiness without rotatory vertigo when both vestibular labyrinths have been impaired due to the use of streptomycin. The patient also may interpret the sensation of giddiness or light-headedness, weakness, a blackout sensation, and blurring of his vision as dizziness. These symptoms are not caused by disorders of the inner ear.

AURAL PAIN

Aural pain may accompany the onset of hearing impairment and in this regard one immediately thinks of severe earache with acute suppurative otitis media. The patient may vividly remember such an episode and may date the occurrence of his hearing loss without subsequent progression to a single such ear infection in childhood. This type of history is not always reliable, however, because I have operated on many patients with such a history whose conductive hearing loss was a result of otosclerosis and whose middle ear showed no evidence of previous infection. In all probability the patient had had an episode of acute suppurative otitis media, but this was not responsible for the chronic hearing impairment. On the other hand, the onset of unilateral, persistent, severe aural pain with hearing impairment would make one immediately suspicious of the possible presence of a malignant neoplasm of the external auditory canal or middle ear.

Severe deep aural pain and facial pain in the distribution of the sensory divisions of the fifth cranial nerve may be associated with hearing impairment due to suppurative otitis media when the infection involves the apex of the petrous bone, which is in close proximity to the gasserian ganglion. The abducens nerve may be involved as well, resulting in diplopia, and the combination of pain, aural discharge, and diplopia is known as "Gradenigo's syndrome."

A more superficial but extremely severe aural pain associated with sensori-neural hearing impairment may result from herpes zoster oticus (Ramsey Hunt syndrome). The diagnosis can be established by the presence of the typical vesicles found in the external auditory canal and over the concha of the auricle.

From these brief illustrations it can be seen that a history of aural pain and its characteristics may aid the examiner in determining the cause of hearing impairment.

AURAL DISCHARGE (OTORRHEA)

An aural discharge may consist of a purulent or mucopurulent exudate, blood, or cerebrospinal fluid and can be associated with a conductive, sensori-neural, or mixed hearing impairment. A history of an intermittent or persistent aural discharge over a period of years would point to infection as the probable cause of hearing impairment. On the other hand, hearing loss with a clear aural discharge appearing immediately after a severe head injury would suggest a fracture of the base of the skull and rupture of the tympanic membrane. Transverse fractures through the petrous bone usually result in complete sensori-neural hearing impairment, while longitudinal fractures are often not as destructive and may cause a conductive hearing impairment due to dislocation of the ossicular chain. A bloody aural discharge may result from infection or trauma. Bleeding can occur with chronic suppurative otitis media when hemorrhagic granulation tissue is present in the middle ear and in acute suppurative otitis media at the time that the tympanic membrane ruptures.

AURAL SENSATION OF FULLNESS

Frequently a patient with endolymphatic hydrops will complain of a sensation of fullness or pressure in the ear with impaired hearing. Occasionally this symptom is extremely annoying but usually the patient considers it as relatively minor compared to the vertiginous attacks, and he may neglect mentioning the problem to the examiner. The sensation of fullness may occur intermittently with or without direct relation to depression in auditory acuity and attacks of vertigo, or it can be present constantly. A patient who has a conductive hearing loss due to fluid in his middle ear associated with an infection or who has secretory otitis media also may complain of a sensation of aural fullness. Elaborating on this symptom, a patient may state that he has the sensation of water being present in his ear, and when he speaks it sounds to him as if his head were in a barrel. In addition to the complaint of aural fullness or pressure, patients with any type of hearing impairment due to any cause occasionally complain of a numb or dead sensation in the affected ear. Although there would appear to be a direct relationship between the sensation of fullness and increased pressure in the endolymphatic system of the inner ear in Meniere's disease, the sensation of numbness associated with any type of hearing impairment is more difficult to explain.

INCREASED AURAL SENSITIVITY TO SOUND

Patients with sensori-neural hearing impairment due to an inner-ear disorder such as Meniere's disease may complain of increased sensitivity to noise in the involved ear. In extreme instances the patient may think that moderately loud noise actually causes pain in the ear, although just as in the case of the symptom of aural fullness, this symptom may be ignored in the presence of severe vertiginous episodes and will be discovered only through specific inquiry. The demonstration of recruitment on audiometric testing will establish more concrete evidence of the basis for this complaint. Patients with lesions of the seventh cranial nerve resulting in paralysis of the stapedius muscle also may complain of increased sensitivity to rather loud sounds in the ear on the paralyzed side. This symptom, often referred to as "hyperacusis," usually is associated with normal hearing. In the presence of this complaint, evidence helping to substantiate an impression of paralysis of the stapedius muscle may be obtained by testing with the acoustic bridge.

DISTORTION OF PITCH (DIPLACUSIS)

Another symptom occasionally associated with hearing impairment due to endolymphatic hydrops is DIPLACUSIS. The patient notices that a sound is heard at a different pitch in the ear with the hearing loss from what he hears in the normal ear. This symptom is less frequently a complaint than aural sensation of fullness or hypersensitivity to sound. It requires a rather astute observer to notice and describe diplacusis, and usually the phenomenon is appreciated primarily by musicians or patients with musical talent.

OCULAR DISORDERS

A thorough history of hearing impairment should include inquiry into ocular disorders, for their association can lead the examiner to the cause of a hearing loss. Conductive hearing impairment with diplopia may be due to a nasopharyngeal neoplasm or suppuration in the apex of the petrous pyramid of the temporal bone. Both of these conditions require immediate attention, and the earlier the diagnosis is suspected, the better. A sensori-neural hearing impairment with diplopia may be due to multiple sclerosis, and the examiner should acquire the appropriate examinations and laboratory tests. Sensori-neural hearing impairment in association with uveitis may lead to a diagnosis of sarcoidosis or the Vogt-Koyanagi-Harada syndrome (hearing impairment, nontraumatic uveitis, poliosis, vitiligo, alopecia, and meningeal irritation). Sensori-neural hearing loss and interstitial keratitis may be a result of congenital syphilis or Cogan's syndrome. These are only a few examples which indicate the importance of eliciting a history of an ocular disorder in the patient with hearing impairment and emphasize the necessity of evaluating the patient and not just an ear.

The Examination

The patient with aural symptoms should have not only a thorough examination of his ears but also a complete examination of the head and neck including the nose, mouth, pharynx, larynx, vasculature of the head and neck accessible to palpation, and evaluation of the function of the cranial nerves and cerebellum. The examination of the patient, the complaints, and the preliminary findings determine how inclusive the examination must be, what laboratory tests should be ordered, and whether or not he should be examined by experts in other specialties, such as ophthalmology, neurology, neurosurgery, and internal medicine. Although the otologist is responsible for performing most of the examinations and interpreting the tests, the audiologist should be familiar with these investigations.

The examination begins when the otologist or audiologist first sees the patient. Does the patient respond to a normal voice? Does he appear alert, underdeveloped, or mongoloid? Are there any gross motor defects or abnormalities in gait? Does the patient appear depressed, suspicious, or have an air of "la belle indifference"? Is the voice quality normal, or is there a monotonous quality to it, suggesting that the patient has had severe sensori-neural hearing impairment of long duration? These simple initial observations can help immensely in the overall assessment of the patient.

AUSCULTATION

A stethoscope and occasionally even an ear-to-ear tube (Figure 3.1) can be of aid in examining the patient who complains of hearing a pulsatile noise or a click in the ear. In the case of an arteriovenous fistula or atherosclerotic plaque in the carotid arterial system, a bruit may be heard

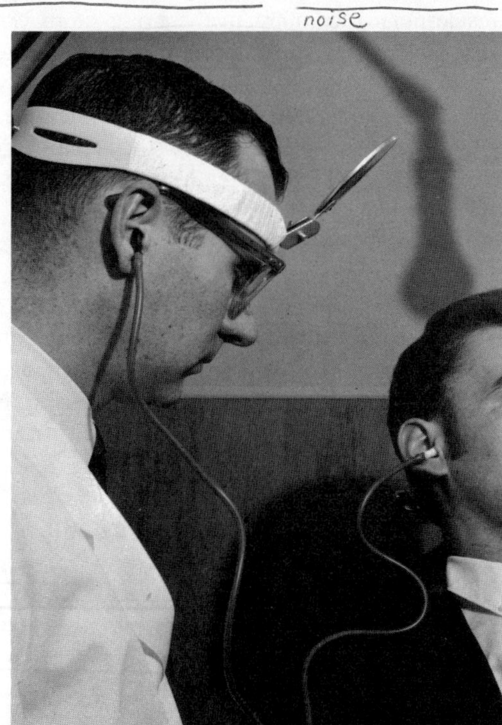

FIGURE 3.1 Ear-to-ear tube.

in the vicinity of the ear and may help to establish the diagnosis. A repetitive click in the patient's ear that is distinctly heard by the examiner can lead to a diagnosis of palatal myoclonus resulting from a brain stem lesion.

AURAL INSPECTION AND PALPATION

The auricles and external auditory canals should be inspected for acquired abnormalities and congenital malformation. A microtic auricle with atresia of the external auditory canal would indicate that the defect occurred in the first trimester of pregnancy. A normal auricle with congenital atresia of the external meatus would indicate that the defect occurred later in fetal life, with an excellent possibility of an intact and functional ossicular chain and approximately a fifty per cent chance of an intact tympanic membrane (35). In such a situation, inspection has helped to define the relative difficulties that would be anticipated during an operative attempt at reconstruction for useful auditory function. Inspection and palpation of the auricle may reveal defects in the cartilage that have resulted from trauma, infection, or chronic relapsing polychondritis and may be related to a disorder in the middle or inner ear. Inspection and palpation of the mastoid process may reveal swelling, discoloration, fluctuation, and tenderness due to suppurative mastoiditis. Pressure on the tragus can cause considerable discomfort in the presence of external otitis and can produce nystagmus and vertigo when there is a fistula into the horizontal semicircular canal (positive fistula test) resulting from cholesteatoma. Palpation over the carotid artery may reveal a thrill associated with a complaint of pulsatile tinnitus. Palpation of the superficial temporal artery may elicit induration, beading, and tenderness due to arteritis which has caused visual impairment, headache, and loss of hearing.

OTOSCOPIC EXAMINATION

Examination of the external auditory canal and tympanic membrane can be performed with an otoscope (Figure 3.2), head mirror and ear speculum (Figure 3.3), Siegle's otoscope (Figure 3.2), or binocular dissecting microscope (Figure 3.4). The use of the simple speculum will reveal most abnormalities of the external auditory canal, such as impacted cerumen, abrasions, infections, and tumors. It is obvious that for a satisfactory examination all cerumen, debris, and pus must be removed from the external meatus. Before doing this, however, when pus is present a specimen should be obtained for culture of organisms and antibiotic sensitivity studies. The tympanic membrane may appear normal, scarred, thickened, flaccid, bulging, discolored, or perforated. In secretory otitis media a fluid level may be discernible in the middle ear space behind an intact tympanic membrane, and sometimes air bubbles are apparent in the fluid. If one is uncertain as

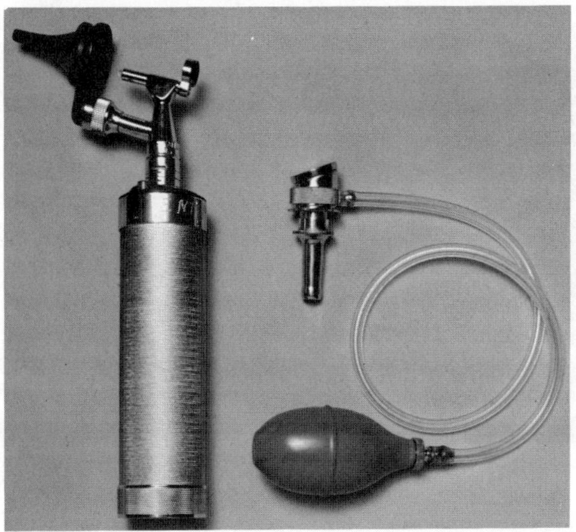

FIGURE 3.2 Left, otoscope. Right, Siegle's otoscope.

to the presence of fluid in the tympanic cavity, diagnostic myringotomy can be performed.

In active chronic suppurative otitis media, in addition to a purulent exudate, hemorrhagic granulation tissue may be seen growing through the rupture in the tympanic membrane, or a cholesteatoma may be evident in an attic defect. Siegle's otoscope is of particular value in testing the mobility

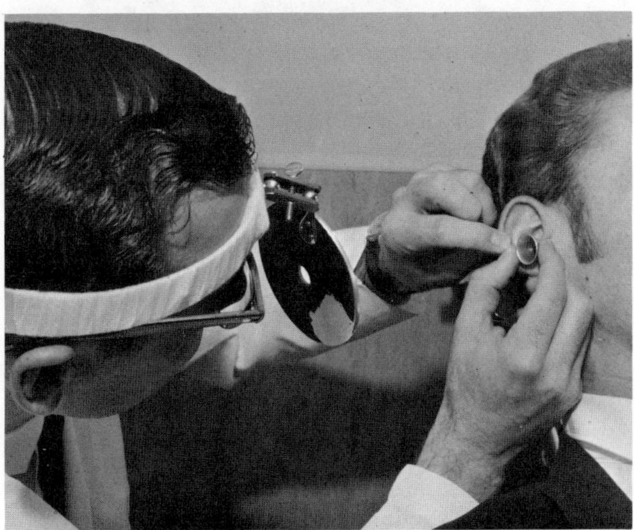

FIGURE 3.3 Examination with head mirror and ear speculum.

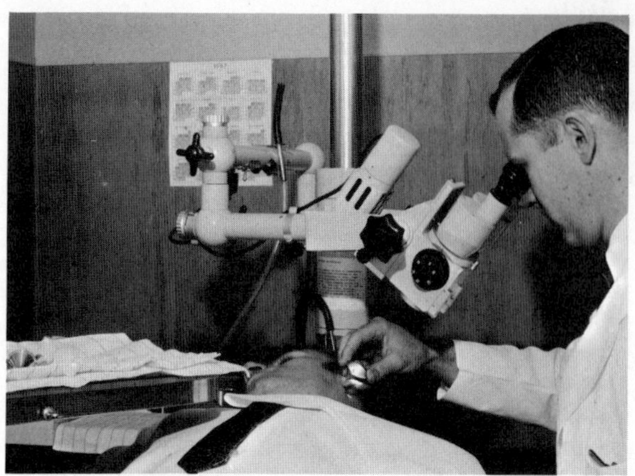

FIGURE 3.4 Examination with binocular dissecting microscope and ear speculum.

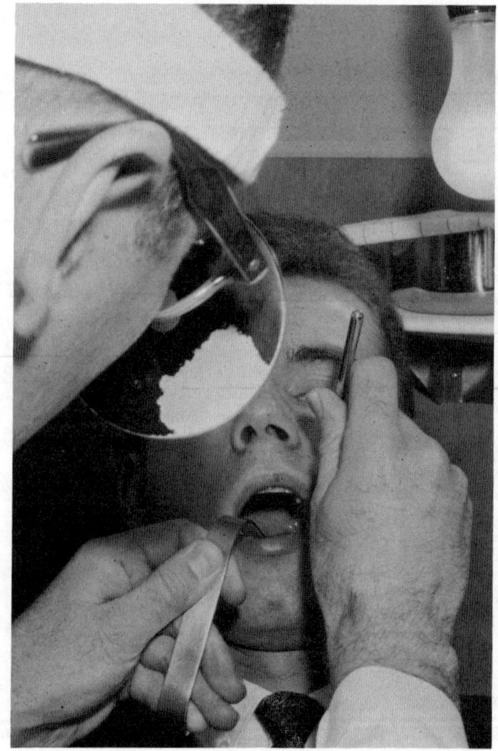

FIGURE 3.5 Use of nasopharyngeal mirror in examination of nasopharynx.

of the tympanic membrane and in sucking secretions through a perforation because the examiner, when inspecting the tympanic membrane, can exert positive and negative pressures on it. Siegle's otoscope can also be used to test for a fistula in the horizontal semicircular canal. Examination of the tympanic membrane or tympanic cavity with the microscope facilitates inspection and palpation with a probe and often provides knowledge of the extent of pathologic involvement of the middle ear that otherwise is unobtainable.

FUNCTION OF EUSTACHIAN TUBE

Evaluation of the function of the eustachian tube begins during the routine otoscopic examination. If the patient complains of a plugged feeling in one ear and of hearing his own voice and breathing excessively loudly in this ear but states that his symptoms are relieved by lying down, the examiner may observe the tympanic membrane moving in and out in rhythm with the patient's breathing. This finding indicates that the eustachian tube is abnormally patent. No aural investigation is complete without a thorough examination of the nasopharynx. With the nasopharyngeal mirror (Figure 3.5), a thorough systematic visual inspection of the nasopharynx is made; any area showing even the slightest abnormality should be biopsied. Often when it seems highly probable that unilateral secretory otitis media is the result of a nasopharyngeal neoplasm but no tumor can be seen, multiple blind biopsies must be taken.

Normal function of the eustachian tube is necessary for successful myringoplasty. The patency of the tube can be tested by the Valsalva or Politzer maneuvers. With the Valsalva maneuver, the patient closes his mouth, holds his nose so that air will not escape, and blows, forcing air into the eustachian tube; with the Politzer maneuver the patient swallows water while air is forced into one nostril with the Politzer bag or Senturia apparatus and the other nostril is clamped (Figure 3.6). Ordinarily, with these maneuvers a normal eustachian tube will inflate readily. When these methods have failed, the pharyngeal orifice of the eustachian tube can be catheterized directly with a cannula inserted through the nose. Air is forced through the tube and used for inflation. The necessity of using a cannula to inflate the eustachian tube usually implies some defect in function.

CRANIAL NERVES

Although the otologist is not responsible for performing a complete neurologic examination, during a routine otolaryngologic examination it should be automatic to test, in addition to the acoustic nerve, the function of several other cranial nerves. Protrusion of the tongue with deviation to one side of the midline indicates either a supranuclear or an infranuclear

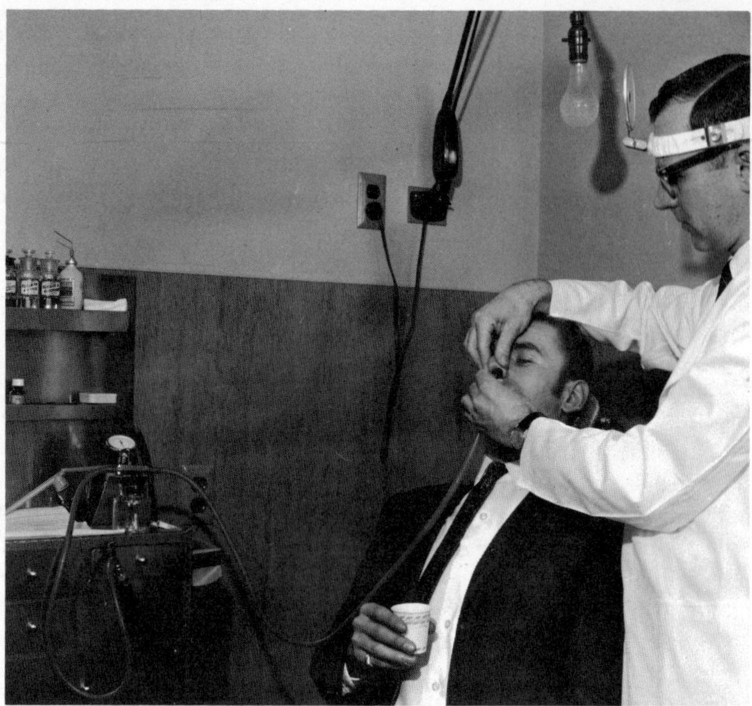

FIGURE 3.6 Politzer method of inflating eustachian tube. Senturia apparatus is being used.

paralysis of the hypoglossal nerve (twelfth cranial nerve) on the opposite side. In the event of long-standing paralysis, the muscles on the paretic side will be atrophied. Deviation of the soft palate to one side and fixation of the vocal cord on the opposite side indicate paralysis of the vagus nerve (tenth cranial nerve) on the side of the nonfunctioning vocal cord. These defects may be the result of lesions in the cerebellopontine angle or at the jugular foramen. A chemodectoma of the jugular foramen may involve the ninth, tenth, eleventh, and twelfth cranial nerves and, in addition to obvious paralysis of the tongue, palate, and vocal cord, there would be decreased pharyngeal sensation to touch (ninth cranial nerve) and weakness of the sternocleidomastoid and trapezius muscles (eleventh cranial nerve) on the same side as the lesion.

Severe unilateral weakness of the muscles of expression is readily discernible, but to elicit a minimal defect both careful testing of the strength of the frontalis, orbicularis oculi, and orbicularis ori muscles and comparison of the function of these muscles on each side of the face are necessary. A peripheral lesion of the facial nerve results in paralysis of the entire ipsilateral side of the face, while a central lesion does not result in paralysis of the frontalis muscle and usually involves the orbicularis oculi muscle to varying degrees in different patients. The paralysis is most evident below the eye. Paralysis of the stapedius nerve, a branch of the facial nerve that supplies the stapedius muscle, occasionally will result in complaints of increased sensitivity to loud sounds in the ear on the paralyzed side (hyperacusis). Often this muscle will be paralyzed, however, without the patient complaining of hyperacusis. More information can be obtained on the function of this muscle by use of the acoustic bridge.

The nervus intermedius (Wrisberg's nerve) is closely associated with the motor facial nerve from the brain stem to the geniculate ganglion and supplies parasympathetic fibers to the ipsilateral lacrimal gland (greater superficial petrosal nerve) and submaxillary and sublingual glands (chorda tympani nerve) and carries gustatory fibers from the ipsilateral anterior two-thirds of the tongue (chorda tympani nerve) to the brain stem. A proper evaluation of the facial nerve involves, in addition to evaluation of function of the muscles of expression, testing tear formation and taste. Formation of saliva in the submaxillary gland also can be tested but is not generally done routinely in clinical practice.

When the motor nucleus itself is diseased, paralysis of the facial muscles will be evident and may be associated with paralysis of the lateral rectus muscle. The abducens nerve (sixth cranial nerve) is in close proximity to, and partially loops around, the facial motor nucleus. Lacrimation and taste are not affected. The patient may complain of hyperacusis. A lesion of the facial nerve in its course from the brain stem to the geniculate ganglion, such as may be seen with fractures of the petrous bone or an acoustic neuroma, causes ipsilateral paralysis of the muscles of expression, lack of tear formation, and loss of taste in the anterior two-thirds of the tongue. A lesion of the facial nerve in its course through the tympanic cavity does not affect lacrimation. The geniculate ganglion is located at the genu of the facial nerve before its entrance into the tympanic cavity, and the parasympathetic fibers supplying the lacrimal gland leave the ganglion and are carried by the greater superficial petrosal nerve. The stapedius nerve arises from the facial nerve as it leaves the tympanic cavity and begins its descent to the stylomastoid foramen and its emergence from the skull. The chorda tympani nerve usually arises from the facial nerve at the stylomastoid foramen or a few millimeters above this level. In Bell's palsy, the lesion of the nerve is most commonly at the foramen and extends a centimeter or more proximally. In such a situation when the chorda tympani nerve is involved, taste will be absent from the anterior two-thirds of the tongue, but the patient will not complain of hyperacusis and tear formation will be normal. These brief examples should illustrate that a few minutes spent in evaluating function of the facial nerve often can provide the examiner with knowledge as to the site of the lesion. This information is of special significance when surgical therapy is contemplated.

A search for spontaneous nystagmus should be made in all patients with audio-vestibular complaints. Observing eye movements may reveal that one eye does not move laterally beyond the midline, and indicates lateral rectus paralysis due to involvement of the abducent nerve by a neoplasm arising in the nasopharynx or infection involving the petrous apex. This is the time to test the sensitivity of the corneal reflexes. A unilateral hypoactive corneal reflex or absence of the reflex may be encountered with a large acoustic neuroma and always is the first indication of involvement of the trigeminal nerve (fifth cranial nerve). When such involvement is indicated, the portions of the scalp and face supplied by the ophthalmic, maxillary, and mandibular divisions of the trigeminal nerve should be tested for tactile, pain, and thermal sensation. Palpation of both temporal and masseter muscles while the patient clenches his teeth readily reveals unilateral paresis of the motor division of the fifth cranial nerve.

CEREBELLUM

The primary function of the cerebellum is the coordination of motor activity. Differentiating a labyrinthine lesion from a cerebellar problem occasionally may be difficult. A short but helpful evaluation of cerebellar function starts with an observation of a patient's gait and determining whether or not the patient has a tremor. The gait of the patient with a vestibular lesion may be drunken and reeling, while the gait of the patient with cerebellar disease may be characterized by apparent looseness of the extremities. In minor involvement of the cerebellum, this ataxia may be apparent only on tandem gait. Cerebellar disease may be associated with a gross tremor on voluntary movements. Coordination can be tested by the finger-nose-finger test in which the patient is instructed to touch alternately the examiner's finger and then his own nose. A defect is manifested by varying degrees of terminal incoordination. Inability to perform rapid alternate movements (adiadochokinesia) is tested by asking the patient to perform rapid alternate pronation-supination of the hand. These simple observations can aid the examiner in the differential diagnosis of an inner-ear disorder.

VESTIBULAR TESTING

The acoustic nerve (eighth cranial nerve) has two main divisions: the cochlear nerve and the vestibular nerve. In general, advances in testing the auditory system have far outstripped those made in vestibular testing. It is commonly possible to differentiate between a cochlear and a retrocochlear lesion with audiometric tests, and sometimes even a central lesion can be distinguished; it is usually impossible to differentiate between a lesion of the vestibular labyrinth and a retrolabyrinthine or central lesion with vestibular tests. Audiometric tests are described in Chapters 6, 7, and 10; therefore only the evaluation of the vestibular system follows.

Each vestibular labyrinth consists of the utricle and three semicircular canals: the anterior or superior vertical, posterior or inferior vertical, and the horizontal or lateral semicircular canal. There is a great deal of controversy as to whether the saccule has any function and, if so, whether the function is concerned with balance, hearing, or both. Experimental studies (29) have indicated that the utricle is stimulated by the forces of gravity, centrifugal force, linear acceleration in any direction, and angular acceleration about a horizontal axis. No adequate methods for clinically testing utricular function are known, however, and the role the utricle plays in various human vestibular disorders has not been clarified. Clinical tests are available, however, for the semicircular canals. These canals can be stimulated by several means and the response is measured primarily by the duration and characteristics of the nystagmus elicited.

CALORIC TESTS

The most useful method of testing vestibular function is by caloric stimulation. With this method the function of the vestibular labyrinth of each ear can be evaluated. The simplest test is the modified Kobrak cold caloric test (Figure 3.7), and ordinarily in clinical practice only the horizontal canal is studied. The head is placed 60° backward from the vertical position, and the horizontal canal on each side is thereby brought into a vertical plane with its ampulla above. Introduction of ice water into one external

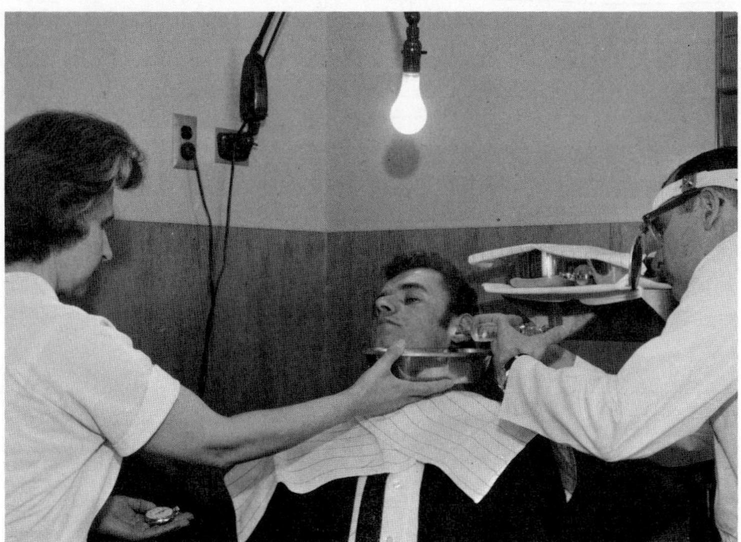

FIGURE 3.7 Modified Kobrak cold caloric test.

auditory canal causes a temperature change in the inner ear and results in a convection current in the endolymph of the horizontal semicircular canal directed away from the ampulla. When vestibular function is normal, the patient experiences vertigo; there is nystagmus with the fast component away from the ear that is stimulated; and there is past-pointing toward the side that is being tested. Results of the modified Kobrak cold caloric test may be as follows: both labyrinths may respond normally; one labyrinth may be less active than the other; both labyrinths may be hypoactive; one or both labyrinths may not respond to caloric stimulation. Cold air can be used as a stimulus when it is undesirable to introduce water into the ear.

The bithermal caloric test was introduced by Fitzgerald and Hallpike in 1942. It consists of stimulating each ear alternately with cold (30° C) and warm (44° C) water. In addition to being able to determine whether or not one labyrinth is more active than the other, one can demonstrate the presence or absence of directional preponderance (the two stimuli which produce nystagmus to one side elicit a greater reaction than do the stimuli which produce nystagmus to the other side). Directional preponderance is found in 20 per cent of the normal subjects who are tested (22), however, so its clinical value is doubtful.

ELECTRONYSTAGMOGRAPHY (ENG)

Electronystagmography (ENG) is an objective method of measuring spontaneous nystagmus, positional-induced nystagmus, and nystagmus evoked by caloric stimulation of the ears or rotation of the patient. Clinically, an electronystagmogram is frequently obtained before, during, and after bithermal stimulation of the patient's ears (Figure 3.8). The duration of the nystagmus and usually its maximum intensity (mean eye speed in the

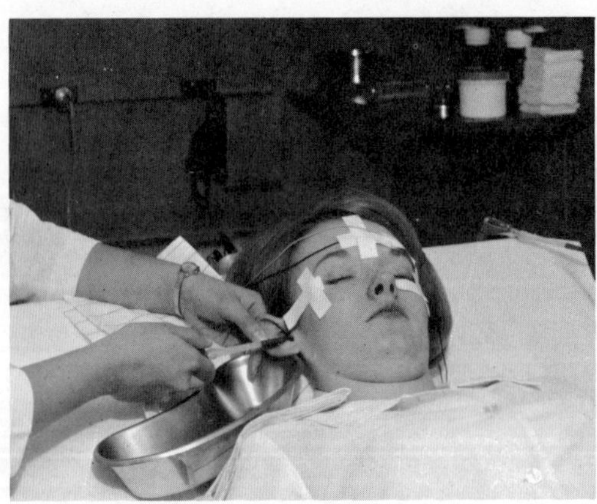

FIGURE 3.8 Electroynstagmography.

slow or fast phase of the nystagmus during a ten-second period at the peak of the reaction) are determined (39). Occasionally in clinical work only the maximum intensity is established. The major advantages of electronystagmography are that it provides an objective measurement of nystagmus, and this can be accomplished while the patient's eyes are closed, thus avoiding reduction in the intensity of vestibular nystagmus due to ocular fixation, as well as when they are open (spontaneous nystagmus of cerebellar origin may disappear with the eyes closed); corrections for spontaneous nystagmus during the bithermal caloric test can be easily made, yielding a more accurate assessment of semicircular canal function; and a permanent record of nystagmus is available for future studies.

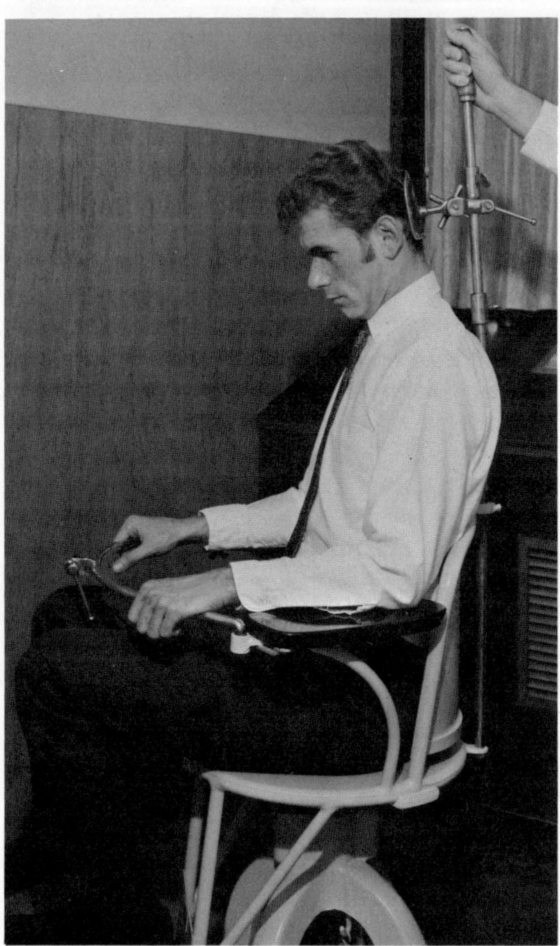

FIGURE 3.9 Rotation test.

ROTATION TESTS

In the simplest test, the horizontal semicircular canals are stimulated by rotating a patient whose head is positioned 30° forward from the vertical position and the horizontal semicircular canal is then parallel to the floor (Figure 3.9). After ten turns of the rotating chair in twenty seconds, it is suddenly stopped, and the postrotatory nystagmus is observed. Because both labyrinths are stimulated, less information can be gained from this test than from the caloric tests. The rotary test is of some use in evaluating certain patients, such as those who, as a result of toxic reactions to streptomycin, show no response to 30 ml of ice water in either ear and in whom the test may reveal a slight amount of residual labyrinthine function. Cupulometry, which as yet has no practical clinical value, is a refinement of the simple rotation test.

In addition to thermal changes and changes in acceleration, the vestibular labyrinth also may be stimulated by a galvanic current or loud noises, but so far this knowledge has not provided a useful clinical test.

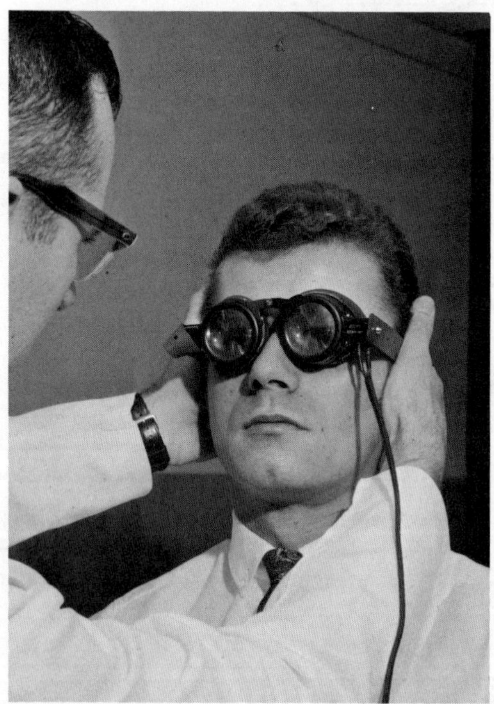

FIGURE 3.10 Nylen test (testing for positional nystagmus). Frenzel glasses are being worn by the patient in order to avoid eye fixation and to aid the examiner in observing eye movements. The patient is about to be placed in a supine position.

POSITIONAL NYSTAGMUS

Vertigo on sudden change in position is not an uncommon complaint and may or may not be associated with hearing loss. Such vertigo associated with nystagmus frequently can be elicited by rapidly placing the patient's head in various positions (Figure 3.10). From a sitting position the patient is rapidly moved into a supine position. The test is repeated with the head turned to the right and left and with the head hanging over the edge of the examining table. The test can be particularly helpful in a patient who has posttraumatic postural vertigo. Eliciting positional nystagmus provides objective evidence of dysfunction in some part of the vestibular system. When positional nystagmus is produced after a short latent period, stops in a few seconds, and diminishes on repeated testing, the cause is thought most commonly to be due to disturbance in the vestibular end-organ, but this is by no means always the case. Sustained positional nystagmus is usually associated with disorders of the central nervous system (2). In the sustained central type of positional nystagmus, the patient may experience only mild vertigo or none.

RADIOLOGIC EXAMINATION

Many special roentgenographic views of the skull can aid in the differential diagnosis of hearing impairment. The history and physical examination will determine the necessity for these studies and what particular views should be obtained. Roentgenograms can show the degree of pneumatization of the mastoid process (Figure 3.11) and may reveal a rarefaction resulting from a cholesteatoma (Figure 3.12). Appropriate views may show an

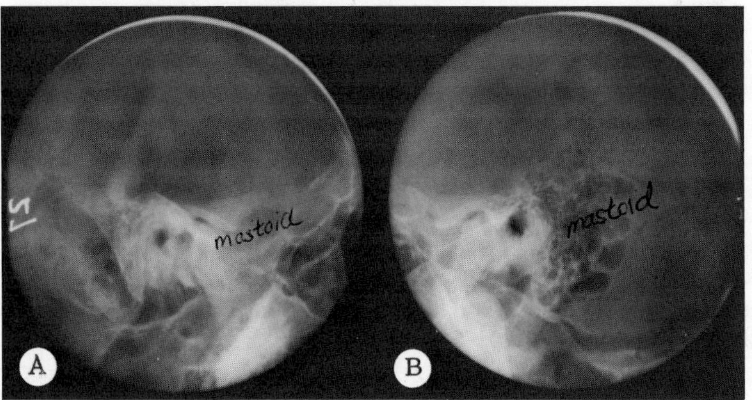

FIGURE 3.11 Law view. (A) The left mastoid process is poorly aerated and sclerotic. (B) The right mastoid process is normally pneumatized.

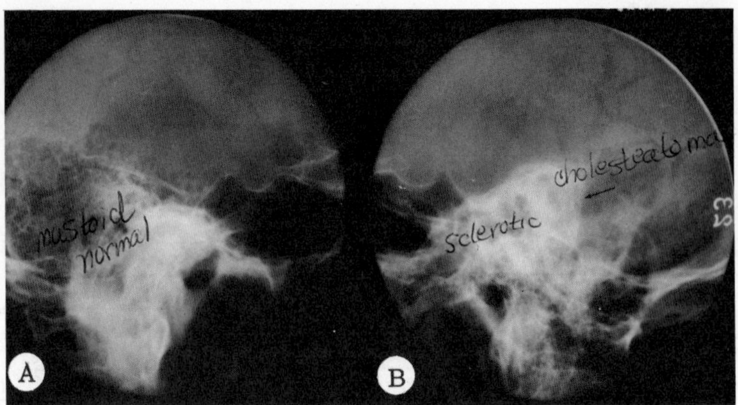

FIGURE 3.12 Law view. (A) The left mastoid process is normal. (B) The right mastoid process is sclerotic, and the arrow points to a large area of rarefaction due to cholesteatoma.

enlarged internal auditory meatus or eroded petrous pyramid due to an acoustic neuroma (Figure 3.13A and B) and other tumors (Figure 3.14). Tomograms of the petrous bone can be particularly helpful in the diagnosis of labyrinthine otosclerosis, in defining a fracture, and in identifying ossicles (Figure 3.15). Pantopaque myelography of the posterior fossa can be of great aid in the diagnosis of a small acoustic neuroma, and selective external and internal carotid arteriography is helpful in defining the extent of a tumor of the glomus jugulare. These few examples indicate some of the many values of roentgenograms to the otologist. Roentgenographic studies as well as all the tests that have been briefly discussed are aids of limited value; the final otologic assessment is determined by fitting together into a logical story all the clues derived from the history, the physical examination, and the laboratory tests.

Specific Disorders Causing Impairment of Hearing and Their Treatment

A large and extremely important part of the treatment of hearing impairment concerns prevention and rehabilitation. Prevention deals with such factors as adequate prenatal, natal, and neonatal care; avoidance of ototoxic drugs and excessive exposure to loud noise; a proper program of immunization for the child; and early and aggressive treatment of middle-ear infections. Rehabilitation involves extensive education of the patient and his relatives; the use of hearing aids; and instruction in speech-reading, auditory training, and sign language. Both prevention and rehabilitation are covered in Chapters 4, 5, and 8 of this book. The hearing disorders discussed in this chapter will be those that, once they have occurred, can be treated by either medical or surgical means.

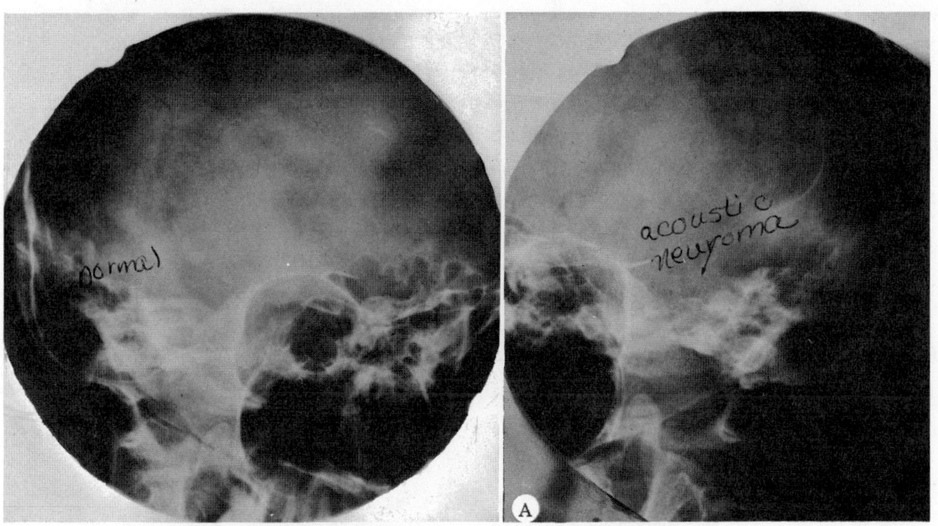

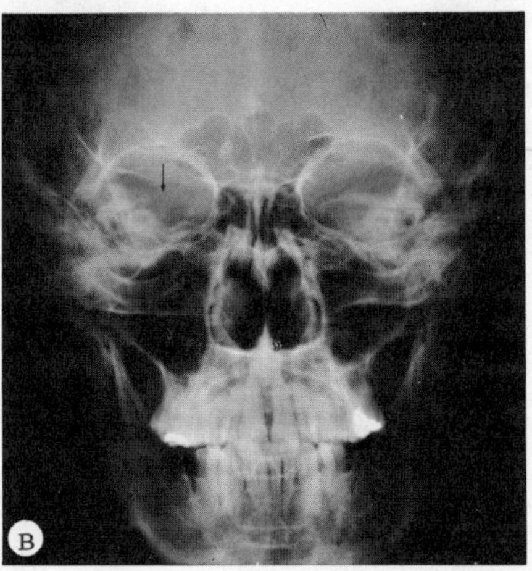

FIGURE 3.13 (A) Stenver's view. On the left, the left petrous pyramid is normal. On the right, the arrow points to an area of erosion of the superior portion of the right petrous pyramid as a result of an acoustic neuroma. (B) Caldwell view. Same patient as in (A). Petrous pyramid eroded on the right.

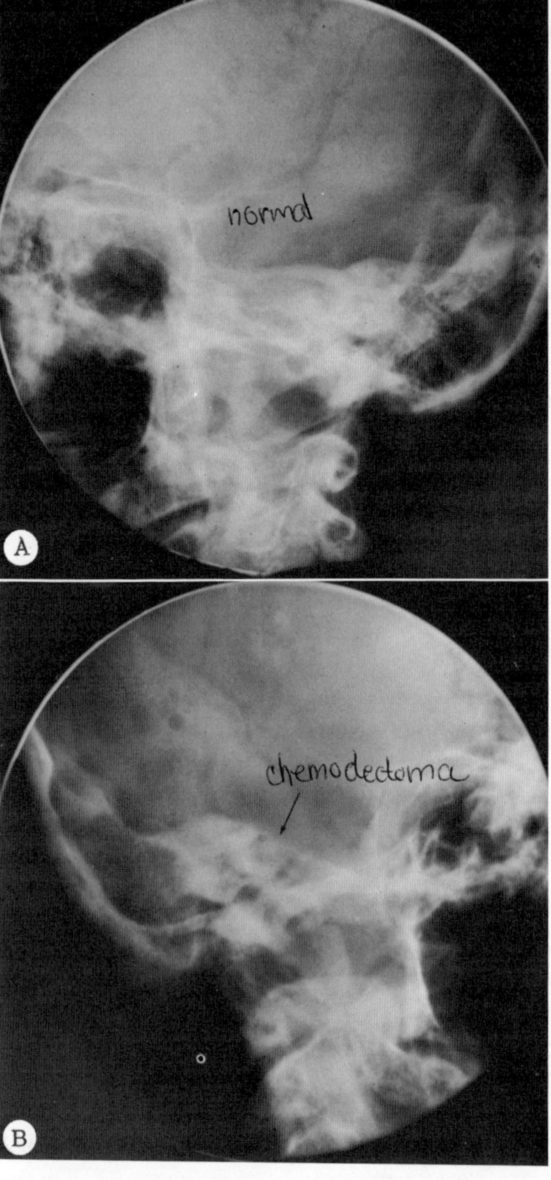

FIGURE 3.14 Stenver's view. (A) The right petrous pyramid is normal. (B) The arrow points to an area of destruction of the tip of the left petrous pyramid as a result of a chemodectoma.

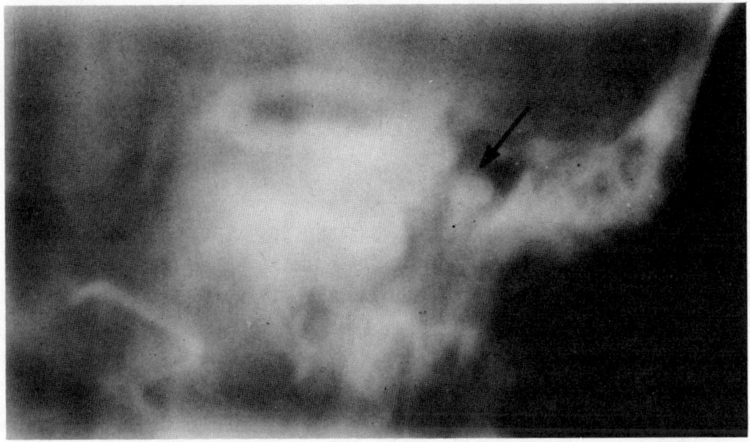

FIGURE 3.15 Tomogram: Arrow points to malleus.

EXTERNAL AUDITORY MEATUS

The Collapsible Meatus. Many diversified problems can result in occlusion of the external auditory canal and a conductive hearing impairment. Most of these conditions are readily apparent. However, unless the examiner is familiar with the possibility of a collapsible external meatus, he can be presented with a puzzling conductive hearing impairment. For example, a child has a conductive hearing loss of 20 to 30 dB in one ear. Otoscopic examination reveals a slightly narrowed external meatus and a normal tympanic membrane. The patient has had no recent ear infections, and there is no family history of congenital deafness or otosclerosis. Suspecting that the tissues of the orifice of the external meatus are flaccid enough to collapse from the pressure of the earphones, the examiner places a small polyethylene tube in the canal to hold the orifice open and repeats the audiogram. The second audiogram shows normal hearing and clarifies the problem. No treatment is necessary.

Foreign Bodies. It is hard to imagine that a foreign body impacted in the external meatus would not be recognized as the cause of a conductive hearing loss, but this does happen. I once saw a woman who had a mixed type of hearing impairment and, on the advice of her physician, had worn a hearing aid for several months. Removal of impacted cerumen resulted in elevating the air-conduction threshold into the socially adequate range and eliminated the need for a hearing aid. This patient was put to a great deal of needless expense because a satisfactory otoscopic examination had not been performed.

External Otitis. Infections in the external meatus causing redness and edema of the skin and exudate in the canal may result in meatal occlusion with a conductive hearing impairment. The etiologic organism is usually a bacterium and rarely a fungus; culturing the pus will establish which of these it may be. Repeated thorough cleansing of the canal, avoidance of placing water in the ear, and local administration of an appropriate antibiotic usually bring complete relief. External otitis of long duration may require considerable perseverance to bring it under control.

Tumors. Osteomas of the bony external auditory canal are not uncommon, are usually small, and do not affect hearing. Occasionally, an osteoma will become large enough to occlude the external meatus. In such instances the patency of the canal can be reestablished by the removal of a sufficient amount of bone. Malignant neoplasms of the external auditory canal, such as epitheliomas and cylindromas, require aggressive treatment in an attempt to save the patient's life, and auditory acuity is of secondary importance.

Meatal Atresia. Atresia of the external auditory canal may be acquired or congenital. The most common acquired form results from surgical procedures, particularly mastoidectomy, and, less commonly, from removal of the skin of the canal in myringoplasty. Atresia of the external auditory meatal orifice complicating a modified radical or radical mastoidectomy can be corrected surgically. Congenital atresia of the external meatus may involve one or both ears and may be membranous or bony, partial or complete. As has been mentioned previously, this malformation may be associated with a normal, deformed, or absent auricle, an intact, defective, or absent tympanic membrane, and a normal or defective ossicular chain. When unilateral atresia exists and the second ear is normal, surgical reconstruction of the meatus is not an emergency measure, since the child will be able to communicate normally. A relatively minor defect such as a membranous flap occluding the canal can be corrected at any time. Complete bony atresia, however, is best left until at least the teens before surgical reconstruction is considered. At that time, if there is little chance of restoring auditory acuity to within 20 to 30 dB of the normal ear, surgical treatment has little to offer the patient and should not be attempted.

The child who has bilateral bony external meatal atresia has a much more serious problem. His auditory acuity is not sufficient for him to function satisfactorily, and precious time may be lost if steps are not taken to improve his hearing capability. A bone-conduction type of hearing aid can be used with benefit by these children and should be employed as early as possible. The age of attempted surgical reconstruction is somewhat controversial. Livingstone (26) is convinced that the child should undergo plastic repair of at least one external meatus between one and two years of age in order to use an air-conduction hearing aid.

Although combinations of inner-ear and external-middle-ear congenital malformations are rare, they do occur, and it has been impossible in the past to obtain accurate air-conduction thresholds in these infants, let alone bone-conduction thresholds. The introduction of cortical audiometry (6, 8) (*see* Chapter 12) however, offers the promise of aid in the otologic assessment of these infants, but even with better knowledge of the cochlear reserve, there is still the considerable problem of wearing a mold in a surgically constructed external auditory meatus. If the cochlear reserve can be determined accurately in the infant, then perhaps this will become the ideal time to attempt total unilateral reconstruction of the defective external and middle ear. At the present time most otologists wait until the child can be tested reliably by conventional audiometric methods before total surgical reconstruction is attempted. Naturally, the opportune age will depend on the child and his family.

TYMPANIC CAVITY

Disorders of the middle-ear transformer mechanism can be a result of sterile fluid in the middle ear, otosclerosis, trauma, infection, neoplasms, tumefactions, and congenital anomalies. In the discussion of the following disorders, when not otherwise specified, it will be assumed that the cochlear reserve is sufficient to expect usable hearing to result from reconstructive surgery.

Secretory Otitis Media. Chronic SECRETORY OR SEROUS OTITIS MEDIA is frequently seen in the young child and less often but not uncommonly in the adult. One of the major causes is blockage of the eustachian tube followed by absorption of air in the tympanic cavity and a resultant negative pressure. In turn, the negative pressure acting on the mucosal vessels results in a transudate into the tympanic cavity and a conductive hearing loss. It is obvious, however, that this is not the only cause of secretory otitis media, for some patients with this condition may have a readily inflatable eustachian tube. Many times the defect seems to concern lymphatic drainage.

In children, typically, there may be repeated episodes of acute suppurative otitis media which are controlled by antibiotic therapy, but between attacks, the middle-ear space remains filled with fluid. Hypertrophied adenoids that cause obstruction of the eustachian tube frequently are the primary cause. A trial of oral decongestants and tubal inflations is worthwhile and in many patients, adenoidectomy and myringotomy can be avoided. When conservative measures fail, adenoidectomy and removal of the fluid in the middle ear through a myringotomy incision are indicated. Occasionally, allergy may play a part in the etiology, but in my experience one rarely can incriminate allergy with any degree of certainty, either in the child or adult, as the cause of secretory otitis media. When a mechanical obstruction from a hypertrophied adenoid coexists with an allergic problem, the adenoids should be removed along with the institution of the necessary allergic precautions and treatment. Occlusion of the eustachian tube due to scar tissue as the result of a poorly performed adenoidectomy can result in permanent secretory otitis media. Nasopharyngeal neoplasms as the etiologic factor are commonest among adults. Secretory otitis media, not infrequently, may appear first in the adult after a mild upper respiratory infection and may persist despite conservative therapy.

In many instances, however, extensive investigation does not show any etiologic factor, and in many others the condition persists despite all available therapeutic measures. These patients can be greatly benefited by the insertion of a polyethylene tube through a myringotomy incision (Figure 3.16A and B). The polyethylene tube will plug up in time, but it restores hearing (Figure 3.17) while it functions, which may be for as long as a year. The daily introduction of a drop or two of mineral oil into the external meatus helps to keep the tube open. Daily introduction of a drop or two of cortisone solution will often aid in keeping the tube functioning when the secretions are thick and tenacious (glue ear). The patient must not get water in the ear, for this will invariably result in acute suppurative otitis media. Many patients can be greatly benefited by this relatively simple surgical procedure.

Otosclerosis. OTOSCLEROSIS is a hereditary disease resulting in an abnormal growth of bone in the otic capsule. In a histologic study of the temporal bones from 1,161 patients, Guild (14) found that this abnormality occurred in 7.5 per cent of the white population and 0.9 per cent of the Negro population. Histologic otosclerosis was diagnosed in eighty-one ears, but in only ten of these was there ankylosis of the stapes footplate (clinical otosclerosis). The hearing loss is primarily of the conductive type but, not uncommonly, sensori-neural hearing impairment also may be present. The hearing loss most commonly begins at thirty years of age and is progressive. Hearing impairment may be apparent in only one ear, but usually both

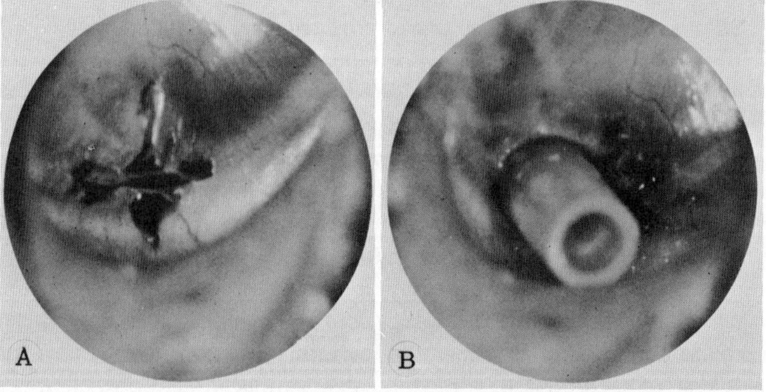

FIGURE 3.16 (A) Incision in tympanic membrane. (B) Polyethylene tube introduced through myringotomy incision.

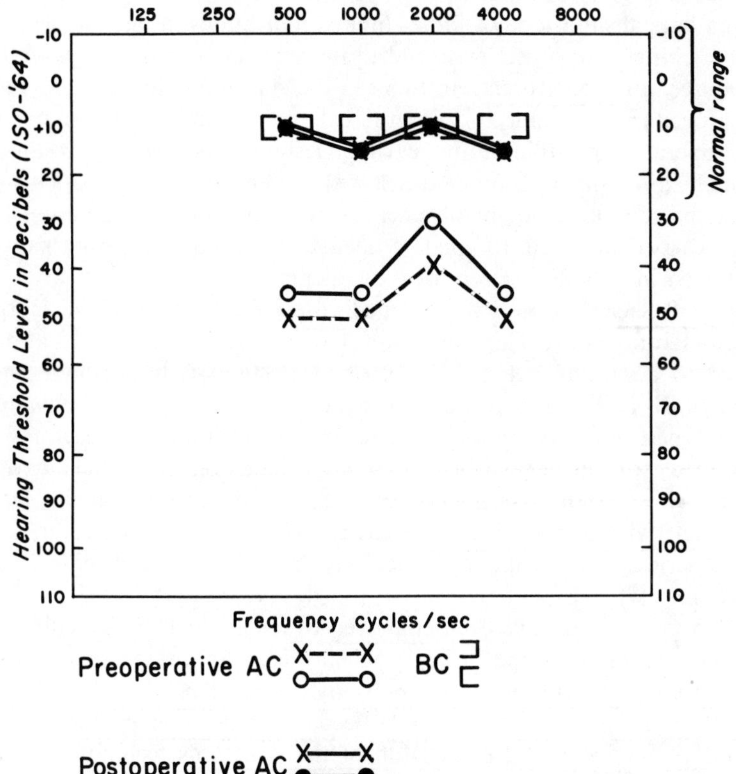

FIGURE 3.17 Audiograms of a five-year-old boy with bilateral secretory otitis media. Six months after bilateral myringotomy and insertion of polyethylene tubes, the air-bone gap remained closed.

are involved. Occasionally a red hue (Schwartze's sign) from the promontory is seen on otoscopic examination.

The first successful treatment for ankylosis of the stapes footplate by otosclerotic bone was the one-stage fenestration of the horizontal semicircular canal introduced by Lempert in 1938. Many modifications of this operation were introduced over the next few years, and Shambaugh reported in 1949 that a socially adequate hearing level could be expected in 80 per cent of the ideal cases by the end of the first postoperative year. To obtain socially adequate hearing, cochlear function had to be essentially normal, since the operation bypassed the transformer mechanism of the middle ear, and the best result would only achieve a closure of the air-bone gap to within 25 dB. In addition to the limited gain in hearing, the fenestration operation left the patient with a large mastoid cavity which required continual care. Despite these drawbacks, the operation has helped a great number of selected patients and today still has limited indications in patients who have massive obliterative otosclerosis and those requiring certain tympanoplastic procedures. In 1953 Rosen reintroduced the stapes mobilization operation. This procedure was done through the external auditory canal, eliminating a postoperative mastoidectomy cavity. Despite good hearing results immediately after the operation in selected patients (in many patients who had extensive otosclerotic involvement of the footplate, the operation could not be carried out), the footplate tended to refix, and a hearing gain was maintained in only 30 per cent of the patients.

In 1958 Shea described total stapedectomy for fixation of the footplate by otosclerotic bone. This operation has resulted in the restoration of hearing to a socially adequate level or in closure of the air-bone gap to within 10 dB in a high percentage of patients. The two main disadvantages of the fenestration operation were overcome in that stapedectomy can result in closure of the air-bone gap and, therefore, offers help to many patients who do not have normal cochlear function, and it avoids leaving the patient with a mastoidectomy cavity. The operation, however, is not without serious complications, particularly those that result in sensori-neural hearing loss (7).

Many techniques have been employed to reconstruct the ossicular chain after removal of the stapes. Shea originally used an autogenous vein graft to cover the oval window and a polyethylene strut between the lenticular process of the incus and the graft. Because of a tendency for avascular necrosis of the incus and dislocation of the strut, this technique has been abandoned by most otologists. Prostheses of stainless steel or tantalum wire attached to fatty connective tissue (34) or a vein (24) have been used successfully and have been the most satisfactory at the Mayo Clinic (7) (Figure 3.18 A, B, and C). Partial stapedectomy (17), an absorbable gelatin sponge-wire prosthesis (18), and a piston prosthesis (28) also have been employed.

In considering patients for stapedectomy, the ear with the greatest hearing loss should be selected because of the risk of further sensori-neural hearing impairment. The patient should be made fully aware of this risk, and also of the maximal gain that can be anticipated with a successful result. For instance, the operation may be undertaken to improve the patient's hearing-aid capability, and he should understand this before the operation is performed.

Trauma. A foreign body, introduced purposely or accidentally into the external auditory canal, can result not only in abrasion of the canal skin but also in perforation of the tympanic membrane and disruption of the ossicular chain. A head injury, particularly a blow on the auricle, may result in a tear of the tympanic membrane and an ossicular chain defect. The commonest abnormality of the ossicular chain is dislocation of the incus. The extent of the injury will determine the severity of the conductive hearing impairment. When a traumatic perforation of the tympanic membrane has occurred, immediate realignment of the margins of the perforation with the aid of the dissecting microscope is usually sufficient to assure

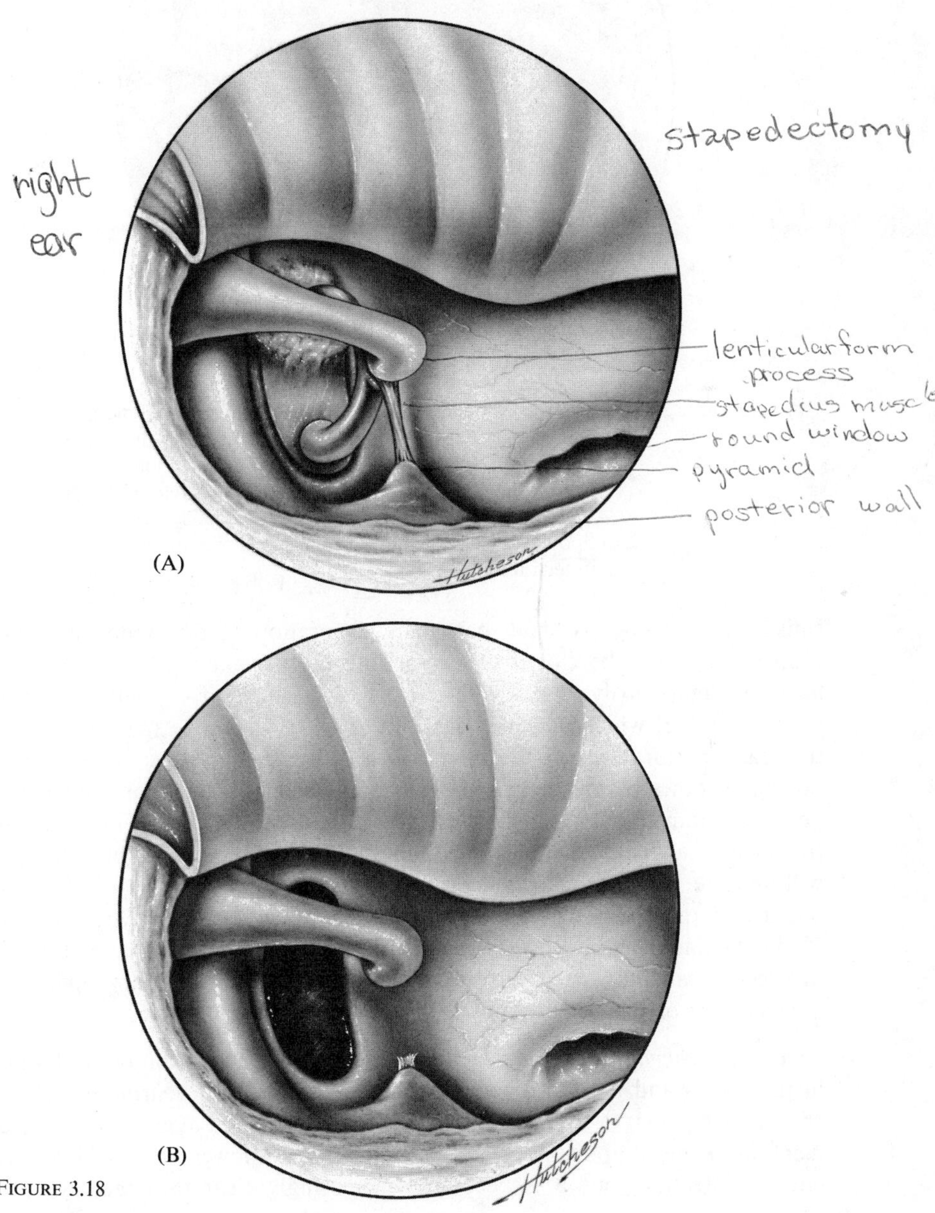

(A)

(B)

FIGURE 3.18

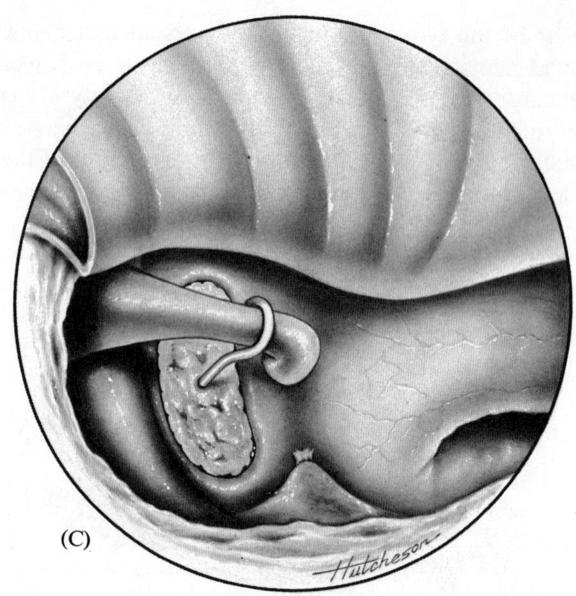

FIGURE 3.18 (A) Stapedectomy. Transcanal exposure of right middle ear. The stapes is fixed by an otosclerotic focus involving the anterior portion of the footplate. (B) The tendon of the stapedius muscle has been cut and the stapes removed. (C) A prosthesis consisting of postauricular subcutaneous adipose tissue attached to a stainless steel wire has been substituted for the stapes.

satisfactory healing. A small persistent perforation of the tympanic membrane usually can be closed by cauterizing the margins with trichloracetic acid and temporarily covering the hole with a patch of cigarette paper or silicone rubber, which acts as a scaffold. This conservative management of traumatic perforations of the tympanic membrane may have to be carried out many times before complete healing has been obtained or until it has been ascertained that the hole cannot be closed by this method. These treatments can be performed on adult patients in the office, but children will require a general anesthetic. A persistent perforation despite conservative management can then be handled adequately only by myringoplasty. If an ossicular problem coexists, reconstruction of the chain can be performed in selected patients, along with myringoplasty or as a secondary operation after closure of the perforation.

Chronic Suppurative Otitis Media. Despite the introduction of antibiotics in the 1940's and increased focus of public attention on hearing disorders, chronic SUPPURATIVE OTITIS MEDIA still occurs. Early and aggressive management of acute suppurative otitis media helps to lower the incidence of chronic infection, but it is becoming increasingly clear that factors other than infection also may play an etiologic role. A persistent negative pressure in the tympanic cavity resulting in the retraction of Shrapnell's membrane and an attic defect has long been incriminated as a cause of cholesteatomas (23). In certain ears, an unusual characteristic has been observed in which the skin in the superior canal wall next to the tympanic membrane has invaded the attic with consequent formation of a cholesteatoma (33). Also, primary congenital cholesteatomas do occur (5). For these reasons, oftentimes the patient's attention is first attracted to the ear because of an infection that is secondary to an insidiously expanding cholesteatomatous tumor.

Whatever the cause of chronic suppurative otitis media may be, once the disease has occurred, the problem is how to manage it. Management depends to a large extent on whether the disease is active or inactive. When the disease is active, the foremost goal is to eradicate the infection and, if present, cholesteatoma. When the disease is inactive, the attention focuses on prevention of flare-up in infection and on reconstruction of the transformer mechanism of the middle ear.

The primary concern of the otologist faced with active chronic suppurative otitis media is to eradicate the disease. Management depends to a certain degree on whether cholesteatoma is present and, of course, on whether there are complications, such as facial nerve paralysis, meningitis, and brain abscess.

When examination proves that cholesteatoma is not present, a strenuous effort is made to bring the infection under control by medical therapy. Culture frequently reveals an organism, such as *Pseudomonas*, which is very resistant to treatment. Careful daily cleansing of the ear and insufflation of antibiotic powder may control the infection. Once a dry ear is obtained, the primary goal of management is to prevent further flare-ups of infection and to restore auditory acuity. For those ears that continue to drain despite medical therapy, surgical eradication of infection will be necessary. To obtain a dry ear, simple or modified radical mastoidectomy is performed, depending on the particular problem, and reconstruction of the tympanic membrane is attempted. If an ossicular chain defect exists, this can be dealt with at a secondary operation after the ear is dry and healed.

If cholesteatoma exists, whether it is acquired or congenital in origin, surgical treatment is indicated. Unless the cholesteatoma is well defined and easily removed in its entirety, modified radical mastoidectomy should be performed. Perforations of the tympanic membrane can be closed, but if there is active infection, ossicular reconstruction in most instances should be postponed for a secondary operation.

In inactive chronic suppurative otitis media, the ears are dry or the infection has been controlled as a result of medical or surgical therapy but a defect in the transformer mechanism of the middle ear will still remain. Treatment then concerns the repair of perforations in the tympanic membrane, reconstruction of the ossicular chain, or both. If a reconstructive operation for hearing is contemplated, there must be adequate cochlear reserve, a functioning eustachian tube, and a mucosal-lined middle ear.

Congenital Anomalies. In addition to congenital atresia of the external meatus and an absent or defective tympanic membrane, many anomalies in the tympanic cavity may occur. The oval window may be absent or there may be congenital ankylosis of the stapes footplate. Although a stapedectomy can be performed satisfactorily in the latter situation, the former anomaly is a much more difficult technical problem, since the facial nerve usually lies over the site of the oval window. If the danger of injuring the facial nerve is excessive, fenestration of the horizontal semicircular canal can be performed. The long process of the incus may be absent, the incus and malleus may be fused, or the malleus may be ankylosed. Almost every

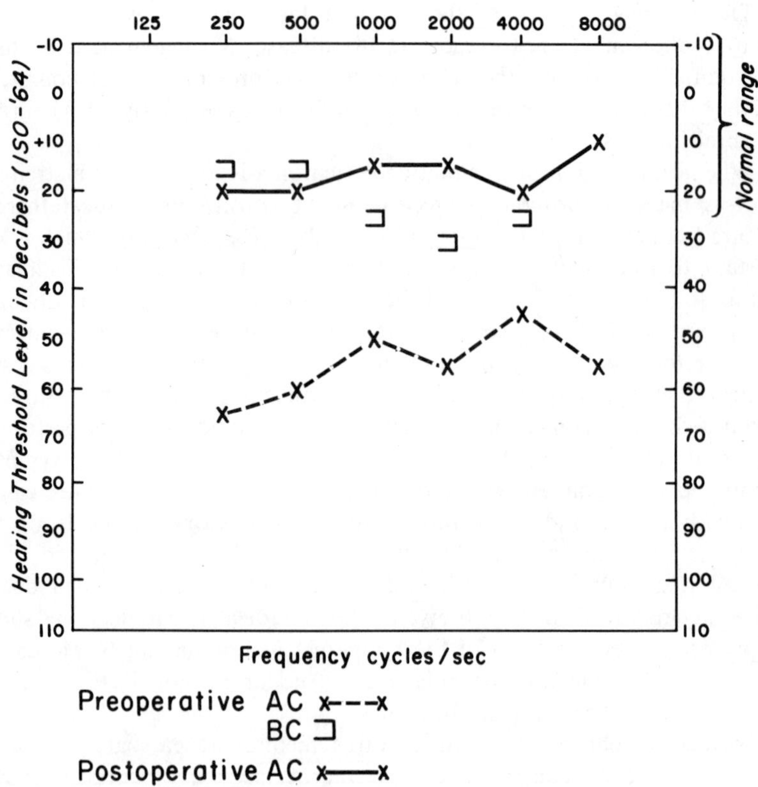

FIGURE 3.19 Left ear audiograms made before and after postauricular skin graft myringoplasty.

ossicular anomaly imaginable has been described, and with the selection of the correct surgical procedure, hearing can be improved in a high percentage of the patients.

Repair of the Tympanic Membrane (MYRINGOPLASTY). The tympanic membrane may be absent or only partially intact as a result of congenital malformation, trauma, or infection. Many surgical techniques have been suggested for repairing the tympanic membrane. Zöllner (41) and Wullstein (40) advocated placing the graft on the lateral surface of the drumhead, while Austin and Shea (1) recommended placing the graft on the medial surface. Grafting is usually not successful in the presence of infection, so every effort should be made to eradicate active infection and have a dry middle ear for at least six weeks before myringoplasty is attempted. Over the years, postauricular skin, canal wall skin, vein, and fascia have been used as the graft material. After having used all these materials, I have found that temporalis muscle fascia provides the most satisfactory autogenous tissue graft. The technique in dealing with most perforations has been to denude the remaining margins of the tympanic membrane of all epithelium. In the marginal perforation, canal skin also is removed from the bony canal wall for a few millimeters next to the tympanic membrane. The graft is then introduced over the lateral surface of the tympanic membrane remnants and held in place with Gelfoam; the packing is not disturbed for four weeks. When there is a very large perforation or an initial graft has not taken, a double fascial graft is used, one on the medial surface of the annulus or drumhead margins and one on the lateral surface. This technique has provided excellent results in the most difficult cases.

During myringoplasty the tympanic cavity is explored for disease and the ossicular chain is checked for any defect. If there is concomitant fixation of the stapes by otosclerotic bone, an opening into the inner ear should not be made, as the risk of sensori-neural hearing loss is great. After the tympanic membrane has healed, stapedectomy can be performed. Defects of the incus and malleus can be dealt with at the time of myringoplasty, but in most instances, I prefer to reconstruct the ossicular chain as a secondary procedure. Figure 3.19 shows air-conduction and bone-conduction thresholds in the left ear before the operation and the air-conduction threshold five years after operation in a fourteen-year-old boy who had a large perforation of the left tympanic membrane as a result of infection. It was possible to obtain a dry ear with medical management and a postauricular skin graft was used to close the perforation. Figure 3.20 shows the auditory threshold of the left ear of a thirteen-year-old boy before and after an operation for a large perforation of the left tympanic membrane as a result of trauma. After medical therapy a dry middle ear was obtained, and the perforation was closed with a graft of temporalis muscle fascia. In both of these patients the ossicular chain was intact and the air-bone gap was closed.

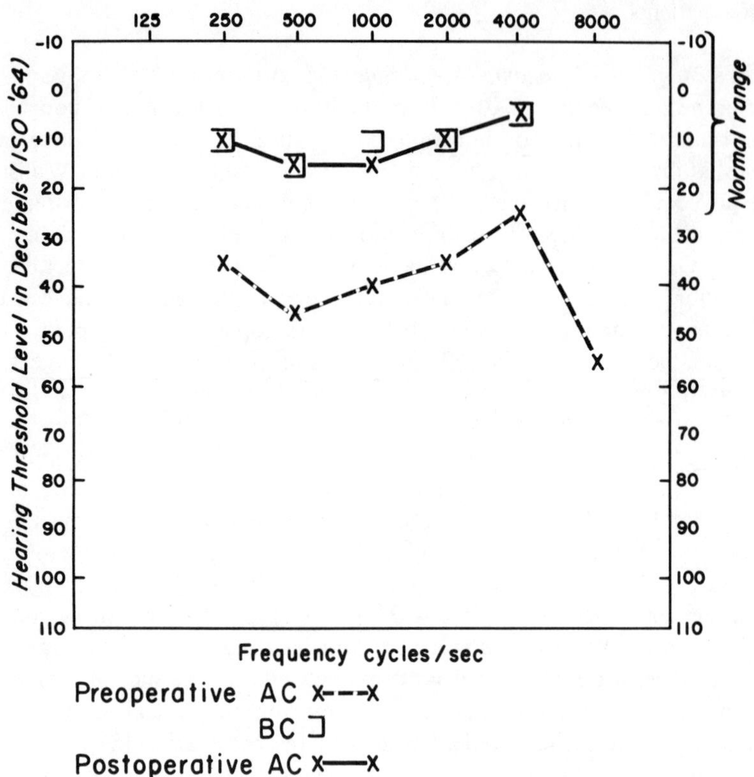

Preoperative AC X---X

BC]

Postoperative AC X—X

FIGURE 3.20 Left ear audiograms made before and after fascial graft myringoplasty

Repair of Defects of Ossicular Chain. Stapedectomy for fixation of the stapes by otosclerotic bone has already been discussed. The results are excellent, and occasionally the patient is fortunate enough as a result of surgical treatment to have considerable overclosure of the air-bone gap (Figure 3.21). An overclosure cannot be predicted before operation, and at the time of this writing there is no satisfactory explanation as to why this phenomenon occurs. Stapedectomy can be used successfully in patients who previously had a fenestration operation followed by initial improvement in hearing but who subsequently experienced closure of the fenestra. In this situation the incus has been removed at the first operation so that the loop of the tissue-wire prosthesis is attached to the manubrium of the malleus. This same technique can be employed when the incus and superstructure of the stapes have been destroyed by disease, but the oval window must never be opened in the presence of infection.

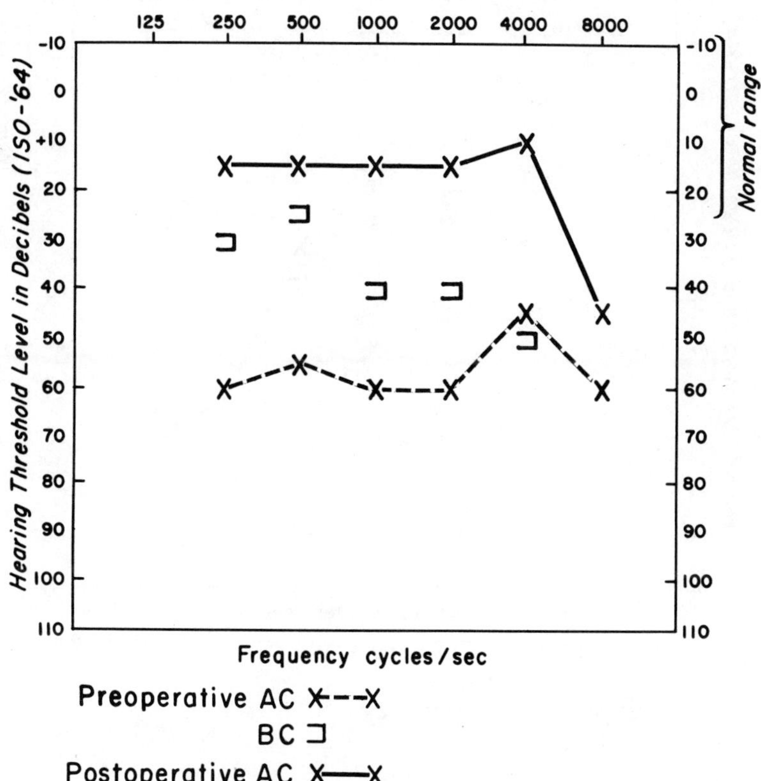

FIGURE 3.21 Left ear audiograms made before and after stapedectomy for otosclerosis. Considerable overclosure has occurred in air-bone gap.

When the long process of the incus is absent but the stapes and malleus are normal, a wire with one end looped around the head of the stapes and the other end looped around the handle of the malleus can produce an excellent hearing gain (Figure 3.22). If the body and short process of the incus are present, the incus can be used as a strut between the stapes and malleus. In addition, pieces of mastoid cortex can serve as a strut, and the use of an incus homograft has been advocated by House and associates (21). When the stapes is normal but the malleus and incus are absent, the tympanic membrane may be placed down against the head of the stapes. The medial surface of the drumhead and the head of the stapes are excoriated and placed in apposition, and if there is a satisfactory union, good hearing improvement will occur. Figure 3.23 shows the audiometric results of a stapediomyringopexy (type 3 tympanoplasty) which was performed in conjunction with a

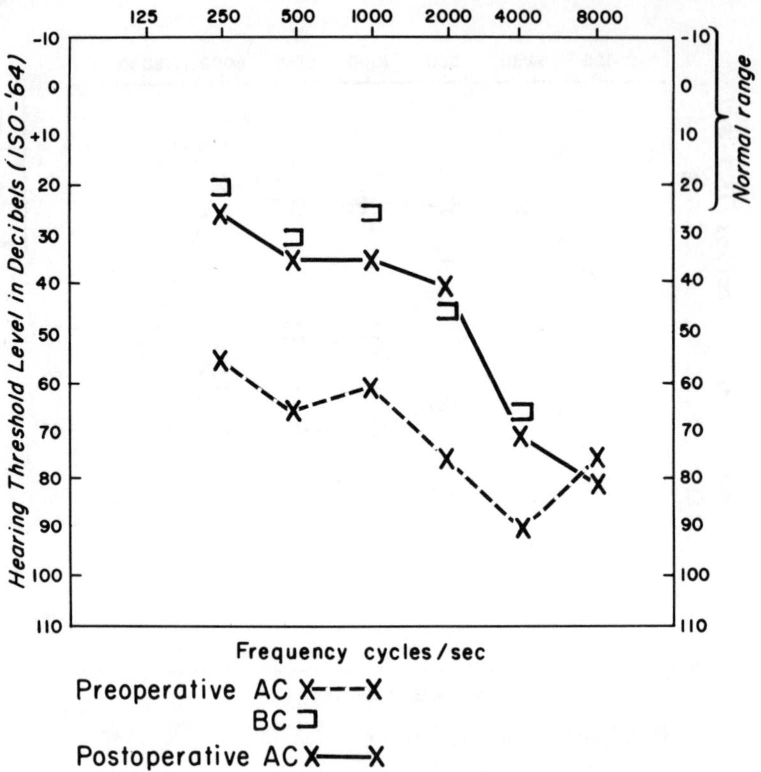

FIGURE 3.22 Left ear audiograms made before and after reconstruction of ossicular chain for defective incus.

modified radical mastoidectomy for chronic suppurative otitis media with an extensive cholesteatoma.

These are just a few examples of the management of defects in the tympanic membrane and ossicular chain. The importance of careful selection of patients for surgical treatment should be emphasized, and if the risk of cochlear damage is excessive, the patient should be encouraged to use or to continue to use a hearing aid.

INNER EAR AND AUDITORY NERVE

While advances have been rapid in the treatment of conductive hearing impairment, little progress has been made in treating sensori-neural hearing loss. The best approach to the management of sensori-neural hearing impairment is in the field of prevention. Once severe loss of hearing has

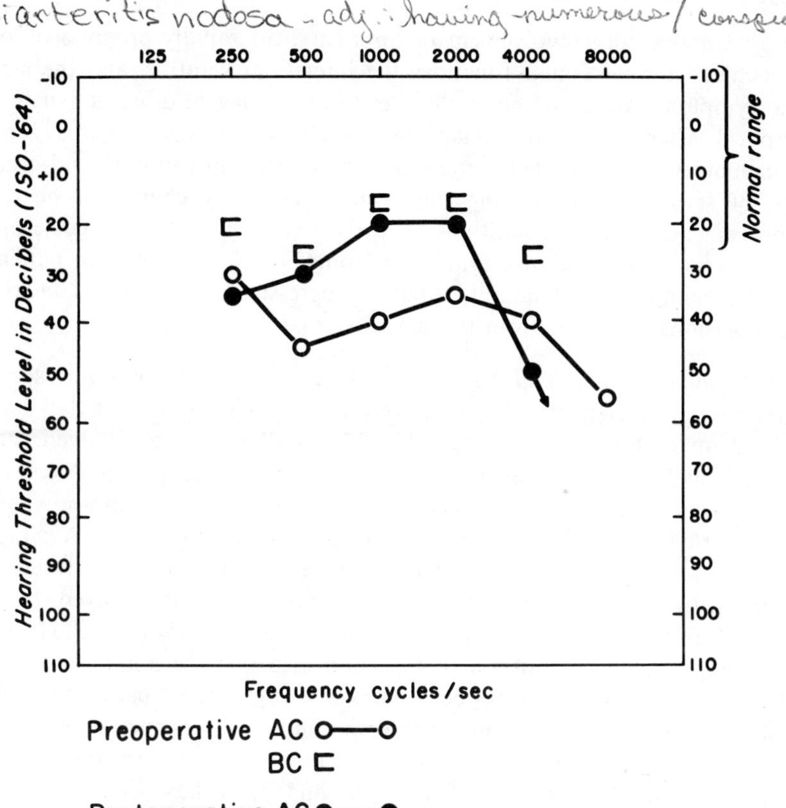

FIGURE 3.23 Right ear audiograms made before and after stapediomyringopexy (type 3 tympanoplasty).

occurred, management usually consists of rehabilitation, for only the patients whose sensori-neural hearing loss is due to a few isolated and relatively uncommon causes can benefit from medical or surgical therapy.

Collagen Diseases. COGAN'S SYNDROME consists of nonsyphilitic interstitial keratitis associated with audio-vestibular symptoms (11). Both ears are involved, and although there may be some fluctuation in the severity of the hearing loss early in the course of the disease, the outlook is for rapid progression to complete deafness. Vestibular function also is rapidly lost. Many of the patients show signs and symptoms of disease in other systems, and present knowledge suggests that Cogan's syndrome is just one manifestation of periarteritis nodosa (10). Some evidence suggests that early treatment with relatively high doses of corticosteroids for a short time will arrest hearing deterioration. The hearing loss in Cogan's syndrome is of the end-organ type and can be differentiated from Meniere's disease by the almost simultaneous involvement of both ears, the rapidly progressive loss of cochlear and vestibular function, the interstitial keratitis, and the signs and symptoms of a systemic disease. Other collagen diseases, such as temporal arteritis, chronic relapsing polychondritis, disseminated lupus erythematosus, and Wegner's granulomatosis, also can cause an end-organ type of sensori-neural hearing impairment. The only chance of hearing improvement in these conditions is early treatment with corticosteroids (38), just as in the case of Cogan's syndrome. In addition, certain patients who have idiopathic, bilateral, rapidly progressive sensori-neural hearing loss occasionally benefit from the use of steroids.

Congenital Syphilis and Sarcoidosis. Audio-vestibular symptoms sometimes develop in patients who have congenital syphilis long after they have had adequate treatment for syphilis (15). Both ears are involved, and although auditory acuity fluctuates at first, rapid progressive deterioration in both cochlear and vestibular function follows. The symptoms and audiometric findings are characteristic of endolymphatic hydrops. Available experimental evidence suggests that the inner-ear disorder is a result of hypersensitivity (27). The only medical therapy that has proved to be beneficial in these patients is the use of corticosteroids (15) or ACTH (30). Depending on the circumstances, penicillin also may be administered. In my experience, however, it has been necessary to give these patients courses of steroids at increasingly shorter intervals until maintenance depends on constant use of the drug, whereupon, symptoms of hypercortisonism tend to arise. Preliminary studies of Perlman and Leek have indicated that these patients may benefit from surgical decompression of the labyrinth.

Occasionally, SARCOIDOSIS will be responsible for sensori-neural hearing impairment. The treatment is the same as for the hearing loss occurring with the collagen diseases and latent labyrinthitis associated with congenital syphilis. In all these conditions, hearing improvement, if it is going to occur, usually will be evident during the first week of use of corticosteroids.

Hypothyroidism. End-organ sensori-neural hearing impairment is encountered in association with three types of thyroid disorders: endemic cretinism, Pendred's syndrome (deaf-mutism with goiter), and adult myxedema. All patients with endemic cretinism and Pendred's syndrome have hearing impairment which is usually severe and for which there is no treatment (3). Sensori-neural hearing loss associated with adult myxedema, however, may be improved by correction of the disorder (31).

Vascular Accidents. Occlusion of the internal auditory artery or cochlear artery may result in sudden severe or total sensori-neural hearing loss. The only other condition that may be difficult or impossible to differentiate from loss of hearing on a vascular basis is the sudden impairment of hearing due to viral labyrinthitis. If the accident occurs in an elderly patient who has cardiovascular disease but who has not had a recent infection of the upper respiratory tract, one can be reasonably justified in assuming that the hearing loss is due to vascular embarrassment of the inner ear. Vasodilators generally are recommended, but some evidence by Bolognesi (4) suggests that anticoagulation during the first few hours after the accident is most likely to result in improvement or restoration of hearing.

Meniere's Disease. MENIERE'S DISEASE consists of end-organ sensori-neural hearing loss, attacks of vertigo, tinnitus, and a sensation of pressure or fullness in the involved ear. Early in the course of the disease, the hearing impairment is characterized by fluctuation in severity, but the overall outlook is for progressive deterioration. The histologic changes consist of dilatation of the endolymphatic system, particularly of the cochlear duct and the saccule (16). In 65 to 85 per cent of patients who have this disease, the vertiginous episodes can be controlled by medical therapy consisting of vasodilators, low-salt diet, diuretics, Lipoflavonoid, antimotion sickness drugs, tranquilizers, anticholinergics, and sedatives, but it is doubtful that medications prevent deterioration of hearing. This observation is particularly important when one considers that in approximately 10 per cent of the patients, endolymphatic hydrops will develop in both ears. Preliminary investigation indicates that surgical decompression of the labyrinth (12, 19, and 9) will control vertigo without vestibular destruction and without loss of the remaining hearing. Improved hearing can be expected if a surgical procedure is performed early in the course of the disease.

Meniere's disease must be differentiated from acoustic neuromas (20). These neuromas usually arise from the vestibular nerve near Scarpa's ganglion in the internal auditory meatus and, consequently, vestibular function may become depressed before auditory acuity and is relatively more severely depressed than in early endolymphatic hydrops. The audiometric finding of a temporary shift in threshold is usually indicative of a retrocochlear lesion, but this shift may not be demonstrated if the tumor is small. The diagnosis is then made on the basis of the history, vestibular tests, and roentgenographic studies. Occasionally, a small tumor can be removed by a middle fossa approach to the internal auditory meatus (20) with preservation of residual hearing.

At this stage of our knowledge, means of managing sensori-neural hearing impairment are extremely limited. However, once a sensori-neural hearing loss is evident (and depending on the circumstances), the earliest possible institution of preventive measures, treatment, and rehabilitation offer the patient the greatest chance of significant benefit.

Bibliography

1. Austin, D. F., and J. J. Shea, Jr. "A new system of tympanoplasty using vein graft." *Laryngoscope*, **71**:596–611, (June) 1961.
2. Barber, H. O. "Positional nystagmus: Testing and interpretation." *Transactions of the American Academy of Ophthalmology and Otolaryngology*, **52**:248–60, 1964.
3. Batsakis, J. G., and R. H. Nishiyama. "Deafness with sporadic goiter: Pentred's syndrome." *Archives of Otolaryngology* (Chicago), **76**:401–6, (November) 1962.
4. Bolognesi, A. V. B. "Sudden deafness: Five cases treated with anticoagulants." *Archives of Otolaryngology* (Chicago), **72**:31–40, (July) 1960.
5. Cawthorne, T. "Congenital cholesteatoma." *Archives of Otolaryngology* (Chicago), **78**:248–52, (September) 1963.
6. Cody, D. T. R., and R. G. Bickford. "Cortical audiometry: An objective method of evaluating auditory acuity in man." *Mayo Clinic Proceedings*, **40**:273–87, (April) 1965.
7. Cody, D. T. R., O. E. Hallberg, and K. M. Simonton. "Stapedectomy for otosclerosis: Some causes of failure." *Archives of Otolaryngology* (Chicago), **85**:184–91, (February) 1967.
8. Cody, D. T. R., D. W. Klass, and R. G. Bickford. "Cortical audiometry: An objective method of evaluating auditory acuity in awake and sleeping man." *Transactions of the American Academy of Ophthalmology and Otolaryngology*, **71**: 81–91, (January–February) 1967.
9. Cody, D. T. R., K. M. Simonton, and O. E. Hallberg. "Automatic repetitive decompression of the saccule in endolymphatic hydrops (tack operation): Preliminary report." *Laryngoscope*, **77**:1480–1501, (August) 1967.
10. Cody, D. T. R., and H. L. Williams. "Cogan's syndrome." *Laryngoscope*, **70**:447–78, (April) 1960.
11. Cogan, D. G. "Syndrome of nonsyphilitic interstitial keratitis and vestibuloauditory symptoms." *Archives of Ophthalmology* (Chicago), **33**:144–49, (February) 1945.
12. Fick, I. A. van N. "Decompression of the labyrinth: A new surgical procedure for Meniere's disease." *Archives of Otolaryngology* (Chicago), **79**:447–58, (May) 1964.
13. Fitzgerald, G., and C. S. Hallpike. "Studies in human vestibular function. I. Observations on the directional preponderance ('Nystagmusbereitschaft') of caloric nystagmus resulting from cerebral lesions." *Brain*, **65**:115–37 (June), 1942.
14. Guild, S. R. "Histologic otosclerosis." *Annals of Otology, Rhinology, and Laryngology*, **53**:246–66, (June) 1944.
15. Hahn, R. D., P. Rodin, and Harriet L. Haskins. "Treatment of neural deafness with prednisone." *Journal of Chronic Diseases*, **15**:395–409, (April) 1962.
16. Hallpike, C. S., and H. Cairns. "Observations on pathology of Meniere's syndrome." *Journal of Laryngology and Otology*, **53**:625–54, (October) 1938.
17. Hough, J. V. D. "Partial stapedectomy: A physiological approach to stapedial

ankylosis." *Journal of the American Medical Association*, **187**:697–702, (March 7) 1964.

18. House, H. P. "The prefabricated wire loop-Gelfoam stapedectomy." *Archives of Otolaryngology* (Chicago), **76**:298–302, (October) 1962.
19. House, W. F. "Subarachnoid shunt for drainage of endolymphatic hydrops: A preliminary report." *Laryngoscope*, **72**:713–29, (June) 1962.
20. House, W. F. "Monograph: Transtemporal bone microsurgical removal of acoustic neuromas." *Archives of Otolaryngology* (Chicago), **80**:601–756, (December) 1964.
21. House, W. F., M. E. Patterson, and F. H. Linthicum, Jr. "Incus homografts in chronic ear surgery." *Archives of Otolaryngology* (Chicago), **84**:148–53, (August) 1966.
22. Jongkees, L. W. B. "Value of the caloric test of the labyrinth." *Archives of Otolaryngology* (Chicago), **48**:402–17, (October) 1948.
23. Jordan, R. E. "Secretory otitis media in etiology of cholesteatoma." *Archives of Otolaryngology* (Chicago), **78**:261–65, (September) 1963.
24. Kos, C. M. "Vein plug stapedioplasty for hearing impairment due to otosclerosis." *Annals of Otology, Rhinology and Laryngology*, **69**:559–70, (June) 1960.
25. Lempert, J. "Improvement of hearing in cases of otosclerosis: A new, one-stage surgical technic." *Archives of Otolaryngology* (Chicago), **28**:42–97, (July) 1938.
26. Livingstone, G. "The establishment of sound conduction in congenital deformities of the external ear." *Journal of Laryngology and Otology*, **73**:231–41, (April) 1959.
27. Magnuson, H. J., E. W. Thomas, S. Olansky, B. I. Kaplan, L. De Mello, and J. C. Cutter. "Inoculation syphilis in human volunteers." *Medicine* (Baltimore), **35**:33–82, (February) 1956.
28. McGee, T. M. "The stainless steel piston: Surgical indications and results." *Archives of Otolaryngology* (Chicago), **81**:34–40, (January) 1965.
29. McNally, W. J. "The otoliths and the part they play in man." *Laryngoscope*, **54**:304–23, (July) 1944.
30. Perlman, H. B., and J. H. Leek. "Late congenital syphilis of the ear." *Laryngoscope*, **62**:1175–96, (November) 1952.
31. Ritter, F. N., and M. Lawrence. "Reversible hearing loss in human hypothyroidism and correlated changes in the chick inner ear." *Laryngoscope*, **70**:393–407, (April) 1960.
32. Rosen, S. "Mobilization of the stapes to restore hearing in otosclerosis." *New York Journal of Medicine*, **53**:2650–53, (November 15) 1953.
33. Ruedi, L. "Acquired cholesteatoma." *Archives of Otolaryngology* (Chicago), **78**:252–61, (September) 1963.
34. Schuknecht, H. F. Film: "Stapedectomy and graft-prosthesis operation." *Acta Oto-Laryngologica* (Stockholm), **51**:241–43, 1960.
35. Shambaugh, G. E. *Surgery of the Ear*. Philadelphia: W. B. Saunders Co., 1959.
36. Shambaugh, G. E., Jr. "Fenestration operation for otosclerosis: Experimental investigations and clinical observations in 2,100 operations over a period of ten years." *Acta Oto-Laryngologica* (Stockholm), Suppl. **79**:1–101, 1949.

37. Shea, J. J., Jr. "Fenestration of the oval window." *Annals of Otology, Rhinology and Laryngology*, **67**:932–51, (December) 1958.
38. Simonton, K. M., and D. T. R. Cody. "Efectos de los corticosteroides en ciertos casos de sordera sensorio-neural." *Revista Otolaryngologica*, **7**:268–75, 1965.
39. Stahle, J. "Electro-nystagmography in the caloric and rotatory tests: A clinical study." *Acta Oto-Laryngologica* (Stockholm), Suppl. **137**:1–83, 1958.
40. Wullstein, H. "Theory and practice of tympanoplasty." *Laryngoscope*, **66**:1076–93, (July) 1956.
41. Zöllner, F. "The principles of plastic surgery of the sound-conducting apparatus." *Journal of Laryngology and Otology*, **69**:637–52, (October) 1955.

4

Psychological and Psychiatric Aspects of Profound Hearing Loss

McCay Vernon, Ph.D.
Eugene Mindel, Ph.D., M.D.

In recent years, the major shift in services for handicapped persons of all types has been from custodial care to rehabilitation. An enlightened public now makes more demands for enlightened services. Despite this, there is no formal organization of community health resources. Interdisciplinary professional cooperation is most often a random process proceeding primarily by "word-of-mouth." To render complete service to clients, a total pooling of the knowledge of specialists from many fields is necessary.

Hearing and speech clinics no longer serve only diagnostic and speech therapy functions. Following diagnosis, professionals are called upon for counseling and assistance in making future plans for total rehabilitation, especially in the case of children who have been found to be deaf. To offer recommendations for amplification and aural training is an important professional service, but the implications for altered psychosocial function due to the loss of hearing must not be ignored. Empathetic and intelligent counseling by speech and hearing specialists is possible only when such professionals understand the kind of unique life adaptation the individual with a profound hearing loss must make. It is a disservice to project the expectancies and baseline behaviors of subjects with normal hearing as the standard for, or the desired behavior in, deaf youth. In certain aspects of his functioning the deaf client is meaningfully compared only against a community of other deaf persons. In other respects there is no reason why he should not equal or excel the person with normal hearing.

This chapter is an attempt to provide hearing and speech specialists with the kind of information needed to place deaf clients into an appropriate life perspective. Some of the material will be regarded by many as controversial and, in some circles, heretical. The more the writings in this area are reviewed, the more one is seized with a sense of urgency in regard to improving the services offered to deaf children. Society's demands for academic and vocational performance are increasing. Deaf persons are not going to be able to meet these demands unless the professional services they are offered become geared to the realities of their problems.

In recognition of this fact and in acknowledgement of the lack of understanding on the part of its members about certain behavioral aspects of deafness, the American Speech and Hearing Association has recently set up a series of conferences between its members and other specialists in deafness. These conferences enable relevant disciplines to share their specialized areas of knowledge. It is the intent of this chapter to further the interdisciplinary method by extracting from psychiatric and psychological literature and professional experience information that will be valuable to those in the speech and hearing fields who will serve youth with profound hearing loss.

The entire area of the psychology of deafness rests primarily on the answer to one question: *What is the effect of the deafness variable on human development and behavior*? Granted that environmental influences are major determinants of personality structure, it follows that a condition such as profound hearing loss which drastically alters a person's perceived environment will have significant psychological consequences. Persons sharing this common alteration of their perceived environment would logically be expected to share common patterns of reacting, i.e., common behavioral patterns.

This chapter will examine behavioral aspects of deafness and other factors frequently associated with it. Several approaches will be used. One will be to examine mental illness in the deaf population. Significant insights about groups of people are gained by determining the prevalence and nature of the pathology they present. Another approach will be to examine some characteristics of normal adjustment to deafness. Environmental and organic influences that have special relevance to the psychology of profound hearing loss will be described. Finally, an overview of psychological and psychiatric assessment techniques will be given to provide professionals, parents, and others with a concise understanding of what is known about the psychological aspects of deafness and about their measurement.

In order to do this in a way that reduces unnecessary confusion, certain basic terms will be defined as they are to be used in this chapter. These terms are related to hearing loss insofar as it constitutes a continuum that cannot be conceptualized in "either-or" categories.

1. PRELINGUAL DEAFNESS. A hearing loss which occurs before the child has acquired normal language patterns (two to three years of age) and which is severe enough to render impossible the understanding of conversational speech in most normal situations with or without a hearing aid.

2. POSTLINGUAL DEAFNESS. A hearing loss which occurs after normal language patterns have been established and which is severe enough to make impossible the understanding of conversational speech in most normal situations with or without a hearing aid.

3. HARD-OF-HEARING. A hearing loss in which connected speech can be understood well enough to permit understanding of most of what is said under optimal conditions with or without the use of a hearing aid.

It is important to note that while these definitions are the most meaningful psychologically, others may be more appropriate in discussing areas such as audiology or hearing-aid evaluation.

Psychological Development

PSYCHOSOCIAL FACTORS

The most important psychosocial influences on the deaf child are his parents, the extent to which he communicates, and the educational process he is so dependent upon if he is to partially compensate for his hearing loss. These influences are not mutually exclusive, nor are they independent of other aspects of the child's life to be discussed later. They form, however, the initial environmental determinants of the deaf child's personality structure and will be discussed first to establish a developmental frame of reference for the balance of the chapter.

Parents. Parents exert the most significant, in fact the controlling, influence on the psychological adjustment of their children. This is true whether the children possess normal hearing or are deaf. If deafness is accepted by the parents and realistically understood and interpreted, the child will accept and adjust to his deafness constructively. Healthy adjustment requires that both parents and children perceive and accept areas in which the deaf child must function differently from children with normal hearing as well as the areas in which he has the capacity to function similarly. If the parent denies the deafness by a euphemism such as "he is just like any other child except that he is deaf" or "he will learn to talk and speech-read so well people will not even notice he is deaf," the deaf child is then forced to see his deafness, and therefore himself, as reproachful—an object of guilt and low self-esteem.

To be deaf is to be different in some respects. Those who know the child will recognize and acknowledge this—just as the deaf child himself will become increasingly aware of his differences as he enters into more and more areas of social living. Attempts to deny differences create for the deaf youth a world in which the unrealistic impossible goals and ideals his parents set for him, which he then internalizes, doom him to inevitable failure in their eyes and his own. Like the tall girl humiliated by her height, the intellectual youth ashamed of his studiousness, and the Negro ashamed of his ethnic heritage, the deaf child's shame of his deafness frequently leads to self-destructive psychological patterns. These have their cause in parental rejection, manifested by attempting to make the deaf child something he is not. Parents who do not accept the child as he is lead him to perceive himself as rejected. The fact that much of this proceeds unconsciously, the parents not being fully aware of the motives or significance of their behavior, compounds the problem, making it even harder to deal with. Unfortunately, unconscious denial is the dominant defense for handling the stress of having a deaf child.

In sharp contrast to parents who attempt to deny deafness are those who magnify its implications. They see deafness as almost totally debilitating and react by smothering overprotection. Extreme, but not uncommon, examples are seen in the family which isolates the young deaf child, keeping him home, away from other children and away from the normal activities of growing up. In some instances the youngster is even kept out of school. As the child grows older, dating, further education, driving a car, employment, and general socialization are all denied to him on the well-intended grounds that he is deaf, helpless, and needs protection—that it is unsafe for him to participate in these normal activities.

Both the mechanisms of denial and overprotection often stem from guilt which parents have over giving birth to a deaf child. During most pregnancies parents have mixed feelings about having a child. Sometimes there are fantasies that the child will abort. On occasion, the mother disregards prenatal care and unconsciously hopes that the pregnancy will somehow terminate and relieve her from the additional responsibility of a child. This underlying theme with its many variations and degrees of intensity is normal. When the child is actually born, the everpresent vicissitudes of child-rearing—two o'clock feedings, night-long illnesses and crying, and diaper changing—all contribute to hostile feelings and fantasies as well as feelings of love and tenderness. The discovery of deafness is often unconsciously seen as a realization of hostile fantasies. The resulting guilt often needs to be worked through in counseling. If not, it can manifest itself in denial (i.e., "these fantasies of harm did not really come true") or guilt (i.e., "how can I atone for having brought this defective person into the world?").

Although many parents adjust well to their deaf child, there are significant pathological patterns that are widely prevalent and are often inadvertently reinforced by well-intended but misguided professionals.

Unfortunately, psychology and psychiatry have failed to fulfill their obligation in the critical area of counseling parents when they are faced with the trauma of finding out that their child is deaf. In many physicians' offices and speech and hearing clinics, this responsibility has often been ignored or thrust upon persons whose professional training and experience does not qualify them for the difficult task. Consequently, the parents are either left in helpless despair or else are given some inspirational or vague promise that amplification and speech and speech-reading will make their child "normal." Until more clinics provide intensive counseling for those who have just learned that their child is deaf, both the child and his parents will continue to compound the actual difficulties of deafness by handling the condition in psychologically destructive ways.

One of a number of factors that has contributed to the large number of private, parochial, and public residential schools for the deaf is the recognition by many parents that they themselves are not meeting the needs of their deaf child. The individualized care of a good home situation for very young deaf children is certainly superior to the group living circumstances of a residential school. However, with the young deaf child whose family can not constructively handle its feelings about deafness, residential programs deserve strong consideration. As the child grows older, his parents must decide between part-time group living in a residential facility or attending school and living at home. The decision increasingly depends on the relative quality of the available educational opportunities as well as the nature of parent-child interactions. Unfortunately, in many states this is decided geographically or arbitrarily by persons representing one of the two types of programs. The individual needs of the child are ignored.

In sum, the greatest psychological danger the deaf child faces is not his deafness but the failure of his parents and professional specialists to understand and accept it. This grows from a combination of psychological needs to deny the unpleasant, especially when it is perceived as reflecting negatively on the parent, and from the guilt associated with having a child with a disability.

Communication. No area is more important in the psychological development of a child than effective communication. Psychiatrists and psychologists find that the failure to develop effective communication between children and parents is intimately related to most of the maladjustment in cases they treat. Countless studies are available which demonstrate the correlation between ineffectual and pathologic communication patterns and serious emotional disturbance (19, 47, 92). Of the importance of language to society, Grinker (57) has said that symbol systems are "the genes of culture."

The deaf child, under present approaches to his education, faces unbelievable frustration in communication. If he has had no opportunity for formal preschool education, it is not until he is five or six years old that he even begins to learn verbal language. A prelingually deafened child of this age often does not know his own name, the names of the foods he eats, or the names of the clothes he wears. Those children who have had preschool training may know how to match some simple words with pictures or they may understand fifty or so rudimentary phrases such as "Good morning." By contrast, at the age of five a hearing child knows approximately 5,000 to 26,000 words and has an excellent command of the complex syntax of the English language (106, pp. 495–516).

Not only has the deaf child of beginning school age lost the crucial years of learning and using a language, but even more important, he has lost the opportunity to freely communicate with his parents and peers. This is a psychological loss which can never be fully recovered. These early years have long been known to be the most important for the development of a healthy personality structure. They are now seen as being critical periods for language learning.

Some believe that if speech and speech-reading are effectively taught, most of the communication void will be filled. The available evidence indicates that this is an inadequate solution for most prelingually deaf children for several reasons (16, 21, 50, pp. 210–11, 67, 74, 79, 94, 107, 138, 149, 172). One reason is that 40 to 60 per cent of the words of English are homophonous, i.e., when seen on the lips they appear similar to other words that may convey totally unrelated meanings. Consequently, the maximum possible comprehension is 40 to 60 per cent. In practice, this figure is considerably reduced. Despite contextual clues and redundancy in speech, head movements, protuding teeth, poor lighting, mustaches, pipes, stiff lips, side-of-the-mouth speech patterns, and countless other anatomical and gestural variations render unintelligible much that otherwise could be understood. In addition, conversational shifts from one person to another in a group make it difficult for the deaf individual to locate the person speaking. When located, the speaker may have finished. Consequently, the speech-reader does well to discern 20 or 30 per cent of spoken sounds under relatively ideal social or educational conditions. It is unrealistic to expect a deaf child to learn language when he perceives at most only 20 to 30 per cent of what his teachers, classmates, and others say, and when he has such limited vocabulary and syntax that much of what he can discern on the lips is incomprehensible.

It is a curious and startling finding that people with normal hearing who have had no speech-reading training do better in tests of speech-reading than do prelingually deafened people with many years of training in speech-reading (93, 94, 95). Normally hearing persons fluent in English can more capably fill in words and grammatical patterns not distinguishable through speech-reading. Deaf persons, partly because they are forced to learn English through speech-reading, lack this fluency. The point is that the major factor in speech-reading is the level of language development, not formal training. However, the deaf child is expected to learn language through speech-reading.

Despite the obvious irrationality of this, it remains the fundamental approach used with deaf children.

In addition to the receptive problems of oral speech, i.e., speech-reading, there are great problems in speech production for the deaf child. Unable to hear and monitor the sounds he makes he is definitely restricted in what he can articulate. Imitation, kinesthesia, and tactile approaches are helpful, but they have severe limitations. For example, imagine having to make the pronunciation distinctions between words such as "nose and toes," "top and dub," or "marry and bury," if you could not hear them. The fact is that the task of teaching speech to a congenitally deaf child is almost completely unrelated to the correction of articulation defects in a normally hearing child. The latter has a self-monitoring apparatus available which dramatically comes to his aid in distinguishing sounds; the former has primarily only the inefficient partial monitoring system of speech-reading.

The total impact of deafness on communication can be understood only if one becomes aware of the language-learning task of the deaf school beginner. His situation is analogous to that of a normally hearing person required to wear a soundproof glass helmet and then asked to learn a foreign language without being permitted any reference to or use of English by himself or his teacher. Those who struggled to learn to speak German or French in college can imagine how impossible the task would have been had they been deaf.

The average deaf child lacks a functional use of language at basic literacy levels (50, pp. 14–16). For example, in tests of reading which are the best available measures of the language achievement of deaf children, the average deaf child 10 and 1/2 to 11 and 1/2 years of age reads at grade level 2.7. From then until age 15 and 1/2 to 16 and 1/2 he progresses less than a year in reading acheivement (173). Only 12 per cent of all deaf children ever achieve linguistic competence (50, pp. 14, 15; 173). The Moore's Study (1967) on Cloze procedure shows that even these are overestimates because they assume a basic grammatical proficiency.

Two obvious and critically important conclusions that follow from this information are: (1) under existing educational approaches, deaf children cannot realize their educational potential, a fact already pointed out in the Babbidge Report (5); (2) the difficulties of speech-reading and speaking, the low-level language development, and late onset of language deny to the deaf child the communication crucial for normal psychosocial development. Psychiatrists and psychologists who have worked in close association with deaf children have recognized this and described its pathological effects (7, 43, 50, 125, p. 204; 142).

There is strong evidence to suggest that the early use of manual communication followed or used conjointly with combined oral and manual instruction can compensate for the language deficit and provide more normal communication with parents and others (1, 2, 67, 79, 137, 138, 147, 153, 160). An especially relevant and interesting point to note here is that the effects of this early preschool manual communication give the deaf child an educational advantage which he maintains throughout his academic career (149, 153, 160). By contrast, oral preschool training results in an initial educational advantage at the beginning school level, but this "washes out," and after three years of regular school work. Those who had this special training are equal to those who did not (32, 122). Although educators are mixed in their feelings about using combined oral and manual approaches, psychiatrists and clinically oriented psychologists experienced in deafness are almost unanimous in their support of the use of combined manual and oral methods in contrast to exclusively oral (speech and speech-reading) techniques (7, 43, 50, 125, p. 204; 142). It is significant that those whose training in psychiatry and psychology are the strongest supporters of the combined approach. It is they who see the human misery and waste of a system that does not meet the needs of most deaf youth and their families. Some educators and speech and hearing personnel in whom there is a professional and psychological investment in emphasizing oralism, seem less willing to recognize the evidence that it is possible that finger-spelling and the language of signs may aid rather than inhibit language, speech, and speech-reading, as limited experimental findings suggest (50, pp. 1–44, 202–23; 153, 160).

Feelings on this issue of the supplementary use of finger-spelling or the language of signs sometimes supersede objectivity and result in biased attacks (38) on research findings that do not support a rigid adherence to "pure oralism." Unfortunately, many experts on deafness find that to raise the issue or fully discuss the research on oral versus combined oral-manual approaches is professionally so dangerous that they avoid doing it rather than placing their careers in jeopardy. Among those who have taken a stand on the subject of deafness, perhaps the strong and best documented position is that expressed in *Thinking Without Language* (50) which supports a combined system. *The Deaf* (37) and *Educational Guidance and the Deaf Child* (42) take the "oralism only" position and cite the major statements of this view. Any serious student of deafness must apprise himself of the facts on this crucial issue and make a decision on the relative value of the different approaches. These three books are essential minimal reading.

Under the existing oral methods, communication skills of deaf youths are generally so poor as to prevent normal psychosocial development and to prevent more than an elementary level of educational achievement. Research findings suggest that a combination of oral and manual methods holds promise for overcoming these problems (153, 160). Whereas no one advocates the use of the language signs and finger-spelling only, many educators and speech and hearing practitioners support oral methods that exclude finger-spelling and the language of signs. In no other area of special education is a rigid, restrictive, one-approach-only philosophy advocated in preference to an eclectic use of all potentially helpful procedures. The issue is not whether spoken language and speech-reading are valuable, because there is universal agreement about this. The issues are: (1) the degree to which it is possible to develop speech and speech-reading in the absence of extensive residual hearing in a child whose hearing loss is prelingual; (2) the extent to which early and continued manual communication aids rather than interferes with the development of oral and written communication skills; (3) the psychological and educational effects of the intense frustration of having to learn academic material primarily through the ambiguous medium of speech-reading; (4) the fact that in the past there were many adventitiously deafened youths with already established speech and language patterns who were able to function "orally" (9, p. 151; 108). Most deaf youth today are congenitally or prelingually deaf (160). They lack the potential and the skill in speech, language, and speech-reading that characterized past generations of deaf children; and (5) the advisability of a rigid adherence to either method as contrasted to a mixture of both approaches based on the needs of the child.

Education. It is not long before the newcomer to the field realizes that there are long-standing differences in the educative orientation toward the deaf. These differences have been inflamed by such intense emotionalism that they have yet to be elevated to the level of meaningful dialogue between the factions so that they may lead to rational decisions in the true interest of deaf children. It is hoped that this section will serve as one step toward achieving that goal by providing objective data to those closely associated with the deaf and hard-of-hearing.

It is an unbelievable paradox that among professionals working with deaf children—otologists, speech pathologists, audiologists, psychologists, pediatricians, general practitioners, and even educators of young deaf children—there are few who have a realistic understanding of the educationally handicapping nature of deafness. Rarely do they objectively grasp the limited educational achievement of most deaf youth and adults. This lack of knowledge is a regrettable and inexcusable irony for which the deaf child and his parents pay dearly.

Those who deal professionally with deafness have a responsibility to carefully study the data of a national survey reported by McClure (107) and Boatner (16). Based on a sample of 93 per cent of all pupils enrolled in schools for the deaf in the United States, it was found that of the 1,277 pupils sixteen years of age or older who left school in 1964, *30 per cent were functionally illiterate. Approximately 60 per cent had a 5.3 grade level or below on the Stanford Achievement Test. Only 5 per cent achieved at the tenth grade level or better, most of these being either hard of hearing or postlingually deafened.* Furthermore, by restricting the study to those leaving school at age sixteen, many younger dropouts and students who were ruled ineligible for school were eliminated. These excluded youth represent a large group (160). Thus, despite the dismal educational picture the survey presents, the sample was biased toward representing the educational level of the deaf as being far higher than it actually is. In view of studies (Table 4.1) demonstrating that deaf children have essentially the same intellectual potential (IQ) as hearing children, this represents a skeleton in the American educational closet.

There is a double tragedy represented: first, by the degree of failure of present educational systems and, second, by the fact that this failure is so well concealed. This concealment is the result of many factors. For example, instead of showing the real "achievement" of secondary school-age prelingually deafened children, educators generally demonstrate classes of cute young beginners where the failure of the educational process is not evident. In the few instances in which classes of older students are demonstrated, it is common to use the hard-of-hearing or those deafened late in life who have good speech and to hold them up as examples of what can be done. Children in these classes who were born profoundly deaf and therefore tend to speak poorly soon learn that when visitors come to school, they are never called upon to recite.

The concealment is an important reason why noneducational specialists in deafness and parents often get a grossly unrealistic picture of their deaf child's educational future. Such misconceptions contribute to the predominance of euphemistic denials of the realities of deafness and to the consequent failure to react to the condition in effective ways. So great is the parental need for denial and the often unintentional participation of the educator and other professionals in the delusion, that it is not at all uncommon for parents of an eighteen- or nineteen-year-old deaf youth, whose educational achievement level is that of a third grader, to plan for his matriculation into college. The all-too-frequent practice of informing parents that their deaf child is in a particular grade, when this placement is based merely on chronological age rather than the actual level at which the child is performing, increases the difficulty a parent faces in realistically assessing the academic achievement of his child. Often these youths have been placed in eleventh- and twelfth-grade high school classes with normally hearing students and go through what is for them a depreciation and for their parents a deception. State residential schools, which typically have larger numbers of deaf students and more qualified teachers, are often able to provide more realistic academic and vocational programs for secondary-age youths (169).

It is essential to the understanding of the psychological aspects of deafness that the end results of the present educational system be fully grasped. In order to help parents minimize some of the pitfalls they face, it is critical that specialists in deafness give factual educational counseling. In most cases advice about the choice of school (residential versus day school versus day class) is made by a physician or audiologist, who rarely if ever has observed first-hand many of the facilities about which he is giving advice. Parents should be counseled to personally observe all available school programs.

TABLE 4.1. INVESTIGATIONS OF THE INTELLIGENCE OF THE DEAF AND HARD OF HEARING: 1930 TO 1967*

Reference	*Sample and Age (Yr.)*	*Measuring Device or Test*	*Results*
Peterson, E. G., and J. M. Williams (1930)	466 deaf, 4–9	Goodenough	Average retardation: 1–10/12 yrs
MacPherson, June, and Helen S. Lane (1932)	61 deaf children	Hiskey, Randall's Island Series	Mean IQ's: 116.62 and 113.87, respectively
Meyer, M. F. (1932)	132 deaf, 5–20	Lectometer	Deaf scored slightly lower
Shirley, Mary, and Florence Goodenough (1932)	406 deaf, 6–14	Goodenough, Pintner Non-language	Medians 87.7 and 98.4, respectively
MacKane, K. (1933)*	Deaf children	Grace Arthur, Pintner-Patterson, Drever-Collins, Pintner Non-language	Retardation: 1 yr. or less; Pintner: less than 2 yrs.
Lane, Helen S. (1934)*	43 deaf children	Randall's Performance	Median: 96 (in 1931); 97 (in 1932)
Lyon, V. W. (1934)	Deaf children	Grace Arthur, Pintner Non-language	Medians 92 and 84, respectively
Bishop, Helen M. (1936)	90 deaf and hard-of-hearing	Grace Arthur	Normal distribution
Peterson, E. G. (1936)	100 deaf, 5 7/12–17	Kohs Block Design	Mean IQ: 92.5; range: 54-156; scores clustered around 80 and 100 with 17 per cent at each
Scyster, Margaret (1936)	50 preschoolers	Minnesota Preschool, Merrill-Palmer, Pintner-Patterson	Deaf showed no retardation
Lane, Helen S. (1937 and 1938)*	250 deaf, 5–19	Lectometer, Randall's Performance	Equal ability; median: 97.6
Lane, Helen S. (1938)*	50 deaf preschoolers	Drever-Collins	Deaf mean: 105–122, depending on scoring record

* *Investigator experienced in the area of deafness at the time of the research cited.*

TABLE 4.1—*continued*

Reference	*Sample and Age (Yr.)*	*Measuring Device or Test*	*Results*
Springer, N. N. (1938)	330 deaf, 6–12	Goodenough	Deaf scored appreciably lower, with congenitally below adventitiously deaf
Streng, Alice, and S. A. Kirk (1938)*	97 deaf children	Grace Arthur, Chicago Non-Verbal	Same results as normals; age at onset not a factor
Pintner, R., and J. Lev (1939)	(4th and 5th graders)		
	1,404 hard-of-hearing	Pintner IQ Test	Mean: 94.7
	1,556 normal	Pintner IQ Test	Mean: 101.6
	315 hard-of-hearing	Pintner Nonlanguage	No significant difference compared to normals
Zeckel, A., and J. J. Kalb (1939)	100 deaf children	Porteous Maze	"Backward" IQ
Burchard, E. M., and H. R. Myklebust (1942)*	189 deaf children	Grace Arthur	Deaf IQ is average; no significant difference between congenitally and adventitiously deaf
Johnson, Elizabeth H. (1947)	57 deaf children	Chicago Non-Verbal	Six groups with mean IQ's of 73, 69, 69, 78, 85, and 99, respectively, from pregrade 2 to grade 3
Kirk, S. A., and June Perry (1948)	49 deaf and hard-of-hearing children	Ontario, Nebraska	No conclusion re relative intelligence
Myklebust, H. R. (1948)*	Deaf children	WISC Performance	Mean IQ: 101.8
Glowatsky, E. (1953)	24 deaf and hard-of-hearing, 7.5–15.7	Goodenough	Mean IQ: 98.46
Graham, E. E., and Esther Shapiro (1953)	20 deaf children	WISC Performance	Mean IQ: 96.1
Ross, Grace (1953)	61 deaf, 3–10	Ontario, Hiskey, Vineland	Mean IQ's: 104.6, 104.8, and 94.7, respectively

TABLE 4.1—*continued*

Reference	*Sample and Age (Yr.)*	*Measuring Device or Test*	*Results*
DuToit, J. M. (1954)	289 deaf children from different schools and 180 from same school	DuToit's Nonlanguage Group Test	Mean IQ of "different school" group: 98.53; mean IQ of "same school" group: 99.96
Lavos, G. (1954)	90 deaf and hard-of-hearing children	Pintner General Tests, Chicago Non-Verbal, Revised Beta Examination	Correlation coefficients between tests ranged from 0.58–0.69; statistically significant
Frisina, D. R. (1955)*	3 midwestern schools for the deaf	Grace Arthur	9.2–12 per cent below 79 in IQ
Hiskey, M. S. (1956)	380 normal children, 466 deaf, 4–10	Hiskey	Mean IQ's: normal hearers, 101; deaf, in mid-90's
Goetzinger, C. P., and C. L. Rousey (1957)*	101 deaf, 14–21	WISC Performance	Mean IQ: 101.9
Vernon, M. (1957)	97 deaf children	Goodenough	Mean IQ: 90
Larr, A. L., and E. R. Cain (1959)	248 deaf children	WISC	Mean IQ: 97.8; range: 61–138
	63 deaf children	Ontario	Mean IQ: 98.1; range: 52–129
	77 deaf children	Grace Arthur	Mean IQ: 101.1; range: 61–147
Brill, R. G. (1962)*	312 deaf, 5–16	WISC Performance	Mean IQ: 104.9
Mira, Mary P. (1962)	60 deaf preschoolers, mean age 4.77	Leiter, Hiskey	Mean IQ's: 96.32 and 108.86, respectively
Anderson, R. M., G. D. Stevens, and E. R. Stuckless (1966)*	1,600 deaf children from six residential schools	Performance Scales	19 per cent below 83 IQ
Vernon, M. (1966)* (1969)	66 deaf children	Performance Scales	Genetic deaf mean IQ: 114
	39 deaf children	Performance Scales	Rh deaf mean IQ: 94
	92 deaf children	Performance Scales	Postmeningitic deaf mean IQ: 96
Vernon, M. (1967)*	115 deaf children	Performance Scales	Premature deaf mean IQ: 89
Vernon, M. (1967)*	98 deaf children	Performance Scales	Postmaternal rubella mean IQ: 95

* *Investigator experienced in the area of deafness at the time of the research cited.*

They should be told to speak to the parents of other deaf children who have gone through the different schools. Most important, the parents and professionals should consult deaf adults who have attended the various schools. Although these steps would appear to be self-evident, surprisingly they are seldom followed by parents of young deaf children.

Intellectual Characteristics. Folklore has frequently associated deafness with stupidity. Even today this is part of a common characterization and represents a painful stigma for the deaf. As will be noted from the extensive data cited below, it is a false notion. (*See* also Table 4.1).

Intelligence. The intelligence of deaf children has been extensively studied. In fact it is one of the few psychological aspects of deafness that can be discussed with authority. Based on a wide number of independent research studies, it is possible to state and to support three generalizations. First, the range of intelligence for the deaf population is the same as that for the normally hearing (*see* original reports cited in Table 4.1). Second, the average IQ for those who are deaf is not significantly different than that for those who are not deaf (*see* Table 4.1). Third, certain etiologies of brain damage which also cause deafness result in a slightly higher prevalence of lower IQ's among groups of deaf children with these etiologies (160, 161, 162, 164).

These three generalizations indicate that there is no causal relationship between deafness and intelligence. Only when a brain-damaging condition is present with a hearing loss, does a correlation appear between deafness and a slightly lower mean IQ score. It is brain damage that accounts for the slightly higher prevalence of hearing impairment in mentally retarded populations (78, p. 465; 104, p. 540). Here conditions like maternal rubella or premature birth may lead to the double handicap of low IQ and deafness.

Cognitive Functioning. In recent years research psychologists and linguists have conducted investigations of the cognitive functioning of prelingually deafened persons (13, 15, 39, 50, 63, 71, 131, 164, 174). Most of this work has been directed at determining relationships between verbal language and thought processes.

Prelingually deafened children frequently have no verbal language until they begin school, and they are generally severely retarded in language development even as adults. Consequently, they offer an excellent sample for the investigation of relationships between verbal language and thought. For those interested in the psychological functioning of the deaf, this work is of major importance.

Well-documented studies suggest that language is not a necessary prerequisite for the occurrence of highly developed intellectual processes (50, 131, 132, 162). In fact it appears that verbal language is not the mediating system of thought and that there is no direct relationship between concept formation and the level of verbal language development (50, 73, 132, 163).

Previous theories which had suggested abstract thinking, generalization, and complex conceptualization were impossible in deaf persons who lacked sophisticated language skills are not consistent with current research evidence (50, 131, 132, 167, 174).

The significance of these findings lies in their demonstrating that there is a far greater potential for intellectual growth and cognitive development among prelingually deafened children than had been previously attributed to them. For educators the mandate is clear. Nonverbal means of tapping the intellectual capacities and permitting their growth must be fully utilized and developed in order that deaf children's cognitive potential may be manifested despite their language disability. In an outstanding book on this topic, Furth (1966) has suggested symbolic logic as one approach.

Adult Adjustment Patterns

VOCATIONAL

There have been four major surveys of the work patterns of the deaf population (17, 81, 97, 125). Although the exact figures vary slightly from study to study, the overall pictures they present are essentially consistent. They show that from 60 to 85 per cent of the employed deaf are engaged in unskilled or semiskilled work; these percentages are two to three times those for the total hearing population. Stated somewhat differently, five-sixths of deaf adults are manual laborers of varying skills—contrasted to one-half of the hearing population similarly employed (5). Conversely, 17 per cent of the deaf population are employed in white-collar jobs including professional, technical, managerial, clerical, and sales, as compared to 46.8 per cent of the general U. S. population (34, 97, 133, 158, 159).

Among the employed deaf there is a strong relationship between educational attainment and both income and level of work. However, the percentage of deaf students able to attain college entrance is only about one-tenth the percentage of those with normal hearing who are admitted to college (136); and, this figure may decline with the decrease in postlingual deafness and the increase in multiply handicapped deaf youths (157, 160).

Once employment is found, the deaf are stable in job tenure (17, 97, 125, 133). Employers report satisfactory work records (49). Despite this exemplary work record, it is not uncommon to find employment practices that are discriminatory to deaf applicants (33, 158).

The American Federationist, official publication of the AFL-CIO, has pointed out that automation is eliminating many of the unskilled, semiskilled, and manual jobs in which the overwhelming majority of the deaf have worked in past years (155). Jobs in technical areas, service industries, professions, and management are expanding and this is where the deaf are currently least well represented and (presumably) least well prepared by aptitude and by training (95).

Frequently these facts about the vocational adjustment of deaf adults are unknown to professionals who counsel deaf youths and their families. In the absence of this basic information appropriate educational and vocational planning and counseling are impossible. Frequently the deaf person is expected to be the architect of his own rehabilitation and it is forgotten that not even the most optimal academic and technical accomplishment on the part of the deaf person can overcome prejudicial practices of employers. It would appear that concurrent with attempting to provide maximum education to deaf youth, educators and other professionals must expend as much energy correcting societal misconceptions of the deaf individual's abilities.

Marriage and Sexual Patterns

Only recently have sexual behavior and marriage been examined in depth (75, 103). Unfortunately, deaf persons were not systematically included in these studies. Therefore, the only information available about sex and marriage among the deaf is from surveys and a few limited clinical reports (9, 97, 125). From these sources it is known that marriages between deaf persons are relatively stable if the criterion is a low divorce rate (9, 49, 70, 97, 125, 133). This finding must be qualified by the realization that a significantly greater proportion of deaf men and women remain unmarried (125, p. 93).

A paradox suggesting certain differences between courtship and marriage is that the better the communication skills of the deaf person (oral or manual), the greater the probability of marriage. However, once married, the better the communication skills of the partners, the greater the reported marital discord (125, p. 112). In all but 5 per cent of the marriages both husband and wife are deaf.

The only study of the sexual patterns of deaf persons is the New York research (125). Questions were asked about premarital sexual experiences, homosexual behavior, extramarital activities, and other questions that could have elicited valuable data. However, interviews were conducted in the presence of spouses and children, casting serious doubt on the validity of the responses. The authors acknowledged this limitation but despite the technique they were able to gain some useful insights. They found that there is limited premarital dating, at least an average amount of homosexual experimentation, and glaringly inadequate sex education. Only 6 per cent of those interviewed received sex education at home. This is not surprising when one realizes that only 12 per cent of the parents learned to communicate with their children at even a rudimentary level in the language of signs. The limitations of oral communication and of the verbal language level of most deaf youths preclude the possibility of teaching the complexities of sex other than in the language of signs and finger-spelling.

This lack of parental or school guidance regarding sex is reflected in the disproportionate percentage of deaf patients seen in the New York Psychiatric Institute outpatient clinic for evaluation of sexual maladjustment (125, p. 245). This fact has led to an experimental program (in the language of signs) of counseling, including sexual information, by the New York Psychiatric group in the Fanwood School for the Deaf (124).

ORGANIZATIONS OF DEAF ADULTS

Deaf adults try not to leave responsibility for their welfare in the hands of others. They have formed strong organizations to meet social, psychological, and legislative needs. These groups play an integral part in the lives of the deaf.

The National Association for the Deaf, consisting of over 10,000 members, is the most prominent. There are chapters in every state. There is a permanent office in Washington, D.C., and national meetings are held. Much constructive work is done for deaf people by this organization; for example, it is actively interested in federal and state legislation for the welfare of the deaf and organizes many athletic and social events.

The National Fraternal Society for the Deaf, whose membership also exceeds 10,000, is an insurance company established and managed by deaf people, providing them life insurance at reasonable rates.

The Oral Deaf Adult Section, consisting of about 150 members, is a subgroup of the Alexander Graham Bell Association. It is sponsored by the hearing members of the Bell Association and promotes the teaching of speech and speech-reading. There are also social and athletic clubs in almost all large cities, and every state has a state-wide organization of deaf people.

Parents of deaf children, professionals in the area of deafness, and students preparing for work in this area should meet and participate in the activities of these groups. One of the tragic ironies in the lives of the deaf is that those who have so much to say about their education and status in society almost never consult them or have enough contact with them to grasp the problems of deafness. By analogy, the blind fought for over a hundred years for braille in order that they might read. Sighted people opposed the idea, ignoring the views of the blind themselves, and claimed that the blind must read raised printed letters that were copies of the letters sighted people read. Finally a blind man, Louis Braille, found influential people who would listen to him, and the system of braille was developed. Thus, the blind were enabled to read and to succeed educationally. A breakthrough wherein hearing people attend to the ideas that deaf people have for their own welfare has yet to be achieved. The deaf are still forced to "read raised printed symbols."

By getting to know deaf parents of deaf children, hearing parents can often get help in everyday practical experiences in the discipline, management, and care of deaf children. Certainly teachers should have extensive experience with the adult deaf regardless of the age of the child they are teaching. They rarely do. In fact educators frequently exclude deaf parents of deaf children from preschool parent education programs where they and other parents could meet deaf adults.

Unfortunately, all organizations for deaf adults do not fulfill constructive roles. Semiorganized, quasi-criminal groups exist throughout the United States which promote "peddling." The activity usually involves a deaf person approaching groups of hearing persons in bars and restaurants with cards that show the manual alphabet or with some other trinket to which is attached the message, "I am deaf and cannot work. Please buy this." This form of begging frequently involves organized groups or gangs, many of which travel all over the United States. Generally, the leaders are intelligent but unscrupulous deaf persons who control and exploit weaker or retarded deaf people. Sometimes individual sociopathic deaf peddlers operate independently.

Peddlers gross up to $600 per week. The deaf community holds in contempt these beggars who are unwilling to work and who create a bad impression of other deaf people. The National Association for the Deaf has attempted to encourage legislation against peddling and "professionals" in deafness, and the lay public render a service when they discourage it or report peddlers who operate without a license.

PROFESSIONAL SPECIALISTS IN THE AREA OF DEAFNESS

To audiologists, speech pathologists, otologists, speech therapists, and others whose careers are devoted to the saving or the restoration of hearing and speech, the child with irreversible deafness often represents a failure. One aspect of their frustration is that efforts to teach speech to these children are not as successful as the efforts directed toward most other speech problems.

It is difficult for anyone to accept failure. Failure in a professional endeavor is especially hard to accept. It is understandable that many specialists in hearing and speech do not admit to themselves and do not fully inform the parents of a deaf child that the child has a sensori-neural deafness that cannot be corrected. Consequently, realistic confrontations about incurable deafness are rare and often may be avoided by subtle denial. Denial is implicit in the characteristic comments of those whose responsibility it is to inform parents of their child's deafness—comments such as, "There is no such thing as total deafness," or "Your child has residual hearing which we can help with a hearing aid," or "Beethoven was deaf." While these statements contain truths, they do not offer a totally objective picture of an 80-dB loss (500–2,000 Hz). They do not make clear to parents that speech-reading and a deaf child's speech will never be adequate communication skills for many social and educational activities. Nor do they give reasonable explanations of how the deaf child's life adaption will differ. Whereas Beethoven may have had a hearing loss late in life, analogies to deaf children are ludicrous yet are often a part of the way deafness is presented to parents by professionals.

To a lay person, holding out hope for the recovery of irreversible deafness may seem reasonable and compassionate. However, studies of psychological adjustment to disability indicate otherwise. They are decisive in showing that when information is frankly and fully presented, the handicapped child and his family can and do develop more effective and gratifying ways to cope with the problem (31, pp. 18–52; 59, 168).

When the full implications of an irreversible disability are not clearly conveyed, families and handicapped persons stand waiting for "cures." They persevere in the same ineffectual patterns instead of constructively adapting to the new problem of deafness. In this state of expectation, parents are often easy marks for those who promise grandly but deliver little. A deaf person or the family of a deaf child can be led into believing that amplification and speech training will, for all functional purposes, eliminate deafness and the need to make realistic adjustments to this major problem.

If a handicap is to be handled effectively, its full ramifications must be understood. It is natural for all concerned to want to deny and minimize the unpleasant aspects of this truth. The professional must avoid an unwitting participation in this denial even when his compassion and psychological needs may make him feel like doing otherwise. It is in this critical responsibility that otologists, audiologists, educators, and others are most likely to fail and where their professional services are most in need of improvement.

Psychopathology and Organic Factors of Mental Illness

PSYCHOSIS

One approach to the understanding of deaf people is to examine the nature and the degree of mental illness among them. Studying the pathological is a traditional and effective approach to understanding normal function.

The only extensive study of psychotic illness among the deaf was done in New York State by Rainer, et al. (125). This research group has examined and compared the kinds of psychotic illness among the deaf patients in the state hospitals of New York to that found among the other patients. Their major finding was that schizophrenia, which accounts for over half of all hospitalized psychotic patients, was not significantly more common among the deaf admissions to the hospitals than among the hearing admissions. However, the deaf patients tended to stay in state hospitals longer. Their communication problems made them custodial, not treatment, cases (125, p. 202).

An atypical finding about the deaf psychotic population was that 5 per cent of those in state hospitals were found to have retinitis pigmentosa (Usher's Syndrome), a genetic condition involving deafness, progressive blindness, and aphasoid problems. Sometimes mental deficiency is present as an additional feature of the disease (125, p. 201).

The age-old concept that paranoid schizophrenia and generalized paranoid patterns are more common among the deaf than the hearing was not substantiated (125, p. 201). The low percentage of the deaf having severe endogenous depression was another finding in contrast to folklore about the traits of deaf people (125, p. 201).

Based on this extensive study of a well-selected sample of the New York State deaf population, the basic conclusion was that psychotic processes such as schizophrenia were essentially the same among the deaf as among the hearing. Certain kinds of genetically related organic psychoses, impulse control disorders, and cases of primitive personality development were more common in mentally ill deaf persons. Alcoholism and depressive psychoses were less prevalent.

Matzker (105) in Germany, in contrast to the New York group, found schizophrenia more common among the deaf, but his study was far less complete. Cases of hearing loss associated with the aging process (presbycusis) were also included. They represent a much different group than the persons referred to in the New York study and in this chapter.

Research on psychosis and deafness is beginning at the Psychosomatic and Psychiatric Institute for Research and Training of the Michael Reese Hospital and Medical Center. The clinical impressions from the initial stages of this work indicate that although paranoid schizophrenia may not be more prevalent among the prelingually deaf, it may be more frequent among the post-lingually deaf and the hard-of-hearing than among the general population.

LESSER MENTAL ILLNESSES

Little is known on neuroses, character disorders, and other mental problems not considered psychoses. These kinds of disorders are not easy to identify in a deaf population. Thus far the only effort to do this has been through the outpatient clinic of the New York Project in a series of several related investigations.

One, a study of fifty-one deaf law offenders (125, p. 143), indicated the largest number, nineteen, were sex offenders; eight were charged with assault; seven with disorderly conduct; and the rest were booked for burglary and theft, murder, manslaughter, forgery, and dope peddling. Misdemeanor charges involved vagrancy, reckless driving, shoplifting, and bookmaking. These findings are difficult to interpret meaningfully because the sample is not known to be representative or random, and no baseline data is provided for comparison.

Major problems in the total New York outpatient clinic population were acute psychiatric illness, homosexuality, poor work adjustment, social conflicts, and family problems (125, pp. 156–57). Schizophrenic illness accounted for 57.5 per cent and passive-aggressive personality disorders for 20.4 per cent (mostly of the passive-dependent type). Overt homosexuality, usually in the characterologic framework of a dependent personality, was the predominant feature in 11.4 per cent. Other common syndromes were antisocial reactions, intellectual subnormality, involutional disturbances, situational reactions, and "primitive personality" (125, p. 157). This last category is a nosological term used specifically for certain types of deaf patients where there is normal intellectual potential coupled with an almost total lack of verbal or manual language. The response of these patients to everyday events is as if they were in a continual emergency. Basilier (7), the Norwegian psychiatric authority on deafness, covers this syndrome and a number of other reactions to congenital deafness under a broader clinical rubric, "surdophrenia."

As to the communication difficulties imposed by deafness, the New York psychiatrists and psychologists found that over three-fourths of deaf patients could not even be approached in treatment except by using the language of signs (125, p. 160). This was true despite the fact that a high proportion were college educated (125, p. 163).

Brain damage plays a major role in a significant number of the behavior disorders in deaf persons. Rainer, et al. (125) note its role in psychoses in their discussion of retinitis pigmentosa. Vernon (157, 160, 161, 162, 163, 164), in a series of articles on sequelae of major causes of deafness, has demonstrated that the organic residua of these etiologies account for an appreciable amount of both psychotic and lesser mental disorders.

A few tenuous generalizations can be drawn from the few studies reported and the authors' clinical experience. First, impulse control problems and their related syndromes are more common among the deaf. Second, there is a frequent lack of insight and the blame for psychosocial difficulties is externalized. As a result, conscious anxiety is not present as often and the motivation for treatment sometimes is minimal.

Organic Factors

The leading causes of deafness are also major etiologies of brain damage. This is a critical factor for consideration in any "psychology of deafness" (62, 157). It means that behavior noted as characteristic for deaf persons may not be caused by deafness at all, as has generally been believed. It may be due to central nervous system damage or an interaction between this and the deafness. Apart from the very important theoretical implications (167), an awareness of concomitant brain injury should participate in formulating therapeutic approaches, in interpreting data, and in developing appropriate modifications in standard teaching techniques. For this reason, we shall discuss some of the conditions that cause deafness and the behavioral processes found to be related to these conditions.

MATERNAL RUBELLA

Since the early 1940's, it has been known that MATERNAL RUBELLA (German measles) in pregnancy, especially if it occurs during the first three months, often results in defective children, deafness being the most common handicap (30, 68). Most studies indicate that between 12 and 19 per cent of postrubella children are deaf (30, 68, 102, 144). Because rubella is an epidemical disease, its prevalence as an etiology among deaf school-age children varies from 4 to 20 per cent, depending upon the year reported (162).

The behavioral characteristics most often reported in postrubella deaf youths are restlessness, hyperactivity, distractibility, and impulsiveness (68, 90, 116, p. 36; 162). Vernon (160, 162), in a study of 129 postrubella children, found their psychological adjustment, as determined by individual psychodiagnosis and by teacher evaluations, reflected appreciably more pathology than that of most other deaf children. Eight per cent were found to be psychotic and the mean IQ of the group was significantly below average. One-half of the children were multiply handicapped. Brain damage was present in many, often manifesting itself in aphasoid disorders.

MENINGITIS

MENINGITIS, an inflammatory condition of the protective covering of the brain, is the leading postnatal cause of deafness among school-age children. Its prevalence as a cause of deafness is generally reported as 8 to 16 per cent (6, 35, 58, p. 82; 72, p. 36; 141, 160, 167).

In recent years, improvements in medical treatment have dramatically reduced the mortality rate from 50 to 80 per cent to 13 to 21 per cent, with from 3 to 5 per cent of the survivors having deafness (36, p. 244; 46, pp.

546–80; 154). In addition to a causative role in deafness, meningitis is a major etiology of brain damage with between 15 to 71 per cent of survivors left with major neurological sequelae (36, pp. 243, 253; 57, p. 822; 72, p. 36; 154, 167).

A significant effect of modern and improved treatment is that very young children, especially prematures and full-term neonates who previously died from the disease, now survive but they frequently have severe residua such as deafness and other neuropathology (46, p. 537; 72, p. 4; 118, p. 344; 160, 167). Consequently, the majority of postmeningitic deaf children today lost their hearing prior to acquiring language. A disproportionate number of them are also the victims of other conditions such as aphasia, mental retardation, psychological disturbance, or hemiplegias (167). By contrast, in the past the very young children who had meningitis generally died. The older children who survived had well-established verbal language patterns and no residua other than their hearing loss. The implication of this is that many of the postmeningitic deaf children of today must be evaluated and understood both in terms of profound hearing loss and in terms of other neurological impairment.

In a study of five measures of behavior—intelligence, psychological adjustment, language skills, educational achievement, and psychodiagnostic evidence of neurological impairment—meningitic deaf children were found to be distributed bimodally instead of in the conventional bell-shaped curve. One of these modes contained those with neurological sequelae who demonstrated either pathology or low achievement on the five behavioral measures. The other mode represented the children without brain damage who were average to above average as a group (167).

It has been noted by numerous investigators that meningitis often destroys the vestibular mechanism, which is anatomically related to the auditory system. Consequently, postmeningitic children and adults may have balance disorders (ataxia). For example, in darkness where vision cannot compensate for the absent vestibular function, the postmeningitic deaf person may stagger as if intoxicated. Among postmeningitic deaf children it is not uncommon for those who contracted the disease postlingually to lose the language they had developed before deafness. Furthermore, they sometimes lose the capacity to learn language or they may have to learn it again in the same way congenitally deaf children do, rather than recover it spontaneously. These deaf aphasic children often suffer severe emotional disturbances that result from the double trauma of deafness and aphasia.

Tuberculous meningitis deserves special consideration. Until recently there were no survivors of this disease. The development of new effective antimicrobial medications has changed this (46, p. 580; 118, p. 470). Current research (44, p. 12; 165) indicates that tuberculous meningitis is associated with deafness either as a direct result of the disease (44, p. 12) or as a result of either the disease or the antibiotics used in its treatment (165). Sexual precocity, hemiplegias, aphasia, learning disability, and other neurophysiological residua with behavioral manifestations, have been demonstrated in a high percentage of this group of deaf children (165).

PREMATURITY

Only recently has the strong relationship between prematurity and the behavioral aspects of deafness been revealed (160, 166). It is well known that the mortality rate for prematurely born infants has been greatly reduced (60, 119). These surviving children often have serious neurological, psychological, educational, and communicative disorders (11, 18, 41, 60, 77, 96, 145).

Based on a sample of 1,468 deaf children in California, Vernon (166) indicated that the rate of prematurity in the deaf population (17.6 per cent) is over four times that of the general population. Furthermore, the mean IQ of these children is 89.4 with a 16.4 per cent prevalence of mental retardation. Two-thirds had other major disabilities in addition to deafness, the most frequent of which were cerebral palsy, aphasia, psychological disturbance, and visual pathology. Four broad psychological patterns especially common among the disturbed prematures were schizoid behavior; a high rate of psychosis; a syndrome of immaturity, hyperactivity, explosiveness, and anxiety-ridden impulsiveness; and a combination of average or better IQ and almost total aphasia that resulted in ego disintegration of a type similar to that noted with postmeningitic aphasic deaf youths.

In five per cent of the cases of prematurity, maternal rubella or complications of the Rh factor were a part of the child's medical history. Such children may have both the residua of prematurity and the residua of one of these other two conditions (Vernon, 166).

HEREDITY

It is difficult to establish with certainty the proportion of deafness caused by genetic factors. Estimates vary from 11.5 to 60 per cent (22, 110, 160). Very few studies have been done on the adjustment patterns of youth with genetic deafness. Brill (22) found them to be either very well-adjusted or below average in adjustment with relatively few being average. Birch and Stuckless (10) and Vernon (160) found them to be more satisfactorily adjusted and better academic achievers than most other deaf youth.

From these limited data and from frequently reported anecdotal observations, hereditarily deaf children as a group seem better adjusted than most deaf children. The exceptions to this are youth in which the genetic combinations result in other somatic pathology such as retinitis pigmentosa (Usher's Syndrome).

SEROLOGICAL COMPLICATIONS

Complications of Rh factor (erythroblastosis fetalis) is the foremost perinatal cause of deafness. They account for three to four per cent of the profound hearing losses found among school-age children (29, 128, 160). A recent study (160) indicates that the mean IQ scores of Rh deaf children are lower than those expected in the general population. Overall educational achievement is slightly retarded, with special difficulties in language. Aphasia or aphasoid conditions are often present as complicating factors in language training (54, 115, 130, 160). About half of the youths whose deafness is due to the Rh factor have cerebral palsy. In addition, another one-third give psychodiagnostic indications that suggest brain damage (160). Others have reported similar findings based on their clinical experience (14, 29, 45, 54, 60, 116, 130).

Considering the degree of neuropathology and multiply handicapping conditions present, there is surprisingly little serious psychological maladjustment compared to the other etiological groups of deaf children. However, many almost classically demonstrate the behavior pattern of the Strauss Syndrome (160).

Research has not been done to determine the prevalence and sequelae of other blood incompatibility diseases relative to deafness, although it is believed that ABO complications result in hearing loss and sequelae similar to those associated with the Rh factor.

OTHER ETIOLOGIES

From one-third to one-half of deafness is of unknown origin. Conditions such as head injuries, encephalitis, viral infections, toxins, polio, and common childhood diseases combine to cause about 10 per cent of deafness (162). Some of these, encephalitis and head injuries for example, are known to be associated with chronic brain syndromes, but there is little data on the behavioral manifestations of these syndromes in deaf children.

Etiologies of deafness have been reviewed more carefully than might have been expected in a chapter on psychological aspects of deafness because these conditions have considerable influence on the behaviour of a large number of deaf children. This information can be of great value if correctly used in evaluating and counseling deaf children and their parents. It is frequently misused in two ways: (1) The characteristics or the prognosis attributed to a specific deaf child are based on what is known about common traits for other deaf children having the same etiology of deafness. For example, the mother of an eighteen-month-old prematurely born child may be told that her infant has a low IQ. This prognosis is based not on a careful evaluation of the infant, but on what is known to be a group tendency in premature deaf children. This kind of gross overgeneralization is unfortunately rather common. (2) Certain pathological behaviors are ignored which may be related to the condition that caused the child's deafness. This leads to blaming the parents' child-rearing practices for maladjustments which they did not cause.

Psychological and Psychiatric Evaluation

PSYCHOLOGICAL EVALUATION

It is the purpose of this section to provide psychologists, educators, counselors, and speech therapists with a usable guide to the basic psychological and educational tests most suitable for assessment of deaf children. Information about such tests and testing procedures is especially important today because of the rapid expansion of psychological services that should be utilized with deaf youngsters and that are being made available through school programs and speech and mental hygiene clinics. In many cases, however, the psychologists involved are not familiar with deaf children and are understandably unaware of the psychometric instruments that can be used with success. In like fashion the educators, audiologists, and speech therapists who do understand the ramifications of deafness in children are not always intimately familiar with the various intelligence and personality tests.

By describing and briefly evaluating the basic psychometric instruments found to be appropriate for deaf children, it is hoped that a useful reference will be provided for psychologists and others who are occasionally faced with the task of testing or interpreting the test results of deaf children. At the same time, this information may enable personnel in schools for the deaf (or related agencies), who refer deaf subjects for psychological evaluation, to specify the basic tests they desire to have administered to the child. In this way the probability of obtaining meaningful measurements of deaf youngsters will be substantially increased.

Intelligence Testing

BASIC CONSIDERATIONS IN THE INTELLIGENCE TESTING OF DEAF AND HARD-OF-HEARING CHILDREN

A clear understanding of the following factors should precede any efforts to test or interpret test findings with deaf children:

1. To be valid as a measure of the intelligence of a deaf youngster, an IQ test must be a nonverbal performance-type instrument (28, 86). Verbal

tests with deaf children are almost always inappropriate. They measure language deficiency due to hearing loss rather than intelligence (24, 64, 91, pp. 217–21; 117, 114, pp. 25, 237). An example of the tragic consequence of the incorrect choice of tests was a student formerly at the California School for the Deaf in Riverside who had been given a Stanford Binet (verbal test) and received an IQ of 29. She was committed to a hospital for the mentally retarded, and she remained there five years. Upon reevaluation, using a performance IQ test, this girl was found to have an IQ of 113, which led to her dismissal from the hospital and her enrollment in a school for the deaf. In the California School for the Deaf at Riverside, in 1964 alone there were three deaf children previously misdiagnosed as mentally deficient who were later given performance tests that yielded scores indicative of favorable academic potential, a finding subsequently demonstrated in the classroom.

It should be noted that all nonverbal tests are certainly not appropriate for deaf children. One main reason is that while many have nonverbal items, they may nevertheless require verbal directions (64, 86, 116, p. 62; 170, pp. 159–61; 175, 176).

Hard-of-hearing children may give the impression of being able to understand verbal tests, but this is often an artifact (91, p. 265; 117, 114, pp. 241–42). In testing such children it is essential to begin with a performance measure and then, if desired, to try a verbal instrument. In cases where the score yielded by the former is appreciably higher, the probability is that it is the more valid, and further, that the lower score on the test involving language is due to the subject's hearing impairment and does not constitute a true measure of intelligence.

2. Even more than with hearing subjects, scores on preschool and early school deaf and hard-of-hearing children tend to be extremely unreliable (64, 66). For this reason, low scores in particular should be viewed as questionable in the absence of other supporting data.

3. There is far more danger that a low IQ score is wrong than that a high one is inaccurate (64, 114, p. 241). This is due to the many factors that can lead to a child's not performing to capacity; whereas, in contrast, there are almost no conditions that can lead to performance above capacity.

4. Tests given to deaf children by psychologists not experienced with the deaf or hard-of-hearing are subject to appreciably greater error than when the service is rendered by one familiar with deaf youngsters. The atypical attentive set of the hearing-impaired child to testing, which has been frequently cited in the literature, is felt to be one of the reasons for this (166, 114, p. 239; 175).

5. It must be noted that the performance part of many conventional intelligence tests is only half or less of the test. Therefore, to approach the validity of a full IQ test with a deaf child, it is necessary to give at least two performance scales.

TABLE 4.2. EVALUATION OF SOME OF THE INTELLIGENCE TESTS MOST COMMONLY USED WITH DEAF AND HARD-OF-HEARING CHILDREN

Tests	*Appropriate Age Range Covered by the Test*	*Evaluation of the Test*
1. Wechsler Performance Scale for Children (1949)	9 years–16 years	The Wechsler Performance Scale is at present the best test for deaf children ages 9–16. It yields a relatively valid IQ score, and offers opportunities for qualitative interpretation of factors such as brain injury or emotional disturbance (Wechsler, 1955, pp. 80–1). It has good interest appeal and is relatively easy to administer and reasonable in cost
2. Wechsler Performance Scale for Adults (1955)	16 years–70 years	The rating of the Wechsler Performance Scale for Adults is the same as the rating on the Wechsler Performance Scale for children.
3. Leiter International Performance Scale (1948 Revision)	4 years–12 years (also suitable for older, mentally retarded deaf subjects)	This test has good interest appeal. It can be used to evaluate relatively disturbed deaf children who could not otherwise be tested. This test is expensive and lacking somewhat in validation. In general, however, it is an excellent test for young deaf children. Timing is a minor factor in this test. One disadvantage lies in the interpretation of the IQ scores: the mean of the test is 95 and the standard deviation is 20. This means that the absolute normal score on this test is 95 instead of 100, as on other intelligence tests. Scores of, for example, 60, therefore, do not indicate mental deficiency but correspond more to about a 70 on tests such as the Wechsler or Binet. Great care must be taken in interpreting Leiter IQ scores for these reasons.
4. Progressive Matrices (Raven, 1948)	9 years–adulthood	Raven's Progressive Matrices are good as a second test to substantiate another, more comprehensive intelligence test. The advantage of the Matrices is that it is extremely easy to administer and score, taking relatively little of the examiner's time and is very inexpensive. It yields invalid test scores of impulsive deaf children, who tend to respond at random rather than with accuracy and care. For this reason, the examiner should observe the child carefully to assure that he is really trying.
5. Ontario School Ability Examination (Amoss, 1949)	4 years–10 years	This is a reasonably good test for deaf children within these age ranges.

Table 4.2—*continued*

Tests	*Appropriate Age Range Covered by the Test*	*Evaluation of the Test*
6. Nebraska Test of Learning Aptitude (Heider, 1940; Hiskey, 1955)	4 years–12 years	A test comparable in value to the Ontario, and standardized for both hearing and deaf children.
7. Chicago Non-Verbal Examination (Brown et al., 1947)	7 years–12 years	This test rates fair if given as an individual test; very poor if given as a group test. The scoring is tedious and reliability is rather low.
8. Grace Arthur Performance Scale (Arthur, 1947)	4.5 years–15.5 years	This is a test that is poor to fair because the timing is heavily emphasized; norms are not adequate, and directions are somewhat unsatisfactory. This test is especially unsatisfactory for emotionally disturbed children who are also deaf. With this type subject, this test will sometimes yield a score indicating extreme retardation when the difficulty is actually one of maladjustment. It is also poor for young deaf children who are of below average intelligence because they often respond randomly instead of rationally.
9. Merrill-Palmer Scale of Mental Tests	2 years–4 years	The Merrill-Palmer is a fair test for young deaf children, but it must be adapted in order to be used and would require a skilled examiner with a thorough knowledge of deaf children.
10. Goodenough Draw-A-Man Test (1926)	8.5 years–11 years	Directions are very difficult to give young children in a standardized manner. Scoring is less objective than would be desired, so this test is relatively unreliable. It does, however, have some projective value for personality assessment.
11. Randall's Island Performance Tests (1932)	2 years–5 years	This is one of the few nonverbal instruments available for measuring preschool children. It consists of a wide range of performance and manipulative tasks which, used by a competent examiner, provide diagnostic and insightful information. This test is relatively expensive, but valuable.

6. Intelligence tests for young deaf or hard-of-hearing children (age twelve or below) that emphasize time are not as valid in most cases as are other tests which do not stress time (66, 86). This is because these children often react to the factor of timing by either working in great haste and ignoring accuracy or else disregarding the time factor completely. In either instance, the result is not necessarily a reflection of intelligence.

7. Group testing of deaf and hard-of-hearing children is a highly questionable procedure that, at best, is of use only as a gross screening device (66, 86, 91, p. 221; 117).

EVALUATION OF SOME INTELLIGENCE TESTS MOST COMMONLY USED WITH DEAF AND HARD-OF-HEARING SUBJECTS

In order to evaluate these tests in a concise manner conducive to easy referral, a tabular form has been used. In fairness to both the tests and the reader it should be stated that these evaluations are based on the experience of the authors and the limited literature relevant to this area. For this reason, they are to a degree subjective and open to question. However, the tests described enjoy a wide acceptance and application by psychological personnel in school and agencies who work with hearing-impaired children (22, 91, pp. 222–24; 114, p. 298–302; 116, pp. 69–76, 161–77; 117).

Personality Testing

GENERAL CONSIDERATIONS TO BE MADE IN THE PERSONALITY TESTING OF DEAF AND HARD-OF-HEARING CHILDREN

As in the case of intelligence testing, it is important in the personality measurement of hearing-impaired children to consider certain basic factors prior to evaluating specific tests. These factors are:

1. Personality evaluation is a far more complex task than is IQ testing, especially with deaf children. Because of this, test findings should be interpreted in light of case history data and personal experience with the child. In fact, it behooves educators of the deaf with long experience in the field to view with skepticism results reported by examiners who are unfamiliar with deaf children, when these findings sharply contradict their own impressions of youngsters they know well.

2. Because of communication problems inherent in severe hearing loss, personality tests are more difficult to use with deaf subjects than with the general population (56, 91, pp. 225–26; 117, 114, p. 313; 116, pp. 121–22; 175). Not only do these tests depend on extensive verbal interchange or reading skill, but they also presuppose a rapport and confidence on the

part of the subject that is difficult to achieve when the person examined cannot understand what is being said or written. Paper and pencil personality measures are perhaps suitable for hearing-impaired children with well-developed expressive and receptive language ability, but such youngsters are rare, and even with them the problems of test administration and interpretation make the results highly invalid (56, 91, pp. 225–26; 117, 114, pp. 121–22). The need for fluency in manual communication by the examiner is especially evident in the area of projective testing.

3. There is some question as to whether the norms for the personality structure of hearing people are appropriate for deaf and hard-of-hearing subjects (175, 176). Conceivably, deafness alters the perceived environment sufficiently to bring about an essentially different organization of personality in which the normality would then differ from that in a person with normal hearing (8, 61, p. 256; 114, p. 115–18; 175). Although this is presently an unresolved problem, it is one that is frequently raised by scholars in the field of deafness and should be considered in any discussion of the personalities of those with severe hearing loss.

4. The use of interpreters who express the psychologist's directions in finger-spelling and sign language is a questionable procedure. What is required is an interpreter, fluent not only in manual communication, but also in psychology and testing (176). Obviously, this person would be doing the examining himself and not interpreting it for another. Therefore, results reported where an interpreter is involved are not likely to meet high standards of validity.

EVALUATION OF PERSONALITY TESTS COMMONLY USED WITH DEAF AND HARD-OF-HEARING CHILDREN

Because of the difficulties that have been pointed out above, few personality tests have had wide application with deaf or hard-of-hearing children. Four of the more commonly and successfully used are evaluated in Table 4.3.

Screening Tests for Brain Injury

Because of the high incidence of brain injury among deaf children, especially among those whom a teacher is likely to refer for psychological evaluation, it is appropriate to discuss some tests used to diagnose and measure this condition (157). A thorough assessment of neurological impairment would generally include one or more of these psychological instruments plus neurological and audiological techniques of diagnosis (157). A brief discussion of some tests and items from tests that are useful for detecting brain injury follows.

TABLE 4.3. PERSONALITY TESTS USED WITH DEAF AND HARD-OF-HEARING CHILDREN

Tests	*Appropriate Age Range Covered by the Test*	*Evaluation of the Test*
1. *Draw-A-Person* (Machover, 1949).	9 years–adulthood	This is a good screening device for detecting very severe emotional problems. It is relatively non-verbal and is probably the most practical proiective personality test for deaf children. Its interpretation is very subjective and in the hands of a poor psychologist it can result in rather extreme diagnostic statements about deaf children.
2. *Thematic Apperception Test (TAT) or Children's Apperception Test (CAT)* (Stein, 1955).	Can be used with deaf subjects of school age through adulthood who can communicate well manually or can communicate very well in written language.	This is a test of great potential, if the psychologist giving it and the deaf subject taking it can both communicate with fluency in manual communication. It is of very limited value otherwise unless the deaf subject has an exceptional command of the English language. This test could be given through an interpreter by an exceptionally perceptive psychologist, although it is more desirable if the psychologist can do his own communicating.
3. *Rorschach Ink Blot Test* (Rorschach, 1942).	Can be given to deaf subjects as soon as they are able to communicate fluently manually or if they can communicate with exceptional skill orally.	In order for the Rorschach to be used it is almost absolutely necessary that the psychologist giving it and the deaf subject taking it be fluent in manual communication. Even under these circumstances it is debatable if it yields much of value unless the subject is of above average intelligence. It would be possible with a very bright deaf subject, who had a remarkable proficiency in English, to give a Rorschach through writing, but this would not be very satisfactory.
4. *H. T. P. Technique* (Buck, 1949).	School age through adulthood.	This is a procedure similar to the Draw-A-Person test. It requires little verbal communication and affords the competent clinician some valuable insight into basic personality dynamics of the subject.

1. *Bender-Gestalt* (8). This is probably the most widely used screening instrument for the detection of gross neurological impairment. Standardization of norms is being continued; interpretation requires extensive training and experience. However, the Bender is a valuable part of a test battery for deaf subjects (117).

2. *Wechsler Performance Scale* (170, 171). Quantitative pattern analysis of these scales is of controversial validity as a diagnostic tool for neurological dysfunction. There is fairly general agreement, however, that in the hands of a capable clinical psychologist a partial qualitative type of diagnosis is possible (91, p. 228–29; 114, p. 301).

3. *Memory-For-Designs Test* (56). A relatively new test, this appears to have considerable value. Its precise scoring technique contains controls for variation in age, intelligence, and vocabulary level.

4. *Ellis Visual Designs Test*. This test appears to have definite possibilities, but lacks validation (91, p. 229).

5. *Strauss-Werner Marble Board Test*. This test is potentially excellent, but it is very hard to get. Scoring instructions are inadequate (91, p. 229).

6. *Hiskey Blocks* (64). This test requires a great deal of visualization and abstract ability and is of value for this reason (64, 114, p. 300).

7. *Rorschach* (129). The use of this test requires not only competency in administering the test, but also a fluency in the use of manual communication employed by the deaf. Results reported where these conditions are not met are of highly dubious validity.

8. *Kohs Blocks* (80). These are similar to the block design subtest of the Wechsler Scale, but are more extensive. A qualitative diagnosis is possible, but norms are lacking for organic involvement.

9. *The Diamond Drawing from the Stanford Binet*. This test has good validity, is generally available, and can be easily administered.

10. Various measures of motor ability and development. Among these would be the rail-walking test, tests of laterality, and certain items on the Vineland Social Maturity Scale that pertain to motor development.

Educational Achievement

In many cases it is important to obtain a measure of the educational achievement level of a deaf client. Any of the three tests below are appropriate for obtaining this information. These tests are easy to administer if the examiner makes certain that the client understands and successfully completes the sample items for each subtest. Another *critical* point in using academic achievement tests is to choose a battery that is at a level appropriate to the person being tested.

Recommended educational achievement tests are: (1) The Stanford Achievement Tests, (2) the Metropolitan Achievement Tests, and (3) the Gray-Votaw-Rogers.

In interpreting results of achievement tests with deaf persons, it is important to keep in mind some information stated earlier. Only about 5 per cent of the graduates from day and residential schools for the deaf attain a tenth-grade level; 41 per cent are above the seventh- or eighth-grade in achievement; 27 per cent are around the fifth- or sixth-grade level; and approximately 30 per cent are below this (most of these persons might be termed functionally illiterate by present governmental standards) (107). These figures are given in order to establish some baseline data about the norms to be used in judging the individual educational achievement findings of a particular child.

An Evaluation of Communication Skills

It is in the realm of communication that deafness presents its major handicap. For this reason, it is important that an evaluation include an assessment of communication skills.

There are three aspects of communication that should be appraised in a deaf person. The first and by far the most important is the ability to read and write. It has been found in research (97) that this is the mode most widely used by persons who are deaf in their job setting and general interaction. Therefore, it is obviously important to determine how effective the person is in exchanging ideas in written language. His degree of effectiveness will go a long way toward determining the type and level of education or occupational opportunity open to him.

Speech and speech-reading are the other key aspects of communication to be evaluated. These skills have considerable potential value to a deaf person educationally and vocationally. If he is able to speak understandably, this is especially important and helpful. Speech-reading ability is an asset, but even the most skilled deaf lip-reader generally finds this an inadequate way to get important information and he will usually prefer writing.

One final point must be made clear in evaluating communication skills: Many extremely bright and capable deaf youths lack the ability to speak and to lip-read. It is of critical importance that the clinician *not* confuse difficulty in communication with a lack of intelligence. It is also possible that a congenitally deaf person may have a very high IQ and yet write language that is not sophisticated grammatically. The clinicians must be keenly aware of these factors if they are to be fair and helpful to a deaf client.

Case History Data

The past is still the best predictor of the future. For this reason complete background information on a client, especially if he is deaf and may not be accurately evaluated with regular psychological procedures, is of extreme importance. Illustrative of just how essential case history data are is that the best psychiatric and psychological evaluations are often based 75 per cent upon background information.

SUGGESTED PSYCHOLOGICAL TEST BATTERIES FOR DEAF AND HARD-OF-HEARING SCHOOL-AGE CHILDREN

Because an adequate psychological assessment should properly be based on a series of tests rather than a single instrument, the following test batteries are suggested for the various age groups of a school population:

1. *Preschool.* Measurement of intelligence should be based on at least two of the following IQ tests: the Leiter International Performance Scale, the Merrill-Palmer Scale of Mental Tests, or the Randall's Island Performance Tests.

There are no suitable personality tests or tests for brain injury for deaf preschool children. Clinical judgment, play therapy situations, and medical, audiological, and case history data must be depended on exclusively for evaluation in these areas.

2. *Beginning School Age Through Age Nine.* IQ tests should include at least two of the following: the Leiter International Performance Scale, WISC Performance Scale, Nebraska Test of Learning Aptitude, Ontario Test of School Ability, Goodenough Draw-A-Man Test, or Progressive Matrices. Human figure drawing interpretation and Bender-Gestalt responses should be used to screen for personality deviations and organ brain damage. Educational achievement tests are usually not appropriate yet.

3. *Ages Nine Through Fifteen.* The most appropriate measure of intelligence for this age range is the WISC Performance Scale. It can best be supplemented with Progressive Matrices, the Chicago Non-Verbal Test, or the Leiter International Performance Scale. Human figure drawings and the Bender-Gestalt become increasingly valid measures in this age range and are the best screening techniques for personality disturbance and brain damage. Tests of educational achievement can be started with some of the better nine-year-old students and they become increasingly appropriate as the children get older.

4. *Age Sixteen Through School Graduation.* The WAIS Performance Scale stands out as the superior measure of intelligence for this age range. The second measure for intelligence found most valid is the Progressive Matrices. To the Bender-Gestalt and Draw-A-Person Test can be added or substituted the Memory-For-Designs Test as a screening measure for organic brain damage. Vocational tests should be added at this time. Their selection is a highly individual matter, depending on the subject and available vocational and educational facilities. For a discussion of these tests, Helmer Myklebust's article is most helpful (117).

PSYCHIATRIC EVALUATION

Psychiatric evaluation is essentially an empirical procedure based on interviewing and clinical observation. The resulting psychiatric diagnosis is stated in terms of categories representing certain characterological features that exist in reasonably consistent patterns. These patterns, when compared with rough expectations of normal behavior, represent important kinds of personality differences. Having made these determinations, conclusions follow regarding whether a patient does or does not need treatment, the type of treatment indicated, the motivation of the patient for treatment, and so on. Diagnostic efforts should serve more toward elaborating these kinds of data than simply establishing descriptive labels.

Obviously a major part of psychiatric diagnoses is derived from what a patient says. Though there is much nonverbal data that actively contributes to conclusions, this information is far more difficult to interpret. However, in the case of the deaf person who lacks adequate verbal communicative means, there is a necessarily greater dependence upon these kinds of cues.

Most psychiatrists asked to evaluate deaf people must resort to written communications. The psychiatrist's inability to use the language of signs considerably reduces the amount of communication that is possible. One might be led to the easy conclusion that if a psychiatrist learns sign language, he will then be able to offer psychiatric service to the deaf on a par with that offered to the hearing. Such an overgeneralized conclusion ignores a large number of factors that render many deaf clients different from most hearing clients. This is particularly true in the majority of the prelingually deaf. These persons generally lack the vocabulary and command of syntax required to communicate many concepts that are basic to therapy and diagnosis. The deficiency exists even if sign language is used and is far more pronounced if regular verbal communication is used. Communication through sign language and writing at the level at which most deaf persons express themselves does not contain the variety of rich connotative patterns that can offer clues to current psychodynamic functioning, interpersonal relationships, and developmental differences. However, there is often a more direct expression of affect which is clinically helpful. There is also a more concrete, immediate, and direct quality to sign language. The communication of temporal relationships is more difficult, making it almost impossible to fully relate past events to present behavior. As this is an essential aspect of most forms of therapy, it presents a serious obstacle to the treatment of deaf patients.

The deaf person's limited perception of social relationships and the problem of communicating temporal relationships means that the psychiatrist must work harder to structure the clinical picture of his patient. He cannot assume the same baseline frame of reference for what is "normal." The perceived environment is very particularized. For example, the patient is most likely functioning in a relatively isolated fashion. These factors must be considered in a determination of what really constitutes a healthy personality structure in a deaf client.

The usual psychotherapeutic techniques, which most often assume that certain linguistic and emotional maturity levels have been reached, must be modified. For example, attention has been drawn to motivation for treatment (125, p. 184), which in the deaf is often affected by "conceptual immaturity." The implication is that the deaf person's lack of basic social and cultural information in turn prevents many of them from realizing that the exchange of ideas in a psychotherapeutic relationship is a meaningful way to achieve relief from emotional tension. Consequently, the deaf individual who is disturbed is less likely to seek therapy, and referrals are most often requested by agencies, not the patients.

Psychiatric help for deaf children is a relatively "unexplored field." Research and clinical reports in this area have been limited to a very few studies (62). The deaf child's degree of variance from norms established by observing normal populations of children seems to become greater with maturation up to certain ages. The definition of the difference presents a challenge which has yet to be met. Appropriate modification of the norms caused by deafness have not been worked out. Brain damage (*see* section on Organic Factors) complicates the behavioral picture. And, the lack of language limits access to the child's representational world.

Psychiatric diagnosis of deaf children is a longitudinal process. The child psychiatrist will have to depend on complete information about the child's behavior at home and in school more than he would with a hearing child.

To communicate basic information to one another, deaf children and their families generally develop idiosyncratic nonverbal methods of varying degrees of effectiveness. Though finger-spelling and formal sign language offer an opportunity to circumvent the language handicap, it is not universally recognized as an appropriate language for deaf children due to reasons discussed elsewhere in the chapter. Recent vigorous efforts to modify sign language by linguistic analysis have gone a long way toward generating the grammar of the language, describing it, and making it more isomorphic with English (150, 151). As a means of resolving the problems the average hearing parent encounters in communicating with a deaf child, manual communication offers a worthwhile supplement to the ambiguity inherent in attempts limited to speech and speech-reading. The child psychiatrist will be surprised to find himself reduced to communications of the most primitive and most ambiguous sort when diagnosing a deaf child.

In addition to a general knowledge of the child's functioning in the home and the role communication plays in this, good psychiatric evaluation involves consultation with the child's teacher in order to obtain a knowledge of the child's behavior with peers. Given an understanding of the child's functioning in the home and in a school situation, the child psychiatrist also needs an understanding of the parents' ways of structuring their activities with the child.

The psychiatrist who understands deafness is then able to synthesize this material along with that received from other specialists, such as otologists, audiologists, or psychologists. This, in turn, must be transmitted in usable form to those responsible for the care of the child. Properly done, the diagnostic evaluation will provide useful information for planning for the child's future.

Bibliography

1. Adler, Edna A. "Reading out loud in the language of signs." *American Annals of the Deaf*, **109**: 364–66, 1964.
2. Amoss, H. *Ontario School Ability Examination*. Toronto, Canada: Ryerson Press, 1949.
3. Anderson, R. M., G. D. Stevens, and E. R. Stuckless. "Provision for the education of mentally retarded deaf students in residential schools for the deaf." Unpublished doctoral dissertation. Pittsburgh: University of Pittsburgh, 1966.
4. Arthur, G. *A Point Scale of Performance Tests, Rev. Form II*. New York: Psychological Corp., 1947.
5. Babbidge, H. D. *Education of the Deaf: A Report to the Secretary of Health, Education and Welfare by his Advisory Committee on the Education of the Deaf.* Washington, D.C.: U. S. Department of Health, Education, and Welfare, 1964.
6. Barton, M. E., S. D. Court, and W. Walker. "Causes of severe deafness in school children in Northumberland and Durham." *British Medical Journal*, **1**: 351–55, 1962.
7. Basilier, T. "Surdophrenia: The psychic consequences of congenital or early acquired deafness. Some theoretical and clinical considerations." *Acta Psychiatrics Scandinavica, Supplementum* 180, **40**: 362–74, 1964.
8. Bender, Lauretta. *A Visual Motor Gestalt Test and Its Clinical Use*. New York: The American Orthopsychiatric Association, 1938.
9. Best, H. *Deafness and the Deaf in the United States*. New York: The Macmillan Company, 1943.
10. Birch, J. W., and E. R. Stuckless. "The relationship between early manual communication and later achievement of the deaf." *Cooperative Research Project 1769*. Washington, D.C.: U. S. Office of Education, 1964.
11. Bishop, E. H. "Etiology and the management of prematurity." *Modern Medicine* (April, 1964), 123.
12. Bishop, Helen M. "The testing of deaf and hard-of-hearing children in St. Paul schools with the Arthur Performance Scale." *National Education Association Proceedings*, **74**: 393–94, 1936.
13. Blair, F. I. "A study of the visual memory of deaf and hearing child." *American Annals of the Deaf*, **102**: 254–63, 1957.

14. Blakely, R. W. "Erythroblastosis and perceptive hearing loss: Response of athetoids to tests of cochlear function." *Journal of Speech and Hearing Research*, **2**: 5–15, 1959.
15. Blanton, R. L., and J. C. Nunnally. "Semantic habits and cognitive style processes in the deaf." *Journal of Abnormal and Social Psychology*, **68**: 397–402, 1964.
16. Boatner, E. B. "The need of a realistic approach to the education of the deaf." A paper given to the joint convention of the California Association of Parents of Deaf and Hard-of-Hearing Children, California Association of Teachers of the Deaf and Hard-of-Hearing, and California Association of the Deaf. November 6, 1965.
17. Boatner, E. B., E. R. Stuckless, and D. F. Moores. *Occupational Status of the Young Adult Deaf of New England and the Demand for a Regional Technical-Vocational Training Center*. West Hartford, Conn.: American School for the Deaf, 1964.
18. Bordley, J. E., W. G. Hardy, and Miriam P. Hardy. "Pediatric audiology." Pediatric clinics of North America, 1962, **9**: No. 4 1147–58.
19. Boszormony-Nagy, I., and J. L. Framo, eds. *Intensive Family Therapy*. New York: Harper & Row, Publishers, 1965.
20. Brain, R. *Clinical Neurology*. New York: Oxford University Press, 1960.
21. Brill, R. G. "Problems of communication for the deaf." Paper presented at the West Coast Regional Institute on Personal, Social, and Vocational Adjustment to Deafness. Berkeley, Calif., February 3, 1959.
22. Brill, R. G. "A study in adjustment of three groups of deaf children." *Exceptional Children*, **26**: 42–48, 1960.
23. Brill, R. G. "Hereditary aspects of deafness." *Volta Review*, **63**: 168–75, 1961.
24. Brill, R. G. "The relationship of Wechsler IQ's to academic achievement among deaf students." *Exceptional Children*, **28**: 315–21, 1962.
25. Brill, T. "Mental hygiene and the deaf." *American Annals of the Deaf*, **79**: 279–85, 1934.
26. Brown, A., S. Stein, and R. Rohrer. *Chicago Non-Verbal examination*. New York: Psychological Corp., 1947.
27. Buck, J. "The H. T. P. technique, a qualitative and quantitative scoring manual." *Journal of Clinical Psychology*, **4**, 1948, **5**, 1949.
28. Burchard, E. M., and H. R. Myklebust. "A comparison of congenital and adventitious deafness with respect to its effect on intelligence, personality, and social maturity," (Part I, Intelligence). *American Annals of the Deaf*, **87**: 241–50, 1942.
29. Byers, R. K., R. S. Paine, and B. Crothers. "Extra pyramidal cerebral palsy with hearing loss following erythroblastosis." *Pediatrics*, **15**: 248–54, 1955.
30. Campbell, M. "Place of maternal rubella in the aetiology of congenital heart disease." *British Medical Journal*, **1**: 691–96, 1961.
31. Cholden, L. S. *A Psychiatrist Works with Blindness*. New York: American Foundation for the Blind, 1958.
32. Craig, W. N. "Effects of preschool training on the development of reading and lipreading skills of deaf children." *American Annals of the Deaf*, **109**: 280–96, 1964.

33. Craig, W. N., and N. H. Silver. "Examination of selective employment problems of the deaf." *American Annals of the Deaf,* **111**: 488–98, 1966.
34. Crammate, A. B. "The adult deaf in the professions." *American Annals of the Deaf,* **107**: 474–78, 1962.
35. Danish, J. M., J. K. Tillison, and M. Lexitan. "Multiple anomalies in congenitally deaf children." *Eugenics Quarterly,* **10**: 12–14, 1963.
36. DeGraff, A. C., and W. P. Creger, eds. *Annual Review of Medicine.* Palo Alto: George Banta Co., 1963. P. 255.
37. DiCarlo, L. M. *The Deaf.* Englewood Cliffs, N. J.: Prentice-Hall, Inc., 1964.
38. DiCarlo, L. M. "Much ado about the obvious." *Volta Review,* **68**: 269–73, 1966.
39. Doctor, P. V. "On teaching the abstract to the deaf." *Volta Review,* **52**: 547–50, 1950.
40. DuToit, J. M. "Measuring the IQ of deaf child." *American Annals of the Deaf,* **99**: 237–51, 1954.
41. Eames, T. H. "The relationship of birthweight, speed of object, and word perception and visual acuity." *Journal of Pediatrics,* **47**: 603–6, 1955.
42. Ewing, A. W. G., ed. *Educational Guidance and the Deaf Child.* Manchester, England: Manchester University Press, 1957.
43. Farber, D. J. "Some observations with emotionally disturbed deaf and hearing patients." Paper delivered to the Counseling Center, Gollandet College, Washington, D.C., November 2, 1961.
44. Fisch, L. *Research in Deafness in Children.* London: Blockwell Scientific Publ., 1964.
45. Flower, R. M., R. Viehweg, and W. R. Ruzicka. "The communicative disorders of children with kernicteric athetosis. Part I. Auditory disorders." *Journal of Speech and Hearing Disorders,* **31**: 41–59, 1966.
46. Ford, F. R. *Diseases of the Nervous System in Infancy, Childhood, and Adolescence.* 4th ed. Springfield, Ill.: Charles C Thomas, Publisher, 1960.
47. Friedman, A. S., et al. *Psycho-therapy for the Whole Family.* New York: Springer Publishing Co., 1965.
48. Frisina, D. R. "A psychological study of the mentally retarded deaf child." Unpublished doctoral dissertation. Evanston: Northwestern University, 1955.
49. Furfey, P. H., and T. J. Harte. Interaction of deaf & hearing in Frederick County, Maryland. Washington, D.C.: Catholic University, 1964.
50. Furth, H. G. *Thinking without Language.* New York: The Free Press, 1966.
51. Glowatsky, E. "The verbal element in the intelligence scores of congenitally deaf and hard-of-hearing child." *American Annals of the Deaf,* **98**: 328–35, 1953.
52. Goetzinger, C. P., and C. L. Rousey. "A study of Wechsler Performance Scale (Form II) and the Knox Cube Test with deaf adolescents." *American Annals of the Deaf,* **102**: 388–98, 1957.
53. Goodenough, Florence. *Measurement of Intelligence by Drawings.* Chicago: World Book Co., 1926.
54. Goodhill, V. "Rh child: deaf or 'aphasic'? 1. Clinical pathological aspects of kernicteric nuclear 'deafness.'" *Journal of Speech and Hearing Disorders,* **21**: 407–10, 1956.

55. Graham, E. E., and Esther Shapiro. "Use of the performance scale of the W.I.S.C. with the deaf child." *Journal of Consulting Psychology*, **17**: 396–98, 1953.
56. Graham, Frances K., and Barbara S. Kendall. Memory-for-Designs Test: Revised General Manual, *Perceptual Motor Skills Monograph Supplement* 2-VII, 1960.
57. Grinker, R. R., Sr. "Symbolism and general systems theory." Paper given at the joint meeting of the American Academy for the Advancement of Science and the Academy of Psychoanalysis. December 29, 1967.
58. Grinker, R. R., Sr., P. C. Bucy, and A. L. Sahs. *Neurology*. 5th ed. Springfield, Ill.: Charles C Thomas, Publisher, 1960.
59. Hamburg, D. A. "Psychological adaptive processes in life threatening injuries." Paper presented to the Symposium on Stress, Walter Reed Medical Center, Washington, D.C. March 18, 1953.
60. Hardy, W. G., and Miriam D. Pauls. "Atypical children with communication disorders." *Journal of Children*, **6**: 13–16, 1959.
61. Hathaway, S., and J. McKinley. *Minnesota Multiphasic Personality Inventory Manual*. Rev. ed. New York: Psychological Corp., 1951.
62. Hefferman, Angela. "A psychiatric study of 50 children referred to hospital for suspected deafness." In Caplan, Gerald, ed., *Emotional Problems of Childhood*. New York: Basic Books, 1955. Pp. 269–92.
63. Heider, F., and Grace Heider. "The thinking of the young deaf child as shown in sorting experiments." *Volta Review*, **43**: 111–13, 146, 1941.
64. Heider, Grace. "The thinking of the deaf child." *Volta Review*, **42**: 774–76, 804–8, 1940. (Review from an article in French by R. Pellet.)
65. Hiskey, M. S. "Determining the mental competence levels of children with impaired hearing." *Volta Review*, **52**: 406–8, 430–32, 1950.
66. Hiskey, M. S. *Nebraska Test of Learning Aptitude for the Young Deaf Child*. Lincoln: University of Nebraska Press, 1955.
67. Hofsteater, H. T. "An experiment in preschool education." Bull. No. 3, V. 8, Washington, D.C.: Gallaudet College, 1959.
68. Jackson, A. D. M., and L. Fisch. "Deafness following maternal rubella." *Lancet*, **2**: 124–44, 1958.
69. Johnson, Elizabeth H. "The effect of academic level on scores from the Chicago non-verbal examination for primary pupils." *American Annals of the Deaf*, **92**: 227–33, 1947.
70. Justman, J., and S. Moskowitz. "A follow-up study of graduates of the School for the Deaf." Publ. No. 215. New York: Board of Education, 1963.
71. Kates, S. L., W. W. Kates, and J. Michael. "Cognitive processes in deaf and hearing children." *Psychological Monog.*, **76**: Whole No. 551, 1962.
72. Kelley, V. C., ed. *Practice of Pediatrics*. Hagerstown, Md.: W. F. Prior Co., 1964. IV, 36.
73. Kendler, H. H., and T. S. Kendler. "Vertical and horizontal processes in problem solving." *Psychology Review*, **69**: 1–16, 1962.
74. Kenny, Virginia. "A better way to teach deaf children." *Harper's Magazine* (March 1962), 61–65.
75. Kinsey, A. C., et al. *Sexual Behavior in the Human Male*. New York: W. B. Saunders Co., 1948.

76. Kirk, S. A., and June Perry. "A comparative study of the Ontario and Nebraska tests for the deaf." *American Annals of the Deaf*, **93**: 315–22, 1948.
77. Knobloch, H., R. Rider, P. Harper, and B. Pasamanick. "Neuropsychiatric sequelae of prematurity." *Journal of the American Medical Association*, **161**: 581–85, 1956.
78. Kodman, F., T. P. Powers, G. Weller, and P. Phillip. "An investigation of hearing loss in mentally retarded children and adults." *American Journal of Mental Def.*, **63**: 460–63, 1958.
79. Kohl, H. R. *Language and Educ. of the Deaf.* A publication of the Center for Urban Educ., 33 W. 42nd St., New York, 1966.
80. Kohs, S. *The Block Designs Test.* Chicago: Stoelting, 1923.
81. Kronenberg, H. H., and G. D. Blake. *Young Deaf Adults: An Occupational Survey.* Washington D.C.: Vocational Rehabilitation Administration, Department of Health, Education, and Welfare, 1965.
82. Lane, Helen S. "The use of standardized performance tests for preschool children with a language handicap." *Proceedings of the International Congress on the Education of the Deaf*, 526–32, 1933.
83. Lane, Helen S. "A performance test for deaf children of school age." *Volta Review*, **36**: 657–59, 1934.
84. Lane, Helen S. "Measurement of the mental ability of the deaf child." *National Educational Association Proceedings*, **75**: 442–43, 1937.
85. Lane, Helen S. "Measurement of the mental and educational ability of the deaf child." *Journal for Exceptional Children*, **4**: 169–73, 191, 1938.
86. Lane, Helen S., and J. L. Schneider. "A performance test for school-age deaf children." *American Annals of the Deaf*, **86**: 441, 1941.
87. Larr, A. L., and E. R. Cain. "Measurement of native learning abilities in deaf children." *Volta Review*, **61**: 160–62, 1959.
88. Lavos, G. "Interrelationship among three tests of nonlanguage intelligence administered to the deaf." *American Annals of the Deaf*, **99**: 303–13, 1954.
89. Leiter, R. *The Leiter International Performance Scale.* Chicago: Stoelting, 1948.
90. Levine, Edna. "Psycho-educational characteristics of children following maternal rubella." *American Journal of Diseases of Children*, **94**: 627–32, 1951.
91. Levine, Edna S. *The Psychology of Deafness.* New York: Columbia University Press, 1960. P. 221.
92. Lidz, T. *The Family and Human Adaptation.* New York: International Universities Press, 1963.
93. Lowell, E. L. *John Tracy Clinic Research Papers III, V, VI, and VII.* Los Angeles: John Tracy Clinic, 1957–58.
94. Lowell, E. L. "Research in speech-reading: Some relationships to language development and implications for the classroom teacher." *Report of the Proceedings of the 39th meeting of the Convention of American Instructors of the Deaf.* Los Angeles, California: John Tracy Clinic, 1959. Pp. 68–73.
95. Lowell, E. L. "Higher education for the deaf." In D. Cutter, ed., *Workshop for Baptists on Deafness and Rehabilitation.* Washington, D.C.: Vocational Rehabilitation Administration, Department of Health, Education, and Welfare, 1965. Pp. 28–36.

96. Lubcheno, Lula O., F. A. Horner, Reed, I. E. Hix, D. Metcalf, Ruth Cohig, Helen C. Elliot, and Margaret Bourg. "Sequelae of premature birth." *American Journal of Diseases of Children*, **106**: 101–115, 1963.
97. Lunde, A. S., and S. G. Bigman. "Occupational conditions among the deaf." Washington, D.C.: Gallaudet College Press, 1959.
98. Lyon, V. W. "Personality tests with the deaf." *American Annals of the Deaf*, **79**: 1–4, 1934.
99. Machover, Karen. "Personality projection in the drawing of the human figure." Springfield: Charles C Thomas, Publisher, 1949.
100. MacKane, K. *A Comparison of the Intelligence of Deaf and Hearing Children*. New York: Columbia University Press, 1933.
101. MacPherson, June, and Helen S. Lane. "A comparison of deaf and hearing children on the Hiskey Test and on performance scales." *American Annals of the Deaf*, **77**: 292–304, 1932.
102. Manson, M. M., W. P. D. Logan, and R. M. Roy. "Rubella and other virus infections during pregnancy." *Reports on Public Health and Medical Subjects No.* 101. London: Her Majesty's Stationery Office, 1960. P. 101.
103. Masters, W. H., and V. E. Johnson. *Human Sexual Response*. Boston: Little, Brown and Company, 1966.
104. Mathews, J. "Speech problems of the mentally retarded." In L. Travis, ed., *Handbook of Speech Pathology*. New York: Appleton-Century-Crofts, 1957. P. 540.
105. Matzker, V. J. "Schizophrenia and deafness." *Zeitschrift für Laryngologie, Rhinologie, Otologie ihre Grenzgebiete*, **39**: 1960.
106. McCarthy, Dorothy. "Language development in children." In L. Carmichael, ed., *Manual of Child psychology*. New York: John Wiley & Sons, Inc., 1946. Pp. 476–581.
107. McClure, W. J. "Current problems and trends in the education of the deaf." *Deaf Americans*. (January 1966), 8–14.
108. Meadows, Kay P. "The effect of early manual communication and family climate." Doctoral dissertation. Berkeley: University of California, 1967.
109. Meyer, M. F. "The use of the Lectometer in the testing of the hearing and the deaf." *American Annals of the Deaf*, **77**: 292–304, 1932.
110. Miller, J. R. "Pediatric disorders in communication, IV. Some genetic counseling problems in families with congenital hearing defects." *Volta Review*, **67**: 118–23, 165, 1965.
111. Mira, Mary P. "The use of the Arthur Adaptation of the Leiter International Performance Scale and Nebraska Test of Learning Aptitude with preschool deaf children." *American Annals of the Deaf*, **107**: 224–28, 1962.
112. Moores, D. F. "Some practical and theoretical considerations." *American Annals of the Deaf*. (In press.)
113. Myklebust, H. R. "Clinical psychology and children with impaired hearing." *Volta Review*, **50**: 55–60, 90, 1948.
114. Myklebust, H. R. *Auditory Disorders in Children: A Manual for Differential Diagnosis*. New York: Grune Stratton, 1954.
115. Myklebust, H. R. "Rh child: deaf or 'aphasic'? 5. Some psychological considerations of the Rh child." *Journal of Speech and Hearing Disorders*, **21**: 423–25, 1956.

116. Myklebust, H. R. *The Psychology of Deafness.* New York: Grune Stratton, 1960.
117. Myklebust, H. R. "Guidance and counseling for the deaf." *American Annals of the Deaf,* 370–415, 1962.
118. Nelson, W. E. *Textbook of Pediatrics.* Philadelphia: W. B. Saunders Co., 1959.
119. Nesbitt, R. E. L., Jr. "Perinatal casualties." *Child.,* **6**: 123–28, 1959.
120. Peterson, E. G. "Testing deaf children with Kohs block design." *American Annals of the Deaf,* **81**: 242–54, 1936.
121. Peterson, E. G., and J. M. Williams. "Intelligence of deaf children as measured by drawings." *American Annals of the Deaf,* **75**: 273–90, 1930.
122. Phillips, W. D. "Influence of preschool training on achievement in language arts, arithmetical concepts, and socialization of young deaf children." Unpublished doctoral dissertation. New York: Columbia Teachers College, 1963.
123. Pintner, R., and J. Lev. "A study of the intelligence of the hard-of-hearing school child." *Journal of Genetic Psychology,* **55**: 31–48, 1939.
124. Rainer, J. D., and K. Z. Altshuler. *Comprehensive Mental Health Services for the Deaf.* New York: Columbia University Press, (In press).
125. Rainer, J. D., K. Z. Altshuler, F. J. Kollman, and W. E. Deming, eds. *Family and Mental Health Problems in a Deaf Population.* New York: N. Y. Psychiatric Institute, 1963.
126. *Randall's Island Performance Series, The.* (Manual). Chicago: Stoelting, 1932.
127. Raven, J. *Progressive Matrices.* New York: Psychol. Corp., 1948.
128. Robinson, G. C. "Pediatrics and disorders in communication. I. Hearing loss in infants and young preschool children." *Volta Review,* **66**: 314–18, 1964.
129. Rorschach, H. *Psychodiagnostics.* Berne, Switzerland: Hans Huber, 1942.
130. Rosen, J. "Rh child: deaf or 'aphasic'? 4. Variations in auditory disorders of the Rh child." *Journal of Speech and Hearing Disorders,* **21**: 418–22, 1956.
131. Rosenstein, J. "Cognitive abilities in deaf children." *Journal of Speech and Hearing Research,* **3**: 108–19, 1960.
132. Rosenstein, J. "Perception, cognition, and language in deaf children." *Exceptional Children,* **27**: 276–84, 1961.
133. Rosenstein, J., and A. Lerman. *Vocational Status and Adjustment of Deaf Women.* New York: Lexington School for the Deaf, 1963.
134. Ross, Grace. "Testing intelligence and maturity of deaf children." *Exceptional Children,* **20**: 23–24, 42, 1953.
135. Sank, D., and F. J. Kallman. "The role of heredity in early total deafness." *Volta Review,* **65**: 461–70, 1963.
136. Schein, J. D., and S. Bushnag. "Higher education for the deaf in the U. S.: A retrospective investigation." *American Annals of the Deaf,* **107**: 416–20, 1962.
137. Scouten, E. L. "Helping your deaf child to master English through finger-spelling." *American Annals of the Deaf,* **105**: 227–28, 1960.
138. Scouten, E. L. "Special curriculum needs of the deaf: Secondary level." *American Annals of the Deaf,* **107**: 515–18, 1962.
139. Scouten, E. L. *A Revaluation of the Rochester Method.* Rochester, N. Y.: Rochester School for the Deaf, 1942. (Reprinted 1964.)

140. Scyster, Margaret. "Summary of a four years' experiment with preschool deaf children at the Illinois School for the Deaf." *American Annals of the Deaf*, **81**: 212–30, 1936.
141. Shambaugh, G. E. "Physical causes of deafness." *Archives of Otolaryngology*, **7**: 424, 1928.
142. Sharoff, R. L. "Enforced restriction of communication, its implications for the emotional and intellectual development of the deaf child." *American Journal of Psychiatry*, **116**: 443–46, 1959.
143. Shirley, Mary, and Florence Goodenough. "Intelligence of deaf children in Minnesota." *American Annals of the Deaf*, **77**: 238–47, 1932.
144. Sigurjonsson, J. "Rubella and congenital deafness." *American Journal of Medical Science*, **242**: 712–20, 1963.
145. Silverman, W. A. *Dunham's Premature Infants*. 3rd ed. Springfield, Ill.: Paul B. Hoeber, 1961.
146. Springer, N. N. "A comparative study of the intelligence of a group of deaf and hard-of-hearing children." *American Annals of the Deaf*, **83**: 138–52, 1938.
147. Stafford, Charlotte. "Fingerspelling in the oral classroom." *American Annals of the Deaf*, **110**: 483–85, 1965.
148. Stein, M. I. *The Thematic Apperception Test*. Cambridge: Addison-Wesley, 2nd edition. Revised 1955.
149. Stevenson, E. A. *A Study of the Educational Achievement of Deaf Children of Deaf Parents*. Berkeley: California School for the Deaf, 1964.
150. Stokoe, W. C. *Studies in Linguistics: Sign Language Structure: An Outline of the Visual Communication Systems of the American Deaf*. Buffalo: University of Buffalo Press, 1960.
151. Stokoe, W. C., D. C. Casterline, and C. G. Croneberg. *A Dictionary of American Sign Language on Linguistic Principles*. Washington, D.C.: Gallaudet College Press, 1965.
152. Streng, Alice, and S. A. Kirk. "The social competence of deaf and hard-of-hearing children in a public day school." *American Annals of the Deaf*, **82**: 244–54, 1938.
153. Stuckless, E. R., and J. W. Birch. "The influence of early manual communication on the linguistic development of deaf children." *American Annals of the Deaf*, **111**: 452–60, 499–504, 1966.
154. Swartz, M. N., and P. R. Dodge. "Bacterial meningitis: A review of selected aspects. II Special neurologic problems, postmeningitic complications, and clinicopathological correlations." *New England Journal of Medicine*, **272**: 954–62, 1965.
155. Tully, N. L. and M. Vernon. "The impact of automation on the deaf worker." *American Federalist*, **72**: 20–23, 1965.
156. Vernon, M. "Measurement of the intelligence and personality of the deaf by drawings." Unpublished master's thesis. Tallahassee: Florida State University, 1957.
157. Vernon, M. "The brain injured (neurologically impaired) child: A discussion of the significance of the problem, its symptoms, and causes in deaf children." *American Annals of the Deaf*, **106**: 239–50, 1961.
158. Vernon, M. "What is the future for the deaf in the world of work?" *Silent Worker*, **16**: 7–12, 1962.

159. Vernon, M. "Vocational needs in educational programs for deaf youth." *American Annals of the Deaf*, **111**: 444–51, 1966.
160. Vernon, M. *Multiply handicapped deaf children. Medical, Education, and Psychological Considerations.* Washington, D.C.: Council of Exceptional Children, 1969.
161. Vernon, M. "The relationship of language to the thinking process." *Archives of General Psychiatry*, **16**: 323–25, 1967 (a).
162. Vernon, M. "Psychological education, and physical characteristics associated with postrubella deaf children." *Volta Review*, **69**: 176–85, 1967 (b).
163. Vernon, M. "Tuberculous meningitis and deafness." *Journal of Speech and Hearing*, **32**: 176–81, 1967 (c).
164. Vernon, M. "Prematurity and deafness: The magnitude and nature of the problem among deaf children." *Exceptional Children*, **38**: 289–98, 1967 (d).
165. Vernon, M. "Meningitis and deafness." *Laryngoscope*, **77**: 1856–74, 1967 (e).
166. Vernon, M. "Current etiological factors in deafness." *American Annals of the Deaf*, **115**: 106–15, 1968.
167. Vernon, M., and D. A. Rothstein. "Deafness, the interdependent variable." A paper presented at the World Congress on Deafness. Warsaw, Poland, August, 1967.
168. Visotsky, H. M., D. A. Hamburg, Mary E. Goss, and B. Z. Lebovits. "Coping behavior under extreme stress." *Archives of General Psychiatry*, **5**: 423–48, 1961.
169. Watson, C. W. "The vocational rehabilitation slant in the case of the young deaf person who has reached terminal school status." *West Coast Regional Institute on Personal, Social, and Vocational Adjustment to Total Deafness* (U. S. Office of Vocational Rehabilitation). Berkeley, Calif.: California Department of Education, 1959. Pp. 80–88.
170. Wechsler, D. *Wechsler Intelligence Scale for Children.* New York: Psychol. Corp., 1955.
171. Wechsler, D. *Wechsler Adult Intelligence Scale.* New York: Psychol. Corp., 1955.
172. Williams, B. "Introduction to a symposium on 'Use of Manual Communication'," A paper given at the meeting of the American Speech and Hearing Society. Chicago, October 31, 1965.
173. Wrightstone, J. W., M. S. Aranow, and Sue Muskowitz. "Developing reading test norms for deaf children." *American Annals of the Deaf*, **108**: 311–16, 1963.
174. Youniss, J., and H. G. Furth. "The influence of transitivity on learning in hearing and deaf children." *Child Development*, 533–38, 1965.
175. Zeckel, A. "Research possibilities with the deaf." *American Annals of the Deaf*, **87**: 173–91, 1942.
176. Zeckel, A., and J. J. Kalb. "A comparative test of groups of children born deaf and of good hearing by means of the Porteous Maze Test." *American Annals of the Deaf*, **84**: 114–23, 1939.

5

Public School Hearing Conservation

Jerome G. Alpiner, Ph.D.

Incidence of Hearing Impairment in School Children

The importance of hearing conservation in the public schools has been stressed by many writers. These authors point to the necessity of locating students with hearing loss as early as possible so that appropriate remediation procedures may be conducted. The educational, vocational, and social development of those children with hearing impairment is vital to their present and future status. Data from previous studies make all persons concerned with children cognizant of the importance of public school hearing conservation programs.

Connor (2) in reviewing thirty-one separate studies reported that the number of school-age children with defective hearing ranged from about 2 to 21 per cent. He commented that despite decades of testing and research, it remains almost impossible to reach general agreement concerning the prevalence of children's hearing impairment in the United States. Various groups and individuals have reported on the incidence of hearing loss from 1926 to 1960. Discrepancies in the reports exist because of different calibration procedures and test environments, the multiplicity of hearing tests employed, the qualifications of the testers, and student motivation. The various investigators also have used different criteria to determine what constitutes the normal range of hearing. Samplings of studies cited by Connor (2) from 1926 to 1960 are reported in Table 5.1.

TABLE 5.1. SAMPLINGS OF HEARING LOSS STUDIES (FROM CONNOR, 1961)

Year	*Author*	*Summary of Study as Indicated in Report*	*Per cent with Hearing Loss*
1926	Fletcher and Fowler	Sampling of school children.	14%
1933	Fowler	774,576 New York City school children grades 3 through 9.	3.17%
1941	New York City Bd. of Education	New York City elementary and secondary school children.	1.3%
1945	American Hearing Society	Prevalence rate among school children.	5%
1949	Johnson	School children with hearing losses that are educationally significant.	3%
		Hearing losses that are medically significant.	5%
1952	Fouracre	General population.	6 to 10%
1955	Spekter	School children in elementary grades.	5%
1957	Sandis	1,931,139 school children in Pennsylvania public schools.	2.4%
1959	American Speech and Hearing Association	Results of number of studies of school-age children.	3%
1960	Magary and Eichorn	School-age children.	4 to 5%
1960	Silverman, Lane, and Doehring	Own best estimate from studies of mass tests of school children.	5%

Definition of a Public School Hearing Conservation Program

In its broadest sense, HEARING CONSERVATION includes activities ranging from the identification of a hearing deficit to follow-up rehabilitation procedures. When school children are considered, this includes identification audiometry in the public schools, threshold tests for those who fail the screening, audiologic assessment for those who fail the threshold tests, medical evaluation and treatment if indicated, hearing-aid evaluation depending on the severity and type of the hearing impairment, possible aural rehabilitation[1] procedures which may include speech-reading, auditory

[1] Rehabilitation is used synonymously with habilitation in this chapter.

training, speech (hearing) therapy, counseling, and periodic follow-up testing.

There is some confusion between the terms "hearing conservation" and "identification audiometry," terms which occasionally are used synonymously. Hearing conservation consists of provisions for medical, surgical, audiological, educational, and related services required to prevent and overcome an impairment in hearing. IDENTIFICATION AUDIOMETRY refers to only one aspect of a hearing conservation program. It may be defined as the original discovery of a hearing impairment which results in isolating an individual as one to be watched or examined further (5).

Responsibility for the Hearing Conservation Program

The new speech "therapist"[2] entering the public schools is often confused about his role in the hearing conservation program because the responsibility for the program in the schools is not always clearly defined. There is considerable variation among the states and among the various school systems within each state. One problem concerns the therapist's responsibility in the identification audiometry phase of the program. Some speech therapists do engage in screening, especially in smaller rural areas, although it is generally felt that the therapist should not be burdened with the responsibility of general screening; however, he will want to have audiometric information on all children receiving therapy. The therapist will want threshold air- and bone-conduction results on each of these children in planning therapy. If a recent audiogram done by an audiologist is not available, the therapist may, if qualified, wish to give these children an audiometric test, or refer them to a competent audiologist. This will not be necessary if they have passed a recent screening test. The Ohio Plan (20) indicates:

> The extent to which the speech and hearing therapist participates in the hearing testing program will necessarily be governed by local policies and conditions. The therapist routinely checks the hearing of all children enrolled in speech class. His chief responsibility is to do speech therapy and he should not be expected to do extensive hearing screening. He should be available upon request to retest children whose problems present difficulties. In districts having no adequate hearing testing program, the speech therapist may wish to take the leadership in helping to develop or improve a hearing conservation program. He may ask the superintendent or coordinator of special services to arrange a conference with appropriate health and education personnel.

A second problem concerns the therapist's responsibility for aural rehabilitation, which is related to his training in audiology. In some states,

[2] Title designation depends upon the individual state.

the therapist may be referred to as a speech and hearing therapist, a speech therapist, a speech pathologist, a speech and hearing clinician, a speech clinician, a speech correctionist, or some other title. Some states merely encourage speech therapists to provide therapy for hard-of-hearing children by working with them on the improvement or preservation of good speech. This can be a difficult task if, in addition, the therapist is not permitted to engage in speech-reading and auditory training, which are integral aspects of the total therapy process. The rationale for restricting the therapist's activities this way is that he may not have had sufficient academic training and practicum. Contributing to this problem are the difficulties of selecting those children who should be enrolled in special hard-of-hearing or deaf classrooms with special teachers. Where, for example, should children with a mild or mild-to-moderate hearing loss be placed? Many of these mildly impaired children can function in the regular classroom with assistance from speech therapy, speech-reading, and auditory training.

In Ohio (20), the regulation pertaining to speech and hearing therapists states that they may engage in auditory training if children have "a hearing loss of thirty to fifty decibels[3] in the better ear in the speech range or a prognosis of progressive loss, regardless of benefit derived from a hearing aid." Those children whose losses are greater are candidates for special education classrooms. Although it is important to consider other audiologic measures such as discrimination ability and tolerance problems, the above criteria at least provide some guidelines while considering the dichotomy of responsibility between the professions of speech pathology-audiology, and deaf education.

The determination of responsibility for the speech and hearing therapist in aural rehabilitation therapy is a problem that needs to be discussed and resolved by university training programs in conjunction with state departments of education and health, using the guidelines established by the American Speech and Hearing Association (ASHA). Prospective public school speech therapists should determine their responsibilities in terms of these ASHA requirements.

Laws, regulations, and interpretations have played a major role in the development of public school hearing conservation programs. Harrington (11) reported that in 1943, twenty states had laws for testing hearing or for the examination of the ear. Harrington (12) later reported that there were forty-four states that had explicit laws on the status of hearing testing programs. In forty states having hearing conservation programs, the hearing testing programs were administered through maternal and child health or crippled children's services. A few programs were serviced through departments of public instruction, and at some local levels the responsibility

[3] In an attempt to conform to present standards, all dB references in this chapter are either ISO, or converted to ISO on the basis of a flat 10-dB increase. See Chapter 6 for a complete definition of ISO.

was assumed by individual school districts.

An attempt was made by Zink and Alpiner (37) to discover any major trends in hearing conservation programs. Of twenty-eight responses received from questionnaires sent to all fifty states, twenty-four states reported having hearing conservation programs. Twenty of these states also indicated hearing-aid selection provisions in their states. When the information was reviewed in relation to the usually reported aspects of identification, diagnoses, medical and surgical treatment, and rehabilitation, considerable differences in procedures were noted. For example, one state reported that identification was conducted as a local school function with diagnosis and treatment provided by the state health department. Another reported an extensive medical program. Differences were reported in the screening levels for identification, the types of tests employed in identification, the frequencies used, the personnel involved in the screening procedure, the grades screened, and the personnel involved in follow-up audiometric studies.

In order to assign responsibility for hearing conservation programs in the public schools, it is the author's recommendation that both state departments of education and state departments of health be involved. The state department of education should require the screening of all school children on a periodic basis with education and aural rehabilitation follow-up mandatory. The state department of health's role should be to ensure that identification audiometry, subsequent threshold testing, and medical follow-up are provided for those who fail the screening tests. At the state level, there should be joint coordination between the two departments. Larger school districts can hire certified supervising audiologists to implement the hearing conservation program. The supervising audiologist can then be responsible not only for the identification phase of the program but also for the educational and remediation follow-up. The state department of health should employ supervising audiologists who will cover the smaller urban and rural areas of the state to conduct identification audiometry. This department should also make provision for otologic-audiologic clinics to be held in both the large metropolitan areas and the smaller geographical areas of the state for those children who fail in the identification phase of the program. School nurses would then be responsible for recommendations made by the physicians, and the supervising audiologists would be responsible for educational and aural rehabilitation. The school nurses would also be responsible for including hearing records in the children's health report. Many school systems are now covered adequately for hearing conservation, but if all children are to be served, an attempt toward uniformity must be made. The state should see that all local school districts are served both efficiently and adequately. Those persons conducting aural rehabilitation will be discussed later in the chapter. A schematic of this suggested organizational structure is presented in Figure 5.1.

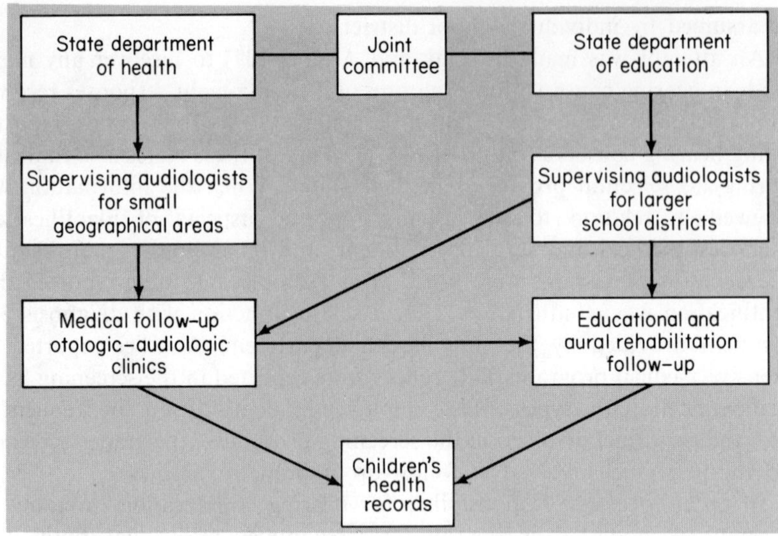

FIGURE 5.1 Recommended responsibility for hearing conservation programs.

Planning Aspects for the Hearing Conservation Program

This first phase of the program should be organization. The audiologist in charge of supervising the screening should make the necessary arrangements with the administrative officer of the school district. The audiologist then will know who to contact in each of the schools in the district. This probably will be the school nurse who is responsible for several schools. She then may establish testing schedules in conjunction with school principals. Testing times and dates are determined, and teachers can be informed about the screening program so that they may schedule their class activities accordingly.

A systematic set of program planning procedures followed in Scott County, Iowa (33), is presented below. The planning procedures for this program are assumed by the audiologist and the nurse. Their responsibilities are as follows:

THE AUDIOLOGIST

1. Establishes awareness of need for the program.
2. Assumes responsibility for and provides leadership in the organization of the program.
3. Interprets purpose to school personnel, P.T.A.'s, and other groups.
4. Plans program requirements.

5. Helps to interpret purpose to related medical professions and health agencies.

6. Prepares necessary forms and instructions.

7. Conducts conference with principals regarding testing environment, facilities required, children to be screened, assistants required, forms and notices needed, testing dates, and explanation of the program and procedures.

8. Advises nurse of plans, if she is unable to attend conferences.

THE SCHOOL NURSE

1. Helps establish awareness of need for the program.

2. Offers mutual cooperation in the organization, execution, and follow-up of the program.

3. Helps interpret purpose to school personnel, P.T.A.'s, and other groups.

4. Estimates her work-load based on previous year's experience.

5. Interprets purpose to related professions and health agencies in the community.

6. Attends principals' conferences.

7. Shares health record information.

8. Evaluates findings to develop the nursing service to meet the health needs of the area.

9. May be asked by the administrator to prepare the class list of children to receive hearing evaluations and an individual hearing record history in accordance with instructions.

10. May be asked by administrator to assist the program by helping maintain a quiet atmosphere, insuring test room and facilities are as they should be, advising the faculty of their responsibilities on the days of testing, recording information for the audiologist, and verifying information contained on forms used in the program.

Although planning procedures, of course, will vary from one program to another, the Scott County pattern described above provides the reader with some idea of the arrangements necessary in setting up a program prior to actual identification audiometry procedures.

TEST PERSONNEL

The question of who should do the initial screening has never been answered definitively. Speech therapists generally do not have time to screen the school children because of their case-loads. Often school nurses, volunteers from women's organizations, mothers, and other interested persons conduct the screening in many school systems. Some of these persons, since they have not received adequate training, are not qualified to administer the tests. In a university community, students in a speech pathology and audiology training program may do the screening under the supervision of the speech and hearing clinic audiologist. Aides are now being considered for assisting in numerous aspects of education and health, and it is possible that, in the future, they will be trained to conduct the screening in a hearing conservation program.

Personnel engaged in screening are referred to as AUDIOMETRISTS or technicians, and they should work under the supervision of an audiologist with ASHA certification in audiology. For maximum effectiveness in the identification phase of the hearing conservation program, these audiometrists should be trained by an audiologist. This training should consist of a short course in which basic information regarding the hearing mechanism and hearing is given. Hopefully, this background information will make the trainees aware of the importance of their role in the hearing conservation program. Audiometrists in training should then be exposed to the instruments used in the screening process and be instructed in the actual screening procedures. Practicum, under the supervision of an audiologist, is necessary. The audiologist conducting the short course may be from either the state health department, the state education department, a university, a community service agency, or a hospital. The training program should produce audiometrists who are capable of doing both hearing screening and individual pure-tone threshold tests. A tentative short course might consist of the following subjects:

1. Background and incidence of hearing impairment.
2. Anatomy and physiology of the ear.
3. Instruments used in screening and threshold tests.
4. Group screening tests.
5. Individual screening tests.
6. Pure-tone threshold tests.
7. Special problems encountered in screening programs.
8. Practicum in administration of tests.

THE TEST ENVIRONMENT

It has been stated classically that the rooms assigned for hearing testing in the public schools have been located next to power plants, gymnasiums, playgrounds, and cafeterias. This, unfortunately, has been the case far too often, and it is a serious problem that must be corrected. A good test environment with low ambient noise levels is a necessity and will do much to eliminate false-failures. From a practical point of view, few school systems can afford funds for sound-treated test rooms. Some state health departments use mobile testing units that are quite satisfactory as a test environment. If ambient noise levels exceed test levels, then the screening program will be unsuccessful and frustrating to all concerned. The audiology supervisor and screening technician will have to judge the test environment themselves. If ambient noise levels are a problem, then noise measurements should be made in the testing rooms.

GRADES TO BE SCREENED

The Committee on Identification Audiometry (5) has stated that in newly established programs, it would be desirable to test all children during the first year. After the initial year, considerable attention should be given to those children in the early school years by implementing annual testing in kindergarten and grades one, two, and three. Less frequent testing may be planned in subsequent years, but no child should experience more than a three-year interval between tests from grades four through twelve. Some screening programs test every other grade each year; for example, grades one, three, five, and seven. There has been a tendency to screen high school students on a referral basis only, but it would be wise to screen high school students routinely every other year since there is always the possibility that otosclerosis may begin to appear in this older group. There exists, also, the possibility of noise-induced hearing loss because some students may be exposed to high-intensity stimuli from overamplified music.

The California State Department of Education (1) makes the following recommendations for selection, in addition to routine screening procedures, in an identification testing program:

1. All pupils who are new to the individual school or to the school district.
2. Pupils discovered by previous tests to have a hearing impairment.
3. Children with delayed or defective speech.
4. Pupils returning to school after a serious illness.
5. Pupils enrolled in adjustment or remedial class programs.
6. Pupils who appear to be retarded.
7. Pupils having emotional or behavior problems.
8. Pupils referred by the classroom teacher for hearing testing for any reason.

Identification Tests

Both individual and group tests are used to identify hearing impairment. The basic philosophy for using a group test is economy of time, that is, more children may be tested in the same time period than with an individual test. Regardless of the type of test used, the major objective is to identify, as completely as possible, all of the children who have potential hearing losses. Realistically, there will undoubtedly be some children who may not be identified and other children who will fail the screening test who have no hearing problem. It is obvious that those responsible for identification should be as accurate as possible. Although no figures are available concerning the number using group screening tests as compared to individual screening, it would appear that many states conduct individual hearing tests. Both types of tests will be discussed in some detail so that the reader may gain insight into the value, advantages, and limitations of each type.

Group Hearing Tests

THE FADING-NUMBERS TEST

One of the earliest group tests employed was the FADING-NUMBERS TEST using a Western Electric 4C phonograph speech audiometer (4). With this test, a maximum of forty children can be screened at the same time. The Fading-Numbers Test uses a record with a woman's voice repeating paired one-digit numbers decreasing in intensity in 3-dB steps from 33 to 0 dB. The examiner explains to the children that the earphone is to be placed first on the right ear and then on the left ear. They are informed that a woman will say two numbers at a time such as "four-two." When the numbers are heard, the children are to write both numbers in the first square on the scoring form with subsequent paired digits written directly in the box under the first one. The children are also told that the woman's voice will become softer as the test proceeds, and that the object of the test is to see how many numbers they can hear. When the numbers can no longer be heard, the children are to wait until they hear the woman's voice on the record tell them that the numbers should now be written in the second column. This procedure continues until all columns have been completed. Modified instructions are given for grades three and four, and for grades one and two. A sample scoring form is illustrated in Figure 5.2. A reported modification of this test is one using fading words with the R. S. Maico audiometric test (31), which employs pictures rather than numbers. The children are presented one word at a time and mark on the scoring form the picture which represents the word they think they hear.

The Fading-Numbers Test requires that the children pass the test at a level of 19 dB in at least one of the four columns in order to be considered as having normal hearing for that ear. Children with essentially normal hearing in the lower frequencies can pass this test by guessing, even though a hearing loss may be present in the higher frequencies. Newby (28) indicated that children with losses as high as 40 to 60 dB at 1,000 and 2,000 Hz have been able to pass the Fading-Numbers Test at the 19-dB level. He also stated that a child who passed the Fading-Numbers Test may not be able to function adequately in conversational situations.

Date:__________ Boy____ Girl________

Name:________________________

Age:____ Birthday:________ Grade:____

Name of School:________________

County:______________________

1. Do you have a cold now?__________
   Do you have many colds?__________
2. Have you ever had an earache?_______
   Once:____ Seldom:____ Frequently:____
3. Have you ever had a running ear?_____
   Once:____ Seldom:____ Frequently:____
4. Have you ever received treatment from a doctor for your ears?__________
5. Have you had your tonsils and adenoids removed?__________
6. Is any member of your family hard of hearing?__________
7. Do you have any difficulty hearing what others say to you?__________

DO NOT MAKE ANY NOISE DURING THIS TEST

	Right Ear				Left Ear			
	1	2	3	4	5	6	7	8
33								
30								
27								
24								
21								
18								
15								
12								
9								
6								
3								
0								

Hearing Loss:______ Hearing Loss:______

Results of this test indicated this child's hearing is:

1. Normal______ 2. Needs Threshold Test_____

FIGURE 5.2 Sample test form used for the Fading-Numbers Test.

Source: Dahl, L. A. *Public School Audiometry: Principles and Methods*. Danville, Ill.: The Interstate Press, 1949.

THE MASSACHUSETTS HEARING TEST

Johnston (15) developed a group pure-tone test which correlated more highly with individual discrete frequency tests recommended by the American Academy of Ophthalmology and Otolaryngology than did the group phonograph speech test. Forty persons may be tested simultaneously with this technique. The MASSACHUSETTS HEARING TEST was designed to simplify scoring procedures in group tests. In addition, the test permits the examiner, because of the reliability and validity of responses, to decide whether or not a medical referral is necessary. Economy of time is an important aspect because in this procedure, threshold testing of all children is not required. Those children who fail the screening are, of course, given an individual pure-tone threshold test.

Figure 5.3 shows a Massachusetts Hearing Test form. After the earphones are placed on the right ears of the children, the examiner calls out a series of numbers ranging from one to six. The children are informed that after each number is called, they may hear a faint tone or they may hear no tone. If the tone is heard, the "yes" opposite the proper number is to be underlined, and if nothing is heard, the children are instructed to underline "no." Practice testing is done at 500 Hz with the children giving verbal responses. The examiner demonstrates the scoring procedures on the blackboard. In testing, the examiner sets up a rhythm like: "One—(3-second interval)—Mark." Intervals are held approximately constant whether or not a tone is presented.

Originally, the children were tested at 500, 1,000, 4,000, and 11,000 Hz, at levels of 30, 35, 35, and 40 dB, respectively. Six tones were presented at each frequency for each ear. Presently, 500, 4,000, and 6,000 Hz are used in the screening process. After the right ear has been screened, the children place the earphones on their left ears, and the procedure is repeated.

A failure is noted if children whose total number of "no" responses differs from the correct number by more than two. These children then are given a second screening test with a different earphone, and those who fail this test are given an individual pure-tone threshold test before a medical referral is made. Using the Massachusetts Test, forty children can be tested and all papers graded in approximately seventeen minutes according to Johnston (15).

A total of 1,496 elementary school children were tested by Johnson and Newby (14) with the Western Electric 4CA group phonograph speech audiometer (Fading-Numbers Test) and by the Massachusetts group pure-tone test method. Children were also given an individual pure-tone sweep-frequency test, and those who failed to hear any frequency at 25 dB were given individual threshold tests. Children whose losses in either ear were 30 dB at two frequencies or 40 dB at one frequency were considered to have medically significant hearing losses. The performance on the individual

MASSACHUSETTS HEARING TEST

Name__________ Grade______ School__________

Example:

1. yes no
2. yes no
3. yes no
4. yes no
5. yes no
6. yes no

I Right Ear				II Left Ear			
A.	1.	yes	no	A.	1.	yes	no
	2.	yes	no		2.	yes	no
	3.	yes	no		3.	yes	no
	4.	yes	no		4.	yes	no
	5.	yes	no		5.	yes	no
	6.	yes	no		6.	yes	no
B.	1.	yes	no	B.	1.	yes	no
	2.	yes	no		2.	yes	no
	3.	yes	no		3.	yes	no
	4.	yes	no		4.	yes	no
	5.	yes	no		5.	yes	no
	6.	yes	no		6.	yes	no
C.	1.	yes	no	C.	1.	yes	no
	2.	yes	no		2.	yes	no
	3.	yes	no		3.	yes	no
	4.	yes	no		4.	yes	no
	5.	yes	no		5.	yes	no
	6.	yes	no		6.	yes	no
D.	1.	yes	no	D.	1.	yes	no
	2.	yes	no		2.	yes	no
	3.	yes	no		3.	yes	no
	4.	yes	no		4.	yes	no
	5.	yes	no		5.	yes	no
	6.	yes	no		6.	yes	no
Total				Total			

FIGURE 5.3 The (original) Massachusetts Group Test scoring form.
Source: Johnston, P. W. "An efficient group screening test." *Journal of Speech and Hearing Disorders*, **20**: 697–703, 1948.

test was the criterion against which the efficiency of the group test was judged. The Western Electric test was found to be less efficient than the Massachusetts Test. The Fading-Numbers Test failed to identify four out of five children with impaired hearing, while the Massachusetts Test failed to discover only one out of five children in the upper grades, and three out of ten in the lower grades. Johnson and Newby (14) indicated that it would be possible to increase the efficiency of the Massachusetts Test by decreasing the intensity of the screening levels employed in the study.

DiCarlo and Gardner (6) recommended a modification of the Massachusetts Test primarily designed for university students, using 500, 1,000, 2,000, and 8,000 Hz. Another modification included five options for each frequency rather than six. Individuals failing at any one frequency were considered to have failed the test. The criterion for failing was 25 dB at two frequencies or 30 dB at one frequency. The authors concluded, as a result of this study, that the Massachusetts Pure-Tone Group Test as modified provided a very efficient testing tool for hearing testing of university populations.

PULSE-TONE GROUP TEST

In the PULSE-TONE GROUP TEST, as many as forty children may be tested at one time using 250, 1,000, 2,000, and 4,000 Hz (32). The frequencies now used for this test are 500, 1,000, 2,000, 4,000, and 6,000 Hz; this is in keeping with the present trend in identification audiometry. The group pure-tone test is calibrated by obtaining a series of threshold measurements with the group audiometer, using sixteen subjects with normal hearing. This is necessary since the output of the audiometer is divided among forty earphones. For example, the normal threshold for 1,000 Hz is 55 dB. Similar adjustments are made for the other frequencies used in the testing procedure. The pure tones are presented, in descending order, at levels of 50, 40, 30, 25, 20, and 15 dB above the normal threshold. The scoring form is illustrated in Figure 5.4.

A light alerts the students to listen for the tones. They are instructed to record in the squares of the columns the number of times the tone is heard each time the light comes on. The tone is presented in one, two, three, or four pulses. The students start recording in the first square of the first column and work down through the entire column. They then move on to the other columns until all columns are completed. The lowest intensity level correctly marked in either of the columns is considered the threshold for that frequency. Failing scores indicate the need for individual testing so that appropriate referral, if necessary, may be made for the children. Newby (28) stated that a loss of 30 dB at any of the test frequencies in either ear is considered to be a test failure. According to Newby, a failure requires an individual test and perhaps a medical referral. The tester may also substitute a screening level of 25 dB for each of the frequencies to be tested, rather than attempt to obtain threshold measurements with this technique. In using this test, the examiner must remember to make the appropriate intensity adjustments as well as to plan the number of pulse-tone presentations at each frequency. Since written responses are required for this test, it is not appropriate for most children below the third-grade level.

Name________________ Age____ Sex____ Earphone No.________

Address________________ Telephone No.________

Tester________________ Date________

Right Ear

Frequencies: ____ ____ ____ ____ ____

1	2	3	4	5	6	7	8	9	10

Left Ear

Frequencies: ____ ____ ____ ____ ____

11	12	13	14	15	16	17	18	19	20

FIGURE 5.4 Scoring form for Pulse-Tone Group Test.

Source: Newby, H. A. "Evaluating the efficiency of group screening tests of hearing." *Journal of Speech and Hearing Disorders*, **13**: 236–40, 1948.

JOHNSTON GROUP SCREENING TEST

Johnston (16) described a group screening test for pure tones in which ten children may be screened at one time. In this test, children as young as grade one can be screened efficiently. A semicircular seating arrangement is used with all ten children facing the examiner. The children are informed that their hearing is going to be tested and when a tone is heard, they are to hold up their hand and lower it when the tone is no longer heard. The children are instructed not to pay attention to what the other children do, since there will be times when the tones are presented to some children and not to others. The earphones are connected to the audiometer by means of a jack arrangement and when screening has been completed in one ear, the child simply places the earphone on the other ear. Once or twice during the testing of the children, the examiner pushes a button that will remove the tone from two of the earphones.

The performance of this group test was initially evaluated in screening 373 elementary school children. Thirty-seven children failed the group test. Of these thirty-seven failures, twenty-seven children subsequently were shown, by means of individual pure-tone threshold tests, to have referrable hearing losses. The new failure rate for the sample group was 7.2 per cent. This was within 1/2 of 1 per cent of the net failure rate found with Massachusetts school children when individual screening tests were used. A minimum of 300 elementary school children can be group-tested in one school day by each examiner with this procedure. According to Johnston, the advantages of this test are:

1. No paper or pencils are used by the children.
2. The tester employs basically the same simple procedure used in individual sweep-check screening tests.
3. The method is much less fatiguing and faster than individual testing.
4. Total equipment consists of an audiometer and a single tray of ten earphones.
5. Accuracy of the test is of the same order as that of individual screening tests.
6. Magnetic receivers and relative simplicity of conversion requirements results in minimum expense.
7. The conversion of an audiometer for the test does not affect the usefulness of the audiometer in individual testing. Neither does it impair the usefulness of the audiometer in giving the group Massachusetts Hearing Test.
8. Testing may be done in nurses', teachers', or other available rooms instead of in a regular classroom.
9. First-grade children may be tested by this method.

The children were originally screened at a level of 25 dB from 125 Hz through 6,000 Hz. The frequencies of 125 and 250 Hz are no longer used in the test. Since the economical magnetic earphones are used in the screening process, it should be emphasized that these earphones should not be used in threshold testing because sound pressure levels in excess of 30-dB HL are not linear. These earphones should be restricted to screening and the more conventional earphones should be used for regular pure-tone threshold testing.

NIELSEN GROUP TEST OF SCHOOL CHILDREN

Nielsen (29) described a group test in which he felt it was important for the children to participate actively. The test consisted of a task in which the children were occupied by writing a series of symbols. The NIELSEN TEST was based on the assumption that it would be easier for the ear to detect an interrupted weak tone than a continuously decreasing tone, since the latter was more fatiguing and the potential for ascertaining threshold was less reliable. Nielsen felt that a pattern of tones enabled the child to identify what he had heard by checking his responses.

A specially constructed audiometer is used in the Nielsen test so that certain patterns of tones can be generated. The pupils record what they hear on printed forms by writing symbols corresponding to the tone pattern. Five pure tones, 250 to 4,000 Hz, are tested in groups of four signals each at 55, 45, 35, 25, 15, and 10 dB. A total of 100 signals is delivered to each ear with nineteen children tested at one time. The total test time required for each group is from fifteen to twenty minutes. This procedure lends itself to a group threshold test rather than a group screening test.

The instructions presented to the children help to clarify the procedures. The examiner tells the children they are to write on the form placed before them on the table. Each time a brief tone is heard, a dot is to be marked in the middle of one of the squares, and each time a long tone is heard, a dash is to be made from one edge of the square to the other. The children are instructed to start on the first line marked "I" on the form and fill in one square after the other from left to right with the tones heard. They are also told that as they approach the end of the line, the tones will get weaker and eventually, if they hear no tones, they are to write nothing in the square. The children mark only the tones that they hear and they must not guess. The examiner demonstrates the dot and dash system on the blackboard as the instructions are given. Binaural earphones are then placed on the pupils and a practice series of dots and dashes is given until they understand what they are supposed to do.

This test would appear to be impractical from several view points. First, a specially constructed audiometer is necessary and most school systems are not likely to use funds for special purchases of this nature. Second, the procedure is time-consuming because it attempts to give threshold tests to all the children. Third, other individual screening or group tests appear to be more practical and just as accurate.

Individual Identification Testing

Many hearing conservation programs employ individual screening procedures. The use of the individual screening procedure continues probably because of the confusion and controversy over which type of screening test is most efficient. The assumption is made that, although additional time is required to screen large numbers of children, the individual test is more effective in identifying those with hearing impairment.

Until uniform standards for identification audiometry are established in the United States, a variety of testing procedures will continue to exist. Even in individual testing, differences in philosophy are prevalent regarding the traditional methods as compared to limited-frequency screening. The traditional individual testing procedure is described in this section as well as the research that contrasts this approach to limited-frequency techniques.

Individual screening is usually conducted at 25 dB at 500, 1,000, 2,000, and 6,000 Hz with a 30-dB level at 4,000 Hz. This is a modification of previous screening procedures where 250 and 8,000 Hz were used in identification audiometry. It is felt that 250 Hz, in addition to being difficult to test in the usual school setting, is of little significance in providing pertinent information for identification. Due to the difficulty of maintaining calibration at 8,000 Hz, this frequency is generally not included in the screening process and 6,000 Hz is substituted. A 20-dB screening level is not realistic unless the testing is done in sound-treated suites and, although desirable, school systems are not likely to provide them.

A routine procedure is to have an entire class come to the designated testing room. In the regular classroom, brief forms are completed indicating the children's names, grades, and teachers. There is a place on the form for the examiner to check either "pass" or "fail." The children are asked to keep silent during the testing, and a volunteer proctor insures that the children do remain silent during the screening process. The entire class is given instructions so that they are aware of what is expected of them. The examiner explains that they are going to hear very soft tones and that each time the tone is heard, they are to raise a hand and then lower it immediately when the tone disappears. The examiner then gives an example by setting the audiometer frequency at 1,000 Hz and presenting it to the class at 100 dB. When it appears that the children understand the instructions, the screening begins at 1,000 Hz and continues to 6,000 Hz with 500 Hz concluding the screening in each ear. If more than one examiner is available, different areas of the room may be used, so that several stations may be in operation in the same screening room. The children who fail the first screening test are rescreened. Those children failing the second screening are given pure-tone air-conduction threshold tests after all children in a given group are screened; the other children return to their classroom. At the conclusion of each day's testing, the recording forms or threshold audiograms are given to the school nurse so that the information can be made part of the children's health records. A separate list is made of those children who fail the threshold tests so that appropriate action may be initiated for them. Considerable time is saved by having all of the children come to the testing room at the same time and by having the identifying information on their report forms completed in their classrooms. Approximately twenty to twenty-five children can be tested each hour by one examiner using the above procedures. The criterion for failure is 25 dB at any one of the frequencies to 500, 1,000, 2,000, and 6,000 Hz; and 30 dB for 4,000 Hz. The same failure criterion holds for the pure-tone threshold test. If a sound-treated room is used, the level for failure may be reduced 10 dB at each of the frequencies.

Identification Audiometry Follow-up

After children have failed both the first and second screening tests and subsequent pure-tone air-conduction threshold tests, the records should be given to the school nurse in order to determine a plan of action. Depending upon the policy of the school district, several things may occur. In some instances the children may be seen at an otologic-audiologic clinic sponsored by the state department of health. The children will receive preotologic audiometric examinations by an audiologist at the clinic. The children then may be given otologic examinations by the otologist to determine if medical or surgical treatment is indicated. If treatment is recommended, the school nurse tells the parents so that appropriate action may be taken by a physician of the family's choice. Occasionally at the state health department clinic discovers the problem to be minor, such as excessive cerumen. Following removal of the cerumen, a postotologic audiometric evaluation at the clinic may reveal hearing to be within acceptable normal limits. Under the circumstances, no further disposition is recommended.

It is imperative, where medical or surgical treatment is needed, that the parents be told. It is not unusual to find some parents who ignore the recommendations. Since the children's educational and health welfare may be at stake, further procedures will have to be instituted. Another member of the hearing conservation team, the school social worker, may have to counsel the parents to follow the prescribed recommendations. Without these follow-up procedures to insure that the medical recommendations have been carried out, the hearing conservation program would be quite ineffective.

At present not all public school hearing conservation programs are under the auspices of state health departments. Some programs are sponsored by regional health departments, some by state departments of education, and some by local school districts. The important consideration is that there may be no otologic-audiologic clinic available after the identification program has been completed. There must be some course of action to insure that recommendations for medical follow-up are carried out by the parents. This responsibility must be designated to a specific individual, as the nurse, the speech therapist, the head of special education, or some other school official. He is also responsible for seeing that competent audiological services are provided for pre- and postmedical examinations. In larger communities, an audiologist may be employed by the school system for this purpose. University and community speech and hearing centers are sometimes used by the school districts for the audiologic assessments. Serious problems may arise in rural areas where no audiologic facilities are accessible, and the only alternative is to send the children to the nearest city where competent audiologic services are available. Travel must be no deterrent when children's health conditions are involved.

If the children's hearing losses are found to be irreversible after all otologic and medical services have been completed, then aural rehabilitation procedures should be considered. Counseling both the parents and the teachers on the seriousness of the hearing impairment and how they may participate in the conservation program is also important. These children should be followed closely and should be retested at least once each year during the testing program, or more frequently if noticeable changes in hearing are observed.

Research Aspects of Identification Audiometry

There have been many studies on various screening procedures, particularly on limited-frequency testing. It is important to consider some of these studies individually in order to make some judgments regarding the past, present, and future directions of identification audiometry. There are almost as many suggestions for procedures as there are studies, and one can only speculate as to the future for this aspect of public school hearing conservation. There are necessarily no "rights" or "wrongs" in some procedures, so long as the basic principles of identification audiometry are maintained. It is mandatory that screening continue despite all of the criticisms leveled at one procedure or another. During this period of continuous research, those responsible for conducting the hearing conservation program must strive to maintain the highest levels of competency to identify those children with hearing losses. It also should be noted that identification audiometry refers to the detection of a hearing impairment and not to the detection of ear pathology. Ear pathology may exist even when hearing sensitivity is well within normal limits, and it is not the intent of this chapter to discuss this phase of hearing, although some of the research deals with the identification of ear pathology.

House and Glorig (13) reported that the usual audiometric screening procedures are not completely suitable for use in the schools, in the military, or in industrial testing programs. In investigating a large number of audiograms, they found that in approximately 99 per cent of the cases, the hearing loss at 4,000 Hz was at least as great as the loss at any lower frequency. On the basis of their findings, it was recommended that testing at 4,000 Hz be used as a screening test. The advantages of such a method, according to the authors of this study, were that ordinary quiet rooms could be used for testing; that the time required was only a few seconds and this prevented fatigue; and that the Oto-chek instrument designed for this test was inexpensive, light-weight, and durable. In this study, 1,500 school children were screened individually at 4,000 Hz. This screening was followed by the usual screening test at 25 dB. All failures were tested by individual pure-tone threshold tests. Of the 1,500 children, 500 were screened at both 2,000 and 4,000 Hz to determine whether a greater accuracy would result when two frequencies were used. Although no increase in accuracy was found, it was felt that if 2,000 Hz was included, fewer unnecessary referrals of school children would be made because of the insignificant "dips" often found at 4,000 Hz.

Lawrence and Rubin (17), in an attempt to evaluate limited-frequency screening, studied two groups of children. Group I consisted of 1,000 school children in grades one through twelve enrolled in the parochial schools in New Orleans; Group II, a different group of 1,000 children with the same grade distribution and school enrollment; and Group III, 536 children for whom case records were available and who had been examined at otological clinics. Children in Group I were given a limited-frequency test at 25 dB at 2,000 and 4,000 Hz with an Oto-chek. Following this test, children were given a routine sweep-check test at 25 dB using 250, 500, 1,000, 2,000, 4,000, and 8,000 Hz. A conventional portable pure-tone audiometer was used. Group II children were given only a sweep-check test at 25 dB at 250, 500, 1,000, 2,000, 4,000, and 8,000 Hz. Children in Group III had originally been selected by a routine sweep-check test from 250 through 8,000 Hz.

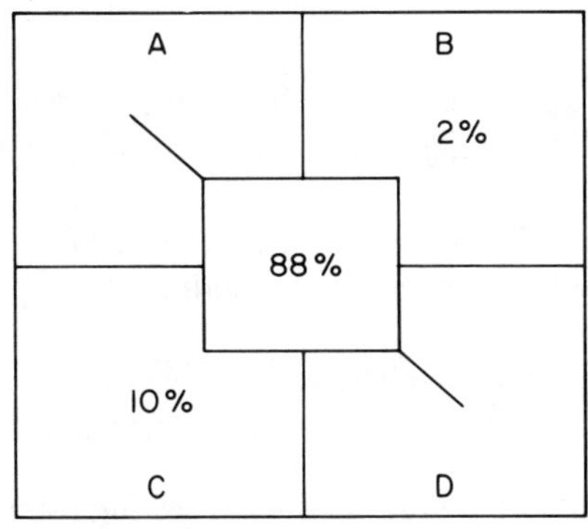

FIGURE 5.5 Tetrachoric method of analysis. *Source:* Reger, S. N., and H. A. Newby. "A group pure-tone hearing test." *Journal of Speech and Hearing Disorders*, **12**: 61–6, 1947.

The analysis of the results compared the testing methods, using the tetrachoric table (Figure 5.5) which had previously been advocated by Newby (27). This method has also been used to compare group and individual screening tests. An effective group test should have a hypothetical distribution of agreements and disagreements as indicated in Figure 5.5. Children either passing or failing both tests should make up a minimum of 88 per cent of the total (Cell A plus Cell D), while a maximum of 2 per cent should be missed by the group test (Cell B) and a maximum of 10 per cent should be unnecessarily referred by the group test (Cell C). The nearer the combined percentages in Cells A and D approach 100 per cent the closer the agreements between the tests being compared.

Lawrence and Rubin (17) reported the following results from this study:

1. Except for results with 4,000 Hz alone in Group II, all limited-frequency combinations would have met hypothetical criteria proposed by DiCarlo and Gardner (1953) for an effective screening test.
2. The number of unnecessary referrals was small (1.5 per cent) when compared with the best group test combination (5.3 per cent).
3. Screening at only 4,000 Hz showed only 66 to 70 per cent agreement with routine sweep-check testing.
4. Screening at 4,000 and 2,000 Hz resulted in some increase in percentage of agreement (76 per cent).
5. Screening at 4,000 and 500 Hz, combined, showed the best agreement (90 per cent) with routine sweep-check testing, and compared favorably with the best group test combination.
6. There was close agreement (95 per cent) when the frequencies 500, 1,000, 2,000, and 4,000 Hz were considered as a form of modified sweep-check in Group II, and this combination of tones was compared with the routine sweep-check. This close relationship, along with other considerations, led to the further comparison of specific frequency combinations with this modified sweep-check test.

This additional information indicated:

1. Screening at 4,000 Hz only agreed more closely with modified sweep-check testing than it did with routine full-range sweep-check testing (80 per cent compared with 66 to 70 per cent).
2. Screening at 4,000 to 2,000 Hz combined, or at 4,000 and 1,000 Hz combined would not materially increase agreement with modified sweep-check testing over screening at 4,000 Hz alone.
3. Screening at 4,000 and 500 Hz combined showed extremely close agreement with modified sweep-check testing (98 per cent agreement).

The authors of this study recommended that a limited-frequency testing using 4,000 and 500 Hz would best meet reasonable criteria for agreement with the standard sweep-check test, although they indicated that further experimental testing was desirable.

The purpose of a study by Ventry and Newby (36) was to determine whether the generality of the single-frequency principle could be extended to include school children. The two null hypotheses they used were: (a) there was no difference between the mean threshold losses from 500 through 8,000 Hz and (b) the mean threshold loss at 4,000 Hz was not different from the mean threshold losses above and below 4,000 Hz. The single-frequency screening was evaluated for school children by giving pure-tone threshold tests on every fourth subject who failed a five-frequency sweep test at levels of 30 dB for 500 and 1,000 Hz and 25 dB for 2,000, 4,000, and 8,000 Hz. All threshold tests were conducted in school rooms that had been used for the sweep-testing. Standard testing procedures were used in the threshold testing. A total of sixty-two subjects (ninety ears) received threshold tests. The children were in grades one, three, and five. Data were analyzed for each of the three grades separately and for all grades combined.

The results of the threshold analyses indicated that there were significant differences between the mean threshold losses from 500 through 8,000 Hz. Further analyses indicated that the mean threshold loss at 4,000 Hz was greater than the mean threshold loss at any of the other four frequencies tested. Ventry and Newby concluded that the validity of the single-frequency principle in his study appeared to be established. In terms of one-frequency screening for determining medically significant hearing losses, they stated that this method needed to be further evaluated.

Norton and Lux (30) compared double-frequency screening at 2,000 and 4,000 Hz to screening at 250, 500, 1,000, 2,000, and 4,000 Hz. Both procedures used a screening level of 25 dB. The study was done on 1,046 subjects from four schools which represented a cross-section of the socio-economic structure of the community. According to this study, the double-frequency method appeared to be less reliable than the five-frequency method, although the double-frequency method was simpler and faster to present. Of special note was the fact that the screening was done in the regular classroom. Norton and Lux felt that this procedure was less distracting for young children and that less advanced preparation was needed in the administration of the testing schedule. It also did not disrupt class schedules. They felt that longitudinal studies would be necessary before any definitive conclusions could be reached as to which screening procedures were the most accurate.

Lightfoot, Buckingham, and Kelly (18) reported the inadequacy of Oto-chek screening in public school programs and physicians' offices. Of 552 ears capable of passing the House-Glorig test, 381 (69 per cent) were found by otological examination to be defective. The tendency to pass an excessively large number of impaired ears reduced its efficiency. Although opposed to this procedure for school children, Lightfoot, Buckingham, and Kelly stated that there were advantages for this procedure for determining the status of persons who work in noisy environments, since the test can be administered easily near the work area, as well as under certain circumstances by physicians. For use by physicians, threshold testing at 500 and 4,000 Hz, rather than Oto-chek screening, could be of value in cases where the physician had on record an audiogram of the patient's threshold. If hearing at 500 and 4,000 Hz was within 5-dB of previously recorded levels, it was assumed that the patient's hearing was probably not undergoing impairment by disease.

Stevens and Davidson (35) took exception to the 4,000 Hz technique of House and Glorig (13). In analyzing the results, Stevens and Davidson noted that there was the possibility that nine children with a hearing loss in every 100 would not be located by the single-frequency method of screening. They further questioned the use of aircraft workers for comparison and the fact that at least two of the groups were entirely male. These groups were prone to the 4,000 Hz dip without accompanying loss at other frequencies.

In a study done by Stevens and Davidson (35) which used audiograms from the Florida State University Speech and Hearing Clinic and the Florida Public Health Department of Leon County, they found that a hearing screening method that used the single frequency of 4,000 Hz or one that used 4,000 Hz combined with any one, two, or even three of the other speech frequencies was not as effective as the standard sweep-check method.

In an attempt to evaluate abbreviated screening procedures, Siegenthaler and Sommers (34) evaluated the results of 14,745 public school children who were given pure-tone individual screening tests by the usual techniques. Three groups were used. All were of school age and were tested with standard pure-tone audiometers using standard audiometric techniques. One of the three groups, 100 consecutive children seen at Pennsylvania State University, were children in kindergarten through twelfth grade. Of the ninety-one children in this group found to have hearing loss, 93.4 per cent failed 4,000 Hz in at least one ear. It was pointed out, however, that these children were seen in the clinic because a physician, parent, or a school hearing test suggested the possibility of a hearing loss. That is, as a group these children were preselected for their ear or hearing difficulties. In the other two groups of school children, over a third of the children did not have hearing losses at 4,000 Hz according to threshold audiograms, but had reductions in acuity at other frequencies. The 4,000 Hz abbreviated sweep-check would not have been adequate to detect hearing loss. If the criteria for hearing loss were modified to at least a 30-dB average for the frequencies 500–2,000 Hz, the 4,000 Hz check would detect an increased number of those with hearing loss. Siegenthaler and Sommers, however, felt that a school hearing conservation program should detect children with less severe hearing losses than this, if it were to be adequate for hearing conservation. They also stated that if both 4,000 and 500 Hz had been used, then about 83 to 94 per cent of those with losses would have been detected. Even with these two frequencies, about 6 per cent of the children would have been missed. A greater number of children with potential hearing losses would be detected as the number of frequencies was increased in the screening procedure.

Although Miller and Bella (25) agreed with the use of the Oto-chek in industrial situations to determine which workers might be susceptible to noise-induced hearing loss, their analysis of 3,630 tests done in the Greenwich, Connecticut school system during a one-year period, indicated that the Oto-chek procedure would not be adequate as a screening method. Miller and Bella offered the following conclusions:

1. The audiometric frequency showing the greatest loss was not at 4,000 Hz in a large portion of the losses found in the population tested.
2. Screening testing limited to the 2,000 and 4,000 Hz frequencies would fail to detect a significant number of children with losses of hearing.
3. A three-frequency test including 1,000, 2,000, and 4,000 Hz was almost as efficient as the complete five-frequency sweep-check, but the amount of time saved was probably negligible.

On the basis of research performed in Australia, Farrant (9) advocated a two-frequency screening test. This procedure has been used in Australian schools since 1951. He recommended screening at 25 dB at 500 and 4,000 Hz. A "moderately" trained audiometrist engaged fully in audiometric screening, including threshold testing on those who failed the screening, could test approximately fifteen children per working hour at the preschool and kindergarten levels, thirty-six children per hour in the first half of primary school, and up to sixty-three children per hour at the secondary school level. Incidence of measurable hearing loss could be expected in about 5 per cent of ears tested or 3 per cent of the children screened, the amount of incidence varying considerably with population characteristics, such as socioeconomic status, and with the seasons, the greatest incidence occurring in winter. Farrant also indicated that most hearing losses detected by screening were monaural, and that most hearing losses were slight to moderate conductive impairments correctable by medical treatment. A considerable proportion of hearing losses occurred in young children who were amenable to eventual spontaneous recovery. Marked binaural losses were relatively rare. To ensure adequate medical, educational, and social treatment of children with hearing loss, it was necessary to interpret and communicate results to parents, teachers, and physicians, and ultimately to inform the community about hearing problems.

In an attempt to discover any relationships between several limited-frequency techniques and various ear pathologies, Maxwell and Davidson (22) analyzed the audiograms and medical records of 161 ears. The limited-frequency tests studied were 4,000 Hz, 4,000 and 1,000 Hz, and 4,000 and 2,000 Hz. If a 4,000 Hz screening test had been used, 79.6 per cent of the pathological ears would have been detected; using 4,000 and 1,000 Hz, detection would have increased to 94.4 per cent; utilizing 4,000 and 2,000 Hz, 90.6 per cent of the pathological ears would have been detected. According to the authors of this study, pathologies of the external ear were the most easily detected and those involving tonsils and adenoids were the least easily detected. It is necessary to caution the reader that the ear pathologies were diagnosed by the physician and were not identified by the screening procedures.

Because of the need for additional data, it was the purpose of a study by Hanley and Gaddie (10) to employ the 4,000 Hz single-frequency screening in a school setting in which (1) a simple, inexpensive, miniature single-tone audiometer would be used; (2) a normal school population would be screened in a public school classroom; and (3) a validation threshold audiogram would be obtained in a "typical sound-proof" testing room on the same day. A transistorized, battery-powered audiometer, capable of producing a 4,000 Hz tone at either 55 or 25 dB was constructed at the University of Washington. A single earphone which could be held in the examiner's free hand and held to each ear of the subject was used. A commercial clinical audiometer, located in a control room adjacent to a sound-treated testing room, was used for the pure-tone individual threshold tests.

The screening was conducted at 25 dB. For the pure-tone threshold tests, the ascending procedure was used. The criteria for the classification "hard-of-hearing" were, for the threshold test, failure either at 25 dB at two frequencies or 30 dB at one frequency. The criterion for failure on the screening was "no response" to the 25-dB test tone. Of the 456 ears tested, 436 were designated as normal and 20 classified as hard-of-hearing by means of the threshold test. From the screening, 97.2 per cent of the normal ears were correctly identified and 2.8 per cent erroneously classified as hard-of-hearing. Of those classified as hard-of-hearing, 90 per cent were correctly identified by the screening procedure and 10 per cent were misclassified. Of the 228 children participating in this study, it was concluded that the 4,000 Hz pure-tone might be used to adequately predict those with hearing loss with a high degree of accuracy. Hanley and Gaddie noted that even though the error in single-frequency testing might be as high as 10 per cent, economy of time is such as to permit the testing of larger numbers of children than with routine screening procedures. Increasing the number screened, because of the time economy factor, would allow for detecting more cases of hearing impairment than is possible with routine procedures that test only every other grade or every third grade. The average time for testing children with the 4,000-Hz screening was under thirty seconds each.

The purpose of a study by Melnick, Eagles, and Levine (24) was to evaluate some of the procedures advocated by the National Conference on Identification Audiometry. The National Conference (5) made the following recommendations:

1. Testing should be conducted in acoustically-treated test rooms.

2. The frequencies recommended for identification audiometry at the school-age level were 500, 1,000, 2,000, 4,000, and 6,000 Hz.

3. The frequencies 500, 1,000, 2,000, and 6,000 Hz should be screened at 20 dB and at 30 dB for the frequency 4,000 Hz.

4. The criteria for failure should be failure to respond at 20 dB at 1,000, 2,000, and 6,000, or at 30 dB at 4,000 Hz.[4]

5. The same failure criteria should apply to both the screening and the pure-tone threshold test.

Eight hundred and eighty children from kindergarten through the eighth grade of four elementary schools in Pittsburgh participated in the study. These children were functioning as normal public school children with no apparent hearing problems at the time of the test. Screening and threshold testing were performed in a double-walled test room. Screening was done at 20 dB at 500, 1,000, 2,000, 4,000, and 6,000 Hz, and at 30 dB at 4,000 Hz. A serial method of limits was used for the threshold tests. Ascending trials were used in determining the threshold hearing levels. The test program was successful in finding those children with a reducing hearing sensitivity. The procedures were not adequate to identify children with otoscopic evidence of active or past ear pathology.

In a report on the dilemmas in screening audiometry, Downs, Doster, and Weaver (7) made the following suggestions:

1. The presently recommended screening level of 20 dB adequately fulfilled the goals and responsibilities of educational programs.

2. The medical aspects of the hearing problems of school children should be attacked vigorously, with special emphasis on obtaining an examination by the otolaryngologist of every child found to have a hearing problem.

3. More intensive search should be concentrated on the lower grades, where the largest percentage of hearing problems occur, and consideration given to relaxing the search in the upper grades.

They indicated that the status quo of screening was not all bad, since the primary concern of education programs was to screen out pupils with deviations in hearing that affected classroom communication. The implication was that screening audiometry had not been successful in identifying active or past ear pathology as reported by Melnick, Eagles, and Levine (24). In this study, 52 per cent of all children were not identified by audiometric procedures, and 70 per cent of those with evidence of past ear diseases were not identified by pure-tone tests. The need for intensive screening in the lower grades was emphasized also as evidenced in a study by Corliss and Watson (3), in which only thirty-one cases of hearing loss identified in the tenth grade had not been detected in the lower grades.

4 The National Conference on Identification Audiometry recommended that only 1,000, 2,000, 4,000, and 6,000 Hz be considered in the criteria for referral.

The Denver Public Schools have decided to test only to the seventh grade, with new students, previous failures, and either parent, physician, and teacher or nurse referrals screened beyond this grade.

According to Lloyd (19), the National Conference on Identification Audiometry, which recommended a 20-dB screening level for most frequencies, seemed an appropriate choice until an air-bone gap screening method became more feasible for use in the school situation. In referring to the limited-frequency tests, he indicated that investigation did not deal with the basic question of what percentage of the children, with medical or communication break-down hearing impairments, would be identified with one-frequency screening. Lloyd rejected the use of one- or two-frequency screening with children except as a last resort. This was supported by studies rejecting the use of 4,000 Hz screening (25, 34, 35, 18). If the one- or two-frequency screening was rejected, a decision had to be made as to how many and which frequencies should be used in screening. Lloyd stated that until further data became available, it seemed appropriate to follow the recommendation of the National Conference on Identification Audiometry using 1,000, 2,000, 4,000, and 6,000 Hz as the criteria for referral (5). He indicated that 500 Hz should be included if low ambient-noise environments were available.

In a study recently conducted by Meissner (23), it was found that the mean time necessary to test four frequencies in both ears was sixty-five seconds. He also concluded that it was not necessary to test 2,000 Hz. Conclusions drawn by Meissner on the procedural advantages of using a newly developed "Automatic Screening Audiometer" are most likely not significant enough to warrant detailed discussion at this time.

Hearing Conservation Follow-up

Children may need hearing-aid evaluation, speech-reading, auditory training, speech (hearing) therapy, or counseling after the medical referral and examination. If the children's losses have been amenable to medical treatment, then no further recommendations are necessary except for periodic hearing rechecks. It is at this phase of the program that children who have hearing impairment must be referred to appropriate aural rehabilitation procedures. Children with a serious hearing problem, as suggested by the Ohio Plan (20), may be referred to a special classroom for the hard-of-hearing or the deaf. It is unlikely that children with severe or profound hearing losses will not have been detected prior to the screening program. In those communities where special classrooms are not available, seriously impaired children may be candidates for a state school for the deaf. Therapy must be made available to children with a mild or moderate loss, with or without amplification, who are not eligible for special education classrooms.

HEARING AIDS

Of the twenty-eight responses received by Zink and Alpiner (37), twenty states reported having hearing-aid provisions as part of their public school hearing conservation programs. Of the twenty states that reported hearing-aid programs, twelve used an audiology center, speech and hearing center, or university clinic as their hearing-aid program resource. Two used state health department clinics and one state used a special mobile unit staffed by the health department. The remaining five states did not elaborate on hearing-aid evaluation procedures except to indicate that an annual evaluation was recommended by the hearing-aid dealer.

An example of a state department of health hearing-aid program is New York's (26) which maintains thirty-one approved hearing centers located throughout the state; the children can usually receive an evaluation close to their homes. The New York policy indicated that hearing-handicapped children should receive the best aid at the lowest price in accordance with their needs, and the assurance of hearing service near their homes. In all instances children must be tested at a center with the selected aid before the purchase will be authorized for state aid under the Medical Rehabilitation Program. Children under age seven must be reevaluated at a center every three months. Beyond age seven, children must be reevaluated every six months. The families and the children must receive at least one interview by the audiologist in the use of the hearing aid. Children also must receive complete reevaluations with each new hearing-aid fitting.

In the state of Maine (21), under Maternal and Child Health and Crippled Children's Services, hearing aids are purchased on recommendation of an otologist. Hearing evaluations may be done by the otologist or an audiologist. The selection of hearing aids is by recommendation of the hearing examiner, and purchase is usually through a hearing-aid dealer. Due to the great size of the state, the hearing-aid dealer may fit the aids; when possible, the audiologist will do it. Regular ENT follow-up is required for children using aids purchased through the department.

The Colorado State Health Department (37) is experimenting with hearing-aid selection procedures. The State Health Department obtains competitive bids from dealers on the desired instruments. These hearing aids are then evaluated on Bruel and Kjaer instrumentation. Hearing aids that appear to have the necessary response characteristics are selected from each manufacturer for evaluation. The budget for hearing aids is limited and those dealers are selected whose bids are the most competitive. The ultimate objective is to obtain hearing aids for children at a cost that will permit fitting all who are in need. The hearing aids that are selected for evaluation are categorized as follows:

1. High amplification body aids with gains between 52 and 80 dB and a minimum frequency range from 330 to 4,000 Hz.

2. Ear-level aids with gains between 44 and 55 dB and a minimum frequency range from 500 to 4,000 Hz.

3. Ear-level aids with gains between 33 and 43 dB and a minimum frequency range from 500 to 4,000 Hz.

4. A distortion level that does not exceed 10 per cent.

The first procedure involves obtaining the children's tolerance limits by plotting the most comfortable levels through pure-tone and speech audiometry. From a stock of approximately twenty hearing aids that have previously been screened, the audiologist selects up to four aids which meet the children's gain and tolerance requirements. The hearing aids are then compared in order to determine which aids appear to be the most satisfactory.

Needless to say, there are several philosophies of hearing-aid selection and fit and they are discussed in Chapter 14. Hearing-aid provisions should be an integral part of a total hearing conservation program and those persons involved in this phase of the program should meet the requirements for clinical certification by the ASHA.

SPEECH-READING, AUDITORY TRAINING, AND SPEECH (HEARING) THERAPY

After all evaluation measures are completed, children may then be considered for speech-reading, auditory training, hearing therapy, or any combination of these rehabilitation procedures. The decision for recommending any of these procedures should be made by the supervising clinical audiologist. The audiologist will necessarily want to interpret the significance of audiological, medical, and educational records before making recommendations for the children. For example, if there is any indication that the hearing loss may be progressive, he may recommend speech-reading and hearing therapy as a precautionary measure. This would insure that the children have the potential for maintaining adequate communication in the event that their hearing significantly deteriorates. Hearing therapy will allow the children to preserve good speech that might otherwise deteriorate due to a progressive loss. These measures would give them the benefit of a doubt as to their future hearing status. It is not necessary to engage the children in an indefinite therapy program. Therapy for a period of six months or one year may be sufficient. These children should also be tested routinely every year as part of the hearing conservation program. The results obtained can help to determine if additional therapy is needed. Auditory training should be considered if the children have reduced discrimination ability with or without amplification. Generally, a discrimination problem will not be present for those with mild impairment although there is no guarantee that this will be the case.

In larger school districts, it is feasible for an audiologist to be employed to supervise the screening program, to conduct audiological assessments for those who fail the screening, and to provide speech-reading, auditory training, and hearing therapy for those children in need of such remediation. If hearing conservation programs are conducted under the auspices of a state department of health, then the supervising audiologist would work in conjunction with these agencies. As increasing numbers of clinical audiologists are employed in larger school systems, it is highly probable that hearing conservation will come under their immediate jurisdiction within the guidelines of this author's earlier recommendations. This solution is practical because the clinical audiologist would have the necessary training and background. In order to help alleviate the shortage of qualified personnel to engage in this type of public school program, Utah State University is pioneering a program in educational audiology. This training program should help a great deal by providing more qualified individuals who are interested in working in the public school systems, since most clinical audiologists do not enter or seek public school employment. It would also help to clarify the present dilemma as to who should provide therapy for mildly impaired children who are not candidates for special education classrooms.

A more serious problem exists in smaller urban and rural communities where the number of children needing hearing therapy is comparatively small. It is not practical for these school districts to employ audiologists. Smaller geographical areas may be adequately covered by traveling audiologists from state health departments, but there is no provision for therapy after the audiological and medical evaluations have been completed. It is the speech therapist's responsibility to provide aural rehabilitation. This problem could be resolved by modifying university training programs so that the student preparing for speech therapy would be given additional training and practicum in aural rehabilitation. This prospective therapist would then be qualified to engage in speech-reading, auditory training, and hearing therapy. Whether or not such a course of action is feasible cannot be determined at this time, but this problem must be resolved. The role of the public school therapist would assume greater importance, although there has been some tendency in the past to minimize his status. The public school therapist, meeting the appropriate determined requirements, would be able to work with both speech- and hearing-impaired children in all school systems, large or small. In any event, there is a need to provide qualified personnel for hearing-impaired children in all school hearing conservation programs. Evaluation alone does not constitute hearing conservation, and without the means for providing aural rehabilitation, the program cannot achieve any degree of success.

COUNSELING

No hearing conservation program is complete without discussing the general problem of counseling and its implications for teachers and parents.

The otologist should assume the responsibility for explaining the medical aspects of the problem, and the supervising audiologist the obligation of counseling the parents on the audiologic and communicative aspects of the hearing problem. Counseling may extend to older children as considered appropriate by the professional persons involved. The school nurse often has an important role in seeing that the parents follow through with the recommendations. If psychological and social problems are evident, then psychologists and social workers must become involved in the hearing conservation program.

It is also important for the nurse or the supervising audiologist to make sure that those children with hearing impairment are retested each year. Adequate records should be kept, and parents should know whom to contact if any problem arises regarding their children's hearing function. Classroom teachers should be told what to look for in children who may have undetected hearing problems and what to look for in changing behavior of children already known to have hearing loss. Duffy (8) describes some of these children's characteristics that should place both teachers and parents on the alert:

1. He fails to pay attention when spoken to casually.
2. He gives the wrong answers to simple questions.
3. He hears better when watching the speaker's face.
4. He is functioning below his potential ability in school.
5. He often asks the speaker to repeat words or sentences.
6. He has frequent earaches and running ears; he also has frequent colds.
7. He has frequent upper respiratory infections like sinusitis and tonsilitis. He has allergies similar to hay fever.
8. He has become a behavior problem at school and at home.
9. He fails to articulate correctly certain speech sounds or he omits certain consonant sounds.
10. He often fails to discriminate between words with similar vowels but different consonants.
11. He is withdrawn and does not mingle readily with classmates and neighbors.

By keeping some of these factors in mind, it is possible to create a greater awareness in parents and classroom teachers, which makes the problem of counseling easier. Informed persons can discuss problems more intelligently for successful follow-up and remediation. In long-range terms, the children should benefit the most. All persons who have contact with children will also benefit because of the increased understanding of hearing impairment and what can be done to help alleviate the magnitude of the communication breakdown.

Bibliography

1. California State Department of Education. *Hearing Testing of School Children.* Sacramento: 1954.
2. Connor, Leo E. "Determining the prevalence of hearing-impaired children." *Exceptional Children*, **27**: 337–44, 1961.
3. Corliss, L., and J. Watson. "A school system studies the effectiveness of routine audiometry." *Journal of Health, Physical Education Rec. of NEA* (March, 1961).
4. Dahl, L. A. *Public School Audiometry: Principles and Methods.* Danville, Ill.: The Interstate Press, 1949.
5. Darley, F. L., ed. "Identification audiometry." *Journal of Speech and Hearing Disorders*, Monograph Supplement Number 9, 1961.
6. DiCarlo, L. M., and E. F. Gardner. "The efficiency of the Massachusetts pure-tone screening test as adapted for a university testing program." *Journal of Speech and Hearing Disorders*, **18**: 175–82, 1953.
7. Downs, M. P., M. E. Doster, and M. Weaver. "Dilemmas in identification audiometry." *Journal of Speech and Hearing Disorders*, **30**: 360–64, 1965.
8. Duffy, J. K. "Report 5: Hearing problems of school-age children." In *Maico Audiological Library Series*, I. Minneapolis: Maico Electronics, 1964.
9. Farrant, R. H. "The audiometric testing of children in schools and kindergartens." *Journal of Auditory Research*, **1**: 1–24, 1960.
10. Hanley, C. N., and B. G. Gaddie. "The use of single-frequency audiometry in the screening of school children." *Journal of Speech and Hearing Disorders*, **27**: 258–64, 1962.
11. Harrington, D. A. "Laws and regulations in identification audiometry: Directions and trends." *Journal of Speech and Hearing Disorders*, Monograph Supplement Number 9, 45–51, 1961.
12. Harrington, D. A. "Hearing conservation programs and controversies." *Journal of Southern Medical Association*, **57**: 1314–16, 1964.
13. House, H. P., and A. Glorig. "A new concept of auditory screening." *Laryngoscope*, **67**: 661–68, 1957.
14. Johnson, K. O., and H. A. Newby. "Experimental study of the efficiency of two group hearing tests." *Archives of Otolaryngology*, **60**: 702–10, 1954.
15. Johnston, P. W. "The Massachusetts Hearing Test." *Journal of the Accoustical Society of America*, **20**: 697–703, 1948.
16. Johnston, P. W. "An efficient group screening test." *Journal of Speech and Hearing Disorders*, **17**: 8–12, 1952.
17. Lawrence, C. F., and W. Rubin. "The efficiency of limited-frequency audiometric screening in a school hearing conservation program." *Archives of Otolaryngology*, **69**: 606–11, 1959.
18. Lightfoot, C., R. A. Buckingham, and M. N. Kelly. "A check on Oto-chek." *Archives of Otolaryngology*, **70**: 103–13, 1959.
19. Lloyd, L. L. "Comment on 'dilemmas in identification audiometry'." *Journal of Speech and Hearing Disorders*, **31**: 161–65, 1966.
20. MacLearie, E. C. *The Ohio Plan for Children with Speech and Hearing Problems.* Columbus: Division of Special Education, 1961.

21. Maine Department of Health and Welfare. Communication received, 1966.
22. Maxwell, R. W., and G. D. Davidson. "Limited-frequency screening and ear pathology." *Journal of Speech and Hearing Disorders*, **26**: 122–25, 1961.
23. Meissner, W. A. "A new automatic screening audiometer." Unpublished M.S. thesis. De Kalb: Northern Illinois University, 1967.
24. Melnick, W., E. L. Eagles, and H. S. Levine. "Evaluation of a recommended program of identification audiometry with school-age children." *Journal of Speech and Hearing Disorders*, **29**: 3–13, 1964.
25. Miller, M. H., and J. L. Bella. "Limitations of selected frequency audiometry in the public schools." *Journal of Speech and Hearing Disorders*, **24**: 402–7, 1959.
26. New York State Department of Health. *Field Memorandum Series*. Medical Rehabilitation Program: Hearing and Speech. Pp. 66–86, 1966.
27. Newby, H. A. "Evaluating the efficiency of group screening tests of hearing." *Journal of Speech and Hearing Disorders*, **13**: 236–40, 1948.
28. Newby, H. A. *Audiology*. New York: Appleton-Century-Crofts, 1964.
29. Nielsen, S. F. "Group testing of school children by pure-tone audiometry." *Journal of Speech and Hearing Disorders*, **17**: 4–7, 1952.
30. Norton, M. C., and E. Lux. "Double-frequency auditory screening in public schools." *Journal of Speech and Hearing Disorders*, **25**: 293–99, 1960.
31. O'Neill, J. J., and H. J. Oyer. *Applied Audiometry*. New York: Dodd, Mead & Co., 1966.
32. Reger, S. N., and H. A. Newby. "A group pure-tone hearing test." *Journal of Speech and Hearing Disorders*, **12**: 61–6, 1947.
33. Scott County, Iowa Schools. "Program and procedures: Hearing conservation program." Correspondence received, 1967.
34. Siegenthaler, B. M., and R. K. Sommers. "Abbreviated sweep-check procedures for school hearing testing." *Journal of Speech and Hearing Disorders*, **24**: 249–57, 1959.
35. Stevens, D. A. and G. D. Davidson. "Screening tests of hearing." *Journal of Speech and Hearing Disorders*, **24**: 258–61, 1959.
36. Ventry, I. M., and H. A. Newby. "Validity of the one-frequency screening principle for public school children." *Journal of Speech and Hearing Research*, **2**: 147–51, 1959.
37. Zink, G. D., and J. G. Alpiner. "Hearing aids: One aspect of a state public school hearing conservation program." *Journal of Speech and Hearing Disorders*, **23**: 329–44, 1968.

6

Pure-Tone Audiometry

Lloyd L. Price, Ph.D.

The primary objective of this chapter is to help the student to an understanding of the concepts underlying pure-tone audiometry. A secondary objective is to present the student with a technique of testing. The relative importance of these objectives makes it imperative to stress concepts and to put relatively little emphasis on any particular methodology or technique. As a result, most of this chapter will be concerned with understanding what pure-tone testing is, and some suggestions concerning a particular test technique will be presented toward the end.

Pure-tone tests for hearing sensitivity[1] are the most basic tests that the audiologist uses. These tests are usually thought of as "routine audiometry" and practically everyone, professional and nonprofessional alike, feels competent in his ability to administer them. As a result, there are many inaccurate audiograms floating around. The administration of valid pure-tone hearing tests requires (a) a basic knowledge of the anatomy and physiology of the auditory system, (b) an understanding of some fundamental

[1] For a discussion of the use of the terms "sensitivity" and "acuity," see Ward (30). Definitions are given in the glossary of this chapter.

concepts about how sounds are generated, transmitted, and controlled, and (c) an understanding of the influence of certain procedural variables and pathologic conditions upon the results of the tests. Some of this information has already been presented in earlier chapters of this text. The present chapter supplies the additional information necessary for a meaningful approach to pure-tone audiometry.

Rationale for Pure-Tone Testing

Since man is seldom called upon to listen to sounds as simple as pure tones, one might ask whether it is reasonable to use such stimuli to test hearing. The answer is yes. Any sound, no matter how complex, can be shown to be a combination of pure tones. This is true of speech, the primary acoustic signal that man must listen to and interpret. A frequency analysis of speech reveals that the greatest concentrations of acoustic energy are between 300 and 3,000 Hz, although frequencies somewhat below and above this range may carry some information. Thus, if an audiologist measures a patient's ability to hear pure tones in the frequency range of about 125 through 8,000 Hz, he has some basis for predicting whether the patient's hearing for speech is normal or impaired.

To establish the threshold for each individual frequency between 125 and 8,000 Hz would be impractical. As a result, two general procedures have been employed in an effort to get an effective sampling of the hearing sensitivity within this range. The first is to select test frequencies at given intervals, to measure the threshold at these frequencies, then to imply, by connecting these threshold points with a line that the hearing follows, an essentially uniform pattern between any two test frequencies. Using this procedure, the frequencies usually tested are 125, 250, 500, 1,000, 2,000, 4,000, and 8,000 Hz. Note that the test frequencies are at OCTAVE intervals with the base at 125 Hz. Many audiometers also have the frequencies 750, 1,500, 3,000, and 6,000 Hz and these frequencies are tested when they fall within an area where sensitivity is changing rapidly as a function of frequency.

The second method for pure-tone testing involves sweeping rather rapidly across all frequencies in the test range and thus establish the threshold for a tone that is continuously changing in frequency. A typical clinical speed is to cross one octave during each two-minute period. The short duration of any given frequency prevents the establishment of more than a trend toward the threshold at that particular frequency and thus the tracing tends to be an averaging process. This smoothed curve tends to approximate the curve that is obtained when using the method of testing discreet frequencies at octave intervals.

In addition to being useful as an indicator of loss of hearing, pure-tone tests are often useful in suggesting the SITE OF LESION (general anatomical location of the pathologic condition). More will be said later in this chapter concerning site of lesion and pathologies of hearing.

The Audiometer

The AUDIOMETER is an electronic device for measuring hearing ability (or lack of it). In its simplest form it is a pure-tone oscillator, an amplifier, and an attenuator. A selection of different frequencies can be obtained by altering the output from the pure-tone oscillator through manipulation of the FREQUENCY SELECTOR SWITCH, and the tone can be turned on and off by pressing or releasing the INTERRUPTOR SWITCH. The attenuator or HEARING LEVEL DIAL controls the intensity of the stimulus. A noise generator is usually included within the unit to provide masking when needed. All clinical audiometers are equipped with a set of earphones and a bone-conduction receiver so that both air- and bone-conduction tests can be carried out.

The types of audiometers available commercially vary from simple screening models to very complex clinical instruments. The deluxe clinical models not only provide for pure-tone testing but are designed so that many of the special tests discussed in Chapters 7 and 10 can be carried out on them. The automatic audiometers have motor-driven frequency and intensity controls in order that the frequency and intensity of the tone can be varied automatically with time. The most widely used automatic audiometer in the audiology clinic is a commercial version of the one developed by Bekesy (4). More discussion will be directed to the use of this instrument later in the present chapter and in Chapter 10.

The Audiogram

Pure-tone sensitivity can be measured by AIR CONDUCTION and by BONE CONDUCTION. The audiogram is a graph showing the hearing sensitivity for air- and bone-conducted sounds. The frequency of the tone in HERTZ (Hz), or CYCLES PER SECOND (cps), is represented along the abcissa, and HEARING LEVEL (HL) in decibels (dB) along the ordinate. Figure 6.1 is a typical audiogram form.

The symbols used on the audiogram are not completely standardized; however, the air-conduction threshold for the right ear is usually represented by a red "O" and the air-conduction threshold for the left ear by a blue "X." Even less agreed upon are the symbols for bone conduction and masking. However, the symbol] is often used for bone conduction in the right ear, and [for bone conduction in the left ear. When masking is used, the amount of masking should be noted somewhere on the audiogram. The individual audiogram must have printed on it a key to the symbols used.

The hearing level numbers along the ordinate are often read as "hearing loss" since they represent not only the level of the tone relative to normal hearing, but also the amount of loss of sensitivity for the individual patient. If a tone must be raised to 40 dB on the dial (HL) in order to reach a patient's threshold, then the patient has a 40-dB hearing loss for that frequency.

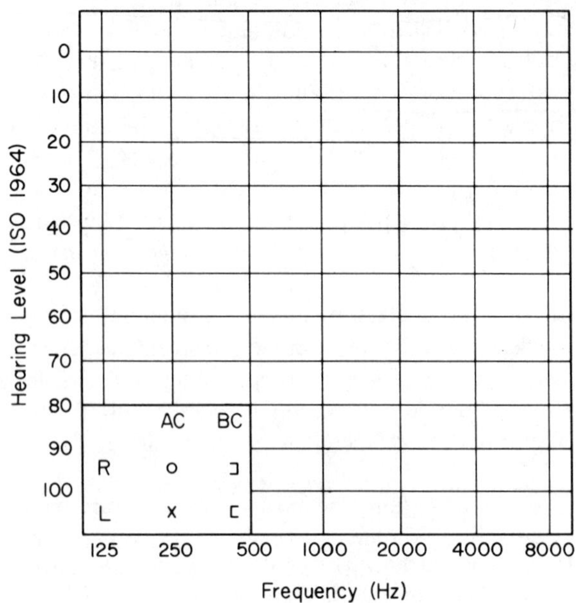

FIGURE 6.1 A typical audiogram form showing frequency along the abcissa and hearing level along the ordinate. Zero represents average normal hearing on the international scale (ISO. 1964).

Reference Levels in Audiometry

Three terms, each referring to a different starting or reference point, are used to specify sound stimulus levels in pure-tone audiometry. These are SOUND PRESSURE LEVEL (SPL), HEARING LEVEL (HL), and SENSATION LEVEL (SL). Since these often prove to be a source of confusion, it is suggested that the student take the time to get them sufficiently clear in his thinking. SPL (sound pressure level) is a physical measure whose reference point is 0.0002 dynes of pressure per square centimeter (dyne/cm^2). This reference point is the same for any and all sounds measured in SPL. When a sound is 25 dB SPL, it is 25 dB above 0.0002 dyne/cm^2.

The ear is not equally sensitive at all frequencies, however, and a 50-dB

SPL tone at 125 Hz will not be nearly so easily heard as a 50-dB SPL tone at 1,000 Hz. Therefore, a weighting system has been developed and built into standard audiometers to make all test frequencies equally loud at a given point that approximates the normal threshold of hearing. This weighting was originally based primarily on Beasley's (2) survey on normal hearing subjects for the U. S. Public Health Service. Figure 6.2 shows the average SPL at each frequency that Beasley found would just elicit a response from the thousands of persons tested. The American Standards Association (ASA) in 1951 took Beasley's data and made it the standard from which to calibrate audiometers and to measure hearing loss. Thus, by ASA 1951 standards, any point on the curve in Figure 6.2 represented 0 dB hearing level at that particular frequency. Note that at 125 Hz, our 50-dB SPL tone would still be below the normal threshold while the 1,000 Hz tone would be about 35 dB above the threshold. Thus, 0 dB HL, the zero on audiometer attenuator dials, is different at each frequency if sound pressure level is measured.

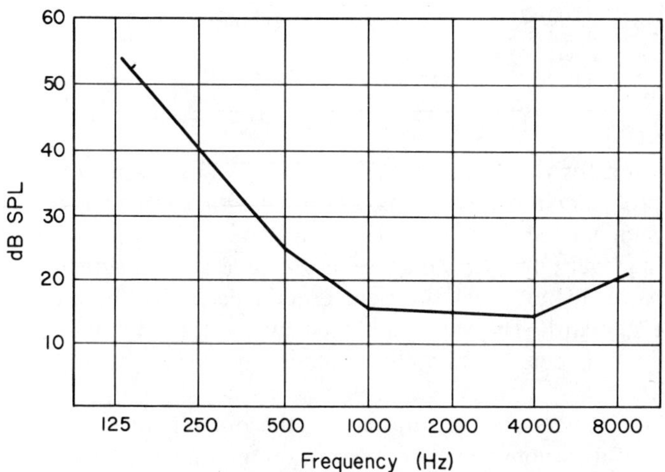

FIGURE 6.2 A curve showing absolute threshold sensitivity in dB SPL for the average ear at different frequencies according to the ASA 1951 standard.

A number of studies carried out in this country and in Europe (26, 8) suggests that the ASA 1951 standard does not properly reflect the average hearing thresholds for young normal hearing adults tested in a laboratory environment. As a result of these studies, Great Britain, and most other European nations, adopted a more stringent standard than that in use in the United States. Because of the discrepancy between American and British standards, the International Organization for Standardization (ISO) reviewed the situation and in 1964 adopted a standard which very nearly approximates Great Britain's. Most other countries of the world have adopted the ISO 1964 standard; however, the American Standards Association has not yet accepted it. The American Speech and Hearing Association (ASHA) and most American medical professional associations have adopted the ISO 1964 standard. As a result, two standards are currently in use in the United States. Table 6.1 shows the ASA 1951 values, the ISO 1964 values (9), and the difference between the two standards.

TABLE 6.1. THRESHOLD OF NORMAL HEARING (DB RE 0.0002 DYNE/CM^2) BY ASA 1951 AND ISO 1964 STANDARDS

Frequency	*ASA 1951*	*ISO 1964*	*Difference*
125	54.5	45.5	9
250	39.5	24.5	15
500	25	11	14
1,000	16.5	6.5	10
1,500	16.5	6.5	10
2,000	17	8.5	8.5
3,000	16	7.5	8.5
4,000	15	9	6
6,000	17.5	8	9.5
8,000	21	9.5	11.5

The reason for the acceptance of the ISO 1964 standard in the United States by professional organizations concerned with hearing and its disorders has been summarized by Glorig (14) as follows: "The original 1951 ASA zero hearing level reference values were obtained from a survey type study and, therefore do not meet the rigid criteria necessary for establishing a worldwide standard. The values accepted by the ISO in 1964 do meet the most rigid criteria possible, and, therefore, are suitable for use as a worldwide standard."

Since these two standards do exist at the present time, the audiologist must be careful to note which he is using on any audiogram that he might make, and to take note of what was used by others when interpreting or comparing his data with previous audiograms. Figure 6.3 is an audiogram showing the same absolute hearing loss plotted against the ASA 1951 and the ISO 1964 standards.

SENSATION LEVEL (SL) refers to the hearing of a given individual at a given instant. Its reference is the threshold of the individual in question. Thus 40-dB SL means 40 dB above the specific threshold, no matter what the threshold might be. The term sensation level is often used in specifying the level at which speech discrimination tests (Chapter 7) and other diagnostic tests (Chapter 10) are administered. For example, a speech discrimination test may be administered at 40-dB SL; that is, at 40 dB above the given individual's threshold for speech.

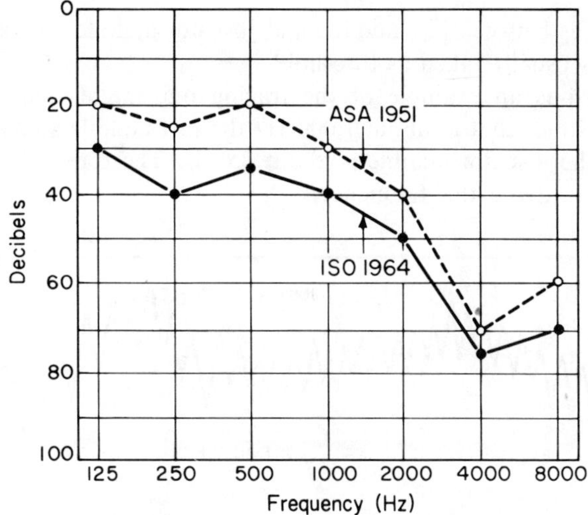

FIGURE 6.3 Audiogram showing same absolute loss of sensitivity as it would be reflected on the ASA 1951 and the ISO 1964 standards.

Psychophysical Methods in Pure-Tone Audiometry

Clinical pure-tone audiometry usually employs one of two psychophysical methods. These are the METHOD OF LIMITS, usually in a somewhat modified form, and the METHOD OF ADJUSTMENT. With the method of limits, the tester has control of the stimulus and the patient simply observes and reports. The tester gradually increases the intensity of the stimulus, usually in serial steps, until the observer reports that he hears the stimulus. This procedure is sometimes referred to as an ASCENDING METHOD OF LIMITS because the intensity of the tone increases or ascends with each stimulus presentation.

A DESCENDING METHOD OF LIMITS is also commonly employed. With this procedure the tester presents a stimulus that is easily heard and serially decreases the intensity with each tonal presentation until the observer no longer reports hearing the tone. In both ascending and descending methods the process is repeated several times and the lowest level at which the observer reports hearing the tone 50 per cent of the time is taken as threshold of hearing at that frequency. Most clinical audiologists use some combination of an ascending and a descending method of limits in their clinical work.

In the method of adjustment, the observer usually has control of the intensity of the stimulus. It is his responsibility to adjust the intensity of the stimulus until it is just barely audible. In general clinical practice, the observer is given a switch which controls a motor-driven recording attenuator. He is instructed to manipulate the switch so that the continuously changing stimulus varies between just audible and just not audible. A mean of these two values is usually taken as threshold.

Figure 6.4 is an example of the tracing one might obtain using this technique. Notice that at about 1,000 Hz the just audible stimulus is about 35 dB and the just not audible is about 25 dB. The threshold then would be taken as 30 dB at this frequency.

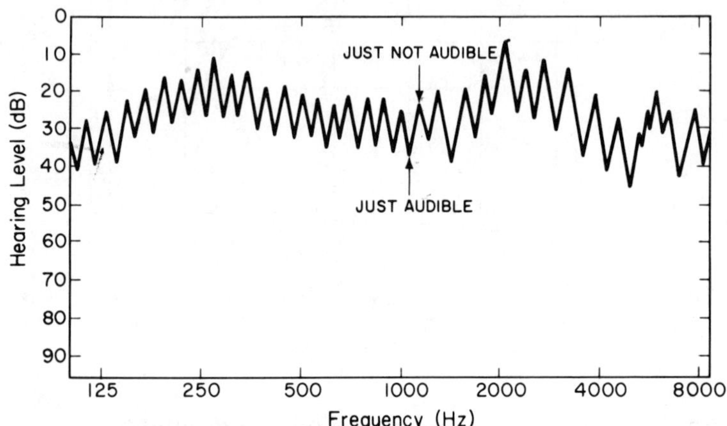

FIGURE 6.4 Example of a threshold tracing using the method of adjustment on an automatic audiometer.

Air-Conduction Hearing

Sounds, as we normally hear them, are the result of air pressure changes that strike the tympanic membrane. These pressure changes move the membrane, to which are attached the ossicles of the middle ear, and set the ossicular chain into vibration. When the footplate of the stapes moves, relative to the oval window of the cochlea, pressure waves are set up in the fluids of the cochlea and the sensory receptors of the inner ear are stimulated. Sounds which enter the external ear canal as air pressure changes are said to be heard by air conduction (*see* Chapter 2).

When we test a patient's hearing by air conduction, we place earphones over his ears and set up pressure changes in the air of the external ear canal by electronically producing a vibration of the diaphragm of the earphone. We determine the smallest change in pressure that the patient can detect 50 per cent of the time and record this as his threshold of hearing for air-conducted sound. The air-conduction threshold tells us how well the entire auditory system is functioning with respect to sensitivity. A malfunction affecting the sensitivity of any part of the auditory system will be reflected as a loss of hearing by air conduction.

Bone-Conduction Hearing

There is an alternative path by which sound can reach the cochlea. When sound vibrations reach an intensity of 40 to 50 dB above the normal air-conduction threshold, they may set the skull into vibration. Since the cochleas are imbedded within the skull, vibrations of the skull also vibrate the cochlea and set up pressure waves in the cochlear fluids.

The works of Bekesy (5) and Kirikae (20) have been especially significant in revealing the sound-stimulated vibrational patterns of the skull. Their work is in good agreement that at low frequencies the skull vibrates as a unit and its movement is parallel to the driving direction of the bone-conduction receiver. At frequencies of about 800 Hz and above, however, the skull begins vibrating in segments such that, as the forehead is driven backward, the back of the head moves forward, and vice versa, producing compressional and flexural forces within the skull. As a result of these two types of vibrational pattern, there are two primary methods by which sounds transmitted by bone conduction stimulate the sensation of hearing. These are INERTIAL and COMPRESSIONAL.

At low frequencies, when the skull is vibrating as a unit, structures which are loosely attached to it will tend to lag behind the skull due to their inertia. This is true of the ossicular chain, the mandible, and probably the cochlear fluids (20) and cranial contents (19). The lagging of the ossicular chain produces movement of the stapes relative to the oval window of the cochlea and stimulates hearing exactly as in air-conduction stimulation. The lagging of the mandible relative to the rest of the skull may help to produce, when the external ear is covered, a phenomenon known as the occlusion effect. This phenomenon will be discussed in more detail later.

Jahn (19) has suggested that the intracranial contents are free to move within the skull and that this relative movement may be transmitted to the cochlea through the internal auditory meatus. Kirikae (20) has pointed out that since there is a difference between the mass of the fluids present on the two sides of the basilar membrane, and since the round window yields more readily to pressure than the oval window (which is filled with the footplate of the stapes), inertia of the inner-ear fluids may cause the fluids to move toward and away from the round window and produce stimulation along the basilar membrane. It should be pointed out that any movement of the basilar membrane relative to the surrounding tissues and fluids may stimulate a sensation of hearing.

In compressional bone conduction, the primary factor is the difference in mobility of the round and oval windows. When the compressional and flexural forces of the skull are transmitted to the inner ear, they act on the noncompressible fluids of the inner ear, vestibule, and semicircular canals and cause these fluids to move toward or away from the more mobile round window, depending upon the phase of the wave. This fluid movement may result in deformations of the basilar membrane sufficient to stimulate the sensation of hearing.

While earlier theory tended to relegate low-frequency hearing exclusively to inertial factors, and high-frequency hearing exclusively to compressional factors, it is now felt that stimulation at all frequencies is probably due to some combination of the two. In all probability, there are additional contributing factors; however, these have not been adequately demonstrated as of yet.

It has been demonstrated (3) that a sound transmitted by air conduction and one transmitted by bone conduction have essentially the same effect at the cochlea. In other words, there are not separate sensory receptor systems for air- and bone-conducted sounds. However, bone-conduction tests are designed to measure a different aspect of hearing than are air-conduction tests. They are an attempt to determine to what extent a given hearing loss is due to an external- or middle-ear breakdown (CONDUCTIVE LOSS) and to what extent the loss is due to an inner-ear or neural system dysfunction (SENSORI-NEURAL LOSS).

In bone-conduction audiometry a bone-conduction receiver is placed either on the mastoid process of the temporal bone or on the forehead. This receiver can be vibrated electronically and will in turn vibrate the skull. Earphones are not used in bone-conduction testing except for delivering a masking noise to the untested ear in the event that masking is needed.

INTERAURAL ATTENUATION (IA) is the term applied to the attenuation in intensity of a sound stimulus when crossing from the ear being tested to the opposite ear. The exact value of the interaural attenuation will vary with the method of testing, the frequency being tested, and the sound conduction characteristics of the head in question. In both air- and bone-conduction tests the sound stimulus which crosses to the untested ear does so by bone conduction (32). The interaural attenuation for air-conducted sound, then, may be essentially the same as the difference in energy necessary to stimulate hearing by air and by bone conduction.

Table 6.2 shows the minimum and maximum values of the interaural attenuation obtained by Liden et al., (22). These authors determined thresholds on seventeen monaurally deaf subjects with the earphone on the nonfunctioning ear. Their values thus reflect the loss of energy of the air-conducted signal in crossing the head by bone conduction to the good ear. From Table 6.2 we see that the minimum interaural attenuation for air is 40 to 50 dB.

For bone-conducted sound the interaural attenuation may vary from a negative value up to about 20 dB. This is due to the fact that in bone conduction, the skull vibrates as a unit to low-frequency sounds, and there is no reason to believe that the two cochleas, both embedded in the same skull, will not be equally stimulated. In the higher frequencies, where the compressional factors become more important, a small interaural attenuation factor can often be demonstrated; however, it is not completely predictable. In clinical practice it is safest to assume that there is no interaural attenuation for bone-conducted sound.

TABLE 6.2. DECIBEL VALUES OF THE RANGES OF THE INTERAURAL ATTENUATION (IA) ACROSS SEVENTEEN MONAURALLY DEAF SUBJECTS AS DETERMINED BY LIDEN ET AL., (22)

	Frequency (Hz)						
	125	250	500	1,000	2,000	4,000	8,000
IA Range	40–75	45–75	50–70	45–70	45–75	45–75	45–80

The Occlusion Effect

As mentioned earlier, the mandible is loosely hinged to the skull and, due to its inertia, may lag behind the skull when the latter is vibrated by bone-conducted sound. Since the condyle of the mandible articulates with the skull just forward of the cartilaginous external auditory meatus, this relative movement of the mandible to the rest of the skull may produce a slight bulging in and out of the canal wall and thus cause air pressure changes in the external ear canal. If the ear canal is open and uncovered, most of the pressure takes the path of least resistance and escapes into the atmosphere. However, if the ear is covered, or OCCLUDED, the path of least resistance may be in the direction of the tympanic membrane and the pressure waves may be of sufficient magnitude to be heard as air-conducted sound.

The occlusion effect should not be thought of as a change in the bone-conduction threshold. The threshold is a point at which the physical energy reaches the level sufficient to stimulate the observer into an awareness of its presence. This level for awareness does not change appreciably as a result of occluding the ear. What does change is the level of the stimulus reaching the inner ear. Thus, the threshold does not change due to the occlusion effect; the observed change in hearing is the result of additional energy being delivered to the sensory receptors of the inner ear.

The occlusion effect may change bone-conduction measures by as much as 25 to 30 dB in the low frequencies with continuously less effect as the frequency is increased. Figure 6.5 shows the approximate values of the occlusion effect reported by Goldstein and Hayes (15). Elpern and Naunton (11) reported average values slightly larger than those of Goldstein and Hayes, and that the effect has a great deal of variability. The occlusion effect is an important factor to be kept in mind when testing by bone conduction and when masking. More will be said about it in the following section on masking.

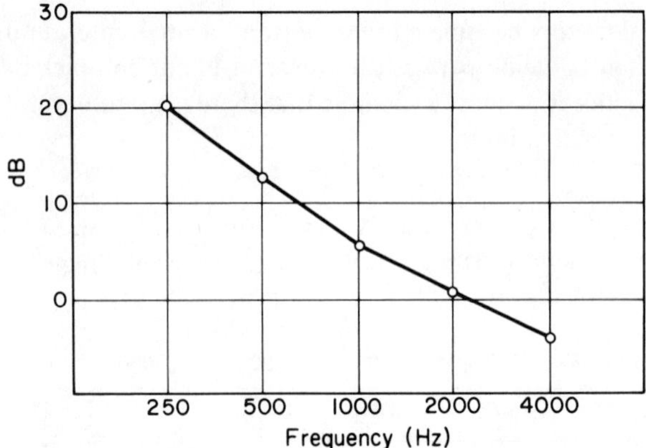

FIGURE 6.5 The amount that bone-conduction measures are enhanced by occluding the ears (from data of Goldstein and Hayes, 1965).

Masking

It is critical that the audiologist test each ear without the participation of the other ear, if he expects to be able to say anything about the hearing of either ear individually. There are test situations in which the primary question involves the patient's ability to use both ears as an integrating auditory system. This is not the case in pure-tone audiometry, however, and the clinician must take every precaution to insure that when he records results from the right ear, he has actually tested the right ear.

The necessity of isolating the test ear becomes obvious if we take another look at bone conduction. You will recall that the skull vibrates as a unit to low-frequency sounds. Thus, the two cochleas, imbedded within the same skull, should be stimulated approximately equally regardless of whether the receiver is on the same (ipsilateral) or opposite (contralateral) side of the head. The necessity for isolating the test ear also arises in air-conduction measures when there is a sizeable difference between the sensitivity of the two ears or when both ears have a conductive hearing loss.

As we have already seen, air-conducted sounds may reach sufficient energy to stimulate the skull directly (bone conduction) at from 40 to 50-dB HL depending upon the frequency of the sound (*see* Table 6.2). Thus, at levels above 40-dB HL, air-conducted sounds may be intense enough to vibrate the skull sufficiently to stimulate the more sensitive cochlea, irrespective of which ear the earphone is covering. Therefore, in both air- and bone-conduction pure-tone testing, some procedure must be employed to prevent the untested ear from participating when the sensitivity of the test ear is being measured. We use a masking noise in the untested ear to accomplish this.

TYPES OF MASKING NOISE

The standard procedure for clinical masking is to place an earphone over the untested ear and introduce a noise sufficiently loud so that if the test tone should cross to that ear, it will not be perceived. The intensity to which the masking noise must be raised depends, in part, upon the effectiveness of that noise in masking the test stimulus.

There are three general types of masking noise available on commercial audiometers today (depending on the make and model of the audiometer). These are (a) complex noise, (b) white noise, and (c) narrow-band noise. The complex noises include sawtooth, square wave, and other similar noises that are composed of a base frequency (often the line frequency of 60 or 120 Hz) and amplified multiples of that frequency. This noise has a buzzing-like quality and masks most effectively in the lower frequencies where its greatest energy is located.

White noise, in its theoretical form, contains all frequencies within the auditory spectrum at equal average energy. The white noise available audiometrically is limited to the band-pass characteristics of the earphone, however, and should more properly be referred to as BROAD BAND NOISE. This broad band noise does contain approximately equal absolute energy at the pure-tone test frequencies, and as a result, is most effective as a masking noise in the middle and upper frequencies where the ear is most sensitive.

Experimentation with narrow bands of white noise in audiometry came about as a result of Fletcher's (13) concepts concerning the CRITICAL BAND. This concept holds that only the energy in the noise in the frequency band

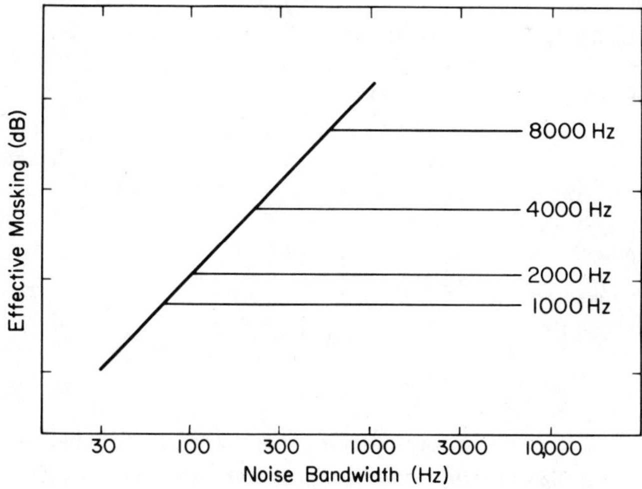

FIGURE 6.6 Curves showing masking effects of noise as a function of noise bandwidth (based on data of Fletcher, 1940).

immediately surrounding the test frequency contributes to the masking of that frequency. Figure 6.6 shows a set of curves, patterned after Fletcher's data, showing the effective masking levels of noise as a function of the noise bandwidth. For example, at 2,000 Hz, note that the effectiveness of the noise increases with increases in bandwidth up to about 100 Hz. As the band increases beyond 100 Hz, however, no further increase in effective masking occurs. Thus, the critical band at 2,000 Hz is 100 Hz wide and is centered at 2,000 Hz. This band contains the energy which actually masks the tone, irrespective of the overall bandwidth of the noise. The energy in the rest of a broad band noise, even though it does not contribute to the masking of the tone, does contribute to the overall intensity level of the noise. When higher levels of masking noise are needed, this excess energy may create a loudness level which is uncomfortable or fatiguing to the patient.

Saunders and Rintelmann (25) measured the effectiveness of three types of noise by putting given levels of the noises into the same ear on which they were determining thresholds for pure tones. Table 6.3 shows an approximation of the effective masking levels which they obtained for the various types of noise, each at 90-dB SPL. It is readily apparent that the narrow bands of noise centered at the test frequency are by far the most efficient method of masking. On the basis of this, and other such evidence (29), many audiologists have begun using narrow bands of noise for clinical masking. Commercial manufacturers have responded to this thinking and as a result, many audiometers now come equipped with narrow-band masking noise. In addition, a number of narrow-band masking generators are available commercially which can be used with any audiometer.

TABLE 6.3. AMOUNT OF MASKING OF PURE TONES PRODUCED BY A 90-DB SPL OF THREE TYPES OF NOISE (AFTER SAUNDERS AND RINTELMANN, 1964)

	Frequency (Hz)				
Noise Type	250	500	1,000	2,000	4,000
Sawtooth	32	32	32	15	11
White	30	43	53	55	62
Narrow-Band	51	59	69	66	73

WHEN TO MASK

Of course, it is not always necessary to mask (only when there is the possibility of cross hearing) and the questions of when to mask and how much masking noise to use are ones that many clinicians find troublesome. A number of authorities have derived formulas for determining the answers to these questions; however, if the clinician understands the concepts involved, and has the data necessary to insert into the formulas, he has the answers already and the use of the formulas becomes largely an academic exercise.

There is some disagreement on what determines the need for masking. The suggestions outlined in this chapter take a conservative approach and may sometimes result in the use of masking when it is not needed. However, the use of masking when it is not needed is a much less serious problem than not using it when it is needed, and adherence to the following suggestions will result in the fewest number of serious mistakes. The question of when to mask can be answered thusly: in air-conduction tests, masking should be used anytime the air-conduction threshold in the ear being tested exceeds the bone-conduction threshold in the untested ear by 40 dB or more. This 40 dB is the *minimum* interaural attenuation. As Table 6.2 suggests, one can often exceed this value considerably without the signal reaching the threshold of the untested ear. However, the conservative approach taken in this chapter would stress working with minimum values, since we have no way of predicting in advance the interaural attenuation for any given patient. In bone-conduction tests, masking should be used anytime bone-conduction thresholds are better than air-conduction thresholds. These statements will be amplified in the following paragraphs.

As already stated, an air-conducted signal may start to stimulate the entire skull by bone conduction at intensities above 40-dB HL. If this happens the untested ear may begin to participate in the test. However, the untested ear can only participate if the sound stimulus is above its threshold. Thus, the threshold value for bone-conducted sound at the test frequency in the untested ear can be added to the 40 dB of attenuation provided by the head. The following example illustrates this point:

	1,000 Hz		*2,000 Hz*	
	A–C	*B–C*	*A–C*	*B–C*
Right Ear	50 dB↘		60 dB	
Left Ear		0 dB		30 dB

At 1,000 Hz this patient's right ear shows an air-conduction hearing loss 50 dB greater than the bone-conduction loss in the left ear. This 50-dB value could very easily be the threshold for bone conduction in the left ear plus the interaural attenuation. Thus, as the arrow suggests, the 50-dB air-conduction signal in the right ear may be heard in the left ear via bone conduction. The only way to determine whether this is happening is to retest the right ear while masking the left.

At 2,000 Hz, however, we can be confident that the threshold of 60 dB for air conduction in the right ear is a measure of the sensitivity of that ear and not a SHADOW CURVE of the left ear. We know that it takes at least 40 dB of air-conducted sound to stimulate bone-conduction hearing, so that the intensity of the bone-conducted sound can be no greater than 20 dB when the air-conducted stimulus is 60 dB. Thus, in this case, the left ear which has a bone-conduction threshold of 30 dB could not be responding to a stimulus that is at least 10 dB below threshold. The air-conducted stimulus in the right ear would have to be at least 70 dB before it could be heard by the left ear. Thus the rule: take the bone-conduction threshold of the untested ear, add 40 dB, and if the air-conduction threshold in the test ear equals or exceeds this sum, the untested ear *must* be masked.

Theoretically, bone-conduction thresholds should never be higher than air-conduction thresholds for the same frequency in the same ear. This is true since air-conduction thresholds reflect the cumulative loss of sensitivity of the entire auditory system, while bone-conduction thresholds reflect the loss of sensitivity of only part of the auditory system. Theory and practice are not always in agreement, however, and the clinician will sometimes see patients who have bone-conduction thresholds somewhat higher than air-conduction thresholds. This is especially true for the lower frequencies. In these cases there is a temptation for the clinician to "fudge" a bit or excessively badger the patient until practice more nearly approaches theory. This is not recommended. To alter one's test results not only raises the question of professional ethics but may also obscure important implications for research, and the uncovering of new theories which better explain the observations.

The air-bone gap in the wrong direction, i.e., bone conduction poorer than air conduction, is not an indication that masking is needed when testing by bone conduction. The air-bone gap which shows air conduction poorer than bone conduction does indicate the need for masking. Let us illustrate this with another example:

	1,000 Hz		*2,000 Hz*	
	A–C	*B–C*	*A–C*	*B–C*
Right Ear	60 dB	10 dB	70 dB	20 dB
		↑ ↓		↓ ↑
Left Ear	30 dB	10 dB	50 dB	20 dB

It is possible here that the right ear is totally deaf. There is a 50-dB difference between the air-conduction measures in the right ear and the bone-conduction thresholds in the left. Thus the patient could be perceiving the air-conducted tone on the right side by the left ear via bone-conduction. The bone-conduction responses in the right ear could also be a reflection of the bone-conduction thresholds in the left ear. You will recall that there is little, if any, loss of energy across the head in bone-conduction hearing. Thus, we could have a mild-to-moderate mixed hearing loss (a loss with both a conductive and a sensori-neural component) in the left ear and as much as a total loss of sensitivity in the right ear.

There is a second very distinct possibility, however. It is quite possible that the right ear has a moderate mixed hearing loss and that the left ear has a mild-to-moderate sensory-neural loss. The bone-conduction values from the left ear could reflect the cochlear sensitivity of the right ear.

Still a third possibility is that both ears have a mixed type of hearing loss. With more definitive testing the hearing levels for the two ears might look like this:

	1,000 Hz		*2,000 Hz*	
	A–C	*B–C*	*A–C*	*B–C*
Right Ear	70 dB	30 dB	80 dB	40 dB
Left Ear	30 dB	10 dB	50 dB	20 dB

There is only one way to learn which of the above possibilities (if either) is the true one. This is to effectively eliminate the untested ear from participating during the testing of the other ear—in other words, to mask.

DETERMINING MASKING LEVELS

The first step in determining how much masking noise to use is to determine the effectiveness of the noise to be used. This can be done by switching both the noise and the pulsing pure-tone signal into the same earphone and by determining the threshold for the tone on several subjects at several levels of the masking noise. Studebaker (27) suggests plotting a median of the obtained data on a graph such as Figure 6.7. Draw a vertical line connecting the abcissa with the plotted line at a point where the plotted line approximates a 45° angle, and then a horizontal line from this intersection to the ordinate. The MINIMUM MASKING LEVEL is defined as the difference between the point on the abcissa and the point on the ordinate marked off by the two lines. In other words, the minimum masking level is the difference between the level of the tone and the noise level just sufficient to mask that tone. The minimum masking level in the example given in Figure 6.7 is 20 dB. This minimum masking level is the level to which the noise must be raised before any masking takes place and therefore must be added to any calculated value of masking needed. As Studebaker (27) has pointed out, in order to just mask the test tone crossing to the masked ear, the noise level reaching the masked cochlea must exceed the level of the test tone reaching the masked cochlea by the amount of the minimum masking level. Determination of minimum masking levels must be carried out for each test frequency, since any given noise may not mask all frequencies equally.

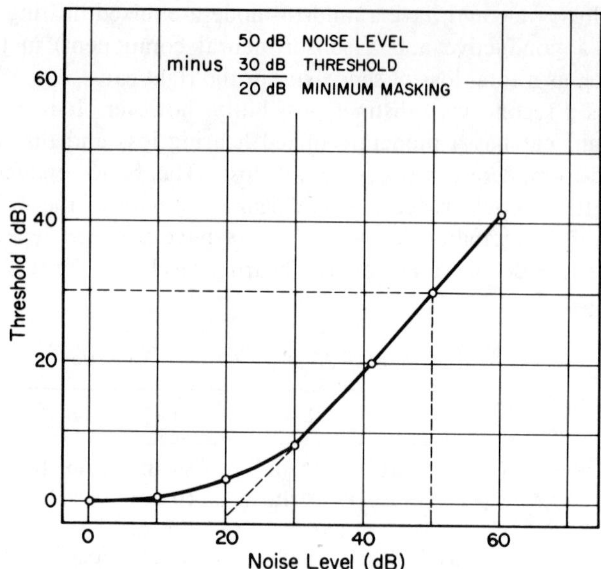

FIGURE 6.7 Relationships between threshold for a pure tone and the level of the masking noise to the same ear. The minimum masking level in this example is 20 dB.

The term EFFECTIVE MASKING should be introduced at this point. Suppose, for example, that we wished to mask a 40-dB tone of 1,000 Hz and that we had previously determined the minimum masking level to be 20 dB at 1,000 Hz. We must add the 20 dB to the 40 dB in order to get the desired amount of masking. Thus we have 60 dB of masking noise, but only 40 dB of effective masking. The overall level of the noise minus the minimum masking level gives effective masking level.

In order to determine the proper level of masking for a particular test situation, one must add the level of the test tone reaching the cochlea of the untested ear to the minimum masking level. For example, if the tone is reaching the untested ear at 30 dB and the minimum masking level is 20 dB, it will take an overall noise level of at least 50 dB to prevent the untested ear from participating in the test. In addition, any factor that strengthens the test signal reaching the untested ear (such as the increase in signal strength in the untested ear resulting from covering that ear with the masking phone, i.e., the occlusion effect) or interferes with the strength of the masking noise reaching the cochlea of the untested ear (such as a conductive hearing loss in the untested ear) must be taken into consideration.

Studebaker (27) has pointed out that it is the signal-to-noise ratio of the two stimuli (test tone and masking noise) at the cochlea of the untested ear that must be considered. A sensori-neural hearing loss (bone-conduction loss equal to air-conduction loss) in the untested ear will not change the signal-to-noise ratio since the signal and the noise will be equally attenuated. A conductive loss (bone-conduction hearing better than air-conduction hearing) in the untested ear, however, will affect the signal-to-noise ratio. This is due to the fact that the signal is being heard by bone conduction, which is not affected, while the noise is being presented by air conduction, which is. This change in the signal-to-noise ratio can be compensated for by adding the amount of the air-bone gap (air-conduction threshold minus bone-conduction threshold) to the level of the masking noise.

The occlusion effect generally is not observable in the ear with a conductive loss of hearing. This is due to the fact that the small changes in air pressure in the external ear canal caused by the occlusion effect are not sufficiently intense to overcome the conductive component of the hearing loss. For example, a 20-dB signal in the external ear canal will not be heard if there is a breakdown in the sound-conducting apparatus of the middle ear that results in more than a 20-dB hearing loss. As a result, the occlusion effects and the air-bone gap usually do not occur simultaneously and thus do not need to be compensated for in the same ear.

We can summarize by stating that the proper level of the masking noise should be the minimum masking level plus the level of the tone reaching the cochlea of the untested ear plus the amount of the occlusion effect if the untested ear is normal or has a sensori-neural hearing loss. If the untested ear has a conductive hearing loss, the level of the noise should be the minimum masking level plus the level of the tone reaching the cochlea plus the amount of the air-bone gap.

The above method for determining the level of masking works well when one knows or is able to determine the values of all the variables involved. Unfortunately, these variables are not always easily determined and a more clinically useful method of finding the proper masking level is needed. The most satisfactory approach is based primarily on the suggestions of Hood (18) and Studebaker (27) and is sometimes referred to as "plateau seeking."

In plateau seeking, one introduces the masking noise at the minimum masking level and then measures the threshold. Then the noise level is increased in 10-dB steps and a measure of the threshold taken at each step. Initially, if the tone is being heard in the untested ear, the threshold measures in the test ear should increase as the noise levels in the untested ear are increased. At some point, however, the threshold should stop increasing with increases in the masking noise, and at a somewhat higher intensity of the noise, the threshold should again show increases with increases in the noise. Thus one obtains a curve with a plateau similar to that shown in Figure 6.8.

The point at which threshold stopped increasing with increases in the masking noise is the smallest amount of masking that will effectively mask the signal crossing to the untested ear. The point at which threshold again started increasing is the maximum amount of masking that can be used without danger of overmasking. Any level between these two values should be a safe level of masking for the particular frequency for which the curve was established. If hearing levels in both ears are relatively flat across frequencies, and if the noise is calibrated in effective masking units, this one level may prove adequate for testing all frequencies in that ear. If the hearing on either each changes much as a function of frequency, however, or if the noise is not equally effective at masking all frequencies, the proper level of masking must be determined for each frequency.

The width of the plateau established by the above technique is equal to the interaural attenuation minus the occlusion effect, if the mask ear is normal or has a sensori-neural hearing loss. In the mask ear with a conductive loss, the width of the plateau is equal to the interaural attenuation minus the air-bone gap. Both the occlusion effect and the air-bone gap raise the minimum noise level necessary for effective masking, but neither raise the maximum permissible masking. This is true since the minimum necessary masking is a function of the untested ear while the maximum permissible masking is a function of the test ear. If the air-bone gap in the mask ear exceeds the interaural attenuation, the plateau is not detectable and the use of masking becomes questionable. In this case the validity of test results is suspect.

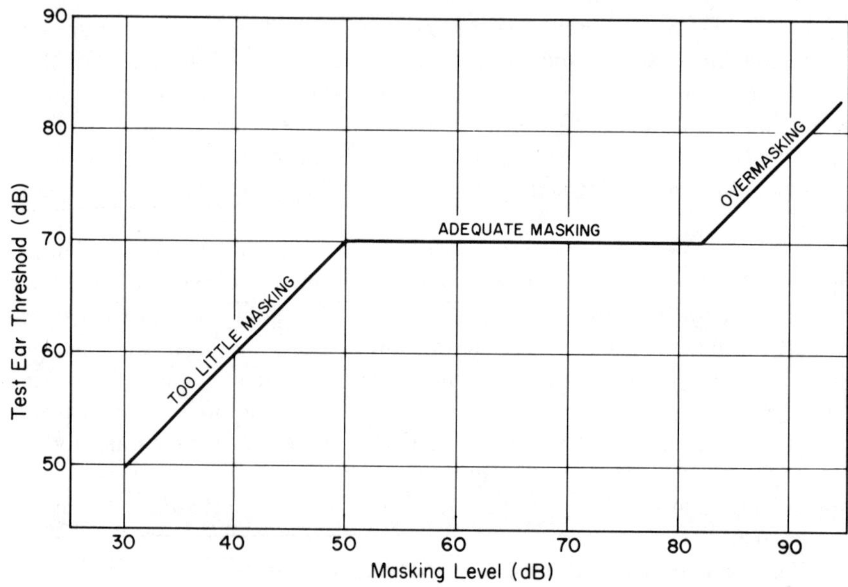

FIGURE 6.8 Effects on threshold of the test ear of masking in the untested ear.

OVERMASKING

When a masking noise reaches an intensity sufficient to stimulate hearing by bone conduction, it may be heard in either ear (or both) if bone-conduction thresholds are normal. If the masking noise level exceeds the interaural attenuation by the minimum masking level, and if the ear under test has a normal bone-conduction threshold, it is possible that the ear under test is also being masked. This is an especially troublesome problem in bilateral conductive hearing losses, where it sometimes proves impossible to mask one ear without masking the other. The following example illustrates this point:

	A–C	*B–C*
Right Ear	50 dB	0 dB
Left Ear	50 dB	0 dB

According to our rule about when to mask, we should use masking in this instance since there is more than a 40-dB difference between the air-conduction threshold of one ear and the bone-conduction threshold of the other. However, the masking noise will not be heard until it reaches at least 50-dB HL, and at this level, it is heard by bone conduction. Thus, the masking noise may reach both cochleas with equal effectiveness and both ears may be equally masked.

There is no simple solution to this dilemma although one possible approach has been suggested by the works of Feldman (12), Littler et al., (21), Studebaker (28), and Zwislocki (32). These investigators have shown that the interaural attenuation can be increased about 15 dB by reducing the area of contact between the earphone and the head. The usual procedure for doing this has been to use insert-type earphones—that is, small hearing-aid type receivers that fit onto a mold of the external ear and canal. This extra 15 dB of interaural attenuation could reduce substantially the number of cases where masking proves to be impossible.

The major problem involved with using insert phones is the matter of calibration. There are no standards for calibration at the present time and the audiologist would have to rely on clinical calibrations, using normal hearing subjects to establish his own norms. This presents a substantial roadblock to the use of inserts for introducing the test stimulus. However, there should be no real drawback to using an insert phone for delivering the masking noise to the untested ear. The minimum masking level could be determined as well for the insert phone as for the standard phone. This, of course, would not increase the interaural attenuation for the test tone, but it would allow the use of about 15 dB more masking before overmasking occurred, and would permit the effective use of masking in a number of cases where it might not otherwise be possible.

In those instances where it proves impossible to mask, the audiologist must rely on all his skill, experience, and knowledge of special tests in his attempts to determine accurate estimates of hearing sensitivity. Above all, he must be prepared to record any questions he may have concerning the validity of his findings and be able to say "I don't know" when all else fails.

Factors Influencing Threshold Measures

There are a number of factors which can influence measures of the pure-tone threshold. The clinician should be aware of these and take the necessary steps to minimize them or compensate for their effects.

INSTRUCTIONS TO THE PATIENT

Many patients are reluctant to admit the presence of a tone until it becomes loud enough to be easily heard. Others guess wildly and almost drive the tester to madness with "false" responses. It is important that we make the criteria for judgment as nearly alike in all patients as possible. This can be done through careful counseling during the instruction period just prior to testing. The exact phrasing of the instructions are not as important as making sure that certain concepts are understood. The clinician should use whatever means are necessary, including pantomime and example, to get the following ideas across:

1. The sounds will be very soft but the patient is to report each one that he hears or thinks he hears.
2. The patient is to report when the tone comes on and when it goes off. The usual procedure is for the patient to raise a finger when the sound comes on and lower it when the sound goes off.
3. The patient is to indicate the ear in which he hears the sound. He should signal with the right hand for the right ear, the left hand for the left ear, and with both hands if he hears the sound but cannot definitely localize it to either ear.

In order to make sure that the patient understands what he is to do, the audiologist should ask him to repeat the instructions. The time spent in instructing the patient and in making sure that he understands what is expected of him pays off handsomely in improved reliability and validity of test results.

DURATION OF STIMULUS

The ear, and particularly the ear with neural pathology, will adapt to a prolonged pure tone. This means that a tone which is audible when first presented, if left on for a prolonged period of time, will gradually become less audible because of adaptive changes in the auditory system. This ADAPTATION occurs much less noticeably if the stimulus is changing, and especially if this changing is of an "on" and "off" nature. It is suggested, therefore, that an unchanging tone never be left on for more than one second at a time. In fact, it is preferable to test using a pulsed tone. Most clinical audiometers have a switch setting which automatically pulses the tone when the clinician introduces the signal with the interrupter switch.

TEST ENVIRONMENT

Needless to say, any test of hearing should be carried out in as quiet an environment as possible. Noise in a test room will appear to raise the threshold because of the masking effects of the noise on the test ear. In addition to a quiet room, the clinician should eliminate as many other distractions as possible. Excessive heat due to poor ventilation in sound-treated rooms may make the patient uncomfortable or drowsy. Unusual visual stimulation may also prove distracting. For best results, keep the test environment simple, quiet, and cool.

METHOD OF OBTAINING THRESHOLD

When the method of limits is used for establishing the threshold, one finds some difference between a descending and an ascending approach to the threshold. This difference is not large on the average but usually the threshold established by a descending method is lower, provided a short duration or pulsed tone is used (17). This is likely due to perseveration to the descending, and inhibition to the ascending stimulus.

In automatic audiometry (method of adjustment), the rate of attenuation affects threshold. For a pulsed tone an attenuation speed of about 2.5 dB per second appears to yield a threshold that is in good agreement with threshold established by the method of limits (24). This may not apply to a nonpulsed tone, however. In fact, there is often a difference between thresholds for a pulsed tone and a threshold for the same tone when presented as a continuous stimulus. This difference is particularly marked in certain pathological conditions of the auditory system, and thus may have important diagnostic significance. This possibility will be discussed in considerable detail in Chapter 10.

BONE RECEIVER PLACEMENT

By far the most commonly employed placement of the bone-conduction receiver is on the mastoid process of the temporal bone: right mastoid for right-ear tests and left mastoid for left-ear tests. There is, however, a growing number of clinicians who advocate forehead placement of the bone-conduction receiver. Their argument is based in part on the findings of Hart and Naunton (16) and Studebaker (29) that thresholds measured at the forehead exhibit less intersubject variability, and that forehead measures are less affected by middle-ear pathologies. Naunton (23) also points out that the mastoid placement too often leads both tester and patient to assume that the ear on the side of the bone-conduction receiver is the one being stimulated when, in fact, the interaural attenuation for bone-conducted sounds is near zero and both ears may be stimulated equally by a receiver on either mastoid.

Both Studebaker (29) and Naunton (23) report that it takes more energy to reach threshold from the forehead placement than from the mastoid, and that this reduces the maximum amount of loss that can be measured using presently available audiometric equipment. Naunton, however, feels that this loss of energy is a small price to pay for the advantages gained. He recommends forehead placement of the bone-conduction receiver.

CENTRAL MASKING

When a noise is presented to the mask ear, even if at a level insufficient to affect the threshold of the test ear directly, one often sees a small change in the threshold of the test ear. This phenomenon has been labeled "central masking" (31) on the assumption that the shift in threshold is a function of the central nervous system. The values for central masking are small, usually ranging from 5 to 10 dB (10). The effects are present whether threshold is being measured by air- or by bone-conduction. When recording threshold values obtained with masking in the contralateral ear, 5 dB should be subtracted from the attenuator reading to correct for central masking.

Pathologies of Hearing

The disorders of hearing are many and varied. Many of these disorders have already been covered in Chapter 3. However, certain information provided by pure-tone tests are of diagnostic significance and insofar as this holds, this chapter will discuss pathologies.

There are three general classifications of hearing losses. These are *conductive*, *sensory*, and *neural*. Conductive pathologies are those that interfere with the mechanical transmission of sound from the external ear to the inner ear; sensory pathologies are those that affect the sensory systems of the inner ear which convert mechanical energy into electrical; and neural pathologies are those that interfere with the orderly transmission of this electrical energy through the acoustic nervous system to the cerebral cortex. Since pure-tone audiometry cannot usually differentiate between sensory and neural deficiencies, we shall follow the generally accepted practice and refer to all losses of hearing that are not conductive as sensori-neural losses.

The conductive hearing loss is due to a malfunction of the external or middle ear. The cochlea is thus not affected and any stimulus reaching the cochlea may stimulate a sensation of hearing. Since air-conducted sound passes through the external and middle ear, while bone-conducted sound by-passes the external and middle ear, a conductive hearing loss should show a loss of hearing by air-conduction tests and normal hearing by bone-conduction tests.

In the sensory-neural hearing loss, the disorder is within the cochlea or the neural pathways or both. Thus, transmitting a signal directly to the cochlea via bone conduction has no particular advantage. As a result, thresholds for bone-conducted sounds will be approximately the same as threshold for air-conducted sounds of the same frequency. The first major diagnostic cue obtained from pure-tone testing, then, is the relation of bone-conduction thresholds to air-conduction thresholds. If bone conduction is normal and air conduction shows a loss, the loss is conductive; if bone conduction and air conduction both show equal losses, the loss is sensori-neural; and if both show a loss but the loss for air-conducted sounds is greater than that for bone-conducted sounds, the loss is a mixed hearing loss, that is, a conductive and a sensori-neural loss in the same ear.

EXTERNAL-EAR CONDUCTIVE LOSSES

Pathological conditions of the external ear and ear canal often do not impair hearing. Unless the ear canal becomes completely blocked there is little loss of hearing sensitivity. The four conditions of the external ear and canal which sometimes result in hearing loss are (a) an excessive build-up of wax (*cerumen*) which blocks the canal, (b) foreign bodies blocking the canal (children sometimes push small objects into their ears), (c) infections that result in the canal being swollen shut, filled with pus, etc., and (d) congenital malformations of the external ear and canal.

The external problems, when they cause a hearing loss, show up as a mild-to-moderate conductive impairment. Figure 6.9 shows an audiogram which one might obtain from a patient with a hearing loss due to external ear dysfunction. Note that the air conduction shows a mild loss while bone conduction is normal or better than normal. Blockage of the external canal may produce an occlusion effect and make bone-conduction thresholds appear better than they actually are.

MIDDLE-EAR CONDUCTIVE LOSSES

Middle-ear problems, on the other hand, very often do result in impaired hearing. These can generally be categorized into (a) perforations of the

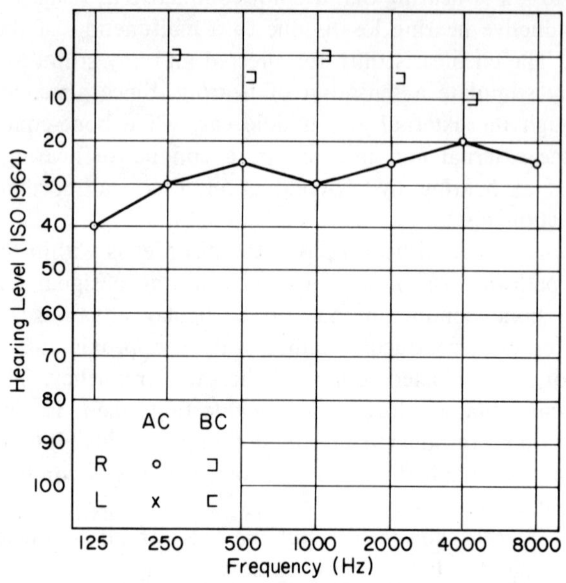

FIGURE 6.9 Audiogram showing type of loss due to impacted wax.

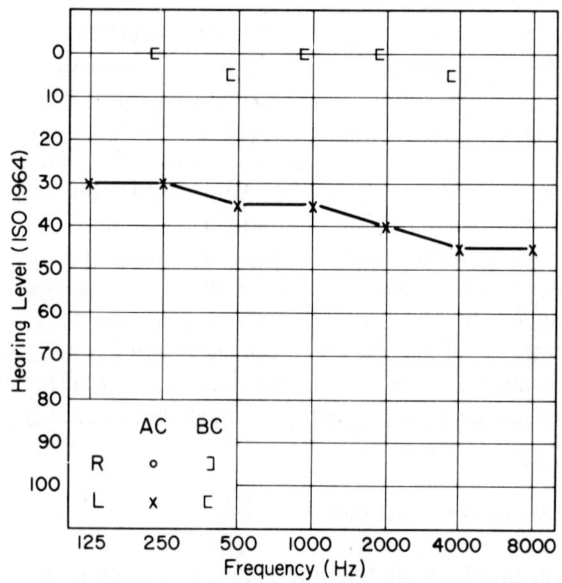

FIGURE 6.10 Audiogram showing type of loss due to otitis media.

tympanic membrane, (b) infections (OTITIS MEDIA), (c) interruptions in the sound-conducting ossicular chain, and (d) fixation of the stapes in the oval window of the cochlea.

Perforations in the tympanic membrane vary in their effect on hearing depending upon the size and location of the perforation. The loss is seldom in excess of 30 to 40 dB, however, provided there is no additional pathology. Perforations of the tympanic membrane may sometimes be the result of foreign bodies being poked into the ear canal or to a concussion type trauma to the head (such as a fall from water skis), but most often they are the result of a rupture due to the building up of pressure in an infected middle ear. Most ruptures of the tympanic membrane heal spontaneously provided the damage is not too extensive and the tissues are healthy. In many cases of chronic infections, however, repeated ruptures, slow healing, and the development of scar tissue may result in permanent holes in the eardrum.

Otitis media is a general term which is used to describe any inflammation or infection of the middle ear. Such infections are the most common cause of conductive hearing losses in children and are frequently seen in adults as well. Middle-ear infections are often due to, or are in conjunction with, a malfunctioning eustachian tube and, as a result, the secretions of fluids, which accumulate in the middle ear due to negative pressure, or the infectious processes are trapped and cannot drain down the tube. Thus, the fluid pressure may continue to build up causing an "earache" and eventually result in a rupture of the tympanic membrane.

Otitis media produces hearing losses which vary to the degree that the disease process interferes with the mobility of the eardrum and ossicular chain. Losses may range from no measurable loss to a maximum conductive loss. At 40 to 80 dB, an air-conducted sound reaches a level sufficient to stimulate hearing by bone conduction. Thus, a conductive loss can be no greater than 40 to 80 dB. Figure 6.10 shows an audiogram which might be obtained on a patient with otitis media.

Occasionally there may be an interruption of the ossicular chain as a result of congenital malformations, trauma to the head or ear, or to infectious processes. Such interruptions usually result in a maximum conductive loss for the impaired ear. This condition is usually unilateral (one ear only).

A fairly common otologic disorder causing conductive hearing losses in young adults is a disease called OTOSCLEROSIS. In this disorder, a bony growth forms around the footplate of the stapes and fixes the stapes against the bony cochlear capsule so that the stapes cannot move relative to the cochlea. Otosclerosis is usually progressive and the hearing loss may vary from a mild loss in the early stages to a maximum conductive loss in the later stages. If the otosclerotic process invades the cochlea, there may even be some sensori-neural loss added to the conductive component. The audiogram in Figure 6.11 shows a profile which one might see on a patient

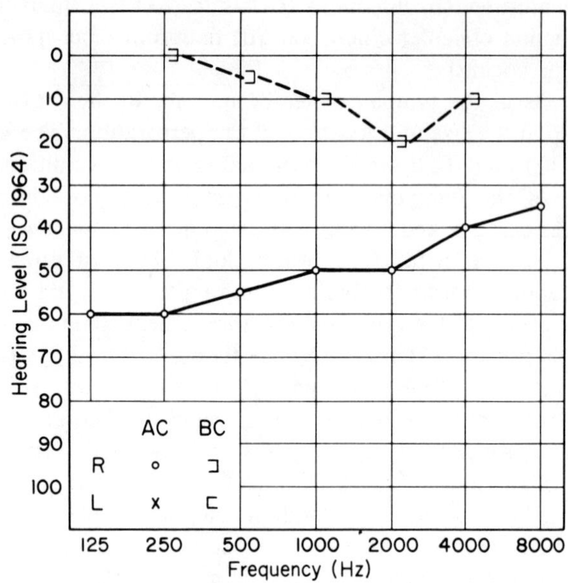

FIGURE 6.11 Audiogram showing type of loss due to otosclerosis.

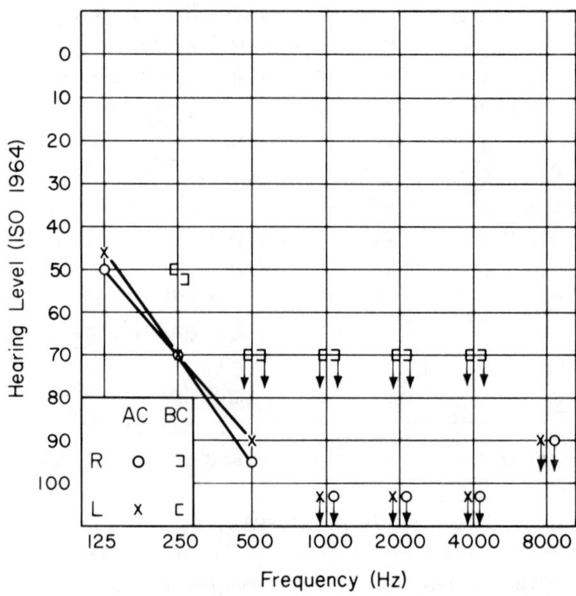

FIGURE 6.12 Audiogram showing profound type of loss due to congenital defects, ototoxic drugs, and viral infections.

with otosclerosis. Note that the bone-conduction threshold is 0 dB at 250 Hz, 5 dB at 500 Hz, 10 dB at 1,000 Hz, 20 dB at 2,000 Hz, and 10 dB at 4,000 Hz. This bone-conduction configuration was found by Carhart (6) to be present in many cases of otosclerosis and is known as "Carhart's notch."

Most of the conditions which cause conductive hearing losses are amenable to medical or surgical treatment. Needless to say, all patients found to have a conductive hearing impairment should be referred for medical attention.

SENSORI-NEURAL LOSSES

Sensori-neural losses may be the result of congenital defects (hereditary or acquired), certain viral infections such as mumps, ototoxic drugs, noise exposure, diseases of the auditory system, vascular disorders, aging, and a number of other pathologic conditions.

Figure 6.12 shows the profound type of losses which often are seen in congenital problems, ototoxic drugs, and some viral infections. Although there is some sensitivity to low-frequency tones, this patient should be considered as educationally deaf.

Figure 6.13 shows the type of loss which frequently results from exposure to intense noise. Note that the major damage occurs in the region around

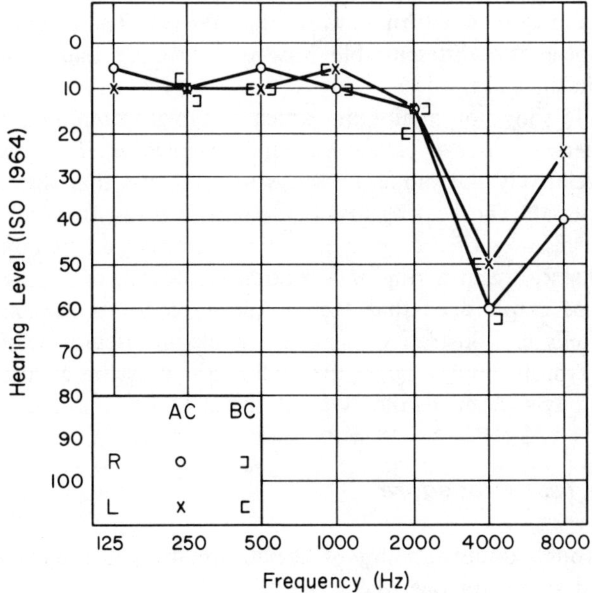

FIGURE 6.13 Audiogram showing type of loss due to noise trauma.

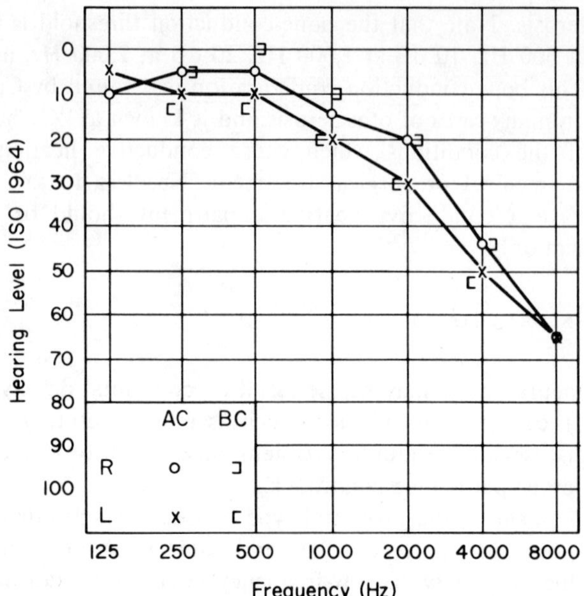

FIGURE 6.14 Audiogram showing type of loss due to presbycusis.

4,000 Hz, with less impairment around 8,000 Hz. Figure 6.14 is an audiogram showing the effects on hearing of the aging process (presbycusis). This loss appears somewhat similar to noise-induced hearing loss, except that the threshold curve does not turn upward at 8,000 Hz. These types of audiograms are not always differentiable, however, since age and noise exposure often go hand in hand.

Figure 6.15 shows an audiogram which one might obtain from a patient with an inner-ear disease called Meniere's Syndrome. This disorder can result in a relatively flat moderate sensori-neural loss that fluctuates. It is usually unilateral. The hearing loss is thought to result from an imbalance in the fluid pressures of the inner ear. It is accompanied by complaints of dizziness (VERTIGO) and a ringing sensation (TINNITUS) in the ear.

It must be emphasized that the sample audiograms presented in this chapter are only for illustrative purposes. While an attempt has been made to present "typical" audiograms, the audiologist must be cognizant of the fact that he may seldom see the "typical" patient.

Pure-Tone Test Procedure

With a thorough understanding of the information already presented in this text, and some practice, the student should be able to obtain a valid pure-tone hearing test. However, in order that the beginning clinician may have a point from which to start, and to help illustrate how the foregoing information can be utilized, the following outline of a step-by-step procedure is given. The pure-tone portion of the procedure is based largely on the Modified Hughson-Westlake technique (1959).

AIR-CONDUCTION TESTS

Step 1. Check the equipment to insure that it is functioning properly. Listen to both earphones and to the bone-conduction receiver while switching across frequencies and increasing and decreasing the attenuation. Use the interrupter switch to turn the tones on and off in order to check for audible switching "clicks."

Step 2. Instruct the patient, then ask him to tell you what he is supposed to do. If he cannot, repeat your instructions. Ask him which is his better ear.

Step 3. Place the earphones on the patient, making sure that both ears are snugly covered. Be especially careful about putting the right phone over the right ear and the left earphone over the left ear.

Step 4. Introduce a pulsed 1,000-Hz tones of a moderate intensity level to the better ear. If the patient responds, turn off the tone and reduce the attenuator dial by 10 dB and again present the tone. Continue this descending procedure until a level is reached where the patient does not respond. Then increase the intensity of the tone in 5-dB steps until a response is again obtained. Continue decreasing the tone in 10-dB steps each time the

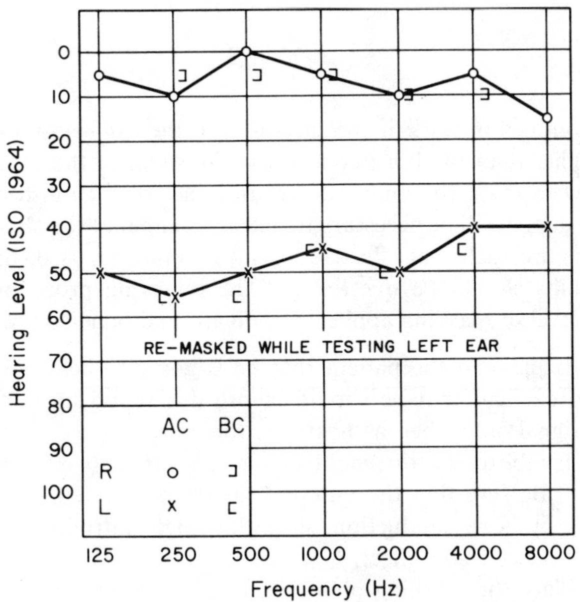

FIGURE 6.15 Audiogram showing type of loss due to Meniere's disease.

patient responds, and increasing it in 5-dB steps each time he fails to respond, until a level is found where the patient responds approximately 50 per cent of the time. Record this level as the threshold for that ear at 1,000 Hz.

If the patient does not respond to the initial presentation of the tone, turn the tone off, increase the intensity by about 20 dB, and present the stimulus again. Continue going up in 20-dB steps until a response is obtained and then follow the procedure already outlined for establishing threshold. Be sure that the tone is always off before shifting the attenuator setting from one position to the other

Step 5. Move on to the other frequencies to be tested and repeat the above procedures for each of them. The order in which these frequencies are tested is unimportant; however, after the last frequency has been tested, a retest of 1,000 Hz should be carried out as a check on reliability. If the second test of 1,000 Hz varies by more than 5 dB from the first test, reinstruct the patient and retest the entire frequency range on that ear.

BONE-CONDUCTION TESTS

Steps 1 and 2. These are the same as Steps 1 and 2 for air-conduction tests.

Step 3. Place the bone receiver on the mastoid of the ear with the better air-conduction threshold. Make sure that the receiver is not touching the pinna.

Step 4. Establish the threshold as in Steps 4 and 5 of air-conduction testing.

MASKING

In air-conduction tests, if the threshold in the ear being tested is 40 dB or more higher than the bone-conduction threshold of the other ear, it will be necessary to mask the untested ear. In bone-conduction tests, if there is an air-bone gap, it will be necessary to mask. In either of the above situations, if conditions are such that effective masking cannot be used, the validity of the test results should be questioned. The following procedure for determining the level of masking applies to both air- and bone-conduction testing.

Step 1. Explain to the patient that he is going to hear a loud noise in his untested ear and that he should ignore this sound insofar as possible. He should signal only when he hears the tone.

Step 2. Establish the threshold in the test ear with no masking in the untested ear. Be sure that the untested ear is not covered by the earphone when testing by bone conduction, since this might introduce the additional problem of an occlusion effect.

Step 3. Place the masking phone over the untested ear and introduce a masking level which is 40 dB plus the minimum masking level plus the bone-conduction threshold of the ear being masked, and redetermine threshold for the test ear. If no threshold shift results (10 dB or less), the unmasked threshold established in Step 2 represents the true threshold for the test ear. If, however, the threshold shifts by more than 10 dB, one can assume that the original responses in Step 2 were the result of cross hearing to the untested ear. If a threshold shift occurs, increase the masking by 10 dB and take another threshold measure. If the threshold does not change due to this increase in masking noise, the first level of masking is the proper level for this frequency in the ear under test. If threshold does shift again as a result of increasing the noise by 10 dB, a plateau-seeking technique should be employed to determine whether it is possible to mask the untested ear, and if so, how much masking noise is needed.

When masking in bone conduction, the earphones should be placed so that only the ear being masked is covered. Never cover the ear being tested since this may cause an occlusion effect in the test ear and result in a faulty measure of threshold. The earphones will fit comfortably with the masking phone covering the untested ear and the other phone resting on the temple in front of the ear being tested.

Tuning-Fork Tests

Before the advent of the electronic audiometer, tuning forks were used in the assessment of the patient's hearing sensitivity for pure tone. These fork tests were usually performed by the otologist, who frequently developed considerable skill in their use. Many otologists still use tuning forks in their preliminary examination and as a check on audiometric results. There was and is a problem of standardization, however, and it is only through long practice that the physician learns to use and interpret his tuning-fork tests in a relatively meaningful manner.

The audiologist is rarely, if ever, called upon to use tuning forks today. However, some of the pure-tone tests performed with the audiometer are based upon much the same principles as the tuning-fork tests and some mention of the more frequently used fork tests seems pertinent.

RINNE TEST

This test compares the patient's hearing by bone conduction with his hearing by air conduction. The fork is struck and the handle placed on the patient's mastoid. He is asked to signal when he can no longer hear the tone. At the patient's signal the tester quickly places the tines of the fork about an inch from the opening of the external ear canal. The information on which the otologist must make his diagnosis is whether the patient hears the tone longer by air than by bone (or the converse) and how much longer the patient hears by one than the other. In addition to the problem of striking the fork in a "calibrated" manner, this test is open to all the pitfalls encountered in pure-tone audiometry when masking is not used. There is no assurance that the right ear is the one responding to a tuning fork placed on the right mastoid process.

SCHWABACH TEST

This test compares the hearing of the patient with that of the tester. It is a bone-conduction test in which the otologist strikes the fork, holds its handle to the patient's mastoid until the patient reports that he no longer hears the tone, then places it to his own mastoid and determines how much longer he can hear the tone than did the patient. In addition to the same problems encountered in the Rinne Test, the Schwabach user must make the assumption that his own hearing is normal for bone-conducted sound.

WEBER TEST

This test is one that may be somewhat useful to the otologist and audiologist even today. It can be performed with either tuning forks or audiometer. The handle of a tuning fork, or the bone-conduction receiver of an audiometer, is placed on the forehead of the patient and the patient asked to report in which ear he hears the tone. Since the impeding of sound from its passage through the external and middle ear often appears to enhance bone-conduction thresholds in that ear (due to the occlusion effect, and to the fact that a conductive loss reduces the ambient noise reaching the inner ear and thus reduces the masking effects of this noise), the test tone will tend to LATERALIZE to the poorer ear if the loss is conductive, and to the better ear if the loss is sensori-neural. The otologist uses the Weber Test most often in order to determine whether a unilateral loss is conductive or sensori-neural. The audiologist, however, may find the test most helpful in deciding which ear to test first by bone conduction. Since the policy of testing the more sensitive ear first is usually followed, some method must be used to determine which ear is most sensitive. The Weber Test, although not foolproof, will often give this information. However, it must be performed at each frequency to be tested, since one ear may be more sensitive at one frequency and the other at a second.

Equipment Check and Calibration

The American Standards Association has set up minimum requirements for pure-tone audiometers These requirements provide guidelines for audiometer manufacturers regarding frequencies to include, intensity ranges, test tone purity, attenuator accuracy, etc. However, even an audiometer which has satisfactorily passed through all phases of inspection before leaving the factory may prove faulty upon arrival at the clinic, or at any time thereafter. For this reason the audiologist should always insure that his equipment is in good working order before testing a patient. Each time the equipment is turned on he should, after giving the equipment several minutes to warm up, put the earphones on himself (or a colleague) and listen to the signals while he switches across frequencies, turns the signal on and off with the interrupter switch, and introduces the masking noise.

The sweep across frequencies is to insure that all frequencies used in the test are being generated and are not noticeably distorted. The attenuator check is to insure that the attenuator has a smooth quiet function. A faulty attenuator will frequently produce a static-like noise when the dial is manipulated. The audiologist should listen carefully when using the interrupter switch to start and stop the tone. The audiometer has a circuit designed to start and stop the tone gradually and smoothly. This eliminates the "pop" or "click" (SWITCHING TRANSIENT) which is audible when a pure tone is switched on or off abruptly. These switching transients, rather than the pure tone, may be the stimuli to which the patient responds if they are present and an audiometer with audible switching transients should never be used to test hearing.

In addition to this daily check on the functioning of equipment, periodic checks should be made on the calibration of the audiometer. Whenever possible these checks should be made electroacoustically. However, good calibration equipment is expensive and many of the smaller speech and hearing clinics do not have access to it. This is especially true for the electroacoustic equipment for calibration of bone-conduction receivers. As a result, the following suggestions for a clinical method of checking calibration are offered.

For checks of air-conduction receivers, obtain thresholds on ten young normal hearing adults. Test both the right and the left ear of each subject, add the results from all the right ears together and the results from all the left ears together, and divide each total by ten. This gives a mean threshold for each ear using that particular audiometer and set of earphones. This mean should agree reasonably well with the zero on the attenuator dial. If there is a discrepancy, the mean thresholds should be taken as the standard and any test results obtained on that audiometer should be adjusted by the difference between the attenuator dial reading and the mean threshold data. Corrections are usually made to the nearest 5 dB.

Bone-conduction calibration checks are more difficult. Normal hearing subjects cannot be used unless the test room is considerably quieter than most clinical test rooms. This is due to the fact that random noise entering the ears by air conduction masks the bone-conducted signal at near-threshold levels for normal hearing subjects. Carhart (6) has suggested a method which avoids this problem of masking by using subjects with sensori-neural hearing losses. He suggests that ten or twelve ears with pure sensori-neural losses be tested by air and bone conduction. In the pure sensori-neural loss, air-conduction thresholds and bone-conduction thresholds should be the same. Thus, if the air-conduction receivers are accurately calibrated, and the losses are purely sensori-neural, a mean of the air-conduction thresholds is the standard to which the mean of the bone-conduction thresholds must be matched.

Another point which the audiologist should check is the linearity of attenuation of the masking level dial. In other words, does increasing the output by 10 dB on the dial actually increase the noise level by 10 dB? This can be checked by taking readings with a vacuum tube volt meter (VTVM) with the masking level dial set at regular increments from high to low. A 10-dB decrease in the dial reading should result in about a 10-dB decrease on the scale of the VTVM.

Audiometer masking dials are sometimes labeled by the manufacturer in decibels of "effective masking." This term is not used in the same meaningful way by audiometer manufacturers as by audiologists, however. At the present time, there are no industry-wide standards for the labeling of masking level dials, and the numbers on these dials should be used only as points to calibrate from. The clinical audiologist must check and determine for himself the meaningfulness, or lack of it, of the numbers on the masking level dial of the particular audiometer that he uses, regardless of how the dial is labeled.

In clinical calibrations, the correction factors (the amount to be added to or subtracted from the attenuator dial reading) can be placed in tabular form on the front of the audiometer so that the corrections can be applied to all clinical tests. However, these clinical calibrations should be regarded simply as checks and should not be used as long-term calibration procedures. All audiometers should be electroacoustically checked and serviced (returned to the factory if necessary) at least once each year and more often if clinical checks reveal or suggest malfunctions.

Glossary

ACUITY This term applies to the ability to discriminate adjacent stimuli. Used when discussing differential thresholds.

ADAPTATION Adaptation is said to occur when a stimulus which at first evokes a response becomes less effective as it continues with time. An apparent reduction in the auditory system's response under sustained stimulation.

AIR-BONE GAP The difference in decibels between thresholds for air-conducted and bone-conducted stimuli of the same frequency.

AIR CONDUCTION The process by which sound is conducted to the inner ear via the air in the external ear canal, the tympanic membrane, and the ossicular chain.

AMERICAN STANDARDS ASSOCIATION (ASA) A voluntary association of manufacturers and consumers which has set up standards for many areas of American industry.

AUDIOGRAM A graph for showing hearing loss or hearing level as a function of frequency.

AUDIOMETRY The art of testing hearing.

AUDITORY SYSTEM The parts of the ear and nervous system that have to do with the processes of detecting and interpreting auditory stimuli.

BILATERAL Two sides. Both ears.

BINAURAL Hearing with both ears.

BONE CONDUCTION The process whereby sound is conducted to the inner ear via the bones of the head.

CENTRAL MASKING When a noise is presented to the untested ear at a level insufficient to affect the test ear directly, a small change in threshold of the test ear may often be observed. This phenomenon is assumed to be a function of the central nervous system and has been labeled "central masking."

CONDUCTIVE HEARING LOSS An interference with the normal mechanical transmission of sound energy from the external ear into the inner ear.

CONTRALATERAL Opposite side.

EFFECTIVE MASKING LEVEL The effective masking level of a stimulus is the amount in decibels that the introduction of that stimulus will shift the threshold of the test signal, when both are applied to the same normal ear.

FREQUENCY The number of compressions and rarefactions per unit of time. In audiometry, frequency is the number of cycles per second (cps) and is referred to in *Hertz* (Hz). For example a 1,000-cps tone has a frequency of 1,000 Hz.

HEARING LEVEL (HL) The intensity of a sound in decibels relative to the average threshold of hearing of young normal adults. May refer to ASA 1951 or ISO 1964 standards.

HERTZ (Hz) *See* Frequency.

INERTIA The tendency for a resting mass to remain at rest and for a moving mass to continue in motion.

INTERAURAL ATTENUATION The loss of energy of a sound stimulus in passing through the head from one ear to the other.

INTERNATIONAL ORGANIZATION FOR STANDARDIZATION (ISO) A volunteer world organization made up of standards groups from countries wishing to participate. The objective of this organization is to standardize standards in the various disciplines.

IPSILATERAL Same side.

LATERALIZATION The impression of the observer that a sound is being heard in one ear or the other. For example, a tone may *lateralize* to the right ear when it is presented at the forehead by bone conduction.

LESION Any injury to, or morbid change in, the structure of organs or parts.

MASKING The process of raising the threshold for a given stimulus by the introduction to a second stimulus.

MINIMUM MASKING LEVEL The level to which the noise must be raised before any masking takes place. Hence, the overall level of a masking noise minus the effective masking level of that noise.

Mixed Hearing Loss A hearing loss which has both a conductive and a sensory-neural component.

Monaural Hearing with one ear.

Neural Hearing Loss A dysfunction in the orderly transmission of electrical energy from the inner ear through the acoustic nervous system to the cerebral cortex.

Octave The interval between two tones which are separated by a frequency ratio of 2:1.

Pure Tone A sound wave whose instantaneous sound pressure is a sinusoidal function of time.

Sensation Level (SL) The intensity of a sound in decibels relative to the given individual's threshold for that sound.

Sensitivity This term applies to the ability to detect the presence of a signal. Used when discussing absolute thresholds.

Sensory Hearing Loss A dysfunction of the sensory system of the inner ear.

Sound Pressure Level (SPL) The intensity of a sound in decibels relative to a pressure of 0.0002 dyne/cm^2.

Threshold Threshold for a stimulus is the lowest level of that stimulus which will elicit a response 50 per cent of the time.

Threshold Shift Any change in threshold in decibels which results from the introduction of, or change in, any variable affecting threshold.

Unilateral One side. One ear.

10-27-75

Bibliography

1. American Standards Association Bulletin. "Specifications for audiometers for general diagnostic purposes." Z 24.5. New York: 1951.
2. Beasley, W. C. *National Health Survey, Hearing Study Series. Bulletin No.* 5. Washington, D.C.: U. S. Public Health Service, 1938.
3. Bekesy, G. v. "Zur theorie deshorens dei der schallaufnahme durch knockenleitung." *Annalen der Physik*, **13**: 111, 1932.
4. Bekesy, G. v. "A new audiometer." *Acta Oto-Laryngologica*, **35**: 411, 1947.
5. Bekesy, G. v. *Experiments in Hearing.* New York: McGraw-Hill Book Company, 1960.
6. Carhart, R. "Clinical application of bone-conduction audiometry." *Archives of Otolaryngology*, **51**: 1, 1950.
7. Carhart, R., and J. F. Jerger. "Preferred method for clinical determination of pure-tone thresholds." *Journal of Speech and Hearing Disorders*, **24**: 330, 1959.
8. Dadson, R. R., and J. R. King. "A determination of the normal threshold of hearing and its relation to the standardization of audiometers." *Journal of Laryngology and Otology*, **66**: 366, 1952.
9. Davis, H., and F. W. Kranz. "The international standard reference zero for pure-tone audiometers and its relation to the evaluation of impairment of hearing." *Journal of Speech and Hearing Research*, **7**: 7, 1964.
10. Dirks, D., and C. Malmquist. "Changes in bone-conduction thresholds produced by masking in the non-test ear." *Journal of Speech and Hearing Research*, **7**: 271, 1964.

11. Elpern, B., and R. F. Naunton. "The stability of the occlusion effect." *Archives of Otolaryngology*, **77**: 376, 1963.
12. Feldman, A. S. "Maximum air-conduction hearing loss." *Journal of Speech and Hearing Research*, **6**: 157, 1963.
13. Fletcher, H. "Auditory patterns." *Review of Modern Physics*, **12**: 47, 1940.
14. Glorig, A. "Audiometric reference levels." *Laryngoscope*, **76**: 842, 1966.
15. Goldstein, D. P., and C. C. Hayes. "The occlusion effect in bone-conduction hearing. *Journal of Speech and Hearing Research*, **8**: 137, 1965.
16. Hart, C. W., and R. F. Naunton. "Frontal bone-conduction tests in clinical audiometry." *Laryngoscope*, **71**: 24, 1961.
17. Hirsh, I. J. *The Measurement of Hearing*. New York: McGraw-Hill Book Company, 1952.
18. Hood, J. D. "The principles and practice of bone-conduction audiometry: A review of the present position." *Laryngoscope*, **70**: 1211, 1960.
19. Jahn, G. "Über die schwingungsfahigkeit des menschlichen felsenbeines im hinblik auf die theorie des knochenleitungshorens." *Zeitschrift für Laryngologie, Rhinologie, Otologie und ihre Grenzgebiete*, **32**: 439, 1953.
20. Kirikae, I. "An experimental study on the fundamental mechanism of bone conduction." *Acta Oto-Laryngologica*, suppl. 145, 1, 1959.
21. Littler, T. S., J. J. Knight, and P. H. Strange. "Hearing by bone conduction and the use of bone-conduction hearing aids." *Proceedings of the Royal Society of Medicine*, **45**: 783, 1952.
22. Liden, G., G. Nilsson, and H. Anderson. "Narrow-band masking with white noise." *Acta Oto-Laryngologica*, **50**: 116, 1959.
23. Naunton, R. F. "The measurement of hearing by bone conduction." In J. Jerger, ed., *Modern Developments in Audiology*. New York: Academic Press, Inc., 1963.
24. Price, L. L. "Threshold testing with Bekesy audiometer." *Journal of Speech and Hearing Research*, **6**: 64, 1963.
25. Saunders, J. W., and W. F. Rintelmann. "Masking in audiometry." *Archives of Otolaryngology*, **80**: 541, 1964.
26. Sivian, L. J., and S. D. White. "On minimum audible fields." *Journal of the Acoustical Society of America*, **4**: 288, 1933.
27. Studebaker, G. A. "Clinical masking of air- and bone-conducted stimuli." *Journal of Speech and Hearing Disorders*, **29**: 23, 1964.
28. Studebaker, G. A. "On masking in bone-conduction testing." *Journal of Speech and Hearing Research*, **5**: 215, 1962.
29. Studebaker, G. A. "Placement of vibrator in bone-conduction testing." *Journal of Speech and Hearing Research*, **5**: 321, 1962.
30. Ward, W. D. " 'Sensitivity' versus 'acuity'." *Journal of Speech and Hearing Research*, **7**: 294, 1964.
31. Wegel, R. L., and G. E. Lane. "The auditory masking of one pure tone by another and its probable relation to the dynamics of the inner ear." *Physiological Review*, **23**: 266, 1924.
32. Zwislocki, J. "Acoustic attenuation between the ears." *Journal of the Acoustical Society of America*, **25**: 752, 1953.

7

Speech Audiometry

Kenneth W. Berger, Ph.D.

Despite the usefulness of pure-tone audiometry, it is limited by its inability to test directly an aspect of behavior which is of the utmost importance to audiologic evaluation: the listener's responses to speech. Speech audiometry, in spite of theoretical and practical difficulties, provides a method by which such assessment can be made, and thus has become one of our most important tools. It is almost too obvious to state that it is not normally necessary to attend to or discriminate among pure-tone stimuli, but rather it is constantly necessary to identify speech units.

Speech audiometry is concerned with answering at least three questions: (1) What is the lowest intensity at which the listener can just barely identify simple speech materials? (2) How well does the listener understand everyday speech under everyday conditions? and (3) What is the highest intensity at which the listener can tolerate speech? At present the first and third questions can be answered fairly accurately, but we fall far short of answering the second.

It is often said that the three measures just mentioned can be determined with the same precision as are pure-tone thresholds. From a theoretical standpoint this simply is not so, and actually the difficulties in measuring the ever-changing speech signal are such that we rarely achieve the desired clinical accuracy, particularly in tests of speech discrimination.

Unlike pure-tone test stimuli, speech changes rapidly within the period of a single word or of an even smaller sound unit. Changes occur in intensity and frequency as well as in rate, rhythm, and duration. Furthermore, materials and methodology in speech audiometric testing are still largely unstandardized. The sources of variability in speech audiometry, thus, far outnumber those in pure-tone audiometry. Therefore, speech audiometry involves many chances for error from such sources as the apparatus, test materials, the audiologist, the environment, and the patient. Describing these potential errors and suggesting ways to minimize them will be one purpose of the present chapter.

The Development of Speech Audiometry

SPEECH DISCRIMINATION

The clinical use of speech in testing for possible hearing impairment undoubtedly preceded the use of discrete tones by many years, but the quantification of speech audiometric tests has been fairly recent. The first systematic use of speech in auditory testing was not concerned with the hearing-impaired population, but rather was used to evaluate the speech-reproducing capabilities of various sound-transmitting and amplifying systems. Fortunately, many of the materials and methods used in these investigations were later found valuable for evaluating hearing function. Figure 7.1 presents in gross form the chain-like factors involved in speech. If, as carefully as possible, we hold all the links in this chain constant but one, we should be able to manipulate the remaining link to determine its relative variabilities.

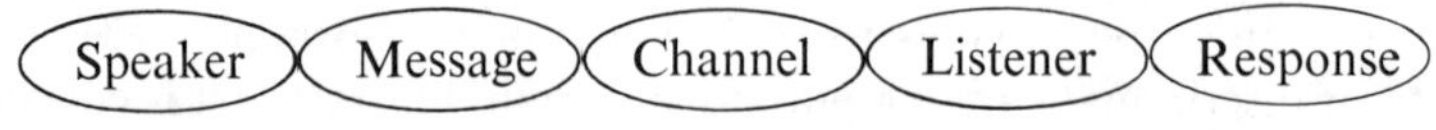

FIGURE 7.1 The speech chain.

In everyday circumstances, and indeed in clinical speech audiometry, the chain of speech is hardly so simple. The variables within each link, as pictured in Figure 7.1, are great and the interaction among links may be significant. Furthermore, the Listener often becomes the Speaker. Speech audiometry, then, is concerned with how well the Listener link of the chain functions under various circumstances.

As noted, the earliest systematic investigation of what is called speech audiometry was concerned with the Channel link as shown in Figure 7.1.

In the 1920's, G. A. Campbell proposed a method of calculating the efficiency of telephone sound-transmitting equipment using nonsense syllables consisting of various consonants followed by the vowel [i]. A group of speakers called these nonsense syllables over communication systems, and in this way the consonant sounds could be evaluated as to how well or poorly they were reproduced by the systems under study. A refinement of the syllable choice was made by Crandall and his associates wherein initial, medial, and final sounds in syllables were obtained by a random selection, and the combination of consonant-vowel was varied in a systematic manner. The result was 174 different lists with fifty nonsense syllables in each. These lists became known as the Standard Articulation Test. J. B. Kelly employed two different speakers and seven or eight listeners at a time to evaluate telephone systems, using the Standard Articulation Test. The efficiency of each test instrument was calculated by assigning to it the percentage of syllables correctly heard (41). Thus arose the "per cent score of articulation" concept, and it is still used today. It is unfortunate that the word articulation has quite another and more common meaning in the broad field of speech pathology and audiology. For this reason the term DISCRIMINATION is usually employed today and is almost synonymous with articulation as used by the workers at Bell Telephone Laboratories.

An advantage of nonsense syllables in testing speech discrimination is their lack of meaning, and thus the listener's vocabulary is not a variable. But this lack of meaning in turn can also be a disadvantage since the listener does not normally need to identify meaningless speech stimuli. Persons trained in such listening tasks manipulate nonsense syllables well, but those untrained generally do very poorly. For these reasons, Fletcher (41) recommended the use of monosyllabic words for testing the deaf as early as 1929.

Although limited use of the Standard Articulation Test was made with the hearing-impaired clinical population, the next major development in speech testing came from Harvard Psycho-Acoustic Laboratory (PAL). Here the need for wartime improvement in communications systems was again the main concern, although the efficiency of the speaker and the message were also examined. Soon the PAL materials and methods were used in army and navy rehabilitation programs at the close of World War II. Egan et al. (33) developed lists of monosyllabic words for such testing. The criteria for word and list selection included: lists must be of equal average difficulty; each list must have a composition representative of English speech, i.e., must be "phonetically balanced"; and the words must be in common usage. Monosyllables used to meet these criteria were drawn from Thorndike's (112) list of the most frequently occurring words in printed English. The resultant test lists are known as the PAL PB–50 Lists, or more commonly the PB–50's. They consist of twenty lists of fifty different words each. In a recorded version of this test, still used in many clinics, the speaker was Rush Hughes, and he spoke the test item number at a set intensity by peaking this as a carrier phrase on the *VU* meter; the key or test word following the item number was spoken at an intensity in relation to the carrier phrase at which it might normally occur ("equal effort"). Note then, that the actual test monosyllables did not all occur at the same level, although it has long been known that small variations in intensity level may cause rather large variations in discrimination for speech (42). Low signal-to-noise ratios also appear to be critical in discrimination test variability.

In response to criticisms of word difficulty and several other factors, a group at the Central Institute for the Deaf (54) amended the PB–50 lists as the CID Auditory Test W–22, and produced the familiar W–22 recordings with Hirsh as the speaker. The speaker followed the procedure of saying a carrier phrase("You will say———")at a set level and allowing the key word to fall at some presumably natural level relative to the carrier phrase. The CID modifications included adding more familiar words to those used in PAL PB–50 lists. The resultant W–22 lists consist of 120 words from the PAL PB–50's plus 80 new words. The 200 test words are divided into four basic lists (numbered one through four) of fifty words each, and these in turn are scrambled in six orders each (A through F). Sample W–22 lists appear in the Appendix, p. 233-34.

The PAL PB–50 lists, the W–22 lists, and to a large extent those test lists developed since, have paid some attention to word familiarity or word difficulty. But note that this familiarity of vocabulary is typically based in whole or in part on the vocabulary studies by Thorndike (112) or by Dewey (29), both of whom were concerned solely with *printed* English. Word length and vocabulary in speech, however, may differ considerably from that of printed English (4, 6). It is also likely that word familiarity changes with time. In this regard, note particularly that the words "inkwell" from the W–1 list and "mew" from the W–22 list, among others, seem out of date. Thus, even if the Thorndike and Dewey lists were representative of English speech—which they are not—they would need revising to account for usage changes since their publication.

The matter of phonetic balance has produced some critics (69, 116). Phonetic balance, like word familiarity, was based on the relative frequency of appearance of various sounds as they occur in English. Again, Thorndike's or Dewey's work with printed materials have been the primary sources. It should also be noted that the balancing of words phonetically within each word list has been concerned only with approximately the first two-thirds of each word. In other words, the initial consonant or consonant blend and following vowel, or initial vowel, have been computed in the phonetic balancing. The usefulness of phonetic balance in discrimination testing has not been demonstrated, regardless of its apparent logic. The "balancing" of vowels within any test, because of some geographic differences in pronunciation, will at best be approximate. It will now be necessary to investigate further the relevance of phonetic balance; and if the concept is found to be useful, the balancing should be done according to speech data rather than according to printed materials. It might well be argued that any sizable sample from *conversational* vocabulary would be, by definition, a phonetically balanced sample of spoken English.

The W–22 word lists and recordings, as we saw, were developed to overcome some of the shortcomings of the PAL PB–50 lists and the Rush Hughes recordings. The resultant recordings contain easier discrimination tasks than their predecessors, although the differences in difficulty between the W–22 and PAL PB–50 lists themselves are not significant (120). Since speech discrimination testing a decade or so ago was an important tool in differential diagnosis in auditory disorders, this difference in difficulty in the recordings was of considerable importance. Today, with a readily available battery of diagnostic audiometric tests for such determination (e.g., loudness balance tests, SISI, Tone Decay, Bekesy patterns, etc.), speech discrimination testing for this purpose is no longer so critical.

The W–22 recordings are the most commonly used recorded speech discrimination tests in present use in the United States. For those clinicians using monitored live voice (MLV) testing, the W–22 lists appear likewise to be the most popular. In spite of their popularity, there have been numerous efforts to further refine or to replace the W–22 records and lists (17, 36, 90, 113, 114).

One modification in the use of the W–22 recordings and lists has been the division of the standard lists into half-lists (16, 35, 46, 47, 94, 101, 116). The user of the recordings or lists simply employs twenty-five rather than all fifty test word items to save time. Using fifty words allows a handy 2 per cent weight for each word correctly identified; using only twenty-five words means each word now has a value of 4 per cent, with the possibility that any single error by the listener or examiner now receives twice the error score as previously; and the variability will be higher. Certainly there is nothing inherently correct in using any particular number of word items in a test. The question really should revolve around whether the W–22 recordings can be just as accurate when using half-lists, and the evidence at hand tends to be positive. Whether the W–22 word lists are just as accurate when used as half-lists with a monitored live voice presentation is less clear.

The original work with the W–22 recordings suggested that no significant differences existed among the four basic lists. More recently it has been shown that there appear to be some differences between them, but these differences are probably not critical in clinical use (34, 58). A decided disadvantage in using the W–22 recordings is that many of the words are nonfunctional. That is, a relatively small number of test words seem to be difficult enough for any listener, except for those having very poor discrimination (20). As with any test, we would like the discrimination task to produce gradations of test scores from superior down to inferior. Another and, in the opinion of this writer, more basic criticism of the W–22 lists and all similar word lists, is that there may be a poor relationship between an individual's performance with them and how well he functions in daily conversational speech demands. Certainly isolated monosyllables are not typical in everyday communication.

What we really wish to know about any listener is how well he can understand everyday speech. Unfortunately little work has been done to determine the structure and content of conversation or the varied sound environments in which we must communicate daily. Worse yet, because of the redundancy of our speech, sentence-length materials are difficult to quantify. Early sentence tests did little more than differentiate gross discrimination problems, and they probably also tested intellectual functioning to a large degree. Furthermore, the sentence tests usually could not be used repeatedly because of memory factors.

In order to more realistically evaluate the listener's understanding of everyday speech there has been a reawakening of interest in sentence tests (44, 51, 27). Initial efforts to use artificial sentences have had a flurry of reports (30, 31, 40, 62, 105, 106, 107, 108, 109, 110), but they seem to have had little acceptance in clinics.

Another approach to discrimination testing has been the use of multiple-choice words (7, 8, 10, 32, 48, 59, 68). In this procedure, printed groups of phonetically similar words are shown the listener but he hears and is to respond to only one word from each grouping. An advantage to this approach is that words of more than a single syllable may be used, so long as each grouping contains words of the same syllable length and stress pattern. A combination of multiple-choice words of similar phonetic content as key words within a sentence may be useful in the clinical setting because they more closely resemble everyday speech discrimination requirements than materials heretofor employed (5). Word familiarity and word difficulty variables are probably less important with multiple-choice tests than with tests employing isolated words.

SPEECH RECEPTION THRESHOLD

The level at which a listener can just barely identify easy speech materials, or the level at which a listener is just barely able to follow continuous discourse with concentrated listening, is called the threshold of hearing for speech, or the Speech Reception Threshold (SRT). The laboratories at Harvard University, in addition to producing the PB materials for speech discrimination, developed spondee[1] lists for measuring SRT (56). The two

[1] Words of two syllables with approximately equal stress on both syllables. It is incorrect to say "spondee words"; the use of "spondaic words" is slightly better, but still redundant.

spondee tests developed at that time are known as Auditory Test No. 9 and No. 14, each consisting of forty-two dissyllabic words with a spondaic stress pattern, which are scrambled into twelve orders or lists. The recorded Auditory Test No. 9 presents the spondees with 4-dB attenuation steps built into the recording. The recorded Auditory Test No. 14 does not include the attenuation, thereby allowing the examiner to attenuate as he desires.

The modifications of the spondee lists were done at the CID laboratories, as were the original PB lists (54). From the original eighty-four spondees, only thirty-six were kept in the CID W–1 and W–2 lists and recordings. These thirty-six spondees are scrambled into six lists and are identified by alphabet letters, A through F. In the W–1 recordings, those words which had been found to be too easy were recorded 2 dB lower than the average, and those that had been found too difficult were recorded 2 dB higher.

The words on the W–1 recording are still far from homogeneous, as has been reported by Bowling and Elpern (14), who suggest that when using the W–1 recordings fourteen of the stimulus words should not be counted in arriving at the SRT. The word differences reported by Bowling and Elpern undoubtedly represent inconsistencies in the W–1 recording and not in the W–1 list, although this still remains to be positively determined.

In this brief discussion of the development of speech audiometry, we have touched on but a few of the test methods and test materials. That inherent differences exist between these methods and materials has not always been considered critical, and this probably accounts for many of the inconsistent results and large variables found in many published studies. We would like to know the relationships among the various test materials, as determined with representative samples of normal hearing and hearing-impaired populations, but data are meager. Reports such as those by Lovrinic et al. (75) and Kopra et al. (67), among others, are a start in this direction.

We shall later discuss in more detail differences between various speech materials when presented above threshold, and the effect of different speakers. Nor should we forget that sophisticated listeners (who usually serve as standardization subjects for such tests) may produce scores considerably better and more consistent than would be found with clinic patients.

In addition to the speech audiometric tests discussed above, several others are occasionally used, particularly in research. These include the Speech Detection Threshold and the Threshold of Speech Perceptibility. For a description and comparison of these thresholds with SRT see Chaiklin (24).

Equipment

Figure 7.2 shows a block diagram of a typical clinical speech audiometric testing setup for a two-room facility. The minimum equipment for speech

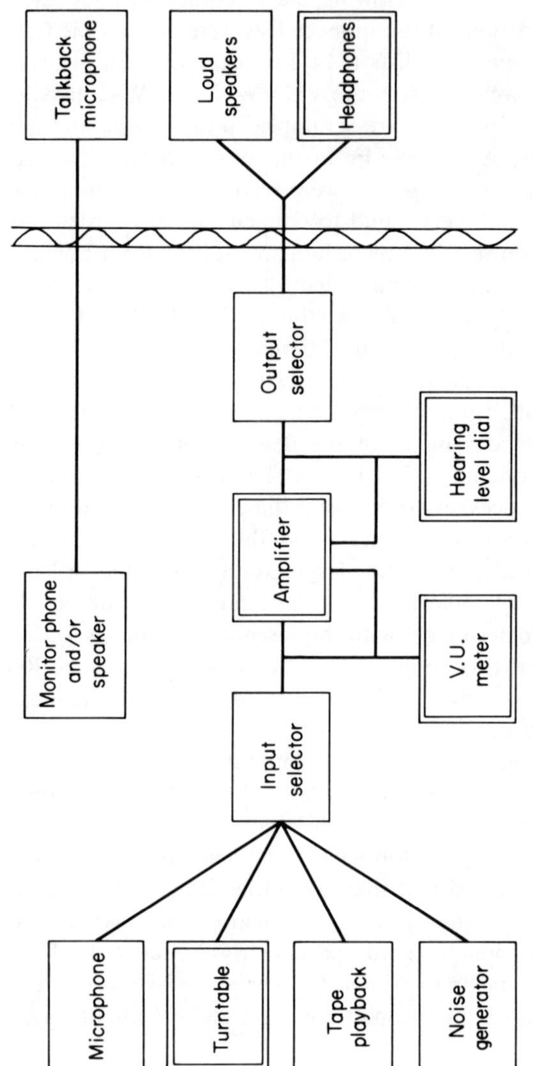

FIGURE 7.2 Block diagram of speech audiometric equipment.

testing, usable in a one-room facility, is indicated in this figure by those blocks marked with double lines. To this diagram could, of course, be added other instrumentation such as two-channel tape playback, filters, and various types of masking noises. The input selector, output selector, VU meter, and hearing level dial (gain control) shown on the diagram would actually be housed in the amplifier cabinet, along with calibration controls for the various inputs.

Whether the clinic purchases one of the commercially available speech audiometers or chooses to construct its own unit, it should take care to meet the technical standards for speech audiometers (118). Depending upon the equipment available at the clinic, the flexibility of the facility used, and the clinician's own biases, various parts of the speech audiometer are likely to be used more than others. The type and degree of hearing loss, along with age and functioning of the listener, often require that modifications be made from normal procedures.

INPUTS

Most speech audiometers have, or have provision for, several speech inputs plus masking noise. If the clinician is using monitored live voice (MLV) stimuli through the microphone, he must first turn the hearing level dial to zero[2] and adjust the input calibration knob until his voice produces peak needle deflections approximating zero on the VU meter. In the case of tape or disk recordings, the proper input selector should be chosen and the 1,000 Hz calibration tone (usually at the beginning of a tape recording, or on the inner groove of a disk recording) is likewise calibrated so that the VU meter needle reads zero. Calibration of the noise for masking or test purposes is done in a similar manner. It cannot be stressed too strongly that whatever input one employs, masking from the noise generator or from one of the available speech inputs, that input must be calibrated to the VU meter of the speech audiometer. Without such calibration the test validity is at best doubtful and probably worthless. Nor is this procedure valid unless the speech audiometer outputs (earphones and speakers) are kept in proper calibration. Clinics usually take great care to keep pure-tone audiometers in calibration, but may not do the same with speech audiometers.

OUTPUT SELECTOR

Most speech audiometers give the clinician some choice and flexibility of outputs. One may choose to direct the stimuli to the listener's right ear or left ear via the headphones, and direct the masking into the same

[2] Calibration procedures performed with the hearing level dial at −10 dB on some speech audiometers cause an error of several decibels.

earphone as the speech stimuli, but more often to the contralateral ear. The clinician may also direct the stimuli through one or more loudspeakers. The use of loudspeakers in a one-room facility precludes the use of monitored live voice testing, and even recorded speech through loudspeakers in a one-room facility may not be satisfactory. The use of loudspeakers provides for FREE FIELD[3] testing, which is essential in the evaluation of amplification procedures, as shall be seen in a later chapter. Furthermore, the evaluation of the listener's function in a free field gives an overall impression that more nearly resembles everyday situations than does monaural testing under earphones.

TALKBACK

In a two-room facility provision must be made for the listener to communicate with the examiner and to repeat the test materials which can then be heard by the examiner. If the speech testing is done under earphones, a monitor speaker or monitor phone may be used by the examiner. In free field testing, the feedback through the microphone during MLV testing may necessitate the use of a monitor phone rather than the monitor speaker, particularly at high-intensity levels.

On many speech audiometers the listener's responses can also be calibrated, thus providing some objectivity to the Lombard Test.

Responses by the Listener

In all routine uses of speech audiometry, the responses by the listener must be recognized and finally quantified by the examiner. In Speech Reception Threshold testing, where the test words are relatively simple and the choices few, the examiner is likely to have little difficulty in determining whether the listener's responses are correct, for the SRT oral responses to the test words are usually quite satisfactory, although for research purposes written responses may be of some value.

For speech discrimination testing, however, the speech stimuli are more difficult and the alternatives much greater in number. In this case the listener's responses place the examiner in the position of being a listener, and thus create an unwanted variable. We have good evidence (82, 117) that this factor can contribute decisively to unreliable discrimination testing. Unless the examiner is interested only in a general impression of the listener's speech discrimination, it is necessary that the responses be clearly received

[3] The writer is aware of the arguments over the terms *free field* and *sound field*. The former term is so restrictive that it might be considered only in a theoretical framework, the latter so general that any room containing sound can be so defined. We shall use the term *free field* since it is a commonly used one, and recognize that its use includes the supposition that the listener's test room is sound treated in such a manner that reverberation and the entrance of extraneous sounds are kept at a minimum.

by the examiner. In spite of the danger, probably the most common practice of clinics in this country is to accept vocal responses, the audiologist apparently being unaware of or unconcerned about potentially large errors.

In tests other than the multiple-choice or word-completion types, to remove or at least lessen the examiner's involvement in the discrimination score, several alternatives are available. The safest procedure is to give the listener a sheet of paper with numbered blanks corresponding to the words he will hear; the listener writes what he hears and the examiner then scores these answers. Of course this may add other problems, inasmuch as the examiner must be careful to accept homonyms (e.g., isle, aisle, I'll) as being correct, and the difficulties may be compounded by the listener's spelling ability and handwriting legibility.

An alternate solution, and one that places much on the experience of the examiner, is to accept spoken responses from the listener but to stop within the test at any point where there is the slightest question about the response. For instance, if the examiner is not certain of a specific word response, he can stop and ask the listener to repeat or to spell that word; if the word can't be spelled, the listener can be asked to use the word in a sentence so as to assure the examiner that it was heard correctly. In MLV testing, this procedure is common; with recorded tests it is more difficult. With tape-recorded tests, the examiner must quickly stop the tape playback and, through the microphone circuit, ask for further identification. In disk-recorded tests, it is most difficult to stop the disk playback and to start it again in the same groove.

The speech materials as well as the response may need to be altered if the listener has a substantial speech disorder or a pronounced foreign accent. In these cases a written response is almost mandatory, or a test should be used that employs multiple choices, where the word presumed to have been heard is checked by the listener.

Likewise, for children with speech disorders, or when a child's interest wanes during testing, an alternate approach must often be tried. For SRT testing, the use of pictured spondees is often useful, in which the child merely points to the picture of the word he heard. It must be remembered that the tests should investigate the listener's hearing function, not his speech production or his mental or physical abilities. Pictures may also be used for discrimination testing, but because of the relatively few choices available, the pictures should probably be changed several times during a test (70, 85, 119). The child, often hyperactive, should be presented with six to nine pictured spondees for SRT testing. With six pictured choices the child has approximately a 17 per cent chance of guessing a single word he hears and approximately a 3 per cent chance of correctly guessing two consecutive words. With nine pictures the chances of guessing are approximately 11 per cent for a single word and 1 per cent for two consecutive words. Lloyd and Reid (74) report good reliability with mentally retarded children, who respond by repeating the spondees or by pointing to pictured spondees.

Less formal testing may have to suffice for children. Instead of a true measure of SRT, we may have to be satisfied to simply note at what level he turns to his name as called by monitored live voice, or to music, or to white noise,[4] all of which probably approximate a level of or just above SRT. For discrimination testing we may use simpler words, such as the familiar (PBF) or kindergarten (PBK) lists. Or we may have to use the few words in the child's vocabulary, either by finding pictures representing these words or by presenting the actual objects for him to point to, such as a toy boat, truck, or car. Having the child repeat alphabet letters or point to them on a chart gives us a fair idea about his speech discrimination performance (60). Still more gross, but often the best we can do, is to ask the child to repeat numbers or hold up the number of fingers for the number he hears. Whenever the examiner departs from "standard" materials or procedures, he should note this fact on the audiogram. The examiner's subjective impression of reliability is often valuable.

Possible variability in kinds of listeners and their responses has been investigated from several standpoints. Many of these studies point up the difficulties in defining populations with which to standardize speech audiometric tests. Farrimond (39) found that persons with lower than average vocabulary, and older subjects performed poorer in speech audiometry than did others. Although the reported mean differences were relatively small, they were significant: 1.5 dB for vocabulary and 4.5 dB for age. Blumenfeld et al. (11) found a fairly high correlation between age and the Rhyme Test of speech discrimination for their over-sixty-year-old group, but the correlation for the younger subjects was low.

Some of the potential variables in pure-tone and speech testing were examined by Jerger et al. (61). They did not find significant differences in SRT in regard to the sex of the listener, or to the right or left ear. There were also no significant differences whether two commonly used procedures were used in arriving at threshold, or whether a single frequency pure-tone threshold was obtained before or after the SRT. A significant difference (3 dB) was found between unsophisticated listeners having prior knowledge of the spondees and those without such knowledge. Differences between SRT's of sophisticated versus unsophisticated listeners were large (5 to 7 dB), and sophisticated listener's SRT's did not change appreciably from test to test. These differences did not occur in pure-tone tests. These latter findings were studied further (115), and they revealed that in normal listeners the practice effect with spondees was negligible, but prior knowledge of the spondee test vocabulary produced SRT's 4 to 5 dB better than when the test words were not known.

[4] Hinchcliffe (53) found a high correlation between the hearing threshold for random noise and the pure-tone average in the speech frequencies. His data, using British Standard, should correspond closely to the ISO 1964 standard.

SRT Procedures

The Speech Reception Threshold is usually obtained by using spondees, but occasionally by using cold running speech.[5] Either of these two materials should produce essentially the same score result in decibels. While often overlooked, it should be remembered that the SRT is, in fact, also a test of speech discrimination; the nature of the task, however, makes the test one of very simple or basic discrimination.

The SRT may be determined by using recorded speech materials or by monitored live voice testing. The poorer ear should be tested while masking the better ear, if the difference in the air-conduction threshold values between the two ears is approximately 40 dB or greater; this follows the same general rules for masking as in air-conduction pure-tone testing which was discussed in Chapter 6. The amount of masking used should be indicated on the audiogram. Either white noise or speech noise (i.e., white noise with slightly greater emphasis in the lower-frequency range) may be used. As with pure tones, approximately a 5-dB central masking effect should be expected on an SRT while masking the nontest ear (79, 81). It is likely that masking during speech discrimination testing should be performed when the difference between the two ears is somewhat less than 40 dB, particularly when using moderate to high sensation levels for test presentation. SRT and discrimination testing via bone conduction has stimulated little research interest, but this might be useful in comparing pre- and postsurgical test scores.

METHOD FOR W–1 RECORD[6]

Before starting the test, present the 36 spondees (or the total to be used) to the listener on a printed list in alphabetical order, so he can briefly familiarize himself with them. Meanwhile, set the input selector to tape or disk as desired. Calibrate the 1,000 Hz tone on the disk or tape to the speech audiometer. Give the following instructions[7] to the listener through the microphone or in printed form:

> You are now going to hear some words which contain two syllables. The words will gradually get softer. Before each word you will hear the phrase "Say the word," which will be followed by the word you are to repeat. Repeat each of the two-syllable words to me even though you have to guess at some of them. Are there any questions?

[5] Connected speech that is informative but is nonemotional in content.

[6] The W–1, W–2, W–22, PAL PB–50, and other test disks are available from Technisonic Studios, 1201 S. Brentwood Blvd., Richmond Heights, Missouri.

[7] Oral instructions for all tests are usually given through the microphone circuit of the speech audiometer, but may be given directly to the listener before the earphones are placed on him. In cases of severe hearing loss, written directions may be needed.

If there are no questions, the examiner is ready to proceed with the test. Usually the examiner will have just completed pure-tone testing and will know the average loss by air conduction. If so, he starts testing with the hearing level dial approximately 20 to 25 dB above the pure-tone average.[8] If the average loss by pure tones is unknown, he can start the testing at a level about 25 dB above the presumed SRT. After choosing the initial presentation level, the examiner starts the tape playback or places the phonograph tone arm at the start of the recording. After the listener correctly responds to several words, the examiner attenuates the level by 4 dB[9] and again determines if the listener can readily repeat the next spondees. After each level where the listener accurately repeats two or three spondees, the examiner continues to turn the hearing level dial down in 4-dB steps until the listener begins to respond incorrectly to the spondees or does not respond at all. The experienced clinician will note a slight hesitancy in responses or other slight changes in the listener's vocal response as the threshold of hearing for speech is approached, and at this point he may want to attenuate by 2-dB steps. The threshold for speech, like the threshold for pure tones, is the lowest level at which the listener responds correctly to 50 per cent of the test stimuli.

In practice, the 50 per cent criterion is not always met. Sometimes the listener responds at a given level to more than 50 per cent of the spondees and, at the next lower level, to less than 50 per cent. In this case the higher reading from the hearing level dial should be accepted. Thus, the threshold for speech often becomes the lowest level at which 50 per cent *or more* of the spondees are correctly identified.

During the testing, the examiner may follow the order of the spondees from a printed list which accompanies the recordings or from one of several textbooks. The experienced examiner will, however, know the spondees, and since he is also monitoring the recording, he will not need the printed list.

After the lowest level has been determined, the hearing level dial should be advanced approximately 10 dB and the same procedures repeated. If there is a difference between the two trials, the lower of the two dial readings should be accepted. Unlike pure-tone testing, where an ascending approach is usually recommended, the SRT is most often determined with a descending approach. An exception to the use of a descending approach is when there is any suspicion that the listener might have a nonorganic hearing loss; in this case an ascending approach to the SRT should be followed and so noted on the audiogram.

An important caution should be noted in recording the SRT on the audiogram after using the W–1 recording. The calibration tone on this

[8] As we shall see, the W–1 spondees are actually about 10-dB lower than the dial reading, thus this setting is really 10 to 15 dB above the listener's average hearing level.

[9] For audiometers having a hearing level dial with 5-dB detents, the attenuation in each instance will be 5 dB.

recording is at approximately the level of the recorded carrier phrase; the spondees, on the other hand, are approximately 10 dB lower than either. Thus, when completing the procedures above, the examiner must subtract 10 dB from the dial reading for the SRT. For example, if a listener correctly repeated all spondees presented at 50 dB, and at 48 dB responded correctly to 50 per cent, but at 46 dB responded to less than 50 per cent, the examiner would accept the 48-dB dial reading and from this subtract 10 dB for an SRT of 38 dB.

As each test is completed, the examiner records the score on the audiogram. This is usually recorded on the same sheet as the pure-tone audiogram, since the measurements by speech audiometry seldom exceed six in number (SRT, discrimination, and Threshold of Discomfort for the right and left ears), unless a hearing-aid evaluation is also done. Some clinics have a separate audiogram for speech audiometry.

The inexperienced clinician is likely to start the SRT testing far above the approximate or presumed threshold, and attenuate by small steps only after four or more words are correctly identified at each level. The experienced clinician knows that he can attenuate rather rapidly after each group of words at higher levels, until the listener begins to miss words or shows some hesitancy in responses. Then greater care may be taken in slowly attenuating until the threshold criteria have been met. The nature of spondees as speech stimuli is such that only about 6 to 8 dB separate a 20 per cent from an 80 per cent correct response. Nor does the extra time required to pinpoint the SRT precisely to the nearest 2 dB seem warranted, particularly since we seldom test clinically by pure tones to increments smaller than 5 dB (25). Theoretically, using 2-dB increments will produce SRT's 1.5-dB better on the average than when using 5-dB steps.

After the examiner tests the first ear, he should inform the listener that he will now test the other ear with the same type of words. The procedure for testing the second ear is the same as for the first, but the same word order should not be followed because the listener may remember it. The examiner should select another band on the W–1 recording or another record for the second and succeeding tests with the same listener. If another record is used for subsequent testing, it too should be calibrated to the speech audiometer.

METHOD FOR W–2 RECORDS

The W–2 recordings present the spondees in the same order as do the W–1 recordings. The difference between the two is that the attenuation is built into the W–2 recordings rather than being manually done by the examiner. The presentation level in the W–2 recordings drops 3 dB after each third word, or an average of 1 dB per word. The W–2 recordings seem to be used less in clinics as compared with the W–1 recordings.

The user of these records is cautioned that on some pressings, the W–1 and W–2 recordings appear on the opposite sides of the same disk, and that he should not mistake the two.

Clinicians desiring to use the W–2 records should follow the directions that accompany them. The procedure is similar to that for the W–1 in that the words are presented initially at a level where the listener can clearly hear them; from this point on the hearing level dial is not moved. The test continues until the listener has missed five consecutive words, at which time a count is made of the words correctly identified and this number is subtracted from the reading on the hearing level dial for the SRT in decibels.

METHOD FOR MONITORED LIVE VOICE

This testing is often referred to as "live voice," but the word *monitored* should be included, for it reminds the examiner that unless the live voice testing is monitored on the VU meter, the results can be considered only in a gross manner. In the monitored live voice (MLV) method, the examiner sets the input selector to microphone. With the hearing level dial at zero, he practices several spondees and adjusts the calibration knob so the first syllable of the spondee causes the VU meter needle to approximate zero. It is recommended that the examiner's lips be approximately ten to twelve inches from the microphone, and that he speak across the microphone rather than directly into the diaphragm. For practice, the inexperienced clinician can tape a piece of string, ten to twelve inches long, to the microphone so he can readily determine microphone distance from the mouth.

For MLV testing it is recommended that rather than showing the listener a printed list of spondees, the examiner familiarize the listener with the words by presenting them at a level well above threshold. The audiologist may use the printed spondee list for this purpose, or the spondees can be typewritten, each on a separate card; then after each use, the cards can be quickly shuffled to randomize the order. After going through the spondees well above SRT, the following instructions should be given to the listener: "You are now going to hear those same words again, but this time in a different order. Gradually the words will get softer. You are to repeat the word you hear even though you have to guess at what it is. Are there any questions?"

If there are no questions from the listener, the examiner should begin testing at a level approximately 10 to 15 dB above the pure-tone average and proceed as was indicated above under method for the W–1 record. After each several words are correctly identified, the examiner attenuates the next words, in each instance taking care that he monitors his voice at zero on the VU meter.

In MLV testing, it is not customary to use the carrier phrase, although there is no harm in doing so. Since the examiner calibrated his voice to zero on the VU meter, he does not have to make a correction factor at the conclusion of the test, as was true for the W–1 recording. The final dial reading is the SRT.

Experienced clinicians can obtain the SRT more quickly—and undoubtedly just as accurately—by the MLV method than by using a recording. A decided advantage to the MLV method is that words can be paced to the listener's responses.

METHOD WITH COLD RUNNING SPEECH

The SRT may be determined with cold running speech (continuous discourse) by using a recording or by using monitored live voice. The "Top of the Morning" recording of Fulton Lewis, Jr., has had wide usage for this purpose, but any similar recording containing relatively few great changes in intensity may be used, provided it can be readily calibrated to the speech audiometer. In using MLV, the examiner simply reads or "ad libs" a sample of nonemotional but informative speech in a conversational manner.

Instructions to the listener for the Fulton Lewis, Jr. record are as follows: "You are now going to hear a radio news announcer talking. Gradually his speech will become softer and softer. As you hear the record, you are to quickly repeat back words or parts of sentences that you hear. Are there any questions?"

The examiner starts the recording, after having made the necessary calibration adjustments, at a level 10 to 15 dB above the average pure-tone threshold. As the listener correctly identifies important words or phrases, the examiner turns the level down in 2 or 4-dB steps until he is just barely able to identify the gist of the speech. This is his SRT and no correction factor is involved.

Sophisticated listeners may simply be asked if they do or do not understand any of the speech; in either event, the examiner alters the intensity to the point where with concentrated listening the listener can just barely follow the train of the speech. Obtaining the SRT with Bekesy-type audiometers appears to be feasible (71).

Speech Discrimination Procedures

TEST LEVEL

Speech discrimination is usually tested at some arbitrary level in dB above SRT, but occasionally at MCL (Most Comfortable Level). Less often it is obtained at an arbitrary 60 or 64-dB SPL (the approximate level at which we usually hear faint speech). Discrimination may be tested at almost any level, including just below the Threshold of Discomfort, but SRT plus 25 dB and SRT plus 40 dB are probably the most commonly used levels. The presentation level, as stated earlier, has an important effect on the discrimination of speech. The articulation of the speaker and the choice of speech materials are no less important.

Common use of the SRT plus 40-dB level undoubtedly results from the Rush Hughes recordings of the PB–50 monosyllables. With this recording, the best discrimination scores, often called PB Max[10] are reached for normal listeners at about 40 dB above SRT. What many clinicians seem to overlook is that when they change speakers or speech materials, the PB Max level is also likely to change. Thus, the Hirsh recordings of the W–22 word lists produce a PB Max more nearly approximating SRT plus 25 dB. For this reason, in testing for PB Max many experienced clinicians suggest SRT plus 40 dB as the presentation level for the Rush Hughes recordings and SRT plus 25 dB when using the W–22 recordings or when using MLV. Still other clinicians use a level somewhere between SRT plus 25 and 40 dB. All of these levels are based on data obtained with normally hearing individuals, and since we are primarily concerned with the hearing-impaired population, the level may not be equally appropriate. Even SRT plus 40 dB does not usually produce maximum discrimination with normal hearing groups; scores continue to rise past that level with corresponding decreases in variability, but clinical testing at levels higher than SRT plus 40 dB seems to be of little value.

We desperately need experimental data on the way in which the parameters of speech audiometry influence various hearing loss and age populations. It is quite probable that one type of hearing loss will result in behavior which differs greatly from another type of hearing loss with the same speech audiometric test, and that both will differ from normal. For instance, Rhodes (95) found the speech discrimination of individuals with high-frequency losses to be better than that of normals who heard through filter mechanisms simulating the same high-frequency loss. With one speech discrimination test (49), scores at SRT plus 30 and SRT plus 40 dB with presbycusic patients were not significantly different. The audiologist must not fall into the trap of assuming that normative data from normally hearing populations will automatically apply to persons having various types of hearing losses.

Whatever presentation level is chosen, the examiner will occasionally find, particularly in the case of cochlear pathology, that the listener may report the level to be too high for comfort. In these cases a lower level should be used and so indicated on the audiogram. Furthermore, for a severe hearing loss it is often impossible to test at SRT plus 40 dB, and

[10] *PB Max* is a useful concept but an unfortunate term since it implies that the maximum discrimination needs to be determined with PB words. *Max Discrim* might be a more accurate term to use and would apply to whatever speech materials are used.

occasionally not even at SRT plus 25 dB, because of the output limitations of the audiometer.

The use of a 60 or 64-dB SPL presentation level for discrimination testing, particularly in free field, has much to offer since it more nearly represents daily listening conditions than does an arbitrary level above threshold. The constant level of 60 or 64-dB SPL has not enjoyed wide use (except for hearing-aid comparisons) and it, too, has some disadvantages; for instance, it is of doubtful validity if the listener's hearing loss exceeds 60-dB SPL. The presentation level, and in fact speech discrimination testing in general, depends upon the measurement we seek: (1) maximum speech discrimination, (2) an evaluation of everyday listening circumstances, (3) an evaluation of performance under a low intensity, i.e. difficult, level, (4) a level where unaided and aided performance may be compared with hearing aids, or (4) some combination of these.

The testing level chosen by the examiner with a particular listener, or even with a given clinic population, is probably not so crucial as is maintaining that same level for all comparisons. The lack of a standard level for speech discrimination testing does, however, make comparison in research reports and comparison from clinic to clinic more difficult. In any event, the test level and the speech materials must be known by one clinic if they are to make meaningful comparisons with what was done at another clinic.

With the hearing-impaired population, more so than with the normally hearing group, the use of several test presentation levels has much to offer. It is unfortunate that clinicians often do not consider as worthwhile the time required for several tests at varying levels. As we shall see in Chapter 14, the hearing-impaired individual may reach his Max Discrim in a manner quite different from that of the normally hearing individual.

W–22 RECORD METHOD

The examiner sets the input selector to tape or record. With the hearing level dial at zero, he calibrates the 1,000 Hz tone on the selected disk or tape to the speech audiometer. He then gives the following instructions to the Listener: "You are now going to hear some words containing one syllable. These words will not get any softer. Before each word you will hear the phrase 'You will say,' which will be followed by the word you are to repeat. Repeat each of these words even though you have to guess at what you hear. Are there any questions?"

The examiner must have meanwhile decided at what level he wishes to present the test materials, SRT plus 40 dB, MCL, or whatever level he feels to be appropriate. Whatever level is chosen, the examiner should not alter that level. The examiner should have in front of him, out of the sight of the listener, a printed list of the PB's matching the order in the recording, and as the listener responds incorrectly to any words, these should be checked. If the full fifty words of any list are used, the examiner then subtracts 2 per cent for each error from the total 100 per cent for the Discrimination Score. If half-lists are used, 4 per cent must be subtracted for each error. Enter the discrimination score on the audiogram; it is well also to note on the audiogram the presentation level at which the testing was done.

Instead of merely checking the incorrect responses on his list of PB's, some clinicians indicate (usually phonetically) the specific error response. This takes a little more time than simply indicating errors, and the usefulness of the added effort is far from clear. On the other hand, it is surprising that little experimental work has been done with error patterns; perhaps this is so because such a study would have to include a very large number of them to be meaningful (98). Campbell (18) has suggested error patterns as a predictor of response to PB's from nonorganic hearing loss cases. DeSa (28), using Portuguese PB's, found phoneme error patterns useful in differential diagnosis in adults.

Discrimination testing is usually determined for each ear separately and unaided in free field, if a hearing aid is under consideration. It will be recalled that the W–22 lists and recordings consist of four basic lists of fifty different words, which are numbered one through four. Each of these numbered lists appears in six scramblings, A through F. Thus, it is suggested that the listener be presented with a different *numbered* list for the second ear tested, and still a different numbered test for succeeding tests during a single session. Unless more than four discrimination tests are administered to a single listener at one session, this procedure avoids repeating the same words even in a different order. If instead of having the listener repeat the stimulus word, the examiner wishes him to write it, as we recommended earlier, he must be provided with answer sheets containing fifty numbered blanks.

MONITORED LIVE VOICE METHOD

In testing speech discrimination by monitored live voice, the commonly used materials are the W–22 PB lists. The examiner sets the input selector to the microphone. With the hearing level dial at zero, the examiner should practice saying the phrase "Say the word" or "Write the word" several times and calibrate his speech so the carrier phrase peaks around zero on the VU meter. The directions to the listener, the setting of the test level, and the scoring are the same as for the W–22 recording just discussed.

In using the MLV technique, the examiner should remember that the carrier phrase is peaked at zero on the VU meter and that the stimulus word which follows should be allowed to fall at some level in relation to the carrier phrase that is natural for that word. To avoid the tendency to peak the key word, the examiner might well look away from the VU meter just as he finishes the carrier phrase. The carrier phrase serves to aid the examiner in controlling his vocal intensity and its omission does not seem to cause lower discrimination scores (80).

A decided advantage in MLV testing is that the examiner can pace the stimulus words according to the rate of the listener's responses. If the listener is fairly sophisticated, the test can be completed in less time than that required by record, but if the listener is slow in responding, the pace of the testing can be slowed appropriately. And if extraneous noise (such as coughing) happens to occur during a test word, the word can easily be repeated.

There are some differences of opinion as to the reliability of MLV testing versus recorded testing, and experimental evidence to date on this matter is not convincing. In the hands of a careful examiner, monitored live voice testing is just as reliable as recorded testing. Resnick (94) presents evidence that a single speaker is consistent from list to list but reliability drops when the speaker changes. Brandy (15) has produced results suggesting a significant difference between "live" and "recorded" testing, but his procedures suggest these to be a result of his correcting the intensity of the test words under the "recorded" condition. With one discrimination test Kreul et al. (68) claim to have demonstrated that there was a difference between talkers and carrier phrases but not between the actual word lists; with the same test recordings, however, Beyer et al. (7) could not determine if obtained differences were due to talkers or test lists. Until further evidence is accumulated, we feel that either procedure, MLV or records, will produce about the same reliability when *all* the necessary precautions are taken.

Most Comfortable Level

Many audiologists consider the Most Comfortable Level (MCL) to be a useful measure. Some use it as the level at which speech discrimination testing is performed. It is perhaps surprising that relatively little research has been published on the MCL. One of the earliest studies to investigate test-retest results with MCL was done by Kelley (66) with sentence materials on a group of normal listeners and two groups with hearing losses. His reported test-retest results are considerably better than any similar studies reported since. In fact, LeZak (72), using normal listeners with many retests, found variations from trial to trial as large as 35 dB.

It would appear that the Most Comfortable Level should actually be considered the Most Comfortable Range, since the listener is not likely to repeat the "level" as consistently as he does a threshold measurement. There is some evidence to suggest that persons with a hearing loss, particularly of a sensory type, will more closely repeat the MCL measurement than will persons with normal hearing.

Traditionally the listener is asked only to make the MCL judgment on the basis of comfort, and not on the level at which speech is clear or understandable. At present we have no data to show whether a difference exists when a listener is directed to indicate a comfortable speech level or the level where speech is most understandable. The relationship between these two listening tasks might be of clinical use.

MCL METHOD

The MCL may be obtained with recorded speech materials or by monitored live voice. In either case there does not appear to be any particular difference in the range of comfort, whether one approaches it from relatively high or relatively low levels. Probably the most commonly used stimulus for determining the MCL is the recording by Fulton Lewis, Jr., as was described above under SRT Method with Cold Running Speech. The instructions to the listener should approximate the following: "You are now going to hear me (or, a record of a radio announcer) talking, and gradually the speech will become louder. I want you to tell me when the speech is at the most comfortable level for you, that is, when the speech is at the level you prefer for listening. Are there are questions?"

The record or the talking is started just above the previously determined SRT level, and gradually made louder (increasing the level about 4 dB every 5 seconds) until the listener signals that this is a comfortable level. At this point the audiologist should increase the signal slightly and ask the listener his opinion of this level for comfort, since the listener may prematurely indicate a comfort level without realizing that a slightly higher level might be still more comfortable. This same procedure should be performed again to determine the listener's consistency.

The examiner should avoid making a judgment as to where he thinks the MCL ought to be for the listener. It is quite probable that the examiner can consciously or subconsciously influence the listener's judgment of MCL. MCL may be measured for the right ear, left ear, and in free field. The score should be entered on the audiogram in decibels relative to speech audiometric zero.

Threshold of Discomfort

The Threshold of Discomfort (TD), also sometimes referred to as the Uncomfortable Loudness Level (ULL) is the level at which the listener reports speech as being uncomfortable. The TD may be obtained with pure tones, but this is more time consuming and probably less meaningful than with speech. At about 120-dB SPL (approximately 100 dB re speech audiometer zero) the normal listener usually reports that sound is beginning to evoke another sensation, such as tickling or pressure. At still higher levels the sound actually becomes painful.

The TD has some diagnostic significance, and, as we shall see in Chapter 14, is one important indicator of the prognosis for hearing-aid use. Like the MCL, the Threshold of Discomfort has produced little experimental interest. We seriously lack data on the reliability of this measurement, its variations in different types of hearing losses, and the effect of auditory training on its possible improvement.

TD METHOD

The Threshold of Discomfort is conventionally obtained with recorded speech materials, usually the same materials as used for the MCL, and it is convenient to obtain the TD immediately following the MCL. The instructions to the listener should approximate the following:

> You are now going to hear a (or, the same) recording of a radio news announcer. This time the speech will get louder and louder. I want to see how loud you can stand the speech. If the speech gets so loud that it actually becomes uncomfortable or hurts, you are to raise your hand and I will turn the sound down immediately. Try to tolerate as much loudness as you can. Are there any questions?

The recording is then started slightly above the previously determined MCL. Gradually the sound is increased (perhaps 4 dB every five seconds) until the listener indicates that the speech is uncomfortable, or until the maximum limit of the audiometer is reached. The procedure should be performed several times in each ear unless on the first trial for each ear the listener is able to tolerate the maximum output of the audiometer. The TD score is entered for each ear on the audiogram, in decibels relative to speech audiometer zero.

Several precautions in obtaining the TD should be taken. First, the examiner should make sure the listener clearly understands what he is to do when the speech becomes intolerably loud. It is advisable that the audiologist be able to see the listener rather than depend upon a push-button response. Second, he should assure the listener that should the sound truly become uncomfortable, it will be turned off immediately. Third, he should encourage the listener to wait until the sound has definitely become uncomfortable before signaling, not just unpleasantly loud. The examiner can keep the listener within sight and still be able to turn the hearing level dial down immediately if the dial has detents of 2 or 5 dB; this is done by simply counting the clicks made by the dial from the starting point. Or, the dial can be turned up to the point where the listener signals the TD and then the input turned to a neutral point. The TD may be determined by using MLV, but feedback is often a problem at the higher levels.

Interpretation of Speech Audiometric Tests

We would expect the person with normal hearing to have an SRT of approximately 0 dB (which is 22 dB above 0.0002 dynes/cm^2), an MCL of approximately 40 dB (which is approximately 60-dB SPL), and the TD would be expected to be about 100 dB (which would be approximately 120-dB SPL). Speech discrimination would be expected to be 90 per cent or higher, depending upon the test materials and the presentation level.

In persons with conductive hearing loss, the SRT, MCL, and TD would be moved upward approximately by the amount of the conductive loss. Speech discrimination would be about the same as for normals, so long as the presentation level is well above the SRT. For the person with a sensorineural loss, particularly one involving a cochlear pathology, the SRT would be elevated above normal, but the MCL and particularly the TD are likely to be considerably lower in relation to the SRT than for the normal.

The SRT subtracted from the TD is known as the DYNAMIC RANGE and is a useful concept in fitting hearing aids. The audiogram may have a place to indicate the Dynamic Range separately, however its calculation is simple and no separate indication of it is really necessary.

One purpose of the SRT is to confirm the pure-tone findings. It has been found that there is a good relationship between the average pure-tone loss at 500–1,000–2,000 Hz and the SRT. However, a number of factors complicate this relationship. First, the USASI (118) calibration standards for speech audiometers call for the zero reference level to be at 22-dB SPL for a 1,000 Hz tone. Using this reference and using the USASI 1951 standards for pure-tone audiometer calibration usually produced SRT's which were a little lower (i.e., worse) than the average pure-tone loss. With the ISO 1964 pure-tone standards, the SRT's are likely to be a little higher (i.e., better) than the average pure-tone loss, but in closer agreement than under the older pure-tone standards. Meanwhile, some clinics changed their speech audiometers to levels such as 29-dB SPL for zero, but this practice has not been common. Nor has it been determined if the ISO will recommend a change in the zero reference for speech audiometers, as was done for pure-tone audiometers.[11] In addition, we know that persons who are experienced in SRT testing and who know the test words are likely to have slightly better SRT's than are inexperienced listeners. Thus, comparisons of SRT and pure-tone averages in the speech frequencies remain somewhat confused.

For clinical purposes, using ISO 1964 pure-tone standards for comparison, we should expect the SRT to be within ± 5 dB of the average pure-tone

[11]The 1969 revision of specifications for audiometers calls for speech audiometers to be calibrated at 20 dB for 1000 Hz tone (American National Standard Institute 53.6 — 1969).

loss in the speech frequencies (500–1,000–2,000 Hz). If the pure-tone threshold contour shows a substantial drop toward the higher frequencies, we would expect poorer agreement, and when this happens some clinicians recommend using only 500 and 1,000 Hz in computing the average. If the SRT is much worse (perhaps more than 10 dB worse) than the average pure-tone loss, we will probably suspect that the listener has poor speech discrimination, and we will confirm this by discrimination testing. If the SRT, on the other hand, is much better than the average pure-tone loss, we may suspect some nonorganic component to the hearing loss and will accordingly perform special tests to confirm or rule this out.

If the thresholds of the two ears of a patient are about the same, we would expect the free field SRT to be slightly better (3 to 5 dB better) than that of either ear. We know of no research on this matter for discrimination, but clinically we have not found a similar improvement in free field speech discrimination over discrimination under phones. Another purpose of SRT determination is to use it as a point above which speech discrimination testing is accomplished.

At one time speech discrimination testing was of considerable importance in audiological diagnosis, particularly in the differentiation of conductive or mixed hearing losses from sensori-neural losses, especially where middle-ear surgery was contemplated. Speech discrimination is also used to identify other diagnostic patterns. Its use for differentiation between conductive and sensori-neural losses is now merely confirmatory. As mentioned earlier in this chapter, the need for speech discrimination in the diagnosis of the types or causes of hearing disorders is no longer critical, because a host of other tests have been developed which accomplish this with greater precision. The precision of speech discrimination tests is, unfortunately, still much less than desirable. We don't know, for instance, whether two discrimination scores are significantly different, unless of course they differ by large percentages.

There have been suggestions that differences of 6 per cent between two discrimination scores should be considered significant, but experimental evidence is inconclusive. Clinically, we usually find excellent speech discrimination in cases of conductive hearing loss, relatively poor discrimination in cases of sensory hearing loss, and very poor discrimination in cases of neural loss.[12] Unfortunately, we have no precise definition of excellent, poor, and very poor. Hopefully speech discrimination norms can be determined. Hopefully too, other uses for speech audiometry will be developed or perfected. In this connection we would mention experiments such as the efforts to alter or distort the speech stimuli by increasing its

[12] That speech discrimination tests alone are not useful in differential diagnosis, we only need note that in nine surgically confirmed neurinomas, Shapiro and Naunton (100) found an equal distribution of scores in the 0 to 30 per cent, 32 to 80 per cent, and 82 to 100 per cent ranges.

speed (51, 83, 93), the effects of time compression and expansion (76, 111), and the effects of filtering a speech stimulus and sending parts of the signal to each ear for diagnostic purposes (1, 13, 64, 73). We have also seen efforts to employ speech SAL techniques (43) and speech EDR (24, 63, 97). These and other efforts may furnish us with a variety of clinically valuable tests.

HEARING HANDICAP

Through most of this chapter we have dealt primarily with measuring hearing for hearing *impairment*. We also need to measure hearing HANDICAP, and it seems likely that speech audiometry will offer the best way. Hearing handicap refers to the disadvantage or difficulty in everyday living or working activities resulting from hearing impairment. We have already mentioned that speech audiometry, though helpful, is no longer critical in the diagnosis of auditory disorders, and it could now be used more to evaluate everyday hearing function and needs.

Hirsh (55) suggests that the most valid test of discrimination would be the sentence because it makes use of connected speech. He states, "We sometimes wonder about the relation between articulation scores for lists of isolated words and the 'score' a person would obtain for his ability to understand conversational speech. We should like to know the latter, but we can quantify only the former." Actually we can quantify the "latter" but only with difficulty. Giolas and Epstein (44, 45) compared speech discrimination by employing recordings of connected discourse, the W–22 lists, and the PAL PB–50 lists. Indeed, they did find a poor relationship between discrimination for the word lists as compared with connected discourse, although the W–22 lists more nearly approximated connected discourse than did the PAL PB–50's.

Efforts to relate hearing impairment to hearing handicap date back at least thirty years, but the first systematic effort to quantify hearing handicap in a single score was by Davis (26). Davis' approach was to combine the SRT with the speech discrimination score, resulting in a number that represented the social adequacy of the hearing, and this number was called the Social Adequacy Index (SAI). The SAI was a useful concept but it was seldom employed. One problem was that the speech discrimination part of the score was determined with the Rush Hughes recording and made the use of any other discrimination test of doubtful value. More important, however, the SAI was never, to our knowledge, related to hearing handicap.

One difficulty in relating any audiometric measure or measures to hearing handicap is the lack of a proper test for hearing handicap. A potential tool for such measurement has been developed by High et al. (52), but initial efforts to relate this to audiometric measures (other than the SRT in the better ear) have been disappointing. A decided need in the field of audiology is a standard tool for measuring hearing handicap that would relate it to hearing impairment. Speech audiometry is the most likely means for developing a hearing handicap measure.

Appendix

MATERIALS FOR SPEECH AUDIOMETRY

Below are words used in the CID Auditory Test No. W-1 and W-2. The words are presented here in alphabetical order, but the tests (and the accompanying disk recording) are scrambled into six orders, identified A through F.

1. airplane
2. armchair
3. baseball
4. birthday
5. cowboy
6. daybreak
7. doormat
8. drawbridge
9. duckpond
10. eardrum
11. farewell
12. grandson
13. greyhound
14. hardware
15. headlight
16. horseshoe
17. hotdog
18. hothouse
19. iceberg
20. inkwell
21. mousetrap
22. mushroom
23. northwest
24. oatmeal
25. padlock
26. pancake
27. playground
28. railroad
29. schoolboy
30. sidewalk
31. stairway
32. sunset
33. toothbrush
34. whitewash
35. woodwork
36. workshop

The words below are used in the CID Auditory Test No. W-22. The four basic lists are presented here in alphabetical order, but the tests (and the accompanying disk recording) are scrambled into six orders each (identified by letters A through F), for a total number of 24 test lists.

LIST 1

1. ace
2. ache
3. an
4. as
5. bathe
6. bells
7. carve
8. chew
9. could
10. dad
11. day
12. deaf
13. earn (urn)
14. east
15. felt
16. give
17. high
18. him (hymn)
19. hunt
20. isle (aisle, I'll)
21. it
22. jam
23. knees
24. law
25. low
26. me
27. new
28. none (nun)
29. not (knot)
30. or (oar)
31. owl
32. poor
33. ran
34. see (sea)
35. she
36. skin
37. stove
38. them
39. there (their)
40. thing
41. toe
42. true
43. twins
44. up
45. us
46. wet
47. what (watt)
48. wire
49. yard
50. you (ewe)

LIST 2

1. ail (ale)
2. air (heir)
3. and
4. bin (been)
5. by (bye, buy)
6. cap
7. cars
8. chest
9. die (dye)
10. does
11. dumb
12. ease
13. eat
14. else
15. flat
16. gave
17. ham
18. hit
19. hurt
20. ice
21. ill
22. jaw
23. key
24. knee
25. live (the verb)
26. move
27. new (knew)
28. now
29. oak
30. odd
31. off
32. one (won)
33. own
34. pew
35. rooms
36. send
37. show
38. smart
39. star
40. tare (tear)
41. that
42. then
43. thin
44. too (two)
45. tree
46. way (weigh)
47. well
48. with
49. young
50. yore (your)

LIST 3

1. add
2. aim
3. are
4. ate (eight)
5. bill
6. book
7. camp
8. chair
9. cute
10. do
11. done (dun)
12. dull
13. ears
14. end
15. farm
16. glove
17. hand
18. have
19. he
20. if
21. is
22. jar
23. king
24. knit
25. lie (lye)
26. may
27. nest
28. no (know)
29. oil
30. on
31. out
32. owes
33. pie
34. raw
35. say
36. shove
37. smooth
38. start
39. tan
40. ten
41. this
42. three
43. though
44. tie
45. use (yews)
46. we
47. west
48. when
49. wool
50. year

LIST 4

1. aid
2. all (awl)
3. am
4. arm
5. art
6. at
7. bee (be)
8. bread (bred)
9. can
10. chin
11. clothes
12. cook
13. darn
14. dolls
15. dust
16. ear
17. eyes (ayes)
18. few
19. go
20. hang
21. his
22. in (inn)
23. jump
24. leave
25. men
26. my
27. near
28. net
29. nuts
30. of
31. ought (aught)
32. our (hour)
33. pale (pail)
34. save
35. shoe
36. so (sew)
37. stiff
38. tea (tee)
39. tin
40. than
41. they
42. through (thru)
43. toy
44. where (wear)
45. who
46. why
47. will
48. wood (would)
49. yea
50. yet

Bibliography

1. Balas, R. F., and G. R. Simon. "The articulation function of a staggered spondaic word list for a normal hearing population." *Journal of Auditory Research*, **4**: 285–89, 1965.
2. Beasley, W. C., and M. Rosenwasser. "Determining factors in composing and analyzing speech-hearing tests." *Laryngoscope*, **60**: 658–79, 1950.
3. Benson, R. W., H. Davis, C. E. Harrison, I. J. Hirsh, E. G. Reynolds, and S. R. Silverman. "C.I.D. auditory test W-1 and W-2." *Laryngoscope*, **61**: 838–41, 1951.
4. Berger, K. W. "Conversational English of university students." *Speech Monographs*, **34**: 65–73, 1967.
5. Berger, K. W. *The K.S.U. Speech Discrimination Test.* Kent, Ohio: Kent State University, 1967. Tape recorded tests available from Audiotone, Inc.
6. Berger, K. W. "The most common words used in conversations." *Journal of Communication Disorders*, **1**: 201–14, 1967.
7. Beyer, M. R., J. C. Webster, and D. M. Dague. "Revalidation of the clinical test version of the modified Rhyme words." *Journal of Speech and Hearing Research*, **12**: 374–78, 1969.
8. Black, J. W. *Multiple-choice Intelligibility Test.* Danville, Ill.: Interstate Printers and Pub., Inc., 1963.
9. Black, J. W. "Responses to multiple-choice intelligibility tests." *Journal of Speech and Hearing Research*, **11**: 453–66, 1968.
10. Black, J. W., and C. H. Haagen. "Multiple-choice intelligibility tests, forms A and B." *Journal of Speech and Hearing Disorders*, **28**: 77–86, 1963.
11. Blumenfeld, V. G., M. Bergman, and E. Millner. "Speech discrimination in an aging population. *Journal of Speech and Hearing Research*, **12**: 210–17, 1969.
12. Bocca, E. "Factors influencing binaural integration of periodically switched messages." *Acta Oto-Laryngologica*, **53**: 142–44, 1961.
13. Bocca, E. "Clinical aspects of cortical deafness." *Laryngoscope*, **68**: 301–9, 1958.
14. Bowling, L., and B. Elpern. "Relative intelligibility of items on CID auditory test W-1." *Journal of Speech and Hearing Research*, **1**: 152–57, 1961.
15. Brandy, W. T. "Reliability of voice tests of speech discrimination." *Journal of Speech and Hearing Research*, **9**: 461–65, 1966.
16. Campanelli, P. A. "A measure of intra-list stability of four PAL word lists." *Journal of Auditory Research*, **2**: 50–55, 1962.
17. Campbell, R. A. "Discrimination test word difficulty." *Journal of Speech and Hearing Disorders*, **8**: 13–22, 1965.
18. Campbell, R. A. "An index of pseudo-discrimination loss." *Journal of Speech and Hearing Research*, **8**: 77–84, 1965.
19. Carhart, R. "Basic principles of speech audiometry." *Acta Oto-Laryngologica*, **40**: 62–71, 1951.
20. Carhart, R."Considerations in the measurement of speech discrimination." *USAF School of Aerospace Medicine Report*, 3–65, June, 1965.
21. Carhart, R. "Monitored live-voice as a test of auditory acuity." *Journal of the Acoustical Society of America*, **17**: 339–49, 1946.

22. Carhart, R. "Speech reception in relation to pattern of pure-tone loss." *Journal of Speech and Hearing Disorders*, **11**: 97–108, 1946.
23. Chaiklin, J. B. "The relation among three selected auditory speech thresholds." *Journal of Speech and Hearing Research*, **2**: 237–43, 1959.
24. Chaiklin, J. B. "The conditioned GSR auditory speech threshold." *Journal of Speech and Hearing Research*, **2**: 229–36, 1959.
25. Chaiklin, J. B., and I. M. Ventry. "Spondee threshold measurement: A comparison of 2- and 5-db methods." *Journal of Speech and Hearing Disorders*, **29**: 47–59, 1964.
26. Davis, H. "The articulation area and the Social Adequacy Index for hearing." *Laryngoscope*, **58**: 761–78, 1948.
27. Davis, H., and S. R. Silverman. *Hearing and deafness*. Rev. ed. New York: Holt, Rinehart & Winston, Inc., 1960, Pp. 181–98.
28. DeSa, G. "Audiologic findings in central nerve deafness." *Laryngoscope*, **68**: 309–17, 1958.
29. Dewey, G. *Relativ Frequency of English Speech Sounds*. Cambridge: Harvard University Press, 1923.
30. Dirks, D. D., and D. R. Bower. "Masking effects of speech competing messages." *Journal of Speech and Hearing Research*, **12**: 229–45, 1969.
31. Dirks, D. D., and R. A. Wilson. "Binaural hearing of speech for aided and unaided conditions." *Journal of Speech and Hearing Research*, **12**: 650–64, 1969.
32. Doyne, M. P., and M. D. Steer. "Studies in speech reception testing." *Journal of Speech and Hearing Disorders*, **16**: 132–38, 1951.
33. Egan, J. P. et al. "Articulation testing methods." *Laryngoscope*, **58**: 955–91, 1948.
34. Elpern, B. S. "Differences in difficulty among C.I.D. W-22 auditory tests." *Laryngoscope*, **70**: 1560–65, 1960.
35. Elpern, B. S. "The relative stability of half-list and full-list discrimination tests." *Laryngoscope*, **71**: 30–36, 1961.
36. Fairbanks, G. "A test of phonemic differentiation: The Rhyme Test." *Journal of the Acoustical Society of America*, **30**: 596–600, 1958.
37. Falconer, G. A., and H. Davis. "The intelligibility of connected discourse as a test for a threshold of speech." *Laryngoscope*, **57**: 581–95, 1947.
38. Falconer, G. "The reliability and validity of monitored connected discourse as a test of the threshold of intelligibility." *Journal of Speech and Hearing Disorders*, **13**: 369–71, 1948.
39. Farrimond, T. "Factors influencing auditory perception of pure tones and speech." *Journal of Speech and Hearing Research*, **5**: 194–204, 1962.
40. Feldman, R. M., and R. Goldstein. "Average evoked responses to synthetic syntax sentences." *Journal of Speech and Hearing Research*, **10**: 689–96, 1967.
41. Fletcher, H. *Speech and Hearing in Communication*. New York: D. Van Nostrand Co., Inc., 1953.
42. Fletcher, H., and J. C. Steinberg. "Articulation testing methods." *Bell System Technical Journal*, **8**: 807–09, 1929.
43. Gibson, J. H. "An investigation of the extension of the sensorineural acuity level (SAL) audiometric method of bone-conduction testing into the area of speech audiometry." Masters thesis. Kent, Ohio: Kent State University, 1961.

44. Giolas, T. G. "Comparative intelligibility scores of sentence lists and continuous discourse." *Journal of Auditory Research*, **6**: 31–38, 1966.
45. Giolas, T. G., and A. Epstein. "Comparative intelligibility of word lists and continuous discourse." *Journal of Speech and Hearing Research*, **6**: 349–58, 1963.
46. Grubb, P. "A phonemic analysis of half-list speech discrimination tests." *Journal of Speech and Hearing Research*, **6**: 271–75, 1963.
47. Grubb, P. "Some considerations in the use of half-list speech discrimination tests." *Journal of Speech and Hearing Research*, **6**: 294–97, 1963.
48. Haagen, C. H. "Intelligibility measurement." *Speech Monographs*, **13**: 4–7, 1946.
49. Harbert, F., I. M. Young, and H. Menduke. "Audiologic findings in presbycusis." *Journal of Auditory Research*, **6**: 297–312, 1966.
50. Harris, J. D. "Some suggestions for speech reception testing." *Archives of Otolaryngology*, **50**: 388–405, 1949.
51. Harris, J. D., H. L. Haines, and C. K. Myers. "The importance of hearing at 3Kc for understanding speeded speech." *Laryngoscope*, **70**: 131–46, 1960.
52. High, W. S., G. Fairbanks, and A. Glorig. "Scale for self-assessment of hearing handicap." *Journal of Speech and Hearing Disorders*, **29**: 215–30, 1964.
53. Hinchcliffe, R. "Threshold of hearing for random noise." *Journal of Speech and Hearing Research*, **4**: 3–9, 1961.
54. Hirsh, I., H. Davis, S. R. Silverman, E. G. Reynolds, E. Eldert, and R. W. Benson. "Development of materials for speech audiometry." *Journal of Speech and Hearing Disorders*, **17**: 321–37, 1952.
55. Hirsh, I. J. *The Measurement of Hearing*. New York: McGraw-Hill Book Company, 1952.
56. Hudgins, C. V., J. F. Hawkins, J. E. Karlin, and S. S. Stevens. "Development of recorded auditory tests for measuring hearing loss for speech." *Laryngoscope*, **57**: 57–89, 1947.
57. Hudgins, C. V. A method of appraising the speech of the deaf." *Volta Review* **51**: 597–638, 1949.
58. Huntington, D. A., and M. Ross. "The reliability and equivalency of the CID W-22 auditory tests." *USAF School of Aerospace Medicine Report*, 61–110, February, 1962.
59. Hutton, C., E. T. Curry, and M. B. Armstrong. "Semi-diagnostic test materials for aural rehabilitation." *Journal of Speech and Hearing Disorders*, **24**: 319–29, 1959.
60. Hutton, C., E. T. Curry, and T. H. Fay, Jr. "Auditory confusions among alphabet letters." *Journal of Auditory Research*, **5**: 109–17, 1965.
61. Jerger, J. F., R. Carhart, T. W. Tillman, and J. L. Peterson. "Some relations between normal hearing for pure tones and for speech." *Journal of Speech and Hearing Research*, **2**: 126–40, 1959.
62. Jerger, J. F., C. Speaks, and J. L. Trammell. "A new approach to speech audiometry." *Journal of Speech and Hearing Research*, **33**: 318–28, 1968.
63. Katz, J., and R. J. Connelly. "Instrumental avoidance vs. classical conditioning in GSR speech audiometry." *Journal of Auditory Research*, **4**: 171–79, 1964.

64. Katz, J., R. Basil, and J. Smith. "A staggered spondaic word test for determining central auditory lesions." *Annals of Otology, Rhinology and Laryngology*, **72**: 908–17, 1963.
65. Katz, J. "The use of staggered spondaic words for assessing the integrity of the central auditory nervous system." *Journal of Auditory Research*, **2**: 327–37, 1962.
66. Kelley, N. H. "A comparative study of the response of normal and pathological ears to speech sounds." *Journal of Experimental Psychology*, **31**: 342–52, 1937.
67. Kopra, L. L., and D. Blosser. "Comparison of Fairbanks Rhyme Test and C.I.D. Auditory Test W–22 in normal and hearing-impaired listeners." *Journal of Speech and Hearing Research*, **11**: 735–39, 1968.
68. Kreul, E. J., J. C. Nixon, K. D. Kryter, D. W. Bell, and J. S. Lang. "A proposed test of speech discrimination." *Journal of Speech and Hearing Research*, **11**: 536–52, 1968.
69. Lehiste, I., and G. E. Peterson. "Linguistic considerations in the study of speech intelligibility." *Journal of the Acoustical Society of America*, **31**: 280–86, 1959.
70. Lerman, J. W., M. Ross, and R. M. McLauchlin. "A picture-identification test for hearing-impaired children." *Journal of Auditory Research*, **5**: 273–78, 1965.
71. LeZak, R. J., B. M. Siegenthaler, and A. J. Davis. "Bekesy-type audiometry for speech reception threshold." *Journal of Auditory Research*, **4**: 181–89, 1964.
72. LeZak, R. J. "Some aspects of comfortable loudness." Doctoral dissertation. University Park, Pa.: Pennsylvania State University, 1961. Reported in part in *Laryngoscope*, **73**: 267–74, 1963.
73. Linden, A. "Distorted speech test and binaural speech synthesis tests." *Acta Oto-Laryngologica*, **58**: 32–48, 1964.
74. Lloyd, L. L., and M. J. Reid. "The reliability of speech audiometry with institutionalized retarded children." *Journal of Speech and Hearing Research*, **9**: 450–55, 1966.
75. Lovrinic, J. H., E. J. Burgi, and E. T. Curry. "A comparative evaluation of five speech discrimination measures." *Journal of Speech and Hearing Research*, **11**: 372–81, 1968.
76. Luterman, D. M., O. L. Welsh, and J. Melrose. "Responses of aged males to time-altered speech stimuli." *Journal of Speech and Hearing Research*, **9**: 226–30, 1966.
77. MacFarlan, D. "Speech hearing and speech interpretation testing." *Archives of Otolaryngology*, **31**: 517–28, 1940.
78. MacFarlan, D. "Speech hearing tests." *Laryngoscope*, **55**: 71–115, 1945.
79. Martin, F. N., H. A. T. Bailey, Jr., and J. J. Pappas. "The effect of central masking on threshold for speech." *Journal of Auditory Research*, **5**: 293–96, 1965.
80. Martin, F. N., R. R. Hawkins, and H. A. T. Bailey, Jr. "The nonessentiality of the carrier phrase in phonetically balanced (PB) word testing." *Journal of Auditory Research*, **2**: 319–22, 1962.
81. Martin, F. N. "Speech audiometry and clinical masking." *Journal of Auditory Research*, **6**: 199–203, 1966.

82. Merrell, H. B., and C. J. Atkinson. "The effect of selected variables upon discrimination." *Journal of Auditory Research*, **5**: 279–284, 1965.
83. Miller, G. A., and J. C. R. Licklider. "The intelligibility of interrupted speech. *Journal of the Acoustical Society of America*, **22**: 167–73, 1950.
84. Miller, G. A., G. A. Heise, and W. Lichten. "The intelligibility of speech as a function of the context of the test materials." *Journal of Experimental Psychology*, **41**: 329–35, 1951.
85. Myatt, B. D., and B. A. Landes. "Assessing discrimination loss in children." *Archives of Otolaryngology*, **77**: 359–62, 1963.
86. Newby, H. *Audiology*. New York: Appleton-Century-Crofts, 1958 (1964). See Chapter 6.
87. Oyer, H. D., and M. Doudna. "Word familiarity as a factor in testing discrimination of hard-of-hearing subjects." *Archives of Otolaryngology*, **72**: 351–55, 1960.
88. Owens, E. "Intelligibility of words varying in familiarity." *Journal of Speech and Hearing Research*, **4**: 113–29, 1961.
89. Palmer, J. "The effect of speaker differences on the intelligibility of phonetically balanced word lists." *Journal of Speech and Hearing Disorders*, **20**: 192–95, 1955.
90. Peterson, G. E., and I. Lehiste. "Revised CNC lists for auditory tests." *Journal of Speech and Hearing Disorders*, **27**: 62–70, 1962.
91. Plummer, R. H. "High-frequency deafness and discrimination of high-frequency consonants." *Journal of Speech Disorders*, **8**: 373–81, 1943.
92. Pollack, I., H. Rubenstein, and L. Decker. "Intelligibility of known and unknown message sets." *Journal of the Acoustical Society of America*, **31**: 273–79, 1959.
93. Quiros, J. B. "Accelerated speech audiometry; An examination of results." *Beltone Translations*, No. 17, 1964.
94. Resnick, D. "Reliability of the twenty-five word phonetically balanced lists." *Journal of Auditory Research*, **2**: 5–12, 1962.
95. Rhodes, R. C. "Discrimination of filtered CNC lists by normals and hypacusics." *Journal of Auditory Research*, **6**: 129–33, 1966.
96. Rosenwig, M. R., and L. Postman. "Intelligibility as a function of frequency usage." *Journal of Experimental Psychology*, **54**: 412–22, 1964.
97. Ruhm, H. B., and R. Carhart. "Objective audiometry: A new method based on electrodermal response." *Journal of Speech and Hearing Research*, **1**: 169–78, 1958.
98. Schultz, M. C. "Suggested improvements in speech discrimination testing." *Journal of Auditory Research*, **4**: 1–14, 1964.
99. Schultz, M. C. "Word familiarity influences in speech discrimination." *Journal of Speech and Hearing Research*, **7**: 395–400, 1964.
100. Shapiro, I., and R. F. Naunton. "Audiologic evaluations of acoustic neurinomas." *Journal of Speech and Hearing Research*, **32**: 29–35, 1967.
101. Shutts, R. E., K. S. Burke, and J. E. Creston. "Derivation of twenty-five-word PB lists." *Journal of Speech and Hearing Disorders*, **29**: 442–47, 1964.
102. Siegenthaler, B. A study of the relationship between measured hearing loss and intelligibility of selected words." *Journal of Speech and Hearing Disorders*, **14**: 111–18, 1949.

103. Silverman, S. R., and I. J. Hirsh. "Problems related to the use of speech in clinical audiometry." *Annals of Otology, Rhinology and Laryngology*, **64**: 1234–44, 1955.
104. Silverman, S. R. "Tolerance for pure tones and speech in normal and defective hearing." *Annals of Otology, Rhinology and Laryngology*, **56**: 658–78, 1947.
105. Speaks, C. "Intelligibility of filtered synthetic sentences." *Journal of Speech and Hearing Research*, **10**: 289–98, 1967.
106. Speaks, C., and J. Jerger. "Method for measurement of speech identification." *Journal of Speech and Hearing Research*, **8**: 185–94, 1965.
107. Speaks, C., and J. Jerger. "Synthetic-sentence identification and the receiver operating characteristics." *Journal of Speech and Hearing Research*, **10**: 110–19, 1967.
108. Speaks, C., J. Jerger, and S. Jerger. "Performance-intensity characteristics of synthetic sentences." *Journal of Speech and Hearing Research*, **9**: 305–12, 1966.
109. Speaks, C., and J. L. Karmen. "The effect of noise on synthetic sentence identification." *Journal of Speech and Hearing Research*, **10**: 859–64, 1967.
110. Speaks, C., J. L. Karmen, and L. Benitez. "Effect of a competing message on synthetic sentence identification." *Journal of Speech and Hearing Research*, **10**: 390–95, 1967.
111. Sticht, T. G., and B. B. Gray. "The intelligibility of time compressed words as a function of age and hearing loss." *Journal of Speech and Hearing Research*, **12**: 443–48, 1969.
112. Thorndike, E. L. *A Teacher's Word Book of Twenty Thousand Words Found Most Frequently and Widely in General Reading for Children and Young People*. New York: Teachers College, Columbia University, 1931. Revised and enlarged with I. Lorge as *The Teacher's Word Book of 30,000 Words*, New York, 1944.
113. Tillman, T. W., R. Carhart, and L. Wilber. "A test for speech discrimination composed of CNC monosyllabic words (N. U. Auditory Test No. 4)." *USAF School of Aerospace Medicine Report*, 62–135, January, 1963.
114. Tillman, T. W., and R. Carhart. "An expanded test for speech discrimination utilizing CNC monosyllabic words: N. U. Auditory Test No. 6." *USAF School of Aerospace Medicine Report*, 55–66, June, 1966.
115. Tillman, T. W., and J. Jerger. "Some factors affecting the spondee threshold in normal hearing subjects." *Journal of Speech and Hearing Research*, **2**: 141–46, 1959.
116. Tobias, J. V. "On phonemic analysis of speech discrimination tests." *Journal of Speech and Hearing Research*, **7**: 98–100, 1964.
117. Tweedie, D. "Discrepancies in scoring of responses made on C.I.D. W-22 word lists by trained examiners." *Audecibel*, **18**: 160–65, 1969.
118. *USASI standards specifications for speech audiometers*. Bulletin Z24. 13–1953. New York: United States of America Standards Institute, 1953.
119. Watson, T. J. "Speech audiometry in children." In *Educational Guidance and the Deaf Child*, W. G. Ewing, ed. Manchester, England: Manchester University Press, 1957.
120. Weinhouse, I., and M. H. Miller. "Discrimination scores for two lists of phonetically balanced words." *Journal of Auditory Research*, **3**: 9–14, 1963.

10-27-75

8

Pediatric Audiology

David C. Shepherd, Ph.D

The identification and measurement of auditory dysfunction in neonates, infants, and young children are the most difficult, but perhaps most challenging responsibilities of the clinical audiologist. Logically, it is impossible to accurately differentiate normal from abnormal auditory systems among children, if one is uncertain as to what auditory response behavior is typical of a child with a normal auditory system. Unfortunately, however, the pool of definitive research data supporting predictable laws of auditory behavior in children with normal hearing is quite shallow, compared to our knowledge of how the normal hearing adult will respond to different auditory stimuli and different stimulus parameters. Of course, as the normal hearing child advances in age from neonate (birth to two months) to infant (two months to two years) and from infant to a young child (two to five years), predictable laws of auditory behavior applicable to normal hearing adults become more applicable to him.

In this chapter the focus of the discussion will be on the problems of auditory evaluation in children from birth to five years of age. The child will be viewed as a complex of systems designed to produce auditory responses when exposed to auditory stimuli. Ideally, if the child under test does not produce an auditory response to a particular auditory stimulus that is known to evoke a response from a normal hearing child, it would be assumed that he is a malfunctioning producer of auditory responses due to a breakdown within his systems complex. Because he is not responding appropriately to auditory stimulation, it would be logical to infer that the breakdown involves some or all components of his auditory system. Realistically, however, the audiometric evaluation of the young child is not this simple.

Although the child is considered to be a producer of auditory responses, it should always be realized that he is also capable of producing responses to other sensory stimuli, as well as internal stimuli (i.e., visceral, ideational), if attuned and stimulated appropriately. The human organism, regardless of age, is generally under constant bombardment by external and internal stimuli of differing sources and magnitudes. Therefore, it is quite probable that upon many occasions the auditory stimulus introduced by the audiologist stimulates the child while he is about to respond or is in the process of responding to another stimulus or other stimuli. According to Wilder (95), every stimulus is a second stimulus and every sensation is a second sensation.

The fact that young children are different from older children and adults in many aspects of stimulus-response behavior is not a revolutionary observation. Their attention spans are shorter, while their perception and discrimination abilities are immature. Therefore, the clinical audiologist must, at times, take great pains with his techniques and tools to insure the production of auditory responses. This may be accomplished by his making the auditory stimulus of greater importance to the child than other incidental stimuli that might be competing for the child's attention.

Basically, the clinical audiologist must perform the following tasks when evaluating the auditory system of a child: (1) He must set criteria that will define an auditory response. (2) He must be flexible and imaginative in structuring a measurement procedure that will insure the production of auditory responses from children whose auditory systems are at least partially functioning. (3) He must set response criteria that will differentiate normal hearing children from children with defective auditory systems.

The Auditory Response

A common audiologic test used to detect auditory impairment in neonates and very young infants consists merely of crumpling a sheet of onion-skin paper. This test is simple in construct and fairly easy to standardize. But what tells the audiologist that the child either responds or does not respond to the sound of the crumpling of onion-skin paper? Obviously, the baby produces some distinctive activity following the auditory stimulus that the audiologist records as an auditory response. This activity, however, is distinctive from what? In its simplest form this poststimulus activity is in some way distinctive from the prestimulus activity. Therefore, the audiologist must make one of two observations after the auditory stimulus is introduced before he records either "auditory response" or "no auditory response." The child's activity either changed or it did not change. A change in activity may be considered an auditory response if it meets certain criteria previously set forth for the test design the audiologist is employing.

The type of activity the audiologist is seeking to change with the auditory stimulus and the criteria established for classifying a change as an auditory response are both dependent upon: (1) the response system chosen for the production of auditory responses; (2) the prestimulus activity level of the child; (3) the age of the child being evaluated; and (4) the magnitude of the auditory stimulus.

AUDITORY RESPONSE SYSTEMS

An auditory response system, as referred to in this chapter, involves a complex of neuroanatomic and neurophysiologic structures that mediate the final auditory response. Specific auditory response systems are those that respond only to auditory stimulation. They include the cochlea and the acoustic neural pathways up to, but not including, the cochlear nucleus. Only one study known to this writer has measured auditory responses in children by using specific auditory response systems. Ruben et al., (79) made electrophysiologic measures of changes in the cochlear and eighth nerve action potentials at the cochlear round window as a function of pure-tone and click stimulation in children.

Non-specific auditory response systems are those that include components that lie within the central nervous system, and components that leave from the central nervous system and go to the point where the response is produced. These response systems are called nonspecific because a large number of the components that make up these systems are not specifically tuned to respond only to auditory stimulation.

In general, all auditory response systems, both specific and nonspecific, fall under two major classifications which are determined on the basis of the nature of the final response. These two classifications are behavioral response systems and electrophysiologic response systems.

Behavioral Response System. Auditory responses produced through the behavioral response systems are characterized by some neuromuscular activity of the child under test. This activity occurs after auditory stimulation and can be visually observed or audibly heard by the audiologist. These response systems can produce muscular responses to stimuli other than the auditory stimulus, if such stimuli are of sufficient magnitude and importance to the child. Thus, they are nonspecific auditory response systems.

Behavioral responses range from very archaic muscle reflexes dominated by the subcortical mechanism in neonates to cortically controlled speech utterances in older children. Logically, as behavioral responses move from the primitive reflex end of the continuum to the speech production end of the continuum, they come more under the willful control of the child. Therefore, the audiologist can do much to tune the older child's behavioral response systems to respond to the auditory stimulus by pretest instruction and training, as well as by utilizing appropriate conditioning principles in the design of his test that will maintain the attractiveness of the auditory stimulus to the child. On the other hand, when testing neonates and very young children, the audiologist can do little more than present the auditory stimulus when the child appears relatively inactive or active, depending upon whether the examiner wants to arouse or inhibit prestimulus behavioral activity.

Electrophysiologic Response System (*Electrodermal*). Auditory responses produced through the electrophysiologic response systems manifest themselves as recorded changes in the electrical properties of body structures, as an indirect result of auditory stimulation. To date, the most common electrophysiologic system used in pediatric audiology terminates with recordable changes in the electrical properties of the skin. These changes occur as a direct result of either increased or decreased sweat gland activity. The nerve supply to the sweat glands has been found to be composed exclusively of the sympathetic nerve fibers of the autonomic nervous system (71, 56). Centers for the regulation of the autonomic nervous system have been found at many levels of the central nervous system (22). Therefore, an auditory sensation of sufficient magnitude and importance to a child will indirectly cause an alteration of sweat gland activity by first exciting the auditory system, which in turn excites the central nervous system, which activates the autonomic nervous system, which finally increases or decreases sweat gland activity by way of its sympathetic nerve fibers. The change in the electrical properties of the sweat glands is generally recorded in one of two ways. The Féré technique measures changes in the electrical resistance of the skin to an electrical current, while the Tarchanoff technique measures differences in the electrical potential between two points on the skin. Goldstein and Derbyshire (40) have termed audiometric procedures utilizing this response system as ELECTRODERMAL AUDIOMETRY (EDA) which measures an ELECTRODERMAL RESPONSE (EDR). Originally, the EDR was called the PSYCHOGALVANIC SKIN RESPONSE (PGSR).

The EDR system is a very nonspecific auditory response system. Lindsley (58) mentions that the EDR is highly sensitive to all the sensory stimuli and internal ideational stimuli associated with attitudes of alertness, attention, apprehension, and arousal. Psychophysiologists have been using the EDR as an index of emotional change for many years. To enhance EDR specificity to auditory stimulation in clinical audiology, the auditory stimulus is periodically followed by an unconditioned stimulus such as electric shock, light, or heat. The procedure resembles the Pavlovian classical conditioning paradigm. After several pairings, the auditory stimulus becomes associated with the unconditional stimulus and a response similar to that evoked by the unconditioned stimulus alone is elicited by the auditory stimulus. Of course, it is important that the EDR occur after the auditory stimulus with no unconditioned stimulus before it can be considered an EDR to auditory stimulation.

Electrophysiologic Response System (*Electroencephalic*). Responses evoked by auditory stimuli and produced through the ELECTROENCEPHALIC RESPONSE (EER) system are represented as changes in the ongoing electrical activity at the cortex. This electrical activity is generally recorded from a disc or from needle electrodes placed on the scalp over certain areas of the brain's cortex. Audiologic procedures employing the EER system have been termed ELECTROENCEPHALIC AUDIOMETRY (EEA) by Goldstein and Derbyshire (40).

The EER system might possibly be used as a specific auditory response system depending upon electrode placement on the scalp and the refinement of recording equipment. If it were possible to isolate and record only electrical activity arising from the primary auditory cortex through strategically placed scalp electrodes, then this response system could be considered specific to auditory stimulation. Walter (92) warns, however, that because specific primary auditory areas at the cortex are so small and are surrounded by large tracts of the nonspecific parietal and temporal cortex, auditory responses seen on the scalp records reflect both specific auditory response activity and nonspecific electrical activity arising from these other areas. He is of the opinion that all evoked responses to sensory stimuli measured from the cortex in humans are primarily due to nonspecific electrical activation unless the contrary can be proven. Nevertheless, Goldstein and Rodman (42) have gathered data which suggest the possibility of isolating from scalp recordings the electrical activity from the primary auditory cortex evoked by auditory stimuli through the use of an averaging computer. Until further research confirms this possibility, however, the electroencephalic auditory response system should be considered nonspecific to auditory stimulation.

A source of nonspecific electrical activity arising through the scalp is the stimulated reticular formation in the lower brain stem. Every primary sensory pathway sends collateral nerve fibers to the reticular formation and, therefore, not only transmits message-carrying nerve impulses to its specific cortical areas, but also excites the reticular formation (60). Stimulation of the reticular formation produces fairly diffuse nonspecific electrical acitivity at the cortex (66). Therefore, any sensory stimulus can excite the reticular formation and thus evoke diffuse electrical activity at the cortex, which when recorded through scalp electrodes appears as an evoked response to that stimulus. If the stimulus is auditory then the product is an evoked auditory response. If the stimulus is visual, then this electrical activity is an evoked visual response

Electrophysiologic Response System (*Electrocardiac*). Although not extensively explored for its value to the clinical audiologist, the electrocardiac response (EKR) system has been investigated for many years by the psychophysiologist in his study of human emotions. The EKR is measured as a change upon stimulation in the electrical activity of the heart. This response system is quite nonspecific to auditory stimulation and like the EDR, the EKR is mediated through the autonomic nervous system. Both the EKR and EDR are considered by the psychophysiologists (2, 20, 30, 57) as contributing components in total autonomic response patterns to a variety of emotionally provoking stimuli. Nevertheless, Beadle and Crowell (6) reported data on the use of the EKR system to measure auditory responses in neonates.

PRESTIMULUS ACTIVITY LEVEL

Based upon Wilder's Law of Initial Value (LIV), the nature of the behavioral and electrophysiologic responses evoked from a child is influenced by the activity level of his response systems prior to stimulation. Very high or very low activity levels could result in no response to sensory stimuli even though all sensory and response systems are intact. Wilder (95) states in reference to the LIV:

> The change of any function of an organism due to a stimulus depends to a large degree on the prestimulus level of that function. That applies not only to the intensity (i.e. extent and duration) of response, but also to its direction. The higher this prestimulus level (the initial value), the smaller the tendency to rise on function-raising stimuli, the greater the tendency to drop on function-inhibiting stimuli. With more extreme high or low levels, there is a progressive tendency to "no response" or to "paradoxic reactions," i.e., to a reversal of the type of response: rise instead of fall, and vice versa.

The majority of the research applying the LIV has been accomplished by psychophysiologists in their study of responses of the autonomic nervous system in adults. Nevertheless, the concept of the LIV has important implications to the clinical audiologist for measuring electrophysiologic and behavioral responses to auditory stimuli in children. The prestimulus activity level as used in this chapter is based upon the LIV and includes two interacting conditions. These two conditions are (1), the psychological state, and (2), the readiness of the response systems to respond to auditory stimulation. The psychological state is described as the emotional set of a child that would either increase or decrease his conscious attentiveness to external stimuli. The readiness of the response systems to respond to auditory stimuli is a function of the amount and magnitude of ongoing response activity to incidental external and internal stimuli within the response systems at the time of auditory stimulation. Both of these conditions interacting with each other provide for favorable or unfavorable prestimulus activity levels for the production of auditory response by the child with either intact, or partially intact, auditory sensory and response systems.

It should be realized that prestimulus activity levels are constantly changing within the child as the auditory test progresses. Whether these changes are brought about by previous auditory stimuli or by incidental external and internal stimuli is very difficult for the audiologist to determine. Nevertheless, it is very possible that two responses produced by the same child to two identical auditory stimuli will have different patterns because the two prestimulus activity levels were dissimilar.

Psychological States. Lindsley (1952) correlated his descriptions of psychological states with EEG patterns, state of awareness, and efficiency relative to performing behavioral activity (59). Excluding EEG correlates, the psychological state of STRONG EXCITED EMOTION is accompanied by restricted awareness, divided attention, and confusion which produces disorganized behavior. Based upon clinical experience, this psychological state would be a component of a very undesirable prestimulus activity level and would make auditory measurement with children very difficult. This emotional set of a child does not provide for selective attention to any sensory stimulus, let alone the auditory stimulus. Nor are his nonspecific response systems tuned to respond only to auditory stimulation. It is quite probable that his psychological state is a result of considerable response activity to unidentified stimuli competing within and overloading the nonspecific response systems. This in turn produces random EDR's, EER's, EKR's, and behavioral responses that mask any possible response to the auditory stimulus from the eyes of the audiologist.

According to Lindsley, ALERT ATTENTIVENESS refers to selective attention, concentration, and anticipation which results in good, efficient, selective, and quick reactions. This psychological state would be very favorable for auditory measurement in children, using either the behavioral or the electrophysiologic response systems. The audiologist, however, must be clever in his manner of presenting the auditory stimulus so that the child's attentiveness to the auditory stimulus, and not to other stimuli, will be reinforced.

RELAXED WAKEFULNESS is accompanied by wandering attention and good reaction to routine tasks. This, too, is a favorable psychological state for measuring behavioral and electrophysiologic responses to auditory stimuli. While the child is in this state, however, it is possible to lose his attention to the auditory stimulus if the conditions of the test are not varied appropriately by the audiologist. The observant, flexible, and imaginative audiologist will immediately detect this state and alter the test conditions periodically.

As the child drifts into DROWSINESS then into LIGHT SLEEP and finally into DEEP SLEEP, attempts at conscious behavioral audiometry are obviously fruitless. Lindsley (59) associates progressive movement through these three psychological states with first, a shift from partial awareness and a "dream-like" state, to very reduced consciousness and a dream state, to finally, complete loss of awareness and no memory for stimulation or dreams. Eisenberg and others (31) found that neonates gave a greater percentage of primitive motor reflexes to auditory stimuli as the neonates' psychological state shifted toward deep sleep. The full Moro reflex was evoked most frequently during deep sleep.

As the child drifts from drowsiness toward deep sleep the conditions become more unfavorable for the use of the electrodermal or electrocardiac response systems to measure auditory responses. During sleep the components of the nonspecific response systems, including the hypothalamus within the brain stem which controls the autonomic nervous system, are less responsive and have higher thresholds of excitability (60) to internal and external stimulation. Hardy and Pauls (48) find it necessary to deliberately disturb a child who begins to doze when measuring electrodermal responses to "... enliven these sympathetic reactions." On the other hand, the specific sensory pathways remain open during sleep (60) and auditory-evoked changes in the ongoing electrical activity recorded at the cortex can be measured. In fact the K-complex, which can be evoked by any sensory stimulus, is most prevalent during moderately deep sleep (21, 61). The K-complex has been reported as a complex of sharp waves occurring singly or followed by synchronous high-amplitude activity on the electroencephalogram. It is more difficult, however, to evoke the K-complex during deep sleep (39).

Response System Readiness. As previously described, response system readiness is a function of the amount and nature of response activity to undetermined stimuli within the nonspecific response systems at the time of auditory stimulation. Broadbent (12) conceives of the nervous system as a single communication channel of limited capacity for which sensory stimuli must compete. One might also reason that response systems have limited capacities for which the effects of external and internal stimuli must compete. The Law of Initial Value suggests that if some unknown stimuli prior to auditory stimulation has driven all response systems to an exceptionally high level of excitability, then the effects upon these response systems by the auditory stimulus will be negligible or nonexistent. In other words, all the lines are too busy with responses to stimuli of greater magnitude and importance to the child than the auditory stimulus. At the other end of the continuum, during deep sleep, the response activity within the nonspecific response systems is at a low level, but the thresholds for exciting these systems are very high. In this psychological state one might say that all lines are closed down for the night except for emergencies.

The child in an attentive psychological state with little response activity occurring within his nonspecific response systems is at the most ideal prestimulus activity level for audiometric testing.

AUDITORY RESPONSE AS A FUNCTION OF AGE

In its most primitive form, an auditory response may be represented as merely a change in a child's prestimulus activity level. In more sophisticated form, an auditory response is a change in prestimulus behavioral, or electrophysiologic activity meeting definite criteria, i.e.: poststimulus activity of a required latency relative to stimulus onset; activity of required latency and magnitude revealed by the swing of a pen on an electrophysiologic recording; a specific type of poststimulus muscular activity occurring at a definite time after stimulus onset; and correct speech production of a spoken stimulus word. Logically, the criteria set forth for auditory responses evoked from neonates are much more primitive than what the clinical audiologist might require of a response from a five-year-old child.

Neonates (*birth to two months*). Behavioral reactions of neonates to external stimulation do not occur unless these external stimuli are intense enough to overcome the neonates' high threshold of perception (85). Studies dealing specifically with the measurement of auditory reflexes in neonates support, to some degree, Spitz's observations and have shown that fairly intensive stimuli must be used to evoke behavioral reflex responses, regardless of the nature of the stimuli. Independent of prestimulus activity levels and other stimulus parameters, the sound pressure levels of auditory stimuli that have been successful in evoking some, or all, types of behavioral reflex responses in assumed normal hearing neonates, average 77 dB and range from 50 to 115 dB (29, 31, 46, 68, 88, 93).

The literature includes many descriptions of aural reflex responses that have been observed in normal hearing neonates as a result of fairly intense auditory stimulation. Some of the descriptions are operational definitions while others rely upon commonly accepted terms to describe patterns of reflex activity observed, such as the Moro reflex, the Quasi-Moro reflex, the Auropalpebral reflex (APR), and the Auditory reflex. Other descriptions of reflex activity fall under the general classifications of Arousal reflex activity and Cessation reflex activity.

The MORO REFLEX as defined by Hoerr and Osol (51) is "A concussion reaction normally observed only in newborn infants, elicited by a sudden sharp noise, such as clapping the hands ... In the normal response both legs are drawn up and the arms brought up as in an embrace..." Parmelee

(72) believes that neck movement is essential for a true Moro reflex. Eisenberg et al., (31) found in a study dealing with auditory reflex behavior in neonates, that the full Moro reflex is evoked most frequently during the psychological state of deep sleep, may be observed on occasion in states of dozing, and is never seen when a child is awake. A clacker that produces a very short percussive peak of 55 to 60 dB (SPL) is very effective in stimulating the Moro reflex in four- to five-day-old normal hearing neonates (46). It is very difficult, however, to synthesize from the literature the types of auditory stimuli that are either effective or ineffective in evoking the Moro reflex from neonates, because of the vague descriptions of the stimuli and responses that appear in many of these reports. At best, one might say that the normal hearing neonate should give a full Moro reflex if stimulated by most any sudden, sharp, percussive sound with a peak sound pressure level of 70 dB, while the neonate is in deep sleep.

The QUASI-MORO REFLEX includes motor reflex responses that approximate full Moro reflexes. An example would be the inhibition of ongoing muscular activity with hands pronated and one arm and leg drawn up. It is apparent that many descriptions of motor reflex patterns that are described as full Moro reflexes would be more aptly termed Quasi-Moro reflexes, or in general, startle reflexes. The same type of auditory stimulus that will evoke the Moro reflex will also evoke the Quasi-Moro reflex. Differences in the nature of the response produced may possibly be attributed to differences in prestimulus activity level.

According to Hoerr and Osol (51) the AUROPALPEBRAL REFLEX (APR) is defined as "...contraction of the orbicularis oculi muscle after hearing a sudden, unexpected sound." The APR does not necessarily involve eye blinking as some investigators have inferred. A slight contraction of the orbicularis oculi (muscle encircling the eye orbit) may not result in eyelid closure. In fact, it is not unusual to observe complete eyelid closure change to merely a contraction of the orbicularis oculi muscle with repeated stimulation. Nevertheless, muscle reflexes termed the APR have been found to be the most frequent aural reflexes, among all the muscle reflexes, given by neonates in light sleep (35, 36, 77). The APR is not specific to age and can be evoked from both children and adults by fairly intense, sharp, percussive sounds.

The APR is sometimes confused with the AUDITORY REFLEX which is also known as the ACOUSTIC REFLEX and the COCHLEAR REFLEX. Hoerr and Osol (51) define these reflexes as "...brief closure of the eyes, resulting from eighth nerve stimulation by the sudden production of a sound." According to the letter of this definition, therefore, eye blinking as a result of sudden stimulation by fairly intense auditory stimuli should technically be termed the Auditory, Cochlear, or Acoustic reflex, and not the APR. This is certainly a minor point, however, since the conditions for the stimulation of these reflexes are similar.

AROUSAL REFLEX activity is generally associated with the prestimulus activity levels of deep sleep, light sleep, or drowsiness. If a neonate is awakened by auditory stimulation, then he has produced an Arousal response. Random movements of the limbs, gross body movements, eye movements toward or away, increased inspiration, crying, or generally increased behavioral activity after auditory stimulation could be considered auditory arousal responses.

CESSATION REFLEX activity includes all behavioral cues of either a decrease or inhibition of prestimulus activity as a function of the auditory stimulus. For example, if a baby's prestimulus activity exhibits crying and extreme random limb and body movements and the auditory stimulus serves to inhibit all or some of this activity, then the audiologist may say that the baby responded to the stimulus.

It should be evident that the clinical audiologist is very dependent upon his observations of prestimulus activity levels to properly evaluate post-stimulus activity when utilizing behavioral response systems in neonates. In many instances poststimulus activity, as a function of the auditory stimulus, will exhibit patterns that contain several, and not just one, of the aural reflexes described above. It is also not unusual to find that the neonate will produce a very obvious reflex response to an auditory stimulus when it is first presented, but upon second presentation either the reflex response is diminished or it does not occur at all. This phenomenon has been termed RESPONSE ADAPTATION or RESPONSE HABITUATION.

Electrophysiologic response systems have also been used to determine auditory function in neonates, though not extensively (*see* Chapter 12 for a more complete discussion of electrophysiologic tests).

Infant (*two months to two years*). During the beginning of the infantile period, the development of the child's central steering organization begins (86), and his behavioral responses to stimuli become more coordinated and directed. The responses produced by the infant come more under cortical control, are more purposeful, and require more meaningful stimuli to evoke them. The infant's auditory response systems are less likely to respond to loud percussive sounds, and reflexive auditory responses occur less frequently. After four months of age, the normal hearing infant produces fewer Moro reflexes regardless of the nature and intensity of the stimulus (17, 65). Loud sounds, in general, are no longer disturbing to the infant, and he becomes more accepting of them as he matures (37). The APR, however, can still be evoked by sudden sharp sounds. At two to three months of age, the infant becomes more attentive to the human voice (98) and is apt to respond more frequently to a quiet voice than a loud voice (33).

By three or four months, the disorganized EEG activity arising from the cortical sensory zones, characteristic of the neonate, changes to rhythmic activity of three or four waves per second. Lindsley (60) postulates that this rhythmic activity signals the development of effective perceptual capacity. During the three- or four-month period, infants have been observed attempting to locate the source of the auditory stimulus by moving their eyes or turning their bodies to the direction of the sound (33, 98). Thus begins the onset of the very valuable localization response in normal hearing infants. This auditory response is not fully developed, however, until six or seven months of age, when the infant will definitely turn his eyes and head to the stimulus source (17, 33, 46). Such stimulus-seeking activity does not require loud sound for its initiation. Noises as low as 25 or 30 dB (above audiometric 0 dB) are effective in stimulating localization responses from infants (8).

The localization response is perhaps the most frequently evoked behavioral response in the auditory evaluation of infants. Another type of auditory response produced by infants approximates arousal or cessation reflex activity in neonates. It is commonly considered to be a distraction response and appears when the auditory stimulus distracts the attention of the infant from either a bright toy or play activity. This distraction may result in cessation of play activity and complete immobilization, or it may result in cessation of play activity and a frantic search to identify the source of the stimulus.

As the infant grows older, the design of the audiologist's procedure to evoke various ramifications of localization and distraction responses become more sophisticated. Response criteria also become more stringent. It is stressed, however, that regardless of the age or maturation of the infant, the audiologist must use auditory stimuli that are sometimes novel and sometimes meaningful to the infant. The infant, as he matures, gains more cortical control and thus conscious control over his nonspecific response systems. There is still competition for the response systems by incidental external and internal stimuli. The infant is too young to rationally follow the audiologist's pretest instructions that tell him to respond only when he hears the auditory stimulus. The auditory stimulus must, however, gain and retain importance to the infant over all other stimuli. Prestimulus activity levels should be constantly observed by the audiologist so that he may gain cues that will aid him in deciding the nature and the magnitude of the auditory stimulus he will present next. (*See* Chapter 12.)

Young Child (*two to five years*). A young child from two to five years of age with normal hearing might be considered a neophyte producer of "adult-like" auditory responses. Auditory responses no longer take the form of mere changes in prestimulus activity levels and reflex activity, as they do in the neonate, or fairly unsophisticated localization and distraction activity as seen in the infant. As the child progresses in age, he has control over the activity within his nonspecific response systems, and the experienced clinical audiologist can gain control over the child's psychological state by appropriate instructions and testing techniques. Therefore, if the young child is properly motivated by both the audiologist and the design of the test, the auditory responses become more specific to the parameters of the auditory stimulus.

The two- to three-year-old child is able to understand and carry out simple commands (32, 54). The audiologist can utilize this facility to gain fairly sophisticated behavioral responses to speech stimuli as well as to pure-tones. A command of "Show me the cat" spoken at either high or low intensities, if audible, can stimulate the child to point to the picture of a cat which may be placed among other animal pictures. Bloomer (9) and Myklebust (70) were both successful in teaching young children to associate various pictures with pure tones of different frequencies. For example, the child learned that upon hearing a 250 Hz pure-tone, regardless of intensity, he was to point to the picture of a bear. The literature contains descriptions of a variety of behavioral responses required of numerous techniques that are designed to capture and hold the young child's attentiveness to either pure-tone or speech stimuli. All of these techniques fall under the general classification of PLAY AUDIOMETRY.

It is possible through the use of play audiometric techniques for the clinical audiologist to measure degrees of auditory impairment in young children, whereas he is able only to identify abnormal auditory systems in neonates and in most infants who are not mature enough to produce responses that are specific to the varying dimensions of auditory stimuli.

Auditory Test Designs

The discussion up to this point in the chapter has centered around the dynamics of the normal hearing neonate, the infant, and the young child. It was assumed that these children possessed intact auditory systems and the differences in the auditory responses produced were attributed to their maturity level and, to some degree, the variability in prestimulus activity levels. This section will be concerned with basic test designs used by the audiologist to stimulate auditory responses from children. The effects of certain defective auditory systems and other disorders upon auditory response production will be discussed, if they have been clearly established in the literature.

In general, auditory tests used to evaluate the auditory systems of children from birth to five years of age serve to identify defective systems, or serve to both identify and measure the degree of the defect. The degree of defect is defined as the difference between the stimulus intensity required to evoke responses from the child under test and the stimulus intensity necessary to evoke responses from a normal hearing child. Basically, then, the degree of defect is the difference between a measured stimulus threshold and a normal reference stimulus threshold, just as it is in adult audiometry. In adult audiometry, a 50 per cent response criterion for threshold is standard and is accepted by most clinical audiologists. On the other hand, the audiologist working with certain hyperactive, distractible children will at times use threshold criteria that appear most applicable at the moment.

Audiologic test designs used to evaluate auditory systems in children from birth to five years of age are either "child-directed," or they are "audiologist-directed." Most of these behavioral audiometric designs, however, are child-directed in that they are tailored to the prestimulus activity levels and other behavioral manifestations that are unique to each child. Audiologist-directed designs would remain fairly standard from child to child. All children would be administered the same treatment, regardless of differences in the behavioral manifestations among them.

NEONATES (BIRTH TO TWO MONTHS)

Behavioral tests used to evaluate hearing in neonates are not designed to measure the degree of auditory defect, and therefore auditory thresholds are not obtained. These procedures fall under the classification of SCREENING OR IDENTIFICATION AUDIOMETRY. Clinical test designs used to stimulate auditory responses from neonates are generally child-directed procedures. It is impractical in most instances to stimulate the neonate in an organized fashion which is inflexible to changes in his prestimulus activity levels. In general, the characteristics of reflex responses produced by neonates are dependent upon the psychological state of the baby at the moment of stimulation. For example, several studies have found that the Moro reflex occurs most frequently during deep sleep, the APR and arousal reflexes are most easily evoked during light sleep, and cessation reflex activity is stimulated most often when the neonate is awake and alert (31, 35, 77). Therefore, the audiologist can do very little to control the nature of reflex responses evoked from neonates except to stimulate the baby when he appears in the most ideal psychological state for producing a particular reflex. The stimuli are seldom varied in intensity and are not particularly attractive. However, they must be sudden, percussive, and intense.

A fairly structured test procedure for testing hearing in neonates is described by Aldrich (1). He rang a bell simultaneously while he scratched a sleeping baby's foot with a pin at one-half hour intervals during the night. After about twelve to fifteen trials, the baby was conditioned to withdraw his foot when he heard the bell. The intensity and the frequency response of the bell were not reported. This is an interesting design and it demonstrates that neonates can be conditioned.

Wedenberg (93) developed a test design that requires a state of deep sleep. From his description, the procedure has two phases: One phase involves stimulating the baby with a 105 to 115-dB (SPL) pure tone.

According to this investigator the neonate with normal auditory sensitivity will give an APR to pure tones presented at SPL's from 105 to 115 dB; the other phase requires stimulation by a 70 to 75 dB (SPL) pure tone in an attempt to awaken the baby from deep sleep. A baby with normal hearing will awaken to a state within which tactile stimulation will evoke an APR. Wedenberg believes that this procedure not only identifies abnormal auditory systems, but that it will also differentiate cochlear problems from conductive and retrocochlear problems. For example, if the neonate gives an APR to the 105 to 115-dB pure tone, but will not awaken until the pure tone in the second phase is greater than 75 dB, he has a cochlear problem which exhibits recruitment. On the other hand, if the neonate gives no APR, but awakens to pure tones greater than 75 dB, he has conductive or retrocochlear problems.

An example of an experimental test design that many audiologists approximate when testing neonates in the clinic is the one used by Eisenberg et al., (31). Three trained examiners observed the neonate's pre- and post-stimulus activity. One examiner stood at the head of the baby and presented four different stimuli from calibrated noise-makers. The other two examiners stood on the left and on the right sides of the baby. The examiner positioned at the head presented the four stimuli five times in random order with variable interstimulus intervals in excess of ten seconds each. The twenty-stimuli sequence was interrupted only when necessary. Each of the three examiners recorded both pre- and poststimulus activity according to a standard coding system.

Another approach is to compare, simultaneously, the poststimulus activity of the baby in question with that of other babies suspected of having normal hearing. The examiners should not know which is the baby in question. The problems with this design, however, are that (1) no one can ever be certain that the reference babies have normal hearing and (2) prestimulus activity levels within each baby at the time of stimulation may not be identical. Because of differing prestimulus activity levels, the stimulus might arouse one baby, it might calm another baby, and the other baby may not change at all. The baby that does not change may be deaf or perhaps the level of his prestimulus activity was not conducive to change at the moment of stimulation. Of course, if this baby continues to demonstrate similar behavior upon repeated stimulation over time, then there is a strong possibility that his auditory system is defective.

The various test designs reported in the literature vary in structure, but most designs have one element in common: the stimulus intensity is seldom varied. Usually a constant stimulus of known intensity and frequency response is used within each design. It is assumed, and in many instances it is known, that this stimulus or these stimuli will successfully evoke reflex behavior in normal hearing neonates. Research has shown that most any auditory stimulus of sufficient sound pressure level will evoke reflex activity from normal hearing neonates. Examples of effective auditory stimuli that have been used are: Pure tones at 50 to 60 dB (68); a clacker with a peak from 55 to 60 dB (46); pure tones and a cow's moo at 68 dB (88); white noise at 93 dB and a 2,500 to 3,500 Hz band at 90 dB (29); onion-skin paper, a drum, wooden sticks, and a whistle at 64 dB (31); and a gong at 126 to 135 dB (35). It is assumed that all of these decibel levels refer to 0.0002 dynes/cm^2.

There are many types of auditory disorders that would inhibit neonates' auditory responses during identification or screening audiometric tests. Also, there are nonauditory problems that would interfere with the baby's response behavior, such as psychological and central nervous system disorders. Nevertheless, these tests serve only to screen out neonates who have problems that require further extensive investigation. Further long-range studies structured to follow-up the initial results obtained using Wedenberg's (93) test might confirm his claims that the test can differentiate cochlear problems from noncochlear problems in neonates, which would be of considerable value to the clinical audiologist.

INFANTS (TWO MONTHS TO TWO YEARS)

The majority of behavioral test designs used to evoke auditory responses from infants are structured to screen or identify hearing loss. Very few designs reported in the literature are intended to measure the degree of defect, or the auditory thresholds. These test designs differ from those employed to screen hearing in neonates in the nature of the response evoked and the stimulus intensity required to evoke the response. While the audiologist has very little control over the type of reflex response he may evoke from neonates, except to stimulate it during specific psychological states, he may control the nature of the localization response by appropriately structuring the physical test environment (i.e., speakers placed some distance apart; examiner presents stimuli behind or on either side of the child, etc.). Infants will attend to stimuli of lower-intensity levels and are more selective in the type of stimuli to which they will respond than are neonates.

Ewing and Ewing (33) accomplished one of the first and most thorough investigations of auditory response behavior in infants. Many different types of stimuli were tested for their effectiveness in evoking recognized behavioral responses. All stimuli were presented free field at a measured distance outside the infant's range of vision. This, in essence, is the design of their procedure. The stimuli included noise-makers, (bells, rattles, sticks, rustling of tissue paper, xylophone played quietly, and teaspoon and cup) and simple commands, or the baby's name spoken quietly at three to four feet from either ear. Intensities and frequency responses of these stimuli were not quantified. The Ewings found that the three- to six-month infant tends to ignore intense sound and responds with arousal activity to his mother speaking quietly. After six months of age, the infant localizes most frequently to low-intensity stimuli that are familiar to his environment. Infants older than seven months show a fairly well-developed capacity for selective listening. The Ewings prefer screening infants of seven months or older. This preference is based upon their findings that a number of infants screened with their design did not give positive localization or distraction responses until they reached seven months of age.

The Ewings (33) stress that meaningful sounds are most effective in stimulating responses from infants. According to their definition, a meaningful sound is one that is unique to the child's environment and has acquired meaning as the infant has grown. Based upon this premise, Miller, DeSchweinitz, and Goetzinger (65) were interested in determining whether or not the stimuli used by the Ewings on infants living in England were appropriate for stimulating responses from infants living in the midwestern United States. As was true in the Ewings' study, they did not quantify the parameters of their stimuli. Nevertheless, they studied the responses of ten normal hearing infants elicited by the various stimuli used by the Ewings, as well as stimuli they felt indigenous to midwestern homes. The infants ranged in age from seven to twelve months. Their findings showed that stimuli familiar to the environment of the infant living in midwestern United States evoked quicker responses, while the stimuli used by the Ewings in England were, at times, ignored.

The basic elements of the Ewings' approach to screening auditory disorders in infants have been adopted by many investigators and clinical audiologists. The concept of using stimuli that are meaningful to the infant, but that are not necessarily intense, has gained wide acceptance and is the basis of many audiologic test designs. Too much emphasis, however, has been placed upon the need and value of employing meaningful stimuli (as defined by the Ewings) when testing infants. Sounds need not be indigenous to an infant's cultural environment to evoke responses, if employed by the audiologist in a proper manner. A pure tone is cultural-free, yet it will stimulate responses in normal hearing infants of any nationality or culture if used appropriately by the audiologist.

Hardy et al., (46) refined the Ewings' procedure by using stimuli that were quantified. They separated their noise-makers on the basis of a frequency analysis of the stimulus produced. A certain rattle, some tissue paper, and unvoiced consonants were selected because they produced primarily high-frequency sounds. Middle-frequency sounds were generated by another rattle, a voice, and a spoon and cup. They selected a third rattle, particular vocalizations, a toy xylophone, and a tonnette that produced mainly low-frequency sounds. All of these noisemakers generated sound that averaged 40-dB (SPL). They also used a 90-dB squeaker, a 60-dB clacker and a 60-dB bell, each of which produced noise within a frequency band from 2,000 to 8,000 Hz. The baby was placed in its mother's lap and an assistant sat in front of the baby using interesting toys to distract the baby, while the examiner presented the stimuli from the back, or either side, of the baby. Localization to the examiner, who was the stimulus source, was the only acceptable response.

One might speculate that the assistant used to distract the baby from the movements of the examiner in the Hardy et al., (46) design also serves, through his efforts, to maintain a psychological state of alert attentiveness and to reduce the incidental response activity within the nonspecific response systems of the infant. Although the infant is attracted to the assistant's play activity with the toy, this is the only stimulus activity with which the examiner's stimuli must compete. Of course, if the infant becomes too interested in the assistant's distraction stimuli, then he will not respond to the auditory stimuli.

Suzuki and Ogiba (89) designed a procedure which they termed Conditioned Orientation Reflex Audiometry. It consists of first pairing a visual stimulus with a pure-tone stimulus. The stimuli emanate from various positions around the room and stimulate the infant either to turn his eyes or head toward the source. Eventually the tone is presented without the visual stimulus. If properly conditioned, the infant will localize to the tone whether the visual stimulus follows or does not follow. Pure-tone stimulus intensities were not cited. These investigators attempted such conditioning with 250 normal hearing children. Their findings showed that only 44 per cent of the children under one year conditioned satisfactorily. Eighty-five per cent of the one-year-old children and 87 per cent of the two-year-old children did condition satisfactorily. Children three years and older lost interest in the test and failed to respond appropriately.

There has been concern among some clinical audiologists that pure-tone stimuli are not appropriate in infant test designs. Apparently, it is believed that pure tones have little meaning to the infant and thus are unattractive. Waldon (91) holds this opinion and suggests that the reproduction of a baby cry would have a more universal meaning to all infants. He has reported some success using filtered bands of the baby cry of a six-month-old infant. Murphy (68) disagrees that pure tones are not effective stimuli and furthermore believes that it is unnecessary to use only meaningful stimuli when testing infants. All that is required is that the pure tones, or other sounds, emanate from a visible and meaningful source. By using a small speaker hidden by a doll's face to transmit pure tones, Murphy has been successful in evoking localization responses to pure tones, ranging from 400 to 6,000 Hz at 40 dB, from normal hearing infants six to nine months of age.

Suzuki and Sato (90) utilized recorded animal sounds and localization responses in a test design aimed at measuring thresholds in infants. The recorded stimuli were presented through spaced loudspeakers. Using this approach they measured thresholds that averaged 36.5 dB (hearing level) within a group of infants less than six months of age. Infants of twenty-four months and older produced thresholds that averaged 10.2 dB.

A very carefully controlled test design structured to stimulate localization responses in infants and young children is described by DiCarlo and Bradley (25). Basically, the design includes a control room separate from a sound-treated room. Four pairs of speakers are placed within the sound-treated room with an azimuth difference of 90 degrees. The equipment is designed so that white noise, recorded pure tones, music, and voice materials can be presented through any one of the speakers, and the intensity levels of all stimuli can be varied. The child is placed in his mother's lap directly in the center of the room. The desired behavioral response is localization to the speaker that transmits the stimulus. Other behavioral reactions, however, are accepted.

DiCarlo and Bradley (25) used this design to evaluate fifty children suspected of having hearing disorders. Ages of the children ranged from ten months to three years. The average duration of the test was five minutes for each child. Music proved to be the most effective stimulus for evoking localization responses. At a later date, when each child was four or five years of age, his pure-tone thresholds were measured using standard and play audiometric methods. The findings showed that thirty-one children, who gave definite startle responses at 90-dB (SPL) and localized at 20 dB during the localization test, had normal pure-tone thresholds when retested.

Frisina (34) analyzed the data presented by DiCarlo and Bradley (25) and found that thirteen infants younger than two years of age were included within the total group of fifty children. Of these thirteen infants, eight gave definite localization response to stimuli of 20 dB and produced normal thresholds during later pure-tone measurement. The remaining five infants did not localize at low-intensity levels, but one gave a startle response at 40 dB, two gave startle responses at 70 dB, and two showed some awareness of the presence of sound when it was at 100 dB. Later pure-tone measurements indicated that the two infants that startled at 70 dB had normal bilateral thresholds. The infant that startled at 40 dB produced average thresholds of 20 dB in both ears, while the two that showed only sound awareness had average thresholds of 80 to 90 dB in both ears.

The test designs presented in this section do not include all the designs that are being used to screen auditory disorders in infants. They are, however, fairly representative of the approaches that are currently being followed in most audiology clinics. It is stressed that these designs serve only to screen or identify infants who may possibly have defective auditory systems. Problems other than auditory disorders, however, can inhibit the production of auditory responses during these procedures. For example, Hardy et al., (47) found that thirty-six of sixty-two twelve-month-old infants, who failed to respond to stimuli, were later diagnosed as having neurologic disorders; and twenty-one of these thirty-six infants were suspected of having psychological disturbances. Not one of the failures had a clearly established sensori-neural hearing loss, and only a few had conductive hearing losses.

YOUNG CHILD (TWO TO FIVE YEARS)

Most audiologic test designs used to stimulate behavioral responses from young children are structured not only to identify hearing loss, but also to evaluate or measure the degree of hearing loss. Basically, they are threshold tests. Design and administration of these tests require experienced, observant, imaginative, and flexible audiologists. These designs differ from those used with infants and neonates in that the behavioral response desired (i.e., putting a peg in a board; pointing to a picture; raising a hand, etc.) is established through instruction and training by the audiologist before actual testing begins. The stimulus is varied in intensity until it reaches a level where it no longer evokes a response or until a certain percentage of responses is evoked.

Some audiometry tests used to measure hearing in the young child approximate audiologist-directed tests, if the child remains alert and co-operative. Many tests, however, administered by clinical audiologists are definitely child-directed tests. The audiologist should always let the child's prestimulus activity be his guide. If the child becomes bored with the task at hand, inattentive to the audiologist and auditory stimulus, or generally uncooperative, then steps must be taken to bring the child back into the test situation. Generally, this can be accomplished by (1) changing the nature of the response required; (2) changing the response reinforcement; or (3) changing the pace of stimulus presentation. These tests are rightfully classified as play audiometric procedures and the games must remain interesting and motivating throughout the duration of their administration.

Pure-tone Threshold. Studies using play audiometry techniques have found that most young children two and one-half to three years of age and above can be conditioned to produce behavioral responses to pure-tone and other stimuli at low-intensity levels comparable to the intensity levels that represent average adult thresholds (5, 17, 49, 62, 86, 96) and others. Play audiometry designs are based upon instrumental or operant conditioning principles. Most all these tests can be classified under: (1) stimulus-response-reward designs or (2) stimulus-response designs.

Stimulus-response-reward designs include the presentation of a preselected reward to the child when he produces an appropriate response to the auditory stimulus. The classical example of a stimulus-response-reward design is the Peep Show test devised by Dix and Hallpike (26). The basic apparatus includes a box with a loudspeaker, a stage that is visible only when lighted, pictures, a signal light, and a push-button. During a brief training session, the child learns that when presented with the flashing signal light or a loud tone, he can light the stage and see a colorful picture by pressing the button. During testing the signal light is not turned on with the tone. Therefore, if properly conditioned, the child will press the button when he hears audible tones to obtain the reward of seeing a picture. The designers report success in measuring reliable pure-tone thresholds using the Peep Show test with children who have mental ages of at least three years.

Guilford and Haug (45) felt that the Peep Show test lacked dramatic appeal and that it did not provide for monaural measurements. Therefore, they designed an apparatus called the Pediacoumeter which provided for air-conduction and bone-conduction pure-tone measurements through earphones and a bone vibrator. The Pediacoumeter includes seven Jack-in-the-box heads which the child is taught to associate with seven pure-tones. After training, when the child hears one of the little men shouting (one of the tones associated with one of the heads is presented) he presses a button that will let the little man out of his little house. These investigators report measuring fairly reliable air-conduction and bone-conduction thresholds using the Pediacoumeter with children above two years of age.

The two designs described above represent only a few of the many stimulus-response-reward procedures that have been reported in the literature. Differences among these designs consist primarily in the type of reward or reinforcement that is offered to the child for producing a response at the correct time. Denmark (23) closely replicated the Peep Show procedure except that the child's reward was a revolving bright-colored merry-go-round. Green (44) used automated toys that moved if the child pressed the button when the tone was presented. Knox (55) provided a removal toy that popped up on a stage if the child responded appropriately. The child was allowed to keep the toy. The success of all of these stimulus-response-reward designs, of course, is very dependent upon the desirability of the reward to the child. If the audiologist has no rewards built into his equipment that interest a particular child, then his apparatus and procedure are useless in measuring the auditory systems of this child.

Stimulus-response-reward procedures must use rewards that are interesting to the child. The response is simply pressing a button and is merely a means to an end, which is the reward. On the other hand, designers of stimulus-response procedures are more concerned with making the response interesting to the child, so that the response becomes an end and reward in itself. Therefore, one design is most concerned with the construct of the reward and the other is primarily concerned with the structure of the response. Actually, the differences between the two designs, in principle, is negligible. The child must know if he has made a right or wrong response. He gains this feedback information within a stimulus-response-reward design after he has made his response. If the stage lights up, he is right;

if the stage remains dark, he is wrong. When involved in stimulus-response procedures, the source of feedback information is generally dependent upon the audiologist. For example, if the child begins to perform the interesting task, which is the desired response, and no stimulus has been presented, the audiologist may stop the child before he begins by frowning or holding the child's hand. He may let the child continue with the task while he shakes his head to indicate disapproval. Of course, if the child has made a correct response, the audiologist can shake his head in approval. Both designs resemble instrumental-reward conditioning paradigms.

The design reported by Bloomer (9) is an interesting example of a stimulus-response procedure. A child is first taught to associate each of several different pure tones with a specific animal picture. For example, 250 Hz is associated with a bear, 1,000 Hz is associated with an airplane, etc. When the audiologist feels that the child can consistently make these associations accurately, he instructs the child to place his finger on the animal every time he hears its associated tone in order to stop the tone. Therefore, the response involves more than just pressing a button. The child must select, among several animal pictures, the one that is associated with the frequency of the audible tone. The task requires concentration and attentiveness to the auditory stimulus, and the child's interest in the test is maintained by his desire to make correct choices. Myklebust (70) used a similar tone-picture association design to measure thresholds in sixty-one children ranging in age from two years, one month to five years, six months. Successful thresholds were measured in zero per cent of the two-year-olds, 68 per cent of the three-year-olds, 93 per cent of the four-year-olds, and 83 per cent of the five-year-olds. Geyer and Yankauer (38) employed a modification of the tone-picture association approach and screened 461 preschool children ranging in age from two years, six months to five years, five months. Each child was instructed to drop a cube in a basket when he heard the pure tone that corresponded to the animal picture the examiner held in his hand.

Concerned with the possibility that the pure-tone stimulus is too abstract to interest the young child, Willeford (96) prepared five filtered bands of environmental noises whose center frequencies were 250, 500, 1,000, 2,000, and 5,000 Hz. Though filtered, he felt that noise bands retained their identity for the child so that they still sounded like a car, a dog barking, etc. Pictures were chosen that represented the various noise sources. Therefore, the child was taught to associate each noise with the proper picture. The auditory response consisted of the child pointing to a picture when he heard its associated noise. Willeford reports that, using this design, thresholds obtained from young children are 5 dB lower than those measured with conventional pure-tone audiometry. Downs and Doster (27) used 250 to 750 Hz, 1,000 to 2,000 Hz, and 3,000 to 5,000 Hz bandwidths of familiar sounds to screen preschool children. Associated pictures were used and the response consisted of pointing to the picture that corresponded to the noise. Testing was carried out by nonprofessional volunteers and the screening program was a reported success.

If the variety of rewards is too limited in a stimulus-response-reward design, or the number of different response tasks is too few during a stimulus-response design, then some children, particularly those with problems in addition to auditory dysfunction, will become bored, inattentive, and hyperactive. Interesting rewards can become disinteresting very quickly to some children. Enjoyable response tasks can become boring in a very short time, or they may become too enjoyable, thus motivating the child to continue the task independent of the stimulus or the audiologist's instructions. Therefore, the ideal play audiometry design is one that is not too cumbersome with apparatus or too inflexible to immediate change in structure as the test progresses.

Many clinical audiologists prefer to use simple and flexible stimulus-response designs when administering daily clinical hearing evaluations to young children. Bender (7) mentions a variety of tasks for the child to perform in response to pure tones. Merely placing a peg in a peg-board is effective for some children, while others prefer to place a ring on a dowel. Bender is not adverse to changing tasks at any point in the test if the pre-stimulus activity of the child warrants a change. Children with problems in addition to auditory defect may perform most adequately with specific response tasks. Brown and Knepflar (13), for example, developed a response task that proved to be quite successful when measuring thresholds in children suspected of having brain damage. The response task involved dropping a bead through a hole in a lighted box while sitting in a dark room. A response task that has been found effective to the writer when measuring pure-tone thresholds in aggressive children requires the child to throw a block into a box as hard as he wishes and not merely to place the block in the box. Many other response tasks have been reported in the literature, but it would be pointless to review them further. It is safe to say, however, that the nature of the response task used will vary with the age and personality of the child and the personal bias of the clinical audiologist administering a stimulus-response procedure.

Regardless of the design of the auditory test used, it is important to measure thresholds in both right and left ears if possible. Therefore, it is necessary that earphones be placed on the child to make these monaural measures. Quite often the audiologist will encounter problems in his attempts to place earphones on young children, which result in the child rejecting both the earphones and the audiologist. There are those uncooperative young children regardless of age, who will not accept the earphones no matter what force or enticement is used. Most children, however, will accept the earphones if the audiologist approaches the child in a relatively unforceful, but direct manner as if he never questioned the possibility that the child would not accept the earphones. The child's rejection of the audiologist can be avoided by never using force to place the earphones. It is better to have a cooperative child to measure in a free field than to have an uncooperative child wearing earphones.

Speech Audiometry. Speech measures can provide the audiologist with information about the efficiency or inefficiency of a child's auditory system as a conveyor of messages necessary for the development of his receptive and expressive communication abilities. Pure-tone measures reveal how sensitive an auditory system is to sound, while speech measures demonstrate how functional an auditory system is for communication. The speech stimulus is also more meaningful and thus more interesting to the child than is a pure tone. Logically, however, the value of the speech stimulus is limited when used with the young child who is linguistically delayed or impaired.

Siegenthaler et al., (82) demonstrated that reliable speech reception thresholds can be measured with three-year-old children and that the relationship between speech reception thresholds and pure-tone averages (500, 1,000, 2,000 Hz) obtained with children four years and older are just as strong as they are in adults. In their design, five lists of five monosyllabic words were presented at five different intensity levels. Pictures corresponding to the words were arranged in front of the child in groups of five. Each word was preceded by the carrier phrase "point to the." The child's response was to point to the appropriate picture that corresponded to the word following the carrier phrase. The lowest intensity level at which the child gave a correct response, either 40 or 60 per cent of the time, was considered the speech reception threshold.

Other investigators have used similar picture-identification designs to measure speech reception thresholds in young children (3, 53, 64). These designs vary among each other in the number of words used, the types of words used, earphone or free-field presentation, live voice or recorded presentation, and threshold criteria. Several audiologists (38, 84) prefer to use objects or toys instead of pictures. They are of the opinion that the experience of both seeing and feeling the object or toy is more interesting and thus reinforcing than just seeing a picture.

Speech reception thresholds are of value to the audiologist for providing information of the lowest intensity level at which speech can be heard and understood. It is also important, however, to know how efficiently a child's auditory system can convey speech information when the speech stimuli are presented at higher-intensity levels, which are the most advantageous to clear understanding. Several investigators have designed procedures to obtain such speech discrimination measures in young children. The speech stimuli are generally presented using a non-calibrated live voice at a level that approximates the intensity of normal conversational speech. Pronovost and Dumbleton (75) structured a procedure around a picture-identification approach. Four pairs of pictures associated with four pairs of words were utilized. The four pairs of pictures were arranged in front of the child, and his response consisted of pointing to the pair of pictures that related to the pair of words heard. They used this design with young children between the ages of two and six years. Results of their study showed that the ability to discriminate between pairs of speech sounds increases with age from two years up to at least four and one-half to five years of age. Myatt and Landes (69) used a similar design and also found that as children progressed in age, their ability to perform this discrimination task improved.

A review of the literature suggests that speech discrimination testing with the young child is not currently practiced to any large degree in audiology clinics. Perhaps this is due to the fact that there is no standardized material available to make such measurements with young children two to five years old. It is not possible to develop a scale of speech discrimination ability without standardized material, and a scale is necessary to determine to what degree a measured score reflects abnormal speech discrimination.

In the opinion of the writer, the clinical value of using speech audiometry with young children is based primarily upon the meaningful nature of the speech stimulus compared to that of the abstract pure tone. Many young children who do not perform cooperatively during pure-tone threshold audiometry will cooperate during speech reception threshold audiometry. As discussed above, a strong relationship between pure-tone threshold averages and speech reception thresholds has been established with young children. Therefore, basic information about the sensitivity of the auditory system as measured by air-conduction and by bone-conduction transmission can be gained through speech audiometry, if it cannot be obtained with pure-tone audiometry. Speech reception thresholds do not reveal to the audiologist the particular slope of air-conduction or bone-conduction threshold curves. They can tell the audiologist, however, whether or not the child has a conductive hearing problem by comparing air-conduction and bone-conduction speech reception thresholds. If there is a discrepancy between the two, then a conductive loss is suspected.

Unfortunately, most commercial speech audiometers do not provide for bone-conduction measurement in the design of their circuits. This problem can be overcome by connecting a bone-conduction vibrator into either the right or left air-conduction channels of the speech audiometer. Speech reception thresholds are then measured within a group of normal ears. The average of this group's decibel reading on the hearing level dial corresponds to the lowest intensity level of speech (produced by this particular bone-conduction system) at which the average of the group could hear and understand 50 per cent of the speech stimuli. This reading on the hearing level dial can then be called 0 dB for bone-conduction speech audiometry.

ELECTROPHYSIOLOGIC TEST DESIGNS

The designs of electrophysiologic procedures used to stimulate and measure the production of auditory responses vary with the equipment employed, the types of stimuli used, and the methods of presenting the stimuli. Also, the characteristics of the final response produced through a particular electrophysiologic response system can differ significantly, depending upon the manner in which it is recorded. Regardless of these differences, however, each audiologist administering an electrophysiologic audiometric procedure is attempting to measure the same phenomenon. He is trying to measure whether a change in electrophysiologic activity, which he can state with a high degree of certainty, is caused by his auditory stimulus. This change in activity can then be considered an auditory response.

Electrophysiologic audiometry has been classified as objective audiometry by some audiologists, because the final response is not under the volitional control of the child. Goldstein (39) stresses, however, that audiometry is a procedure and not a response. Although the electrophysiologic response produced by the child may be objective, the procedures used by the audiologist to separate this auditory response from a field of nonauditory responses in an electrophysiologic recording are subject to each audiologist's own bias. Therefore, truly objective clinical audiometry awaits the development of examiner-free electrophysiologic procedures that can be administered in practical clinical settings.

Electrodermal Audiometry (*EDA*). EDA designs used in the clinic are generally structured around one of two psychophysical methods of measurement: the Method of Limits or the Method of Constant Stimuli. Most designs are based upon classical conditioning principles that require the use of an unconditioned stimulus such as electric shock, heat, or light. The unconditioned stimulus is paired with the auditory stimulus during initial conditioning and is used as reinforcement during the actual test. Use of a noxious stimulus such as shock has been questioned in terms of its traumatic effects on a child. Hardy and Pauls (48) stress, however, that only minimal shock should be used and, by handling the child properly, the traumatic effects of shock and the general test situation will be minimal. These audiologists employ a team approach when measuring children. One member of the team operates the EDA equipment and stimulates the child, while the other member attempts to keep the child calm and alert using various toys.

Variations of the Method of Limits, which resemble techniques used to measure behavioral thresholds in the clinic, are also used to measure electrodermal response (EDR) thresholds. Basically, the audiologist attempts to find the intensity level at which a certain percentage of EDR's is evoked. This threshold intensity level lies between a lower level at which no EDR's occur and a higher level at which EDR's may be evoked 100 per cent of the time. Therefore, it is necessary for the audiologist to make one of three immediate judgments of the electrodermal activity, traced by the pen on the recording chart, after each stimulus presentation. He must decide whether or not: (1) the activity has changed significantly from prestimulus activity; (2) the change in activity is a function of the auditory stimulus; or (3) the change in activity is a function of incidental external or internal stimuli. If he judges no change in activity, then he might raise the intensity of the stimulus for the next presentation. A judgment of change due to the stimulus might cause him to present the stimulus again at the same intensity or to reduce the stimulus for the next presentation. If he feels the change was due to incidental stimuli, then he might stimulate again at the same intensity, or in the case of a very active recording, he may wait until the random activity decreases before presenting the stimulus again. The direction that the stimulus presentation will take and the duration of the test are both dependent upon the overall activity level of each child under test and the audiologist's judgments of stimulus and poststimulus electrodermal activity. EDA, using this approach to measure auditory thresholds, is truly child-directed testing and is very subject to audiologist bias.

EDA procedures structured around the Method of Constant Stimuli closely resemble audiologist-directed tests and are less subject to audiologist bias than are Method of Limits designs. A typical design includes a schedule for stimulus presentation. Prior to testing, this schedule is planned and may include auditory stimuli presented at seven different hearing levels. The stimulus will be presented randomly at each of these seven hearing levels six times during the test. Some of these hearing levels may be below 0 dB. This schedule now includes forty-two stimulus events. It has been demonstrated that for maximum reinforcement to provide resistance to response adaptation, one should include the unconditioned stimulus (shock) 40 per cent of the time (50). Therefore, of the forty-two stimulus events in the schedule, seventeen of them should be a tone followed by a shock. In addition to these forty-two stimulus events, six silent-control intervals are scheduled. A silent-control interval represents a recorded time period in which no stimulus is presented. This schedule now includes forty-eight events that are presented at random intervals throughout the test. After a period of conditioning, the presentation of the forty-eight events is begun. If the total time computed from the schedule, which includes stimulus duration and interstimulus interval time, is one hour and thirty minutes, then ideally the test should take no longer than one hour and thirty minutes. No judgments of prestimulus, stimulus, or poststimulus electrodermal activity are made by the audiologist during the test. A pen marks on the recording chart the instant each of the forty-eight events begins and ends, so that the audiologist will know at what point in the record the stimulus may have been presented. After the test, the record is read and the audiologist marks either response or no response in each one of the forty-eight event time periods, depending upon his judgment of whether or not the electrodermal activity after the stimulus onset mark meets certain latency and amplitude response criteria. He next looks at the schedule of stimulus presentation to find which of the forty-eight events included either a stimulus at a certain intensity, a stimulus plus a shock, or a silent control. His judgments of response or no response are then tallied relative to each of the six presentations at the seven hearing levels and the six silent controls.

The value of including silent controls in the test schedule is to provide a zero level for each child, which is a function of the amount of each child's own random electrodermal activity (39). For example, if the audiologist rated the electrodermal activity that occurred during three of the six silent-control intervals as a response, he could not say that the child produced auditory responses at a hearing level that was followed by activity rated as a response only one-half of the time. Using this criteria the response could likely be due to chance. The audiologist might require that electrodermal activity following four or perhaps five of the six stimulus events be graded as a response before he judges that the auditory stimulus was heard by the child. Very seldom will responses occur 100 per cent of the time at each audible hearing level during electrophysiologic audiometry (39). Random activity almost always presents a problem in positive response identification regardless of the prestimulus activity levels of the child under test. Stewart (87) found that the electrodermal activity that occurred during 20 per cent of the silent controls used in an adult study was evaluated as positive electrodermal activity evoked by the auditory stimulus. Several different criteria have been offered for electrodermal activity to be considered positive. Generally, these criteria are based upon amplitude and slope of the pen excursion and stimulus-response time interval (63, 80, 87). or just the stimulus-response time interval (14).

Placement of pick-up and unconditioned stimulus electrodes vary somewhat from audiologist to audiologist. When administering EDA to children, Hardy and Pauls (48) place the pick-up electrodes on either: (1) the palmar and dorsal surfaces of the hand, (2) the sole and dorsal surface of the foot, or (3) the soft pads near the first joint of the second and third fingers of one hand. They feel that these electrodes should be placed on the foot with children under eighteen months. Shock electrodes are placed on the calf of one leg.

Considerable research has been published regarding the value of EDA as a clinical procedure with children since its introduction in 1948 (11). EDR thresholds have been measured in infants as young as four months (10). Barr (5) found that EDR thresholds do not differ significantly from thresholds obtained using behavioral techniques in children ranging in age from two years to six years. Nevertheless, some investigators are concerned about the value of EDA when used with children who have problems in addition to hearing loss. The auditory systems of mentally retarded children (52, 67) and brain-damaged children (83) have been evaluated using EDA with limited success. Moss et al. (67) are of the opinion that most mentally retarded children, who cannot be tested successfully using play audiometry, cannot be tested successfully using EDA techniques. One of the problems that inhibits success involves conditioning difficulties. Goldstein et al. (41) found that of thirty-two normal hearing children, fourteen could not be conditioned adequately for the administration of EDA. Statten and Wishart (86) and Barr (5) encountered problems with young nonverbal children because of their lack of cooperation or intolerance of the test situation. It seems apparent, particularly after reviewing the current literature dealing with clinical audiology studies, that the interest in EDA testing of children has waned over the past several years.

Electroencephalic Audiometry (*EEA*). Audiometric procedures based upon auditory evoked responses from the electroencephalic response systems in children have been receiving a great deal of interest since the introduction of the averaged response computer into the field of clinical audiology. EEA test designs that have been and are currently being used are based upon either the traditional method which does not utilize the averaged response computer, or the averaged-response-over-repeated-stimuli method which does employ the averaged response computer. These designs are not based upon conditioning principles and therefore unconditioned stimuli are not used.

Traditional EEA designs are generally structured around the Method of Constant Stimuli and resemble those used for EDA threshold measurements. Stimulus presentation schedules are preplanned and judgments of electroencephalic activity occurring after each stimulus are not made until the actual testing is completed. EEA procedures, however, can be administered with the child awake or asleep, while EDA tests are unsuccessful unless the child is awake and alert. Nevertheless, a sleeping child is preferable during EEA to reduce the possibility of random electrical activity occurring from muscle movements that might be created by an awake and restless child (39). According to Goldstein (39), the nature of the evoked electroencephalic response (EER) is: (1) independent of age; (2) not different in normals and abnormals; and (3) not different during induced sleep (under anesthesia) and during the same stages of natural sleep. The characteristics of EER's evoked using the traditional method depend upon the appearance of ongoing prestimulus electroencephalic activity. For example, if the prestimulus activity is of large amplitude, then the stimulus may cause a reduction in amplitude. On the other hand, if the prestimulus activity is of small amplitude, then the stimulus may cause an increase in amplitude. Derbyshire and Farley (24) describe other characteristics of electroencephalic activity that may occur instantly at stimulus onset (on response), during stimulation (continuous response), and after stimulation (off response) that may be judged as effects of the auditory stimulus.

Considerable research is presently being directed toward the development of practical clinical test designs which utilize the averaged-response-over-repeated-stimuli method of auditory measurement and the averaged response computer. Current clinical tests that are based upon this method of measurement combine it with variations of the Method of Limits or the Method of Constant Stimuli. Regardless of specific methodological details, however, the manner in which the final evoked response is obtained with the computer differs very little from test design to test design. Basically, the electro-encephalic waveform, which occurs immediately after the presentation of a predetermined number of auditory stimuli, is stored in the memory of the averaging computer. The audiologist can adjust the computer so that it stores 16 msec., 250 msec., 500 msec., or whatever time space he desires, of the electrical waveform evoked by each auditory stimulus and recorded from the scalp. At the end of a series of perhaps twenty-five identical stimulus presentations, the average waveform of the electroencephalic activity that occurred after each of the twenty-five auditory stimuli (within the preselected time space) can be read out from the memory of the computer. Averaged evoked responses over repeated auditory stimuli have been investigated in many different laboratories. Fortunately, reports from these laboratories are consistent in showing that, regardless of the particular equipment used, the averaged evoked response to auditory stimulation is quite definite in its waveform. Latencies and amplitudes of the major peaks have been shown, however, to vary to some degree as a function of: race, sex, and age (74); stimulus intensity (78); and different sleep states and anesthetics (73). The latency and amplitude of the waveform peaks vary to a greater degree between individuals than within individuals (81).

Averaged evoked response thresholds can be measured using an approximation of the Method of Limits approach by evaluating each averaged response immediately after each series of auditory stimuli has been presented at a specific hearing level. If the averaged waveform has all of the major peak components, then it can be assumed that it represents an average of positive auditory responses. The audiologist must then decide whether he wishes to present the next series of stimuli at the same hearing level, at a lower hearing level, or at a higher hearing level. He can continue with this approach until he decides that he has adequately bracketed the auditory threshold.

If the audiologist wishes to employ a variation of the Method of Constant Stimuli in his design, he must first plan a schedule of stimulus-series presentation. He will randomly include, within this schedule, several series of stimuli presented at each of several hearing levels along with silent control intervals. After testing, the averaged responses are judged and tallied for each hearing level and each silent control to determine the auditory threshold.

Scalp electrode placements, as reported in the literature, vary to some degree from investigator to investigator, for both traditional and averaged-response-over-repeated-stimuli procedures. The most popular electrode placement appears to be a monopolar vertex placement (16, 73, 76, 97).

Studies dealing with the traditional approach of recording auditory evoked responses in children have provided information which supports the feasibility of measuring the auditory system by way of the electroencephalic response systems. The traditional methods, however, are cumbersome and as subjective as the EDA procedures. Although still in its early stages of development, the averaged-response-over-repeated-stimuli approach has already been shown to be of value in recording fairly objective auditory responses and measuring auditory thresholds in neonates, infants, and young children (4, 15, 16, 18, 19, 43, 73, 76, 94).

Diagnosis of Auditory Communication Disorders

A diagnosis of the nature of auditory communication disorders in neonates, infants, and young children cannot be based purely upon the results of an auditory test. At best, these test results only tell the audiologist how intense a sound, whether pure tone or speech, must be to stimulate the child to produce the appropriate responses. If the sound must be more intense than normal to evoke a response from a child, then the audiologist may suspect that the child has an auditory disorder. At present, however, there are no available auditory tests, or established response patterns obtained with several auditory tests, that can tell the audiologist beyond a reasonable doubt that: (1) this neonate, infant, or young child definitely has a defective peripheral auditory system, but an intact central auditory system; (2) he has a defective central auditory system, but an intact peripheral system; or (3) he definitely has defective peripheral and central auditory systems.

Up to this point in the chapter, there has been no mention of the importance of medical and developmental histories to the identification and diagnosis of auditory communication disorders in neonates, infants, and young children. This was purposefully done so that the organization of the chapter would approximate the writer's proposed sequence of events that should be followed during auditory testing.

The first event involves an intuitive study of the child aimed at predicting what the dynamics of this child may be as an auditory response producer. The age of the child is, of course, important to consider for the nature of the response that can be evoked. The audiologist may ask himself, "Is this child so hyperactive and distractible that random activity will obscure all possible auditory responses except those that are very great?" On the other hand, "Is this child so shy and timid that auditory responses cannot possibly be stimulated until proper rapport can be established?" When testing a neonate, the audiologist may wish to wait, after studying the baby, until the baby is in a psychological state that is most conducive to the production of specific reflex responses. The audiologist may find it necessary to experiment with various response tasks for a child with a motor handicap before he selects and plans the design of the auditory test he will employ. In essence then, the first event involves the time spent by the audiologist to acquaint himself with the sometimes unique behavioral manifestations of the child and to establish a warm and friendly rapport with the child.

The second event is the selection and administration of the appropriate auditory test design. The test design selected is dependent upon the particular response system chosen to stimulate information gained from regarding the behavioral manifestations of the child and the age of the child. During the administration of the test, the audiologist should be prepared to vary the technique, the response tasks, or the rate and direction of stimulus presentation as warranted by the changing behavior or prestimulus activity levels of the child. The second event is terminated when the audiologist has observed all of the reflex behavior from neonates that can possibly be evoked by his noise-makers; when he feels secure that the measurements obtained from infants and young children represent the best estimate of the status of their auditory systems; when he has completed his schedule of stimulus presentation; or when the child becomes so uncooperative that further testing is futile.

The third, but not final event for some children, involves the interpretation and synthesis of the audiologic findings along with all possible medical, developmental, psychological, neurological, and sociological information that may be relevant to a thorough understanding of the dynamics of the child's suspected auditory communication disorder. In the opinion of this writer, the clinical audiologist should have no knowledge of this additional information before testing a child, unless it is necessary for the safety of the child. Audiologists are not immune from entering a test situation with a preconceived diagnosis based upon medical history, developmental history, and other information. These preconceptions can bias the audiologist to observe auditory responses that do not occur, or to ignore auditory responses that do occur.

For children whose auditory communication disorders (identified or measured) stem only from peripheral end-organ impairment and are not caused or compounded by a central nervous system dysfunction, mental retardation, or emotional disorders, the third event can be the final event in diagnosis. In most instances with very young children auditory retests should be accomplished before any final diagnosis is made regardless of how secure the audiologist may be with his first diagnosis. Children suspected of having communication disorders in addition to or in place of auditory dysfunction, should be placed in a diagnostic nursery so that larger samples of the child's behavior may be observed and possibly measured. All young children, for that matter, ranging in age from two to five years of age with auditory communication disorders, or any type of communication disorder, should have the opportunity, if mature enough, of being exposed to speech and language training in special preschool nurseries. Some hearing and speech centers use their preschool nurseries for both diagnosis and speech and language training. The preschool nursery is also an excellent environment to determine, under controlled conditions, the benefits children with auditory disorders might gain wearing hearing aids.

In essence then, the clinical audiologist specializing in pediatric audiology plays a very important role in the identification, diagnosis, and habilitation of children with communication problems that stem from auditory dysfunction, central nervous system disorders, emotional disturbances, mental retardation, or problems compounded by all types of neurophysical and psychologic abnormalities. His basic responsibility, however, is to either "rule out" or "rule in" the existence of a defective auditory system within the child in question.

Glossary

AURAL REFLEX An involuntary response, usually muscular, to an auditory stimulus. Common aural reflexes are the Moro reflex, Quasi-Moro reflex, and Auropalpebral reflex (APR).

AUTONOMIC NERVOUS SYSTEM (ANS) A major division of the nervous system which serves to activate and regulate smooth muscle and glandular activity. Although the activities of the ANS are primarily free from voluntary control, they are not totally independent of influence from the brain and spinal cord. The ANS has two divisions: the sympathetic and the parasympathetic.

BRAIN STEM The axial portion of the brain which includes the pons and medulla oblongata; the part left, after the cerebrum and cerebellum are removed.

COCHLEAR ACTION POTENTIAL Change in the electrical potential of the cochlea as a function of auditory stimulation.

ACTIVITY LEVEL Level of neurophysiologic and muscular activity within the behavioral and electrophysiologic response systems.

CORTEX The thin outer layer of the brain.

EIGHT NERVE ACTION POTENTIAL Change in the electrical potential of the auditory nerve as a function of auditory stimulation.

EMOTIONAL SET A more or less temporary facilitating condition of an individual, accompanied by characteristic motor and glandular activity that orients him toward responding to certain environmental or internal stimuli.

EVOKED RESPONSE Any behavioral or electrophysiologic response produced by a stimulus.

IDEATIONAL STIMULI Neural impulses initiated by mental activity. These neural impulses are classified as internal stimuli.

NEUROANATOMY The study of the nerve structure of any of the parts of an organism.

NEUROPHYSIOLOGY The study of the physiologic activities of nerve tissue.

PARIETAL CORTEX The thin outer layer of the brain's parietal lobe.

PRIMARY AUDITORY CORTEX That portion of the cortex which receives neural impulses from the auditory sense organ.

PSYCHOPHYSIOLOGIST One who specializes in the study of the relation of mental activity and change in the physiology of the body.

RETICULAR FORMATION A dense network of neurons forming a central core in the brain stem extending from the medulla oblongata to the thalamus in the mid-brain.

SENSORY STIMULI A form of physical energy, i.e. sound, light, pressure, etc., affecting a sense organ.

TEMPORAL CORTEX The thin outer layer of the brain's temporal lobe.

Bibliography

1. Aldrich, C. A. "A new test for hearing in the newborn: The conditioned reflex." *American Journal of Diseases of Children*, **35**: 36, 1928.
2. Ax, A. F. "The physiological differentiation between fear and anger in humans." *Psychosomatic Medicine*, **15**: 433, 1953.
3. Bangs, T., and J. E. Bangs. "Hearing aids for young children." *Archives of Otolaryngology*, **55**: 528, 1952.
4. Barnett, A. B., and R. S. Goodwin. "Averaged evoked electroencephalographic responses to clicks in the human newborn." *Electroencephalography and Clinical Neurophysiology*, **18**: 441–50, 1965.
5. Barr, B. "Pure-tone audiometry for preschool children." *Acta Oto-Laryngologica*, Supplement 121, 1955.
6. Beadle, R., and D. Crowell. "Neonatal electrocardiographic responses to sound: Methodology." *Journal of Speech and Hearing Research*, **5**: 112, 1962.
7. Bender, R. "Evaluation of a child's hearing." *Maico Audiology Library Series*, Report 2, 1964.
8. Bergman, M. "Screening the hearing of preschool children." *Maico Audiology Library Series*, Report 4, 1964.
9. Bloomer, H. "A simple method for testing the hearing of young children." *Journal of Speech and Hearing Disorders*, **7**: 311–12, 1942.
10. Bordley, J. E., and W. G. Hardy. "A study in objective audiometry with the use of a psychogalvanic response." *Annals of Otology, Rhinology and Laryngology*, **58**: 751–59, 1949.
11. Bordley, J. E., W. G. Hardy, and C. Richter. "Audiometry with the use of galvanic skin-resistance response." *Bulletin of the Johns Hopkins Hospital*, **5**: 569, 1948.
12. Broadbent, D. E. *Perception and Communication.* New York: Pergamon Press, 1958.
13. Brown, E. A., and K. J. Knepflar. "Play audiometry with brain-damaged children." *ASHA*, **4**, 1962.

14. Charan, K., and R. Goldstein. "Relation between EEG pattern and ease of eliciting electrodermal responses." *Journal of Speech and Hearing Disorders*, **22**: 651, 1957.
15. Cody, D. T. R., and R. G. Bickford. "Cortical audiometry: An objective method of evaluating auditory acuity in man." *Mayo Clinic Proceedings*, **40**: 273–87, 1965.
16. Cody, D. T. R., D. W. Klass, and R. G. Bickford. "Cortical audiometry: An objective method of evaluating auditory acuity in awake and sleeping man." *Transactions of the American Academy of Ophthalmology and Otolaryngology*, **19**: 81–91, 1967.
17. Darley, R. L. "Identification audiometry." *Journal of Speech and Hearing Disorders*, Supplement 9, 1961.
18. Davis, H. "Some properties of the slow cortical evoked response in humans." *Science*, **146**: 434, 1964.
19. Davis, H. "Slow cortical responses evoked by acoustic stimuli." *Acta Oto-Laryngologica*, **59**: 179–85, 1965.
20. Davis, R. C. "Response patterns." *Transactions of New York Academy of Science*, **19**: 731, 1957.
21. Davis, H., P. A. Davis, A. L. Loomis, E. N. Harvey, and G. Hobart. "Electrical reactions of the human brain to auditory stimulation during sleep." *Journal of Neurophysiology*, **2**: 500–14, 1939.
22. Dempsey, E. W. "Homeostasis." In S. S. Stevens, ed., *Handbook of Experimental Psychology*, New York: John Wiley & Sons, Inc., 1951.
23. Denmark, F. "Development of the peep-show audiometer." *Journal of Laryngology and Otology*, **64**: 357, 1950.
24. Derbyshire, A. J., and J. C. Farley. "Sampling auditory responses at the cortical level: A routine for EER audiometric testing." *Annals of Otology, Rhinology and Laryngology*, **68**: 675, 1959.
25. DiCarlo, L. M., and W. H. Bradley. "A simplified auditory test for infants and young children." *Laryngoscope*, **71**: 628–46, 1961.
26. Dix, M. R., and C. S. Hallpike. "The peep show: A new technique for pure-tone audiometry in young children." *British Medical Journal*, **2**: 719, 1947.
27. Downs, M. P., and M. E. Doster. "A hearing testing program for preschool children." *Rocky Mountain Medical Journal*, **56**: 37, 1959.
28. Downs, M. P., M. E. Doster, and M. Weaver. "Dilemmas in identification audiometry." *Journal of Speech and Hearing Disorders*, **30**: 360, 1965.
29. Downs, M. P., and G. Sterritt. "Identification audiometry for neonates: A preliminary report." *Journal of Auditory Research*, **4**: 69–80, 1964.
30. Dykman, R. A., W. G. Reese, C. R. Galbrecht, and J. Thomasson. "*Psychophysiological* reactions to novel stimuli: Measurement, adaptation, and relationship to psychological and physiological variables in the normal human." *Annals of New York Academy of Science*, **79**: 43, 1959.
31. Eisenberg, R. B., E. J. Griffen, D. B. Coursin, and M. A. Hunter. "Auditory behavior in the human neonate: A preliminary report." *Journal of Speech and Hearing Research*, **7**: 245–69, 1964.
32. Ewing, A. W. G., ed., *Educational Guidance and the Deaf Child.* Manchester: Manchester University Press, 1958.
33. Ewing, I. R., and A. W. G. Ewing. "The ascertainment of deafness in infancy

and early childhood." *Journal of Laryngology and Otology*, **59**: 309–33, 1944.

34. Frisina, D. R. "Measurement of hearing in children." In J. Jerger, ed., *Modern Developments in Audiology*. New York: Academic Press Inc., 1963.
35. Froding, C. "Acoustic investigation of newborn infants." *Acta Oto-Laryngologica*, **52**: 31–40, 1960.
36. Froeschels, E., and H. Beebe. "Testing the hearing of newborn infants." *Archives of Otolaryngology*, **44**: 710, 1946.
37. Gesell, A., and C. Armatruda. *Developmental Diagnosis*. New York: Harper & Law, Publishers (Hoeber), 1948. 2nd ed., 1964.
38. Geyer, M., and A. Yankauer. "Detection of hearing loss in preschool children." *Journal for Exceptional Children*, **72**: 723, 1957.
39. Goldstein, R. "Electrophysiologic audiometry." In J. Jerger, ed., *Modern Developments in Audiology*. New York: Academic Press Inc., 1963.
40. Goldstein, R., and A. J. Derbyshire. "Suggestions for terms applied to electrophysiologic tests of hearing." *Journal of Speech and Hearing Disorders*, **22**: 696, 1957.
41. Goldstein, R., S. Polito-Castro, and J. T. Daniels. "The difficulty in conditioning electrodermal response to tone in normally hearing young children." *Journal of Speech and Hearing Disorders*, **20**: 26, 1955.
42. Goldstein, R., and L. Rodman. "Early components of averaged evoked responses to rapidly repeated auditory stimuli." *Journal of Speech and Hearing Research*, **10**: 697–705, 1967.
43. Goodman, W. S., S. V. Appleby, and J. W. Scott. "Audiometry in newborn children by electroencephalography." *Laryngoscope*, **74**: 1316–28, 1964.
44. Green, D. S. "The peep-show: A simple inexpensive modification of the peep-show." *Journal of Speech and Hearing Disorders*, **23**: 118, 1958.
45. Guilford, F., and C. O. Haug. "Diagnosis of deafness in the very young child." *Archives of Otolaryngology*, **55**: 101, 1952.
46. Hardy, J. B., A. Dougherty, and W. G. Hardy. "Hearing responses and audiologic screening in infants." *Journal of Pediatrics*, **55**: 382–90, 1959.
47. Hardy, W. G., J. B. Hardy, C. H. Brinker, T. M. Frazier, and A. Dougherty. "Auditory screening of infants." *Annals of Otology, Rhinology and Laryngology*, **71**: 759–66, 1962.
48. Hardy, W. G., and M. D. Pauls. "The test situation in PGSR audiometry." *Journal of Speech and Hearing Disorders*, **17**: 13–24, 1952.
49. Haug, C. O. and F. R. Guilford. "Hearing testing on the very young child." *Transactions of the American Academy of Ophthalmology and Otolaryngology*, **64**: 269–71, 1960.
50. Hind, J. E., A. E. Aronson, and J. V. Irwin. "GSR auditory threshold mechanisms: Instrumentation, spontaneous response, and threshold definition." *Journal of Speech and Hearing Research*, **1**: 222, 1958.
51. Hoerr, N. L. and A. Osol, eds., *Blakiston's New Gould Medical Dictionary*, New York: McGraw-Hill Book Company, 1956.
52. Irwin, J. V., J. E. Hind, and A. E. Aronson. "Experience with conditioned GSR audiometry in a group of mentally deficient individuals." *Training School Bulletin*, **54**: 26–31, 1957.
53. Keaster, J. "A quantitative method of testing the hearing of young children." *Journal of Speech and Hearing Disorders*, **12**: 159, 1947.

54. Knauf, V. H., J. V. Irwin, and C. S. Hayes. "Developmental norms for certain auditory tasks." *ASHA*, **3**: 357–58, 1961.
55. Knox, E. C. "A method of obtaining pure-tone audiograms in young children." *Journal of Laryngology and Otology*, **74**: 475–79, 1960.
56. Landes, G. and W. A. Hunt. "The conscious correlates of the galvanic response." *Journal of Experimental Psychology*, **18**: 506–29, 1935.
57. Lacey, J. I. "The evaluation of autonomic responses: Toward a general solution." *Annals of the New York Academy of Science*, **67**: 123, 1956.
58. Lindsley, D. B. "Emotions." In S. S. Stevens, ed., *Handbook of Experimental Psychology*. New York: John Wiley & Sons, Inc., 1951.
59. Lindsley, D. B. "Psychological function and the electroencephalogram." *Electroencephalography and Clinical Neurophysiology*, **4**: 443, 1952.
60. Lindsley, D. B. "Attention, consciousness, sleep and wakefulness." In J. Field, H. W. Magoun, and V. E. Hall, eds., *Handbook of Physiology, Section* 1*: Neurophysiology, Volume III*. Washington, D.C.: American Physiological Society, 1960.
61. Loomis, A. L., E. N. Harvey, and G. A. Hobart. "Distribution of disturbance patterns in the human electroencephalogram, with special reference to sleep." *Journal of Neurophysiology*, **1**: 413–30, 1938.
62. Lowell, E. L., G. Rushford, G. Hoversten, and M. Stoner. "Evaluation of pure-tone audiometry with preschool age children." *Journal of Speech and Hearing Disorders*, **21**: 292–302, 1956.
63. Meritser, C. L. and L. G. Doerfler. "The conditioned galvanic skin response under two modes of reinforcement." *Journal of Speech and Hearing Disorders*, **19**: 350–59, 1954.
64. Meyerson, L. "Hearing for speech in children: A verbal audiometric test." *Acta Oto-Laryngologica* Supplement 128, 1956.
65. Miller, J. K. and L. DeSchweinitz, and C. P. Goetzinger. "How infants 3, 4, and 5 months of age respond to sound." *Journal for Exceptional Children*, **30**: 149–54, 1963.
66. Moruzzi, G. and H. W. Magoun. "Brain stem reticular formation and activation of the EEG." *Electroencephalography and Clinical Neurophysiology*, **1**: 455–73, 1949.
67. Moss, J. W., M. Moss, and J. Tizard. "Electrodermal response audiometry with mentally defective children." *Journal of Speech and Hearing Research*, **4**: 41, 1961.
68. Murphy, K. P. "Ascertainment of deafness in children." *Audecibel* (Summer, 1966, 89–94.
69. Myatt, B. D. and B. A. Landes. "Assessing discrimination loss in children." *Archives of Otolaryngology*, **77**: 359, 1963.
70. Myklebust, H. R. *Auditory Disorders in Children*. New York: Grune and Stratton, 1954.
71. O'Leary, W. D. "The autonomic nervous system as a factor in the psychogalvanic reflex." *Journal of Experimental Psychology*, **15**: 767–72, 1932.
72. Parmelee, A. H., Jr. "A critical evaluation of the Moro reflex." *Pediatrics*, **33**: 773–88, 1964.
73. Price, L. L. and R. Goldstein. "Averaged evoked responses for measuring auditory sensitivity in children." *Journal of Speech and Hearing Disorders*, **31**: 248–56, 1966.

74. Price, L. L., B. Rosenblut, R. Goldstein, and D. C. Shepherd. "The averaged evoked response to auditory stimulation." *Journal of Speech and Hearing Research*, **9**: 361–70, 1966.
75. Pronovost, W. and C. Dumbleton. "A picture-type speech sound discrimination test." *Journal of Speech and Hearing Disorders*, **18**: 258, 1953.
76. Rapin, I. "Evoked responses to clicks in a group of children with communication disorders." *Annals of the New York Academy of Science*, **112**: 182–203, 1964.
77. Richmond, J. B., H. J. Grossman, and S. Lustman. "Hearing tests for the newborn infant." *Pediatrics*, **11**: 634, 1953.
78. Rose, D. E. and H. B. Ruhm. "Some characteristics of the peak latency and amplitude of the acoustically evoked response." *Journal of Speech and Hearing Research*, **9**: 412–22, 1966.
79. Ruben, R., A. Lieberman, and J. Bordley. "Some observations of cochlear potentials and nerve action potentials in children." *Laryngoscope*, **72**: 545, 1962.
80. Ruhm, H. B. "Rapid electrodermal audiometric procedure for testing adults." *Journal of Speech and Hearing Disorders*, **26**: 130–36, 1961.
81. Shepherd, D. C. "Intrasubject variability of normal hearing adults for patterns of averaged evoked responses to click and light." *ASHA*, **7**: 390, 1965.
82. Siegenthaler, B. M., J. Pearson, and R. Lezak. "A speech reception threshold test for children." *Journal of Speech and Hearing Disorders*, **19**: 360–66, 1954.
83. Sortini, A. J. "Hearing evaluations of brain damaged children." *Volta Review*, **62**: 536–40, 1960.
84. Sortini, A. J. and C. G. Flake. "Speech audiometry testing for preschool children." *Laryngoscope*, **63**: 991, 1953.
85. Spitz, R. A. "Otogenesis: The proleptic function of emotion." In P. H. Knapp, ed., *Expression of the Emotions in Men*. New York: International Universities Press, Inc., 1963.
86. Statten, P. and D. E. S. Wishart. "Pure-tone audiometry in young children: Psychogalvanic skin-resistance and peep show." *Annals of Otology, Rhinology and Laryngology*, **65**: 511, 1956.
87. Stewart, K. C. "Some basic considerations in applying the GSR technique to the measurement of auditory sensitivity." *Journal of Speech and Hearing Disorders*, **19**: 174–83, 1954.
88. Suzuki, T., Y. Kamijo, and S. Kiuchi. "Auditory test of newborn infants." *Annals of Otology, Rhinology and Laryngology*, **73**: 914–23, 1964.
89. Suzuki, T. and T. Ogiba. "Conditioned orientation reflex audiometry." *Archives of Otolaryngology*, **78**: 84–150, 1961.
90. Suzuki, T. and I. Sato. "Free-field startle response audiometry: A quantitative method for determining the threshold of infant children." *Annals of Otology, Rhinology and Laryngology*, **70**: 997–1007, 1961.
91. Waldon, E. "The baby-cry test." *Asha*, **5**: 795, 1963.
92. Walter, W. G. "The convergence and interaction of visual, auditory, and tactile responses in human nonspecific cortex." *Annals of the New York Academy of Science*, **112**: 320–61, 1964.
93. Wedenberg, E. "Objective audiometric tests on noncooperative children." *Acta Oto-Laryngologica*, Supplement 175, **32**: 1963.

94. Weitzman, E. D., W. Fishbein, and L. Graziani. "Auditory evoked responses obtained from the scalp electroencephalogram of the full-term neonate during sleep." *Pediatrics*, **35**: 458–62, 1965.
95. Wilder, J. "Modern psychophysiology and the law of initial value." *American Journal of Psychotherapy*, **12**: 199–221, 1958.
96. Willeford, J. A. "A new approach to measuring hearing in young children." *Asha*, **3**: 357–58, 1961.
97. Williams, H. L., D. I. Tepas, and H. C. Morlock, Jr. "Evoked responses to clicks and electroencephalographic stages of sleep in man." *Science*, **138**: 685–86, 1962.
98. Wolski, W., J. Wiley, and M. McIntire. "Hearing testing in infants and young children." *Medical Times*, **92**: 1107, 1964.

9

The Geriatric Patient

Jack A. Willeford, Ph.D.

Hearing loss that develops as a function of advancing age has been termed PRESBYCUSIS. In spite of the fact that it probably represents the most common cause of auditory deficiency occurring in most adults (41, p. 379; 69, p. 124), at least among sensori-neural disorders, presbycusis has been somewhat neglected in the professional literature. This oto-audiological entity usually occupies little more than a paragraph in most textbooks. At least a part of this neglect is probably due to the complexity of the disorder. The term presbycusis was originally employed to describe diminished hearing in elderly people, but has gradually taken on much broader implications. An expanded concept was inevitable in light of advancing knowledge about the geriatric patient. For example, a great deal more is now known about the myriad of senescent changes exhibited by older people, both in organic structures and emotional patterns, which combine to modify total behavior. Thus, presbycusis has become generally recognized as a considerably more complicated clinical phenomenon than it was a few years ago. In view of this fact, the presbycusis patient should present a fascinating challenge to audiologists and otologists. This chapter was written for the purpose of focusing greater attention on the various aspects of geriatric audiology.

The Nature of Presbycusis

INCIDENCE

Due largely to phenomenal advances in medical science in the last two decades, the number of aged persons in our society has increased steadily.

The United States Department of Health, Education and Welfare (28) estimates that the number of people who are sixty-five years or over presently exceeds 17 million, and that by 1980 this group will number approximately 24 million.

Recent figures released by the Metropolitan Life Insurance Company (60) show that life expectancy in the decade period between 1949–51 and 1959–61 increased for both white males and females in the United States. Although geographic variations in longevity were noted, forty states revealed increases. (Florida showed the greatest longevity for both sexes among its senior citizens—presumably because of the many healthy people who have migrated there upon retirement.) Life expectancy remained unchanged in four states and decreased slightly in eight others. The longevity rate for women actually increased in every state, and only in Utah (where the rates for men and women were the same) did it fail to exceed the gains made by men. Mean increases for the United States during this period were 0.2 years for males (77.8 to 78 years) and 0.9 years for females (80 to 80.9 years). Similar information for nonwhite populations was not made available.

In an earlier report (59), Metropolitan drew on data from the United States National Health Survey to estimate the number of aged persons with impaired hearing. These data are presented in Table 9.1 with the permission of the Metropolitan Life Insurance Company. Of the 5,822,000 people in the United States with some degree of hearing impairment, 2,497,000 are sixty-five years or older. In other words, nearly one-half of

TABLE 9.1. FREQUENCY OF HEARING IMPAIRMENT BY AGE. UNITED STATES NATIONAL HEARING SURVEY, JULY, 1957—JUNE, 1958*

Age Period (Years)	*Number of Cases*	*Rate per 1,000 Persons*
All ages	5,822,000	34.6
Under 25	583,000	7.9
25–44	941,000	20.6
45–64	1,801,000	52.2
65–74	1,244,000	129.2
75 *and over*	1,253,000	256.4

* *Data refer to the civilian noninstitutional population, and include total deafness.*

Source: U.S. National Health Survey, Series B–9, 1959, p. 9.

the American people with impaired hearing are over sixty-five years of age. The incidence rate per 1,000 persons is also very revealing. It may be noted in Table 9.1 that the incidence increases sharply with each age group, and that the values for people sixty-five years and older far exceed the rate for all age groups combined.

If one considers the projected increase in the geriatric population, the importance of communication skills in a society that will become progressively more complex in both its social and technological aspects, the isolation imposed by impaired hearing, and the limited medical and surgical treatment presently applicable to presbycusis, the importance of expanding present audiological rehabilitation services for the geriatric population becomes readily apparent.

ETIOLOGY

Defining presbycusis merely as hearing impairment that accompanies aging fails to represent a number of clinical and theoretical aspects which characterize this phenomenon. For many years the belief was popularly held that prebycusis was due simply to atophy of the organ of Corti and its associated nerve supply—specifically, the spiral ganglion cells (12, p. 67; 27, p. 102). However, it has been common for many authors to concede the possibility of similar changes also occurring in the central nervous system. Recent evidence convincingly confirms the fact that subjects with presbycusis do indeed experience degeneration of tissues in the cochlea and spiral ganglion cells, but that they also incur changes in the external and middle-ear mechanisms as well as deterioration of tissues in the neuron elements of the central auditory pathways and in the auditory cortex. Hinchcliffe (46) has suggested a convenient outline to describe the structural changes that are reported to develop in the ear as a function of age. An outline is presented below which retains all of the features of Hinchcliffe's proposal, but with one modification to include brainstem findings:[1]

A. EXTERNAL EAR:

1. Changes in the pinna.
2. Atrophic changes in the external auditory meatus and tympanic membrane.

[1] It is important to emphasize at this point that all discussion of presbycusis relates to generalizations about the total population of elderly persons with impaired hearing when viewed as a group since there are individual exceptions. For example, it is not unusual for audiologists to see an occasional elderly person who exhibits little or no abnormality in auditory function. It would seem reasonable to assume that: (1) these hardy individuals have incurred only minimal structural changes in their auditory mechanisms, or, (2) the damage is restricted to anatomical structures which do not elevate the auditory threshold. For example, Schuknecht and Woellner (76) found that up to 75 per cent of the spiral ganglion cells in cats must be damaged before threshold elevations occur.

B. MIDDLE EAR:
Nonspecific osteitis and sclerosis of the auditory ossicles.

C. INNER EAR:
1. Neuroepithelial degeneration.
2. Angiosclerosis (arteriosclerotic involvement of cochlear vessels).
3. Calcification of basement membrane in the basal turn.

D. COCHLEAR NERVE:
Degeneration of spiral ganglion cells.

E. BRAIN STEM:
Cellular degeneration.

F. BRAIN:
Cellular degeneration.

STRUCTURAL CHANGES IN THE EXTERNAL AND MIDDLE EAR

Presbycusis is classically considered to be a sensori-neural entity as far as auditory physiology is concerned, and senescent changes in the external ear and the middle ear are presently of little more than academic interest. That is, while anatomical modifications have been observed to occur in the pinna, external meatus, and middle ear, attention has traditionally centered on alterations in the inner ear.

Many audiologists have probably noted that the auricles in certain older patients, males in particular, appear to be unusually large and seem stiff and brittle when compared to the soft and flexible auditory appendages of children. Unusual hair growth may also be observed along the helix, the antihelix, in the fossae, or on other parts of the pinna. Such hairs may be numerous or be quite sparse, and they have a wiry texture like the bristles on a brush. These characteristics naturally attract the audiologist's attention when he places earphones over a patient's ears prior to audiometric testing. With occasional patients it becomes difficult to place the earphones properly or to keep them in position because of the size and structure of the pinnas. Similar experience with younger patients is extremely rare.

Tsai et al. (81) have provided experimental evidence to support some of these observations. In a study of changes in pinna size as a function of age, they selected a sample population of both male and female Taiwanese-Formosans between the ages of twenty and the middle and late fifties. They found that male ears increased 5.13 mm in length and 2.31 mm in breadth, while female ears increased 3.69 mm in length and 2.28 mm in breadth. The assumption was made that the increase in size was caused by relaxation of ear tissue due to senility.

Other writers have made reference to changes in the external and middle portions of the ears of aged persons. Over forty years ago Politzer (65) wrote that diminished hearing in presbycusis was due partially to the frequent development of chronic, insidious inflammation of the middle ear which leads to a thickening of its lining membrane and to rigidity of the ossicular articulations. Magladery (57) states that atrophic changes in the elderly occur in the supporting walls of the external auditory meati, and Crabbe (24) concluded that, in general, presbycusis is the result of total involution of the ear, including sclerosis of the formations of the middle ear. Klotz (54) also refers to sclerosis and rigidity of the ossicular joints in older patients and notes that in individuals who also exhibit chronic rheumatism and arthritis, examination may reveal dry otitis with accompanying sclerotic thickening of a nonreflecting tympanic membrane. Farrior (30) has shown that geriatric patients are also vulnerable to otosclerosis which is thought by many to be a disease of the younger person. In more than a third of the 125 cases he reported, sclerotic stapes fixation developed after fifty years of age.

Glorig and Davis (35) have also reported data which suggests that some pathological condition exists in the conductive apparatus of the auditory mechanism of aged patients. As a part of a larger study, they sought to test the hypothesis that aging induces pure sensori-neural impairment. They tested 164 professional businessmen and some inmates from a home for old soldiers, each of whom had been screened to assure that he had no history of noise exposure. Their ages ranged from twenty-five to eighty. Thresholds were obtained for both air conduction and bone conduction at the frequencies of 500, 1,000, 2,000, and 4,000 Hz. Surprisingly, their results revealed an air-bone gap that increased progressively with higher frequencies and advancing age. In fact, their seventy-nine-year group showed an air-bone gap that approached 40 dB at 4,000 Hz. They concluded that:

> ... Evidently the high-tone threshold shift that occurs with age is not primarily sensori-neural but is largely a conductive loss in the middle ear. We make this general statement without speculating as to the exact mechanism of conductive loss that is greater the higher the frequency. Such a relation is perfectly possible, however, and the conductive presbycusis that is revealed by the air-bone gap ... must be attributed to the middle ear. (pp. 561–62)

The Glorig and Davis data are reproduced in Figure 9.1. In reviewing their unique findings, these authors refer to Mayer's theory that there may be conductive loss in the inner ear if physical changes impede sound at any point short of the hair cell action (and even impede the efficiency of the final step of hair cell bending action). They conclude that one should not term a hearing loss as sensori-neural until recruitment can be demonstrated, until there is a speech discrimination loss, or until hearing is totally lost for very intense sound. In summary, they state:

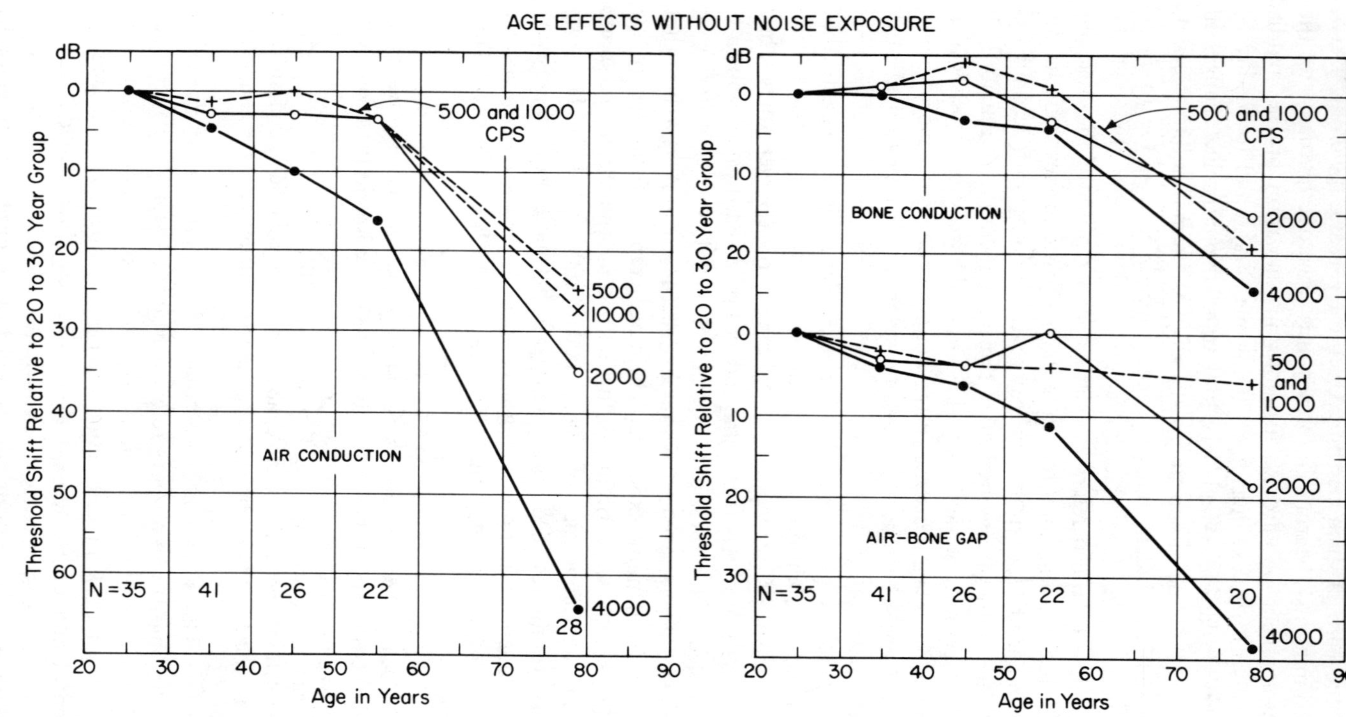

FIGURE 9.1 Comparison of air-conduction and bone-conduction thresholds in 164 men between twenty-five and eighty years of age with a history of no noise-exposure. Note the air-bone gap as a function of age and frequency.

Source: Glorig, A., and H. Davis. "Age, noise, and hearing loss." *Annals of Otology, Rhinology and Laryngology*, **70**: 556–71, 1961.

> . . . Concerning presbycusis, we identify four major age effects. One is central presbycusis. Another is the classical sensori-neural presbycusis which we believe has generally been overemphasized. A third is middle ear conductive presbycusis, and the fourth is inner ear presbycusis, which shows considerable high-tone hearing loss by bone conduction. These age effects may occur in any combination. Strong supporting arguments for the existence of inner ear conductive presbycusis are (1) the complete independence of age effects from noise-induced sensori-neural hearing loss, and (2) the absence of loudness recruitment in many cases of carefully selected inner ear presbycusis. (p. 568)

The length of this discussion of the Glorig-Davis findings may be unwarranted, but it seems justified by the esteem in which these authors are held and by the uniqueness of their findings, particularly since the air-bone gap in this same population was discussed further in a subsequent report by Nixon, Glorig, and High (62). In fact, these results served as the primary motivation for an investigation by Sataloff, Vassalo, and Menduke (71). The latter group studied fifty-five males and females between the ages of sixty-two and eighty-six years, with careful attention given to calibration factors. Their findings failed to reveal the presence of an air-bone gap. On the contrary, their results confirmed the widely held belief that presbycusis involves a reduction in sensori-neural sensitivity.

Rosenwasser (68) has presented a brief, but excellent overview of the physical changes associated with aging. He states:

> Closer study is now being made of the part infectious diseases play in hastening the degenerative processes associated with old age. Those not as yet shown to be due to specific diseases are gradual tissue desiccation; gradual retardation of cell division, capacity of cell growth, and tissue repair; gradual retardation of tissue oxidation rate; cellular atrophy, degeneration, increased cell pigmentation, and fatty infiltration; and gradual decrease in tissue elasticity and degenerative changes in the elastic connective tissue. Although this is by no means a complete enumeration of the structural and functional changes of old age, it is formidable enough. (p. 11)

Among the specific structural changes in the aged ear, Rosenwasser lists ossicular atrophy, particularly in the crura of the stapes; ossification of the incudo-malleolar joint with calcification of the articular cartilage; degeneration and atrophy of the middle-ear muscles; a thin and translucent tympanic membrane; and atrophy and thinning of the skin that lines the external meatus together with loss of elastic tissue elements.

It seems apparent, irrespective of impairment in auditory sensitivity, that substantial changes do take place in the outer and middle ear of the geriatric patient. Indeed, there is no reason why this region should be immune to the aging process as opposed to other portions of the ear and the entire body. However, as noted earlier, presbycusis is usually viewed as a sensori-neural problem. Therefore, attention is normally focused on damage to the sensory and neural mechanisms that are involved in auditory physiology. That is, interest is centered on those structures which are thought to be primarily responsible for impaired hearing. Thus, aside from instances of specific disease in the conducting mechanism, and notwithstanding the isolated reports by Glorig and Davis (35) and Nixon, Glorig, and High (62), the consensus is that no conductive-type hearing deficit is present. It is for this reason, apparently, that conditions in the outer and middle ear are frequently ignored in discussions of presbycusis. Hopefully, this background information will lead audiologists to a broader view of the geriatric patient.

STRUCTURAL CHANGES IN THE INNER EAR AND CENTRAL AUDITORY MECHANISMS

In spite of the rationale presented above, it is still common practice for many writers to dispose of the etiological considerations of presbycusis with a very limited discussion. As suggested previously, it is frequently reported that hearing loss associated with aging is due to the atrophy of sensory cells and their connecting nerve fibers, and of the spiral ganglion cells at the basal end of the cochlea. Such oversimplifications may serve quite adequately for many occasions, but analysis in greater detail is both interesting and enlightening. Reliable evidence is accumulating which suggests that the central auditory pathways and the cortex also sustain structural changes which intimately involve total auditory behavior in the geriatric individual.

Hansen and Reske-Nielsen (43), Schuknecht (73, 74), and Harbert, Young, and Menduke (44), among others, have presented literature reviews and conducted important studies which have provided us with much broader and precise concepts of the sensori-neural involvements.

INNER EAR ALTERATIONS

Using our modification of Hinchcliffe's (46) outline as a guide, the following specific alterations have been documented for the inner ears of patients with presbycusis:

A. COCHLEA:

1. Atrophy and degeneration of both hair cells and supporting cells of the cochlea. In some instances the hair cells are sharply reduced in number or completely disappear altogether, and the supporting cells appear flattened (43, 44, 67, 73, 74, 75).
2. Angiosclerotic degeneration of the epithelial tissues and vessels of the inner ear, including the organ of Corti, basilar membrane, and stria vascularis (43, 51, 73, 74).
3. A marked thinning of the tectorial membrane which may also develop restrictive adhesions (43).

4. Calcification and loss of elasticity of the basilar membrane (67, 73).
5. Reduced nutritional content of the endolymph (43, 74).

B. COCHLEAR NERVE:

1. Degeneration and loss of spiral ganglion cells and their associated nerve fibers (12, 27, 41, 43, 44, 67, 73, 74, 75).
2. Hypertrophy in the base of the internal auditory meatus which leads to increased pressure and subsequent atrophy of the nerve fibers (44, 67).

CENTRAL AUDITORY MECHANISM INVOLVEMENTS

A. BRAIN STEM:

1. Atrophy and degeneration of ganglion cells at all of the principal stations of the central auditory pathways, particularly in the ventral cochlear nucleus and the medial geniculate body. To a lesser degree in the superior olivary nucleus and the inferior colliculus (43, 51, 73, 74).

B. BRAIN:

1. Atrophy and sharp reduction in number of cells in the cortex including the auditory radiation area (10, 15, 43, 72, 74, 75).
2. Cell outlines shrink and become irregular, the cytoplasm becomes discolored, and red blood cells develop dark stains as they do in cases of severe anemia (15).

The foregoing outline summarizes the many changes which are germane to impaired auditory function. When combined with alterations in the structures of the external and middle ear, despite the apparent minimal influence which the latter have on hearing per se, it becomes obvious that presbycusis is indeed a very complicated entity. Moreover, it is likely that it is even more complex than one might envision from the preceding review. One justification for this statement is the fact that very limited attention has been given to the incidence of tinnitus and vertigo in the geriatric patient. Weston (84) reports that there does appear to be a relationship between the presence of these two symptoms and aging which increase in parallel fashion with severity of hearing loss. However, he also found that tinnitus and vertigo may be present together or alone. It would seem that this would be a fruitful area for study, both for further elucidation of symptoms and their incidence, as well as for identifying physical changes in the vestibular mechanisms. More will be said about these factors in subsequent discussion.

Some important information for our presently limited body of knowledge of presbycusis stems from the outstanding contributions of Schuknecht (73). He feels, after detailed study of human temporal bones, that we can now identify at least four types of presbycusis: (1) *sensory presbycusis*, which is characterized by atrophy of the organ of Corti and the auditory nerve in the basal turn of the cochlea. Schuknecht believes that his evidence places the primary site of degeneration in the supporting cells of the organ of Corti, with secondary degeneration involving the acoustic nerve; (2) *neural presbycusis*, which results from loss of neurons in the auditory pathways and cochlea; (3) *metabolic presbycusis*, which involves atrophy of the stria vascularis, thought to be the site of endolymph production and apparently necessary to sustain bioelectrical and biochemical properties of the endolymph and hence cochlear function. The metabolic type affects all regions of the scala media about equally; and (4) *mechanical presbycusis*, which, Schuknecht believes, results from a disorder in the motion mechanics of the cochlear duct that is caused by a stiffening of the basilar membrane or some other, as yet unknown, mechanical problem.

Since structural changes, such as the various types described, occur to varying degrees and in several different anatomical locations, it seems reasonable to expect that still further classifications of presbycusis await discovery. In any event, it is obvious that we can no longer confine our generalized definitions of presbycusis to a sensory cell and spiral ganglion locus.

A final comment regarding etiology is important to our understanding of presbycusis. At the stage of life at which this disorder becomes a clinical problem, it is highly unlikely that the human organism has been able to escape the adverse and cumulative influences of infectious diseases, arteriosclerosis, smoking, alcohol, drugs, and traumatic injuries. All of these factors make it difficult to identify behavioral or physical changes which are solely the result of aging. In addition, postmortem alterations often compound the problem of analyzing and describing histological material. Thus, we undoubtedly have a great deal more to learn about the causes which precipitate presbycusis.

MEDICAL TREATMENT

An interesting aspect of presbycusis is the fact that at the present time it is essentially untreatable. Sataloff (69) and Goodhill (41), both otologists, support this view. The latter states that there is no satisfactory treatment for this condition and that its progression is continuous in spite of all types of medical therapy. The author has heard similar statements made by a number of other otologists. Weston (84) suggests "... the possibilities of attempting to prevent, limit or treat it (presbycusis)—apart from the use of hearing aids—have also remained relatively unexplored." Boies, Hilger, and Priest (12), devote one paragraph to the subject of presbycusis in their textbook on otolaryngology, and omit reference to treatment entirely. Treatment, with vitamins, nicotinic acid, aneurin, and hormones has been attempted (54), but there is still no successful medical treatment. Audiological rehabilitation and psychological counseling remain the major ways of aiding the elderly patient with uncomplicated presbycusis.

In instances where other otopathologies are present in geriatric patients without associated hearing loss, or where they coexist with presbycusis, treatment is usually well defined unless other complicating health factors preclude such treatment. Farrior (30) has shown that stapes surgery may be successfully carried out to the satisfaction of certain geriatric patients. However, the experiences and philosophies of otologic surgeons vary widely where decisions to perform surgery on elderly individuals are concerned (68).

Audiological Manifestations

It has been previously stated that presbycusis means hearing loss that develops concomitantly with aging. Evidence was presented to show that structural changes take place along the entire continuum of the auditory mechanism—from the pinna to the cortex. However, there is little supporting data to suggest that any of the senescent alterations occurring peripheral to the cochlea have an influence on how well the geriatric patient hears unless other pathologies are present. Indeed, research has traditionally and overwhelmingly shown that presbycusis is an auditory disorder of the sensori-neural type which manifests itself in two major ways. First, there is a progressive reduction of sensitivity for pure tones (both air and bone). This diminution is particularly noted for the high frequencies and is bilaterally symmetrical. Second, a decreased ability to discriminate speech is frequently noted even though the pure tone loss may be minimal and speech is presented at a level that is sufficiently loud.

PURE TONE ACUITY AND AUDIOMETRIC PATTERNS

Bunch (16, 17) was the first to describe detailed audiometric characteristics of presbycusis, even though the gross audiological attributes have been recognized since 1899 (74). The common feature is that tonal sensitivity becomes progressively lessened for high-frequency stimuli. This reduction may be particularly observed for frequencies above 1,000 Hz. Considerably less deviation from audiometric zero is exhibited for tones below 1,000 Hz. A number of more recent studies have generally confirmed Bunch's findings. Among the important contributions in the United States, which have shaped our present knowledge of auditory sensitivity as a function of age, have been studies by: Beasley (4); Steinberg, Montgomery, and Gardner (78); Webster, Himes, and Lichtenstein (82); Glorig, Wheeler, Quiggle, Grings, and Summerfield (37); National Health Survey, 1960–1962, data reported by Glorig and Roberts (36); Corso (22, 23); and Klotz and Kilbane (53).

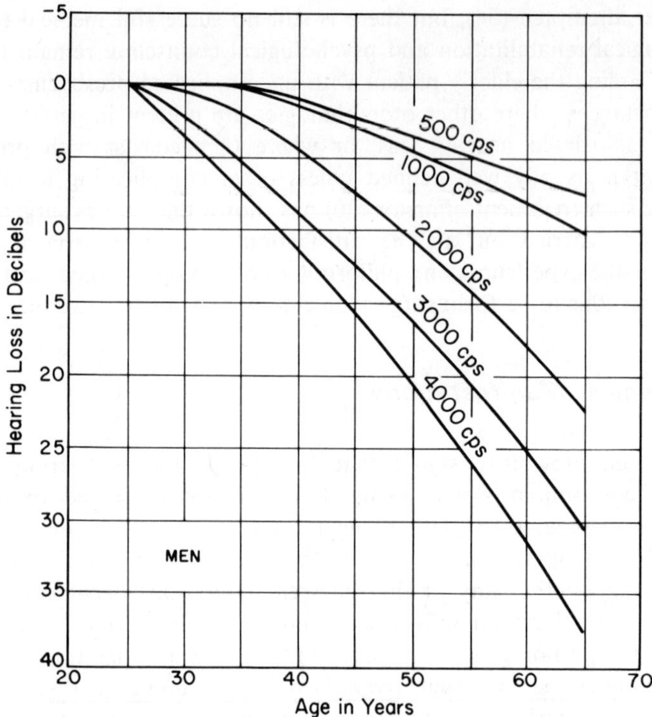

FIGURE 9.2 Presbycusis curves for men: average hearing loss to be expected with age.

Source: ASA Subcommittee Z24-X-2. "The Relations of Hearing Loss to Noise Exposure." New York, 1954.

The American Standards Association (3)[2] established a set of hearing-sensivity curves which were based on a consideration of the data accumulated in the studies prior to 1954. These curves represented the expected hearing levels at 500, 1,000, 2,000, 3,000, and 4,000 Hz for men and women between the ages of twenty-five and sixty-five years. These values, shown in Figures 9.2 and 9.3, are reported in reference to the 1951 American Standards Association values for audiometric zero. In Figure 9.4, however, the curves have been modified to conform with the 1964 standard reference zero suggested by the International Organization for Standardization (26), and represent typical curves for men and women at the age of sixty-five.

A number of other studies, both in the United States and in foreign countries, have shown only minor deviations from the curves illustrated in Figures 9.2 to 9.4. Thus, these curves essentially represent a composite of expected threshold shifts through the age of sixty-five. Such relatively good agreement is interesting in view of the fact that certain experimental

[2] Recently retitled the United States of America Standards Institute (USASI).

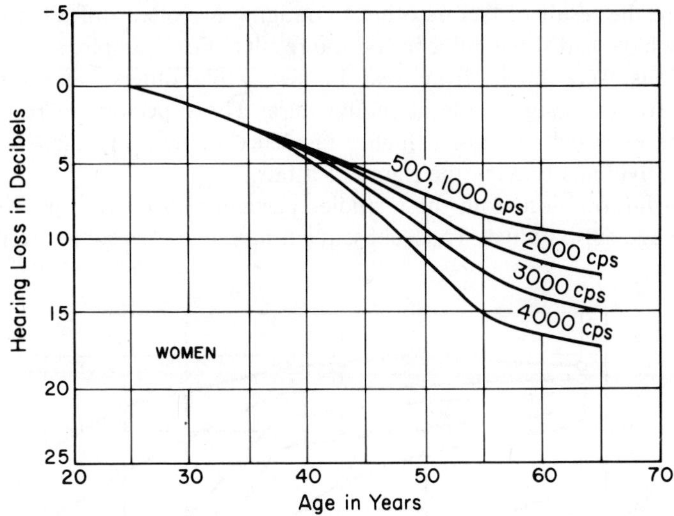

FIGURE 9.3 Presbycusis curves for women: average hearing loss to be expected with age.

Source: ASA Subcommittee Z24-X-2. "The Relations of Hearing Loss to Noise Exposure." New York, 1954.

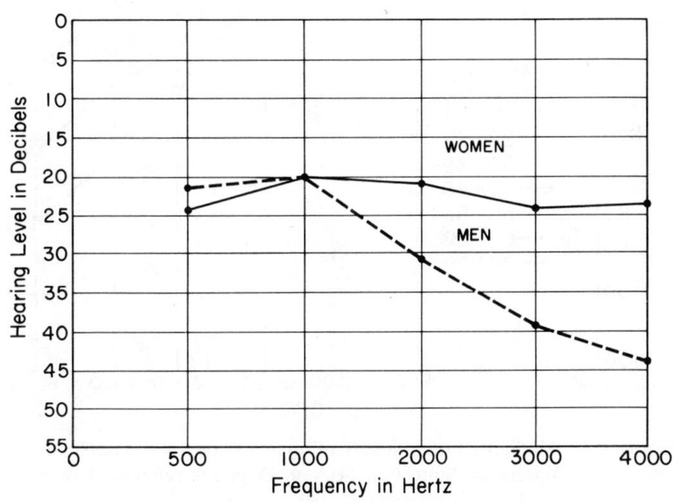

FIGURE 9.4 Presbycusis curves for men and women, at age sixty-five, on the ISO-1964 reference scale for audiometric zero. Curves based on American Standards Association data.

controls varied somewhat in a number of these studies, and since alterations which are the result of factors other than aging are often difficult to isolate and may have had some influence on the results. For example, some sample populations were taken from rest homes, while others were randomly selected from among people attending fairs. Those persons in rest homes would be expected to show a higher incidence of infirmity than the more robust individuals braving the rigors of a fair.

Little information from these studies pertained to hearing performance after the age of sixty-five. Thus, subsequent investigations sought to provide

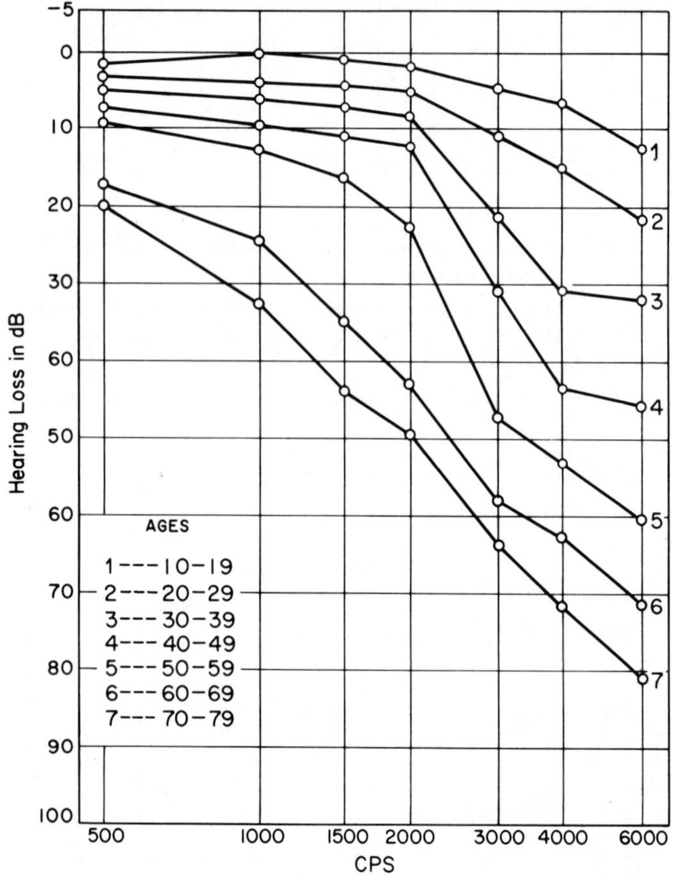

FIGURE 9.5 Median hearing losses of men in the total sample of the Wisconsin State Fair Survey. Data are referenced to ASA, 1951, audiometric zero, left ear only.

Source: Glorig et al. "1954 Wisconsin State Fair Survey." *American Academy of Ophthalmology and Otolaryngology*, 1957.

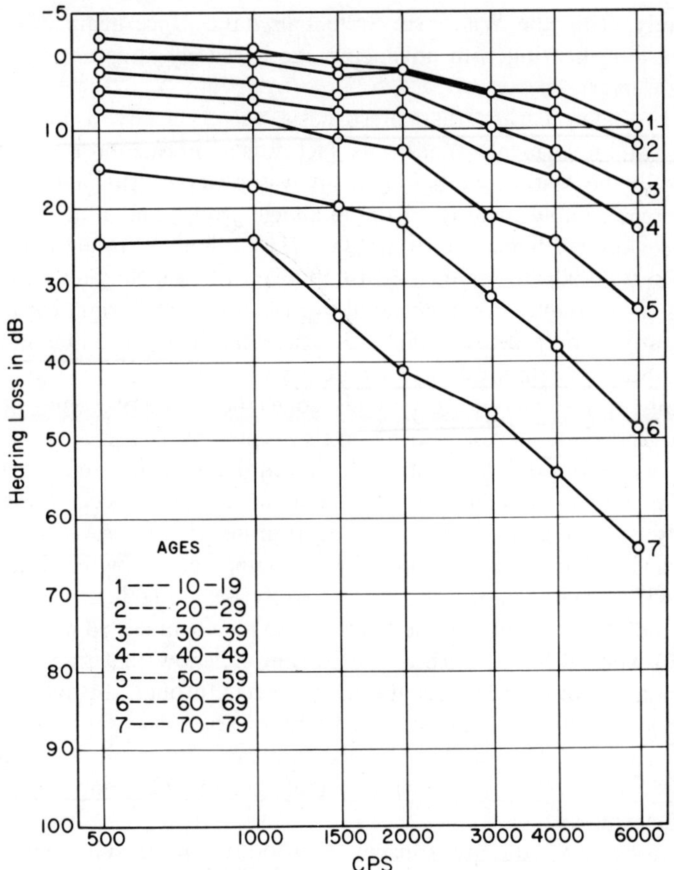

FIGURE 9.6 Median hearing losses for women in the total sample of the Wisconsin State Fair Survey. Data are referenced to ASA, 1951, audiometric zero.

Source: Glorig et al. "1954 Wisconsin State Fair Survey." *American Academy of Ophthalmology and Otolaryngology*, 1957.

such knowledge. Glorig, et al. (37), published data from the Wisconsin State Fair Hearing Survey on men and women up to seventy-nine years of age. They also included the frequency of 6,000 Hz in their examinations. From their results the following conclusions were drawn: (1) hearing losses for persons in their total sample became greater with increasing age; (2) the onset of hearing impairment is more gradual among women than it is among men, except in later years when the reverse becomes true; (3) with each ten-year increase in age for males, the median hearing loss at 6,000 Hz increases approximately 10 dB as compared with only 3 dB at 500 Hz. Figures 9.5 and 9.6 reflect the median hearing losses for men and women, respectively, from the Wisconsin State Fair data. Once again, the pattern of diminishing hearing with advancing age is readily apparent to even the casual observer.

It was stated earlier that presbycusis was typically a bilateral and symmetrical impairment. While this fact was confirmed for all practical purposes in the Wisconsin Fair data, it was observed that left ears show slightly greater impairment for males in all age groups and at all frequencies. Differences ranged from 0.2 dB at 1,000 Hz for men 30 to 39 years of age to 9.1 dB at 3,000 Hz for men 50 to 59 years of age. Similar results were found for women in the frequencies above 1,000 Hz, while right ear averages were slightly poorer below 2,000 Hz. These minimal ear differences were found to bear no relationship to handedness.

A point on which Glorig and his colleagues did not comment is the fact that their data suggest hearing levels in the decade age group 70 to 79 (at least as reported for twenty-fifth percentile, median, and seventy-five percentile points of their distributions) which show decreasing tonal sensitivity by a magnitude that is commensurate with progressive decreases in the earlier decade age groups. This finding agrees with Hinchcliffe's results (45), which demonstrate progressively declining hearing sensitivity through the age of seventy. It also agrees with results obtained by Goetzinger et al. (40) who, although with a limited sample, show that impairment for both men and women becomes gradually greater through the age of eighty-nine, while maintaining the same pattern of loss. The latter study also revealed data at 8,000 Hz, but showed that no measurable level could be obtained in a number of instances so that meaningful group values could not be determined.

The foregoing data are somewhat at odds with results reported by Melrose, Welsh, and Luterman (58), and with those of Sataloff and Menduke (70) from which it was concluded that very little additional loss occurs after age sixty-five. The latter results do reveal, however, that substantial variability in the hearing level is observable in the declining years, as was mentioned earlier in a footnote.

Two other studies are worthy of mention before concluding the present discussion. Corso (22, 23) investigated the influence of aging on auditory thresholds and demonstrated, once again, results which were generally similar to the presbycusis curves established by the American Standards Association (3). However, he noted that a progressive diminution of sensitivity for pure tones of higher frequencies continues beyond the age of sixty years. He also concluded that the rate of deterioration of hearing in women is fairly uniform as a function age, whereas men exhibit marked changes in hearing on the average about every fifteen years.

The most recent study of large magnitude was the Health Examination Survey (36) conducted as part of a national health survey by the United States Public Health Service. This survey was patterned somewhat after, and reported in much the same manner as, the Wisconsin State Fair study. Generally, the results were also comparable. However, when the median data were compared with the Wisconsin findings and those of Beasley (4), it was noted that lower thresholds (better hearing) were consistently demonstrated by the USPHS survey at all ages for both men and women from 500 through 4,000 Hz than in either of the latter surveys. The reasons for this deviation could not be explained, but were likely due to differences in experimental controls.

OTHER CHARACTERISTICS OF PERFORMANCE WITH PURE TONES

Little evidence is available on populations of sufficient size to generalize about the performance of presbycusics for frequencies outside the 500 to 6,000 Hz range. Few of the large-scale studies offered such evidence due to limitations in time, in instrumentation, and in the acoustical environment. However, studies conducted on clinical populations or under laboratory conditions (40, 53, 22, 23) suggest there is little departure from the pattern of hearing thus far described. For example, tonal sensitivity at 250 Hz tends to approximate the levels for 500 Hz, and 8,000 Hz appears to shift in a fashion parallel with or greater than 4,000 and 6,000 Hz, depending on whether the subjects have a history of noise exposure. More will be said about the relationship of noise exposure to presbycusis shortly. Goetzinger et al. (40), as mentioned earlier, found many patients who were unable to respond to maximum audiometer stimulation at 8,000 Hz. This experience is common to clinical audiologists. Corso (22, 23) found that women, who presumably experience less noise exposure than men, have greater threshold shifts with age at 6,000 and 8,000 Hz than they do at 4,000 Hz. The reverse was true for his male population.

Bekesy (5) has presented some interesting knowledge on this subject. He states that:

> On the high-frequency side, the range that the ear covers is remarkable. In childhood some of us can hear well at frequencies as high as 40,000 cycles per second. But with age our acuteness of hearing in the high-frequency range steadily falls. Normally, the drop is almost as regular as clockwork: testing several persons in their 40's with tones at a fixed level of intensity, we found that over a period of five years their upper limit dropped about 80 cycles per second every six months. (The experiment was quite depressing to most of the participants.)

Judging from the rate of deterioration shown by Bekesy's experiment, it seems fortunate that we are endowed with the ability to perceive a great range of frequencies in early life. Klotz and Kilbane's 1962 data on over 200 subjects between the ages of fifty-one and ninety-two years supports Bekesy's statement. They show a progressive decrease in hearing level as a function of frequency through 8,000 Hz.

Information regarding frequencies below 250 and above 8,000 Hz is extremely scarce. Limitations in contemporary clinical instrumentation preclude our seeking information above 8,000 Hz, while the recording of sensitivity at 125 Hz is generally considered to be of insufficient value.

Carhart (19) has provided some provocative observations about low-frequency sensitivity in elderly persons. He reported that the loss at 125 Hz is frequently greater than at 250 Hz, and "... appears as a clearly identifiable feature in the audiograms of many clinical cases, who sometimes yield thresholds 15 dB poorer at 125 cps than at 250 cps."

Carhart also speculates about the reasons for this peculiar finding which will provide interesting supplemental reading for many enthusiasts of hearing theory. In the same publication, Carhart discusses another interesting observation associated with presbycusis which he terms the "Bernero phenomenon" (after Ray Bernero who noted its characteristics in the records of the Hearing Clinics at Northwestern University). This phenomenon is characterized by an abnormal impairment for bone conduction sensitivity at 500 Hz (on the order of 10 to 15 dB poorer than the air conduction threshold at this frequency) which cannot be accounted for by errors in measurement. Apparently the condition is invoked only in instances where the untested ear is masked and, Carhart postulates, is the result of reduced perceptual abilities which accompany aging. He could not explain why the phenomenon was restricted to 500 Hz. Although the Bernero phenomenon presents an intriguing puzzle, it does not alter the large body of evidence which supports the opinion that presbycusis is a sensori-neural involvement. The finding of a conductive element by Glorig and Davis (35), mentioned earlier, stands as a rather marked exception. However, Sataloff (69, p. 128) has presented an unusual observation, apparently as the result of clinical experience and unsupported by experimental data. He states that bone conduction thresholds are usually much worse than those by air conduction, and often cannot be determined with either an audiometer or with tuning forks. He concludes that bone conduction is a particularly poor indication of the sensori-neural potential. Although the Glorig and Davis report and the one by Sataloff represent rather isolated departures from most data on presbycusis, it should be remembered that the majority of studies of any magnitude have dealt primarily with air conduction performance. Thus, a detailed investigation of sensori-neural sensitivity on a sizeable population of geriatric persons seems warranted.

The work of Schuknecht (73) may alter the present concepts of presbycusis when sufficient statistical data accrue. It was mentioned before that Schuknecht (73) has described four types of presbycusis (abrupt high-frequency sensory, neural, flat metabolic, and descending mechanical). He believes that all types reflect sensori-neural involvement. However, he combines audiometric findings with postmortem study of temporal bones to conclude that: (1) sensory presbycusis manifests itself in an abrupt high-frequency pattern of pure-tone impairment; (2) usually there is no practical deterioration in hearing until later in life from neural presbycusis, then it often produces an inordinate loss of speech discrimination ability without a parallel reduction in pure-tone acuity; (3) metabolic presbycusis results in a slowly progressive hearing loss which manifests itself in a flat audiometric curve; and (4) mechanical presbycusis is characterized by a gradually descending audiometric contour which involves slowly progressive hearing loss. It may be that large-scale studies have obscured patterns for individual types of presbycusis, particularly if one type such as mechanical presbycusis is prevalent in geriatric populations, as present evidence would suggest. Reports of the continuing work by Schuknecht should be highly interesting.

PRESBYCUSIS AND NOISE-INDUCED HEARING LOSS

One of the most important factors that clouds our understanding of presbycusis and one that deserves special mention is the contaminating damage which excessive noise exposure produces in the auditory mechanism. This problem, however, is equally disconcerting (perhaps more so) to those authorities responsible for establishing compensation laws and adjudicating claims related to occupational hearing losses (47). The basic question facing those concerned is "How much of an industrial worker's hearing loss is due to aging and how much to noise exposure?" One method for estimating loss that is noise induced is to subtract out the presbycusis curves established for various age groups. However, a series of problems becomes immediately apparent when you do so. First, as shown previously, prebycusis is a phenomenon which varies widely among individuals. Second, one is faced with the problem of which set of presbycusis curves should be used as the reference. As has been shown, a good deal of variability exists here as well. Third, as pointed out in the American Industrial Hygiene Association's *Industrial Noise Manual* (2, p. 48), it should also be noted that the type of deafness which results from aging and excessive noise exposure also results from some intoxications, infections, tumors, and degenerative diseases. Thus, such factors as these also contaminate the diagnostic picture. The manual stresses (p. 50) that while it is necessary to differentiate between hearing loss that is due to aging and that which results from acoustic overstimulation, no satisfactory means for separating them has been found. Contemporary audiological tests have not been sufficiently effective for this purpose.

Glorig (34, p. 141) has suggested an interesting classification of inner-ear hearing loss. It excludes impairment that results from otologic disease, presumably on the assumption that such factors can be isolated through the otologic examination and history. He terms *presbycusis* those impairments resulting from physiologic changes that accompany aging; losses stemming from the noise exposures of our social environment he calls *sociocusis*; and losses induced by occupational noise exposure he classifies as *occupational hearing loss.*

Corso (22) states that:

> If a correction factor for presbycusis is to be used in establishing the degree of hearing loss due to noise exposure, it should be understood that an assumption is involved; specifically, that hearing losses from presbycusis and noise exposure are considered to be additive with no interaction between the two. While this is a reasonable assumption, since both factors probably produce permanent damage to sensory cells and their associated auditory nerve fibers, the possibility exists that the two variables may, in fact, interact to produce multiplicative effects. Such a possibility should be investigated.

A number of investigations have sought to eliminate, through detailed history information, those subjects with minimal noise exposure. However, one particular study reported by Rosen et al. (66, 67) represents a unique approach to the problem. These investigators sought to assess the hearing behavior of a noise-free population insofar as was possible. The objective was to obtain a more accurate evaluation of hearing sensitivity which results from aging alone. Such a population, the Mabaan tribe, was found in a remote area of the Sudan, near the Ethiopian border. These people live in a region which is extremely isolated, and in a state of cultural development equivalent to the late stone age. Thus, they enjoy protection from the damaging acoustic environment of modern civilization. Moreover, the Mabaans were found to be excellent physical specimens. As a group they exhibited a much lower incidence of elevated blood pressure, coronary thrombosis, ulcers, asthma, hypertension, and the like. They presented an ideal population on which to assess changes in hearing sensitivity which were the uncontaminated result of aging.

The results were most interesting. It was revealed that decrement of hearing was extremely slight in comparison with even the best of samples in the outside world that were unexposed to noise. This limited decrement, which also increased as a function of frequency as in the previous studies cited, approached only 23 dB (ASA–1951) at 6,000 Hz in Mabaan males between the ages of seventy and seventy-nine years. In other words, hearing in these primitive tribesmen remains excellent throughout their lives. The authors conclude that we must now begin to assess true presbycusis in terms of these observations.

SPEECH PERCEPTION IN THE GERIATRIC PATIENT

In addition to the progressive deterioration in tonal sensitivity generally attributed to presbycusis, the geriatric patient also typically demonstrates a reduced ability to understand spoken language. This particular auditory function is measured by means of standardized tests of speech discrimination ability. The various instruments at the audiologist's disposal include the

Harvard PAL tests of phonetically balanced word lists, the CID W-22 lists, and the Michigan CNC lists, among others. The slope of the articulation function rises more sharply for some of these materials than it does for others but, regardless of which test or tests one employs, performances can be related with that of normals or with persons having other entities of otopathology.

Abnormally reduced speech discrimination scores with only limited impairment for pure tones is a common clinical observation. However, a number of studies have helped to crystallize our concepts of specific aspects of discrimination problems in the aged.

Gaeth (32) conducted the first study on the discriminatory skills in aged people. It has since become a minor classic reference in the audiological literature even though it was never published. Gaeth's work was the subject of a doctoral dissertation completed at Northwestern University, and was motivated by the observation noted above that certain patients show much greater difficulty in discriminating the phonemic elements of speech than would be expected on the basis of their pure tone scores. Gaeth describes a syndrome for such individuals which he termed "phonemic regression," and which, he stated, is characterized by the following features:

1. Otological and audiological findings indicate a loss of the perceptive (nerve) type, which is either mild or moderate in severity.
2. The threshold shift in hearing for connected speech agrees with the threshold shift for pure tones (512 to 2,048 cps average).
3. There is a greater difficulty in understanding speech, as revealed by appropriate discrimination tests, than the type and severity of the loss would lead one to expect.
4. The patient does not appear to evidence a general decay in mental capacities paralleling his deterioration in phonemic perception.
5. The patient lacks insight into the quality of his discrimination problem, for he tends to blame all his trouble on his deficiency in auditory acuity.
6. These symptoms appear more frequently in adults over fifty years of age than in those younger, but a substantial number of the older individuals with hearing losses do not display the difficulty. Therefore, age alone must be ruled out as a causative factor.

Gaeth selected only those individuals who were fifty years of age or older, and who exhibited a sensori-neural hearing loss which manifested itself during adulthood and which did not exceed a gradually increasing impairment for pure tones of higher frequencies. The performances of each subject on a battery of audiological and psychological tests were then compared.

The results of Gaeth's investigation clearly confirmed that phonemic regression is a characteristic of some elderly people with minimal deterioration in sensitivity to pure tones, even though it may also occur in younger adults as well. Unfortunately, the study did not establish the relationship of reduced discrimination scores to the gradually descending audiometric pattern of presbycusis, except that poorer discrimination does seem to accompany increasing hearing loss. It did, however, serve to stimulate other researchers to seek answers to this peculiar problem. Confirmation of this conclusion, at least as it applies to flat audiometric patterns, has been established by Thompson and Hoel (80).

Pestalozza and Shore (64) sought to further clarify and expand some of the questions raised by Gaeth's investigation. Their population of older subjects conclusively confirmed that discrimination scores are frequently very poor with mild hearing losses, but also become lower as the hearing loss increases. *They also found, as had Bunch* (16, 17) *earlier, that conditions of health do not influence the magnitude of loss in people of the same age group. By implication, then, it would appear that health factors are not of serious consequence in discrimination ability.* Finally, they showed that no significant relationship exists between discrimination loss and audiometric slope. They concluded that their results substantiated the hypothesis that a phonemic regression syndrome is associated with presbycusis.

Melrose, Welsh, and Luterman (58) reported audiological data on a population of Spanish-American War veterans with a mean age of eighty-two years who were chosen for study only when examination failed to reveal evidence of otologic disease. Their results offered additional confirmation that speech discrimination scores in geriatric patients tend to be lower than one would expect on the basis of their pure-tone test performance. However, they also found sufficient individual differences to conclude that phonemic regression is not an invariable consequence of presbycusis.

Studies by Goetzinger and Rousey (39); Goetzinger et al. (40); Olsen (63); and Harbert, Young, and Menduke (44) have since offered further evidence of abnormal inability in discriminating speech among older persons.

The etiological implications for such results may at first seem paradoxical. However, recalling that structural degeneration may take place throughout the aging auditory system, the departure from classical behavior should not be too surprising. A considerable body of evidence accumulated in recent years has substantiated that tumors involving the eighth cranial nerve result in a disproportionate reduction of speech discrimination when compared with sensitivity for pure tones. For example, Schuknecht and Woellner (76) have demonstrated, by quantitative histological and functional studies on cats, and with clinical findings on humans with acoustic neurinomas, that only a small number of cochlear nerve fibers are necessary to conduct impulses of threshold magnitude, while greater numbers of fibers are required to facilitate transmission of the complex neural patterns of speech. In fact, they have shown that up to 75 per cent of the nerve fibers to particular regions of the cochlea may be destroyed without elevating thresholds for the frequencies whose excitation is induced in these regions. Schuknecht (74) also believes it quite reasonable to assume that when thresholds are elevated, there must also be reductions in cell populations at the second-, third-, and fourth-order neuron levels. The fascinating work of Bocca (10) has also demonstrated that on speech tests that have been experimentally modified to reduce the redundancy of the test items, aged persons exhibit behavior which is quite comparable to that of subjects with temporal lobe insults. From such experiments one is unalterably led to conclude that cortical degeneration is at least one of the concomitant aspects of presbycusis, and that these peculiarities in auditory dysfunction unquestionably transcend the simple loss of loudness.

PERFORMANCE ON OTHER AUDITORY TASKS

The auditory skills of presbycusics on "special" audiological measures have also come under experimental and clinical scrutiny, although to a more limited extent. The work of Bocca (10) was alluded to above. Additional brief references by Bocca and Calearo (11) essentially constitute the limited research involving "distorted" speech tests with elderly persons. However, at present one may conclude that, as a result of a deficit in cortical cell population, even those geriatric subjects who perform in a relatively normal fashion on standardized measures of speech audiometry show subpar skill on tasks which require synthesization of complex speech stimuli.

PITCH DISCRIMINATION

The difference limen for frequency has received considerable attention as far as it relates to normal ears, but has been neglected where otopathologies are concerned. Gaeth (32) had noted consistent differences in pitch discrimination which corresponded to phonemic perception abilities in an elderly population, and concluded that further study of this finding was warranted. From among the limited number of subsequent studies that were undertaken on presbycusic subjects, the work of König (55) is a representative report of their observed behavior. In general, older people exhibit larger than normal values for frequency difference limens. Data from König's study are illustrated in Table 9.2 and in Figure 9.7 and support his conclusion that pitch discrimination does deteriorate with age. This finding is particularly noticeable after the age of fifty-five, and is especially true for frequencies above 1,000 Hz. Such results suggest that deterioration in pitch discrimination is a correlate of reduced pure tone sensitivity and speech discrimination skill in the aged person.

LOUDNESS FUNCTION

Since structural changes may occur at all levels of the auditory mechanism, it is reasonable to expect considerable individual variability in the loudness

TABLE 9.2. AVERAGE VALUES OF THE ABSOLUTE DIFFERENCE LIMEN (DF) AS A FUNCTION OF FREQUENCY AND AGE GROUP

Each age group was composed of ten listeners. The standard deviation (SD) of the distribution of individual differences in pitch discrimination performance and the total range of difference limens are also given for each age decade. All the tests were carried out at a sensation level of 40-dB above threshold (after König, 1957).

		Age group (years)						
Frequency (cps)	*Remarks*	*20–29 (cps)*	*30–39 (cps)*	*40–49 (cps)*	*50–59 (cps)*	*60–69 (cps)*	*70–79 (cps)*	*80–89 (cps)*
125	*DF*	1.05	1.6	2.2	3.0	4.4	5.3	7.5
	SD	0.2	0.5	1.0	0.5	0.3	1.5	1.7
	Range	0.75–1.25	1–2.25	1–3.5	2–4	3.5–6	3.25–7	4.5–10
250	*DF*	1.55	2.5	3.2	3.7	5.6	6.0	8.0
	SD	0.35	0.6	1.1	1.0	1.6	1.7	1.9
	Range	0.75–2	1–3.5	2–5	2–6	4.5–9.5	3.75–9	6–11
500	*DF*	2.4	3.7	4.7	5.0	7.1	7.8	9.5
	SD	0.7	1.2	1.9	1.1	1.5	2.4	2.9
	Range	1.8–4	1–5	3–7	3–7.5	5.5–9.5	5–13	6–14
1,000	*DF*	3.6	5.6	6.9	7.8	10.2	11.8	15.4
	SD	1.6	1.7	1.5	1.9	2.3	3.5	4.9
	Range	2–6	2–8	5–9	5–11	6–14	8–20	11–25
2,000	*DF*	6.8	11.2	14.0	16.4	22.2	28.6	38.2
	SD	2.0	3.8	3.1	4.8	7.7	12.8	14.4
	Range	4–13	4–16	10–18	10–24	11–35	14–50	22–70
3,000	*DF*	12.3	17.7	27.0	32.1	39.0	48.0	70.2
	SD	4.8	6.3	8.7	9.3	14.1	21.0	17.7
	Range	6–24	6–25	15–39	12–70	23–60	33–60	40–90
4,000	*DF*	21.2	33.2	53.2	64.0	89.2		
	SD	6.8	16.2	21.2	25.2	45.6		
	Range	12–36	11–60	26–92	28–100	40–150		

function of elderly persons. Indeed, as evidenced by both research data and clinical observation, such is the case. Pestalozza and Shore (64) employed the Reger technique of monaural bifrequency loudness balancing to assess loudness recruitment in twenty-four presbycusic subjects. Fifty per cent showed no recruitment, 30 per cent had partial recruitment, and 20 per cent had essentially complete recruitment. They concluded from these findings that damage to the spiral ganglion cells and the nerve fibers is the most common problem in presbycusis. These results add further support to the present belief that the site of cellular degeneration varies widely in presbycusics, since recruitment is known to be a manifestation only of cochlear lesion.

Goetzinger et al. (40) also addressed themselves to the problem of loudness recruitment in a population of aged subjects. Among eighty male ears tested they found twenty-seven which showed complete recruitment, forty-one with incomplete recruitment, and twelve ears with no recruitment. Among forty female ears tested, seven had complete recruitment, sixteen incomplete, and fourteen with no recruitment. These results may not refute Pestalozza and Shore's conclusion on prevalence with regard to the site of

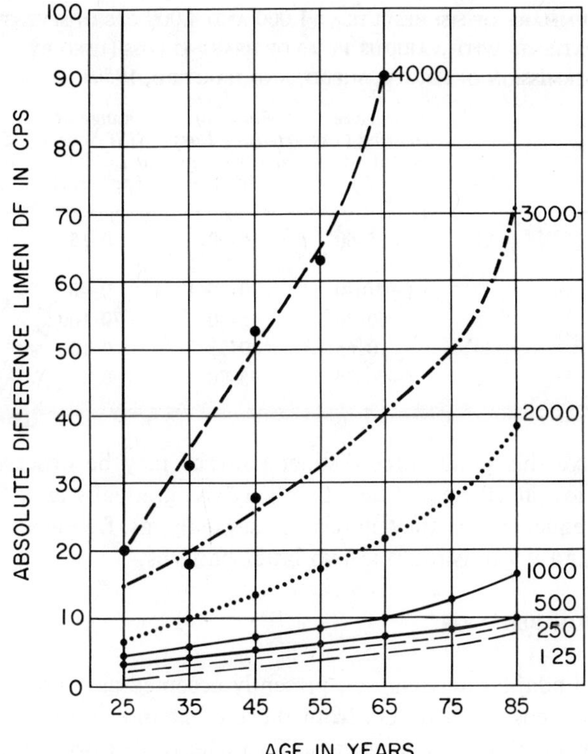

FIGURE 9.7 Absolute difference limen DF as a function of age. Sensation level: 40 dB above threshold. Parameter: frequency in cps.

Source: Konig, E. "Pitch discrimination and age." *Acta Oto-laryngologica*, **48**: 482, 1957.

lesion in presbycusis, but they do suggest that generalizations based on present knowledge are as yet hazardous or at least premature.

This point is further illustrated in a study by Harbert, Young, and Menduke (44). Using monaural loudness balance tests, they found no recruitment in 70 per cent of their fifty subjects. Moreover, recruitment in the other 30 per cent was minimal and of the above-threshold (asymptotic) type. However, they felt the significance of such findings was questionable because of the difficult nature of the monaural loudness matching procedure and the small hearing-level differences in the two-octave range they employed.

Jerger, Shedd, and Harford (49) examined the loudness function in subjects with presbycusis by the use of another method—the Short Increment Sensitivity Index (SISI). One may observe, in Table 9.3, that results ranged from 0 to 100 per cent. These authors note that "... presbycusis appears to be a clinical entity in which the SISI score is quite unpredictable." They suggest further that it is invariably low for frequencies below 1,000 Hz,

TABLE 9.3. SUMMARY OF SISI RESULTS AT 1,000 AND 4,000 CPS IN SEVENTY-FIVE PATIENTS WITH VARIOUS TYPES OF HEARING LOSS (USED BY PERMISSION OF JERGER, SHEDD, AND HARFORD, 1959)

Type of Loss	*No.*	*Range of Hearing Loss at 1,000 Cps (dB)*	*Range of Hearing Loss at 4,000 Cps (dB)*	*Range of SISI Scores at 1,000 Cps (per cent)*	*Range of SISI Scores at 4,000 Cps (per cent)*
Conductive	21	5–60	15–60	0–15	0–15
Noise-induced (acoustic trauma)	9	(−10)–0	30–70	0–40	95–100
Meniere's	8	50–70	45–80	70–100	95–100
Presbycusis	34	0–65	30–75	0–100	0–100
Retrocochlear	3	(−5)–85	45–70	0	0

but that above this point three distinct patterns may be observed: scores may remain low at all frequencies; they may rise gradually as a function of increasing frequency; or they may rise markedly as frequency increases. Figures 9.8 and 9.9 illustrate the two latter patterns.

ADAPTATION BEHAVIOR

Abnormal adaptation (relapse), presently accepted as a useful technique for separating sensory disorders from those of neural origin, is commonly assessed in two major ways. One is the Tone Decay Test originally described by Carhart (18), and the other is by the Bekesy audiometry procedure popularized by Jerger (48).

Little tone decay among presbycusics was observed by Goetzinger et al. (40). The median decibel values of decay for men and women in the 80 to 89 age group were 0 dB at 500 and 1,000 Hz, and 5 dB at 2,000 Hz. The maximum range of tone decay was 0 to 30 dB among females in the 70 to 79 age group. Harbert, Young, and Menduke (44) found slightly higher median values (5 dB for low frequencies and 10 to 15 dB for high frequencies), but found only one case who exhibited as much as 20 dB of tone decay. A direct comparison between these two studies is not really possible, since Harbert's group employed a modified procedure of the tone decay test (total threshold shift in a one-minute time span), whereas Goetzinger and his colleagues utilized the original method advocated by Carhart. The latter technique affords the opportunity for tone decay values of substantially greater magnitude. Thus, results of the two procedures must be interpreted differently. Nonetheless, the results in both studies cited led to the conclusion that the absence of abnormal tone decay in subjects with presbycusis suggests they have only a thinly spread or generalized deterioration of eighth nerve fibers as opposed to the destruction caused by an acoustic tumor.

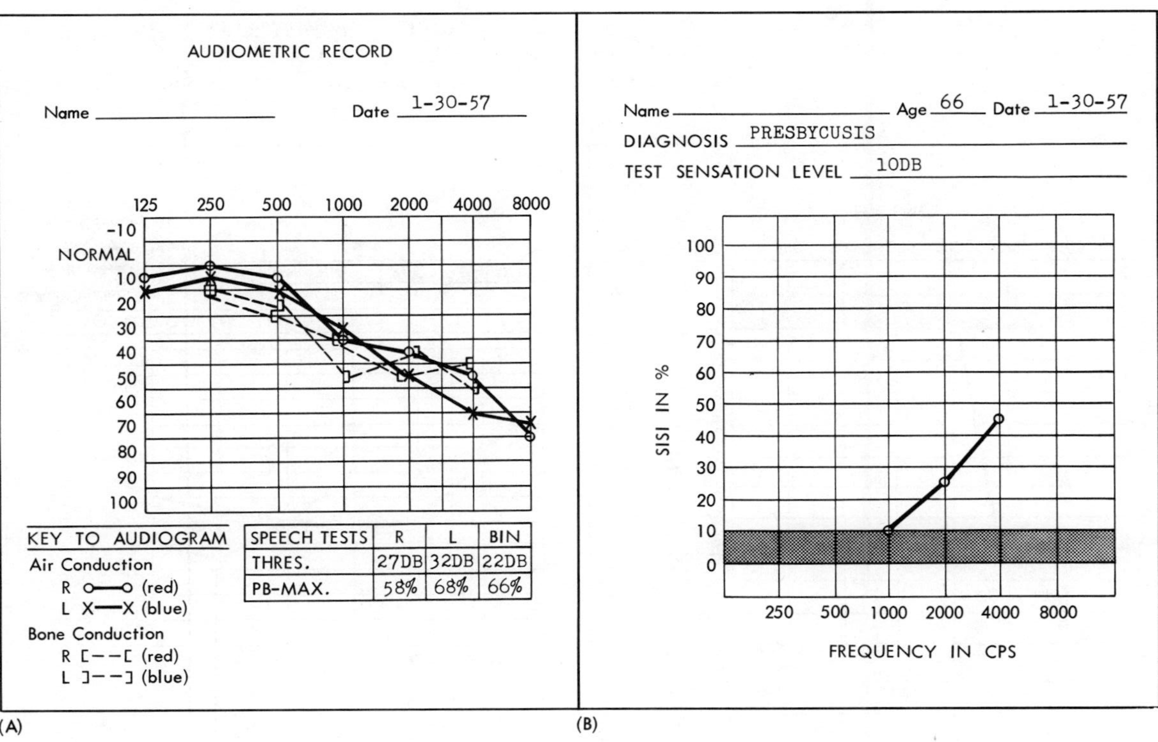

FIGURE 9.8 Audiogram (A) and SISI-gram (B) of a patient with presbycusis.

Source: Jerger, J., J. Shedd, and E. Harford. "On the detection of extremely small changes in sound intensity." *Archives of Otolaryngology*, **69**: 200–11, 1959.

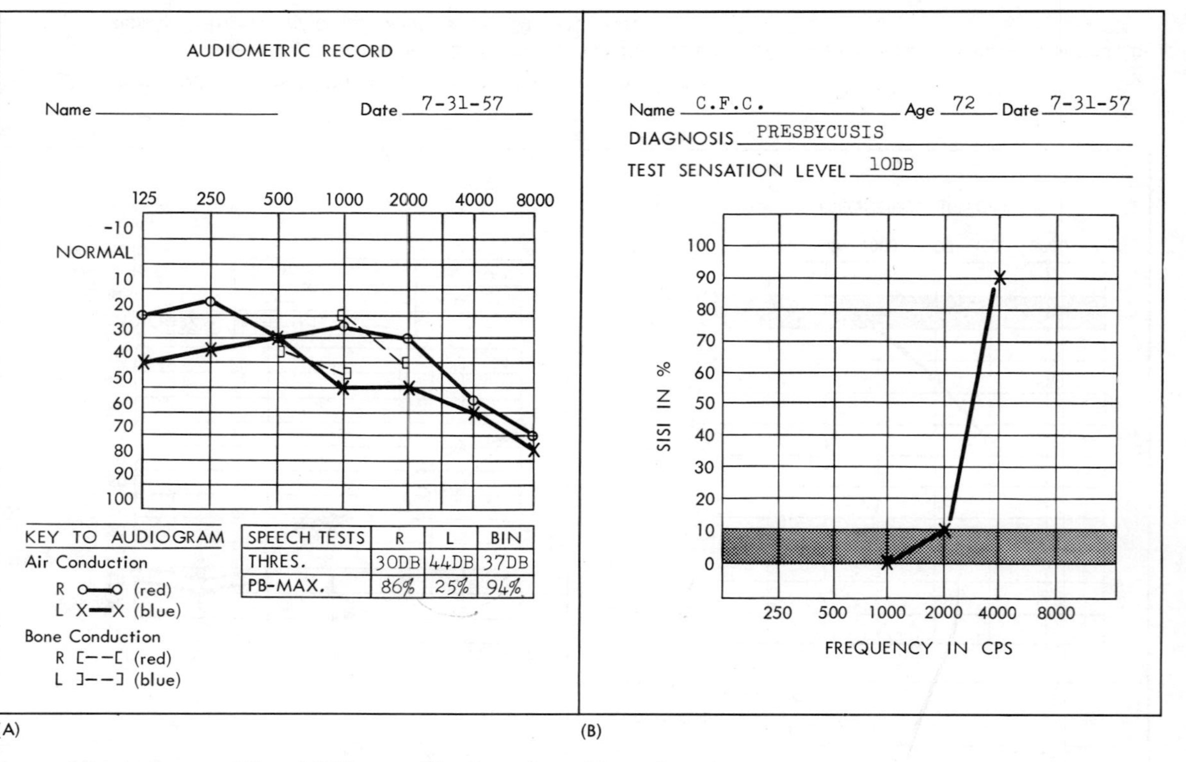

SPEECH TESTS	R	L	BIN
THRES.	30DB	44DB	37DB
PB-MAX.	86%	25%	94%

FIGURE 9.9 Audiogram (A) and SISI-gram (B) of a patient with presbycusis.

Source: Jerger, J., J. Shedd, and E. Harford, "On the detection of extremely small changes in sound intensity." *Archives of Otolaryngology*, **69**: 200–11, 1959.

A somewhat different result was obtained by Willeford (85), who administered Carhart's Tone Decay Test at eight frequencies to a group of eight subjects with presbycusis. His results are shown in Table 9.4. It may be noted that thirty-nine of the sixty-four responses were classified as showing abnormal adaptation, and that fourteen of the twenty-five normal responses were recorded at 250 and 500 Hz. His criterion standard for normal tone decay behavior was established on normal listeners. Both the incidence and magnitude of aberrant responses exceed the findings in the two previously cited studies. Once again, it would appear that the seemingly paradoxical results could be attributed to individual variations among aged persons as these results apply to degeneration at various levels of the auditory system. Another factor that may be responsible for differences encountered on the tone decay tests is the test itself. Many patients report that the stimulus loses its tonal characteristic and subjectively becomes more like a white noise. Others maintain that the stimulus waxes and wanes in intensity, which presents a problem when testing at near-threshold levels. Another criticism arises in instances where the test level reaches the output limits of the audiometer. It is not uncommon for a patient to indicate that the stimulus has faded to inaudibility, but when the stimulus is removed he realizes that it was still audible. While the latter criticism would not apply to the milder impairments found among presbycusics, it does emphasize one of the several questions that has arisen regarding tone decay tests.

Although a less sensitive measure, in the writer's opinion and experience, Bekesy-type audiometry by the procedures recommended by Jerger (48) is probably a more reliable measure of abnormal adaptation. At least the

TABLE 9.4. DISTRIBUTION OF THRESHOLD TONE DECAY RESPONSES FOR PRESBYCUSIC SUBJECTS (AFTER WILLEFORD, 1960)

	Sensation Level at Which Tone Remained Audible for One Minute											*Response Totals*	
Frequency	*0*	*5*	*10*	*15*	*20*	*25*	*30*	*35*	*40*	*45*	*50*	*Normal*	*Abnormal*
250	8											8	0
500	6	1	1									6	2
1,000	2	2	1	2	1							2	6
2,000		3	2		2[a]			1				3	5
3,000				3	1		1[b]	1	1	1		0	8
4,000			2	1	1	1	1[b]	1	1			2	6
6,000			2[c]	1[b]	1	1		2	1			2	6
8,000	1[b]	1[b]			1	2[a]	1	2				2	6
Totals	17	7	8	7	7	4	3	7	3	1		25	39

[a] *One of the two responses reached the limits of the equipment before adequate response was obtained.*

[b] *Reached limits of the equipment before adequate response was obtained.*

[c] *One normal response and one response which reached limits of the equipment without being sustained for a full minute.*

results are more in accord with expectations. Jerger studied a population of forty-six subjects with presbycusis and found that tracing patterns were widely distributed between the various types he recommended for classifying auditory disorders. Numerous reports on Bekesy-type audiometry have appeared since 1960, including a recent investigation by Harbert et al (44), but no author has examined presbycusic behaviour with this technique to the extent that Jerger reported in his original publication. Thus, his findings remain unchallenged and represent a paradigm of both measurement technique and response characteristics of abnormal adaptation in subjects with presbycusis. It seems safe to conclude that abnormal adaptation is minimal in this population, but it is also a quite variable phenomenon among individuals.

TINNITUS AND VERTIGO

The literature relating tinnitus and vertigo specifically to presbycusis is also very limited. Goetzinger et al. (40) make only cursory mention of these factors in their comprehensive study of presbycusis. In response to a questionnaire, twenty-one of their ninety subjects admitted experiencing periodic episodes of slight vertigo. Stevens and Davis (79, p. 352) state that mild, chronic tinnitus of high pitch is the usual finding in subjects of advancing age. However, they do not document the statement.

Weiss (83) has reviewed a small series of studies dealing with changes in vestibular functions as a result of aging. Evidence from these investigations suggests that: vertigo may increase with age, but it is not known if the vestibular mechanism is involved; that postrotary nystagmus is nearly always present in the seventh and eighth decades, but the duration and frequency of nystagmus and the number of beats appears to decrease gradually with age even though the subjective effect is longer; and that side effects such as nausea and headache also decrease. Caloric-induced nystagmus behavior from this review may be summarized as decreasing in incidence, magnitude, duration, and number of beats to cold stimulation, while latency increased. Similar trends were observed with heat stimulation. Most of Weiss' references are rather dated, which suggests that further study of these factors are in order.

Weston (84) has more recently examined the factors of tinnitus and vertigo in a population of 509 subjects with presbycusis. The results are summarized graphically in Figure 9.10. The data show a positive relationship between the incidence of tinnitus and vertigo and the severity of hearing loss. He reported that approximately 49 per cent had tinnitus, 32 per cent had vertigo, 20 per cent had both, and 38 per cent evidenced neither. Tinnitus without vertigo was found to occur more than twice as frequently as the reverse, and more frequently than both together. Sixty per cent of his cases, regardless of their history of tinnitus or vertigo, were found to have

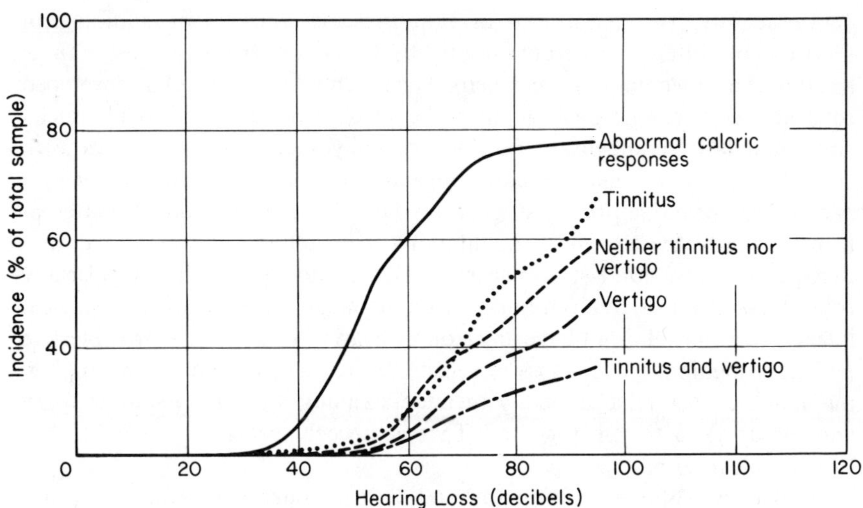

FIGURE 9.10 Relationship between degree of hearing loss and other labyrinthine disturbances.

Source: Weston, T. E. T. "Presbycusis: a clinical study." *Journal of Laryngology and Otology*, **March**: 276, 1964.

abnormal caloric responses. The incidence of such responses also increased as the hearing loss became greater, particularly in cases with bilateral canal paresis. For example, 23 per cent of his cases with hearing levels below 50 dB had abnormal caloric responses, while all subjects with impairments of over 70 dB had abnormal calorics. Weston concluded that, whatever the underlying process, the cochlea appears to be at a considerably greater risk than the vestibule.

A great deal of emphasis has been given to electronystagmography in recent years. As experience and data accumulate with this technique, our knowledge of geriatric vestibular function should increase both quantitatively and qualitatively. Detailed analysis of tinnitus characteristics among presbycusics should be easily available, but this remains to be well documented.

AUDIOLOGICAL DIAGNOSIS AND REHABILITATION

Since little can generally be done for the patient with presbycusis by either medical or surgical treatment, audiological rehabilitation becomes especially important. It is unfortunate, therefore, that many aged persons resist efforts to enroll them in programs that might be of benefit. The reasons for such resistance are numerous and complex because they are related to personality changes, to sociological factors, and to general states of health and well-being.

Frequently, the geriatric individual presents himself for audiological services only after considerable urging by family or friends, rather than as a result of his own desire to seek help. His hearing impairment has developed so insidiously that he has had to make gradual adjustments to his social environment to compensate for his gradually increasing difficulties with communication. He may be philosophical and accept his fate simply as a part of the inevitable process of growing old. However, he may also attempt to place the blame elsewhere, maintaining that he hears as well as ever and that people "just don't speak clearly." He has noted that this is especially true of women and children and will point out to experienced audiological interviewers that "I don't have any trouble hearing you." The more objective patient recognizes that his loss of sensitivity frequently is not handicapping, but that he does have difficulty in understanding speech—it sounds fuzzy and words seem to run together. That is, speech seems loud enough, but it is not clear to him.

A history obtained during the audiological interview is generally unremarkable for its well-established otological etiologies, but the older patient is inclined to elaborate at length on the more dramatic aspects of his medical history which may include a variety of unrelated health problems. The skillful interviewer will adroitly maneuver the discussion in such a way that he can "tease out" pertinent information from that which is superfluous, and he must do so within a reasonable time limit without creating the illusion that he is disinterested in the patient's recitation. Needless to say, rapport established in the interview will add immeasurably to the cooperation and confidence the clinician can inspire in the patient during subsequent planning and implementation of rehabilitation procedures.

Skillful maneuvering is also frequently necessary to avoid problems during the audiological examination. Precise and consistent patterns of patient response must be established if the clinician is to accomplish his goals before the patient tires and begins to exhibit a corresponding decline in response reliability. One example of the types of problems which confront the audiologist often occurs during speech audiometry where many older patients seem compelled to chat about the test items (or even to remind the examiner of some oblique item he forgot to relate during the history interview), rather than to simply respond with the stimulus words. Simple and explicit test instructions prior to the examination are most important for setting an exemplary model of performance. Finally, one must be alert to peculiarities in the patient's reaction time. This is a factor that varies widely among aged invividuals, but Birren (6, p. 111–32) reported that a tendency toward slowing of psychomotor speed is a distinguishing feature of aging. He believes this reduction in speed is most likely due to nerve cell loss, reduced neural excitability, and chemical change at synapse. However, he also feels that the reduction of activity in a given unit of time may also be affected by depressive moods as a primary or additive cause. Thus, the speed and pattern of stimulus presentations must be geared to a pace that is commensurate with the patient's abilities.

Counseling the patient following the examination is another matter of considerable importance. A simple explanation of the patient's audiogram and the implications of the combined audiological results can be very useful. It provides the patient with insight into his problem, reduces his anxiety by removing the mystery of the unknown, and provides him with a basic vocabulary with which to discuss his problem with others. Effective education of the patient is a good part of the battle. When he understands his problem and can verbalize it, he can begin to deal with it somewhat appropriately. This kind of educating is equally helpful to the patient's spouse and other members of the family. Their insight into the patient's auditory limitations can assist substantially in lightening his burden in the home and in supporting the audiologist's rehabilitation plan for him.

In recent years considerable literary attention has been given to the physical, psychological, and social changes that occur in the aging individual (6, 7, 8, 9, 13, 14, 29, 50, 86). Acquaintance with this kind of background literature can be most helpful to clinicians who deal with presbycusic populations.

The use of amplification is a rather controversial issue where the patient with presbycusis is concerned. Some professionals feel that the older patient simply cannot profit sufficiently from a hearing aid to justify the investment, particularly when the individual's speech discrimination ability is impaired. Part of this philosophy is based on the common knowledge that, as a rule, hearing aids may make speech louder but not necessarily clearer. Others, taking a more idealistic position, feel that the declining years should be made as pleasant as possible, regardless of cost, and that if the patient can adjust to amplification, an instrument should be provided. Basic considerations for both philosophies, or modifications of either, include: the patient's age and general state of health; a hearing level of appropriate magnitude to warrant amplification; the benefits obtained with, and the patient's adjustment to, an instrument; the individual's attitude and motivation—his acceptance of the limitations of amplification and a willingness to undergo a program of hearing-aid orientation and other auditory rehabilitation procedures; and the ability of the patient or his family to assume the financial investment.

The key to the successful use of amplification and participation in programs of hearing therapy is motivation, all other factors notwithstanding. Thus, the audiologist's skill at "salesmanship" and the family's supporting role can be an effective combination in overcoming the resistance of aged persons to rehabilitation.

Much of the discussion just presented may also be applied to speech-reading and auditory training programs. Once the patient is persuaded to engage in such activities, the instruction must be sufficiently stimulating and profitable to maintain his interest. Although limited vision (which would seriously restrict his speech-reading efficiency) and other physical ailments of a serious nature may necessarily preclude a patient's participation in rehabilitation regimes, excuses such as "I'm simply too old to learn" should not be accepted without a concerted effort on the part of the audiologist to change the patient's attitude. When he can, and the person does enroll for such instruction, many geriatric individuals become apt and enthusiastic students. Moreover, they extend their social boundaries through the establishment of interpersonal relationships with other elderly people having a common problem.

Studies by Kleemeier and Justiss (52); Grossman (42); Sherer (77); Coleman and Fine (21); Coleman (20); Gaitz and Warshaw (33); Alpiner (1); and others have explored various aspects of auditory rehabilitation in the aged. In all instances, the problem of motivation and general factors of personality are found to be unequivocably related to the degree of participation in, and benefits obtained from, rehabilitation procedures. Thus, the audiologist should be challenged to seek a better understanding of the geriatric personality and to extend greater effort toward rehabilitating this burgeoning population.

Birren (6, p. 223–51) states that due to the variety of theories and measurements, personality characteristics are difficult to define, but that, in general, certain distinctive patterns of behavior occur in later life which include: a reduction in drive levels; a reduction of spontaneous physical activity and sexual behavior; declining social activities and interpersonal relationships, many of which are socially induced by retirement; affective detachment (reduced ego energy); and relative fixation of habit systems so that behavior requiring novel adaptations become less frequent. These behavioral shifts, of course, represent an incomplete listing of psychological changes that occur with aging. Others are related to vocational and social levels achieved during one's life span, and all are undoubtedly modified by auditory impairment. Thus, the patient with presbycusis presents a fascinating challenge to professional workers concerned with auditory function because it is impossible to isolate and work with audition processes as an entity apart from the individual.

The population of senior citizens continues to increase in number, and the span of human life is steadily lengthening. A common corollary of these processes is a gradual diminution in auditory function. Consequently, there is a growing need for greater understanding of presbycusis and other geriatric phenomena. Understanding is essential if we are to deal effectively with the complex problems of the aged. The prospect of infirmity, with its accompanying structural and behavioral changes, is in store for most of us eventually. Therefore, the geriatric patient should be viewed in a framework that transcends a narrow clinical interest in impaired audition. It should be remembered that the aging individual resents his diminishing productivity and the increasing dependency on others that it brings. This process, even though it is an inevitable transition, can be retarded and substantially alleviated in many instances if auditory skills are maximized. Useful hearing can be an effective agent in restoring the geriatric patient's self-esteem.

Glossary

ETIOLOGY The study of the causes of diseases.

GERIATRICS The science of the diseases and the medical treatment of aged persons.

PHONEMIC REGRESSION Abnormally reduced speech discrimination skill in the presence of limited pure-tone impairment.

PRESBYCUSIS A defect of audition incident to advancing age.

Bibliography

1. Alpiner J. "Diagnostic and rehabilitative aspects of geriatric audiology." *ASHA*, **7**: 455–59, 1965.
2. American Industrial Hygiene Association. *Industrial Noise Manual.* 2nd ed. Detroit: American Industrial Hygiene Association, 1966.
3. American Standards Association. *American Standards Subcommittee X24-X2 Report: The Relations of Hearing Loss to Noise Exposure.* New York: American Standards Association, 1954.
4. Beasley, W. "Generalized age and sex trends in hearing loss." *Hearing Study Series Bulletin No.* 7. National Health Survey. Washington, D.C.: U.S. Public Health Service, 1938.
5. von Bekesy, G. "The Ear." *Scientific American*, Reprint 44: 1–12, 1957.
6. Birren, J. *The Psychology of Aging*. Englewood Cliffs, N.J.: Prentice-Hall, Inc., 1964.
7. Birren, J., ed. *Relations of Development and Aging*. Springfield, Ill.: Chas. C Thomas, Publisher, 1964.
8. Birren, J., ed. *Handbook of Aging and the Individual.* Chicago: University of Chicago Press, 1959.
9. Birren, J., H. Imus., and W. Windle, eds. *The Process of Aging in the Nervous System.* Springfield, Ill.: Chas. C Thomas, Publisher, 1959.
10. Bocca, E. "Clinical aspects of cortical deafness." *Laryngoscope*, Special Issue, 301–9, March, 1958.
11. Bocca, E. and C. Calearo. "Central hearing processes." In J. Jerger, ed., *Modern Developments in Audiology*. New York: Academic Press, Inc., 1963.
12. Boies, L. R., J. A. Hilger, and R. E. Priest. *Fundamentals of Otolaryngology.* Philadelphia: W. B. Saunders Co., 1964.

13. Bondareff, W. "Morphology of the Aging Nervous System." In J. Birren, ed., *Handbook of Aging and the Individual.* Springfield, Ill.: Chas. C Thomas, Publisher, 1959.
14. Braun, H. "Perceptual Processes." In J. Birren, ed., *Handbook of Aging and the Individual.* Springfield, Ill.: Chas. C Thomas, Publisher, 1959.
15. Brody, H. "Organization of cerebral cortex: III. A study of aging in the human cerebral cortex." *Journal of Comparative Neurology*, **102**: 511–56, 1955.
16. Bunch, C. "Age variations in auditory acuity." *Archives of Otolaryngology*, **9**: 625–36, 1929.
17. Bunch, C. "Further observations on age variations in auditory acuity." *Archives of Otolaryngology*, **13**: 170–80, 1931.
18. Carhart, R. "Clinical determination of abnormal auditory adaptation." *Archives of Otolaryngology*, **65**: 32–39, 1957.
19. Carhart, R. "Audiometry in diagnosis." *Laryngoscope*, Special Issue, **68**: 253–77, 1958.
20. Coleman, F., Jr. "Some attitudes of unsuccessful hearing aid users." *E.E.N.T. Digest*, **40**: 405–9, 1961.
21. Coleman, F., Jr. and A. Fine. "Some attitudes of successful hearing aid users. *E.E.N.T. Digest*, **38**: 1027–31, 1959.
22. Corso, J. "Age and sex differences in pure-tone thresholds." *Archives of Otolaryngology*, **77**: 385–405, 1963.
23. Corso, J. "Aging and auditory thresholds in men and women." *Archives of Environmental Health*, **6**: 350–56, 1963.
24. Crabbe, F. "Presbycusis." *Acta Oto-Laryngologica*, Supplement 183, 24–26, 1963.
25. Davis, H. "Hearing and deafness." In H. Davis and S. R. Silverman, eds., *Hearing and Deafness.* Rev. ed. New York: Holt, Rinehart & Winston, Inc., 1960.
26. Davis H. and F. Kranz. "The international standard reference zero for pure-tone audiometers and its relation to the evaluation of impairment of hearing." *Journal of Speech and Hearing Research*, **7**: 7–16, 1964.
27. Davis, H. and E. P. Fowler, Jr. "Hearing and deafness." In H. Davis and S. R. Silverman, eds., *Hearing and Deafness.* Rev. ed. New York: Holt, Rinehart & Winston, Inc., 1960.
28. Department of Health, Education, and Welfare, Vocational Rehabilitation Administration. *Information Service Series No.* 63–11. Washington, D.C.: 1963.
29. Eisdorfer, C. "Rorschach rigidity and sensory decretment in a senescent population." *Journal of Gerontology*, **15**: 188–90, 1960.
30. Farrior, J. B. "Stapes surgery in geriatrics. Surgery in the nerve-deaf otosclerotic." *Laryngoscope*, **73**: 1084–98, 1963.
31. Fowler, E. "The aging ear." *Archives of Otolaryngology*, **10**: 475–80, 1940.
32. Gaeth, J. "A study of phonemic regression associated with hearing loss." Unpublished doctoral dissertation. Evanston, Ill.: Northwestern University, 1948.
33. Gaitz, C. and H. Warshaw. "Obstacles encountered in correcting hearing loss in the elderly." *Geriatrics*, **19**: 83–86, 1964.
34. Glorig, A. *Noise and Your Ear.* New York: Greene and Stratton, 1958.

35. Glorig, A. and H. Davis. "Age, noise, and hearing loss." *Annals of Otology, Rhinology and Laryngology*, **70**: 556–71, 1961.
36. Glorig, A. and J. Roberts. "Hearing levels of adults by age and sex. United States 1960–1962." *Public Health Service Publication*, N.1000-series, 11-No.11. Washington, D.C.: 1965.
37. Glorig, A., D. Wheeler, R. Quiggle, W. Grings, and A. Summerfield. "1954 Wisconsin State Fair Hearing Survey." *Monograph, American Academy of Ophthalmology and Otolaryngology*, 1957.
38. Glorig, A., W. Grings, and A. Summerfield. "Hearing loss in industry." *Laryngoscope*, Special Issue, **68**: 447–65, 1958.
39. Goetzinger, C. and C. Rousey. "Hearing problems in later life." *Medical Times*, 771–80, (June, 1959).
40. Goetzinger, C., G. Proud, D. Dirks, and J. Embrey. "A study of hearing in advanced age." *Archives of Otolaryngology*, **73**: 662–74, 1961.
41. Goodhill, V. "Pathology, diagnosis, and therapy of deafness." In L. E. Travis, ed., *Handbook of Speech Pathology*. New York: Appleton-Century-Crofts, 1957.
42. Grossman, B. "Hard of hearing persons in a home for the aged." *Hearing News*, **23**: 11, 12, 17, 18, 20, 1955.
43. Hansen, C. and E. Reske-Nielsen. "Pathological studies in presbycusis." *Archives of Otolaryngology*, **82**: 115–32, 1965.
44. Harbert, F., I. Young, and H. Menduke. "Audiologic findings in presbycusis." *Journal of Auditory Research*, **6**: 297, 312, 1966.
45. Hinchcliffe, R. "The threshold of hearing as a function of age." *Acoustica*, **9**: 303–8, 1959.
46. Hinchcliffe, R. "The anatomical locus of presbycusis." *Journal of Speech and Hearing Disorders*, **27**: 301–10, 1962.
47. Hoople, G. "Diagnosis, presbycusis, and susceptibility." *Laryngoscope*, Special Issue, **68**: 477–86, 1958.
48. Jerger, J. "Bekesy Audiometry in analysis of auditory disorders." *Journal of Speech and Hearing Disorders*, **3**: 275–87, 1960.
49. Jerger, J., J. Shedd, and E. Harford. "On the detection of extremely small changes in sound intensity." *Archives of Otolaryngology*, **69**: 200–11, 1959.
50. Kastenbaum, R., ed. *Contributions to the Psychobiology of Aging*. New York: Springer Publishing Co., 1965.
51. Kirikae, I., R. Sato, and T. Shitara. "A study of hearing in advanced age." *Laryngoscope*, **74**: 2, 1964.
52. Kleemeier, R. W. and W. A. Justiss. "Program of the seventh annual meeting of the Gerontology Society." *Journal of Gerontology*, **9**: 479–80, 1954.
53. Klotz, R. and M. Kilbane. "Hearing in an aging population." *New England Journal of Medicine*, **266**: 277–80, 1962.
54. Klotz, P. "La surdité du troisième âge." *Readaption*, **102**: 27–31, 1963.
55. König, E. "Pitch discrimination and age." *Acta Oto-Laryngologica*, **48**: 475–89, 1957.
56. Luterman, D., O. Welsh, and J. Melrose. "Responses of aged males to time-altered speech stimuli." *Journal of Speech and Hearing Research*, **9**: 226–30, 1966.
57. Magladery, J. "Neurophysiology of aging." In J. Birren, ed., *Handbook of Aging and the Individual*. Chicago: University of Chicago Press, 1959.

58. Melrose, J., O. Welsh, and D. Luterman. "Auditory responses in selected elderly men." *Journal of Gerontology*, **18**: 267–70, 1963.
59. Metropolitan Life Insurance Company. *Statistical Bulletin*, **40**: October, 1959.
60. Metropolitan Life Insurance Company. *Statistical Bulletin*, **48**: February, 1967.
61. Miller, M. "Audiological rehabilitation of the geriatric patient." *Maico Audiological Library Series*, **2**: Report One, 1967.
62. Nixon, J., H. Glorig, and W. High. "Changes in air- and bone-conduction thresholds as a function of age." *Annals of Otology, Rhinology and Laryngology*, **74**: 288–98, 1962.
63. Olsen, I. "Discrimination of auditory information as related to aging." *Journal of Gerontology*, **20**: 394–97, 1965.
64. Pestalozza, G. and I. Shore. "Clinical evaluation of presbycusis on the basis of different tests of auditory function." *Laryngoscope*, **65**: 1136–63, 1955.
65. Politzer, A. *Diseases of the Ear*. Philadelphia: Lea & Febiger, 1926.
66. Rosen, S., M. Bergman, D. Plester, A. El-Mofty, and M. Satti. "Presbycusis study of a relatively noise-free population in the Sudan." *Annals of Otology, Rhinology and Laryngology*, **71**: 727–43, 1962.
67. Rosen, S., D. Plester, A. El-Mofty, and H. Rosen. "High frequency audiometry in presbycusis. A comparative study of the Mabaan tribe in the Sudan with urban populations." *Archives of Otolaryngology*, **79**: 18–32, 1964.
68. Rosenwasser, H. "Otitic problems in the aged." *Geriatrics*, **19**: 11–17, 1964.
69. Sataloff, J. *Hearing Loss*. Philadelphia: J. B. Lippincott Co., 1966.
70. Sataloff, J. and H. Menduke. "Presbycusis." *Archives of Otolaryngology*, **66**: 271–74, 1957.
71. Sataloff, J., L. Vassalo, and H. Menduke. "Presbycusis: Air- and bone-conduction thresholds." *Laryngoscope*, **75**: 889–901, 1965.
72. Schuknecht, H. "Perceptive hearing loss." *Laryngoscope*, Special Issue, **68**: 429–39, 1958.
73. Schuknecht, H. "Further observations on the pathology of presbycusis." *Archives of Otolaryngology*, **80**: 369–82, 1964.
74. Schuknecht, H. "Presbycusis." *Laryngoscope*, **65**: 402–19, 1955.
75. Schuknecht, H. and M. Igarashi. "Pathology of slowly progressive sensorineural deafness." *Transactions of the American Academy of Ophthalmology and Otolaryngology*, **68**: 222–42, 1964.
76. Schuknecht, H. and R. Woellner. "An experimental and clinical study of deafness from lesions of the cochlear nerve." *Journal of Laryngology and Otology*, **69**: 75–97, 1955.
77. Sherer, A. A. "Rehabilitation of the hard of hearing." *E.E.N.T. Digest*, **36**: 573–76, 1957.
78. Steinberg, J., B. Montgomery, and M. Gardner. "Results of the World's Fair Survey." *Journal of the Acoustical Society of America*, **12**: 291–301, 1940.
79. Stevens, S. and H. Davis. *Hearing: Its Psychology and Physiology*. New York: John Wiley & Sons, Inc., 1938.
80. Thompson, G. and R. Hoel. "Flat sensory-neural hearing loss and PB scores." *Journal of Speech and Hearing Disorders*, **27**: 284–85, 1962.
81. Tsai, Hsi-Kuel, Fong-Shyong Chou, and Tsa-Jung Cheng. "On changes in ear size with age, as found among Taiwanese-Formosans of Fukienese extraction." *Journal of the Formosan Medical Association*, **57**: 105–11, 1958.

82. Webster, J., M. Himes, and M. Lichtenstein. "San Diego County Fair Hearing Survey." *Journal of the Acoustical Society of America*, **22**: 473–83, 1950.
83. Weiss, A. "Sensory functions." In J. Birren, ed., *Handbook of Aging and the Individual.* Chicago: University of Chicago Press, 1959.
84. Weston, T. "Presbycusis—A clinic study." *Journal of Laryngology and Otology*, **78**: 273–86, 1964.
85. Willeford, J. "The association of abnormalities in auditory adaptation to other auditory phenomena." Unpublished doctoral dissertation. Evanston, Ill.: Northwestern University, 1960.
86. Zinberg, N. and I. Kaufman. *Normal Psychology of the Aging Process.* New York: International Universities Press, Inc., 1963.

10

Differential Audiology

Noel D. Matkin, Ph.D.
Wayne O. Olsen, Ph.D.

Differential Audiology

A number of existing audiological tests have been found to yield differential information on the function of an impaired auditory mechanism. To explain, the auditory behavior observed during certain audiological measurements can be of assistance in localizing the site of lesion underlying a hearing disorder since it appears that some of these measures are more sensitive than others to particular types of involvement. On this basis, various tests have been grouped to form test batteries. One such grouping, sometimes referred to as the *peripheral auditory test battery*, can be utilized to differentiate conductive from sensori-neural hearing impairments and may further help in localizing a sensori-neural loss to either the cochlea or to the eighth cranial nerve. Other tests have been evolved for the study of auditory deficits in the central auditory system. Still another battery of audiologic procedures is designed to detect nonorganic hearing disorders. While the profile of findings from these batteries may be of assistance when establishing a medical diagnosis, it must be kept in mind that differential auditory measures cannot be used to establish the disease process underlying an auditory disorder.

There is no uniform terminology within the field of audiology to label the area of testing described above. The type of audiological evaluation under consideration here is most aptly named, in our judgment, "differential audiology," since selected tests are considered to yield differential information as to site of lesion. From our point of view, such terms as "diagnostic audiometry" or "medical audiology" are not appropriate when one considers the current stage in the development of audiological measures as discussed in the following sections of this chapter. In other words, considering our present state of knowledge, a battery of auditory tests, in and by itself, will not yield information by which a hearing disorder can be attributed to any one specific etiology. In the same vein, selected tests may identify pseudohypocusis, but they cannot be expected to differentiate malingering from psychogenic hearing problems. Thus the findings from any audiological study must be viewed as contributory to the diagnostic workup deemed necessary by the managing physician in reaching his final diagnosis.

The intent of this chapter is to highlight the current status of differential audiology through a brief discussion of various special auditory tests and of the findings obtained from such measures in cases with various hearing disorders. Considering the breadth of our topic, it is not possible to describe in detail either the instrumentation or the specific procedures for the administration of the many audiological tests. Similarly, an in-depth discussion of the interpretation of the findings from each of the many differential measures is not feasible. However, an extensive bibliography is appended which will enable the interested reader to acquire good insight into the many facets of differential audiology.

Assessment of Conductive Hearing Impairment

One of the most common differential problems faced by the clinician is to determine whether the patient's auditory response indicates deficits in the conductive or the sensori-neural mechanism. As discussed in Chapter 6, which deals with pure-tone audiometry, the initial identification of a hearing loss as of the conductive or sensori-neural type is most commonly derived from a comparison of the listener's response to air-conducted and bone-conducted stimuli. Thus, routine pure-tone audiometry remains the basic clinical tool for initiating a differential audiological study.

Beyond a general classification of the hearing loss as conductive, the causal factor can also be inferred in some instances from a scrutiny of the bone-conduction configuration. It is widely recognized that an average depression of the bone-conduction responses of 5 dB at 500 Hz, 10 dB at

1,000 Hz, 15 dB at 2,000 Hz, and 5 dB at 4,000 Hz may result from mechanical factors rather than from actual sensori-neural involvement (2, 3). Specifically, such a bone configuration has come to be known as the "Carhart notch" and it may indicate possible stapes fixation (*see* Figure 10.1). Evidence supporting the fact that this so-called Carhart notch is mechanical in origin is found in data from postoperative audiometry following stapes surgery (36). In contrast to the bone-conduction response pattern associated with stapes fixation is the effect of fluid in the middle-ear cavity. Figure 10.2 illustrates the enhanced sensitivity to the lower test frequencies for pure tones presented via bone conduction. Again, this response pattern is mechanically induced due to changes in the middle ear since such a configuration is no longer observed when the condition of the middle ear returns to normal (5). From these two examples, it can be seen that a routine audiometric measure such as bone-conduction testing should be considered as a differential audiological tool. The most basic of the audiologist's tests may yield much important information which is, as yet, not fully appreciated or, in some instances, not even recognized.

The air-conduction audiogram may also convey information of importance to the final otologic diagnosis. As has been pointed out by Carhart (3), "... air-conduction curves are sufficiently typical in some types of hearing loss so that the audiometric pattern suggests a possible etiology to the

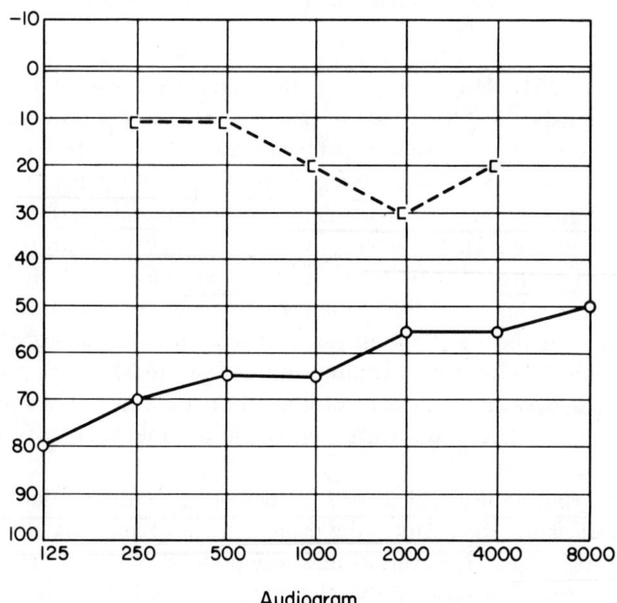

FIGURE 10.1 An audiogram for the right ear of a patient with otosclerosis. Note the configuration of the bone-conduction thresholds reflecting the "Carhart Notch."

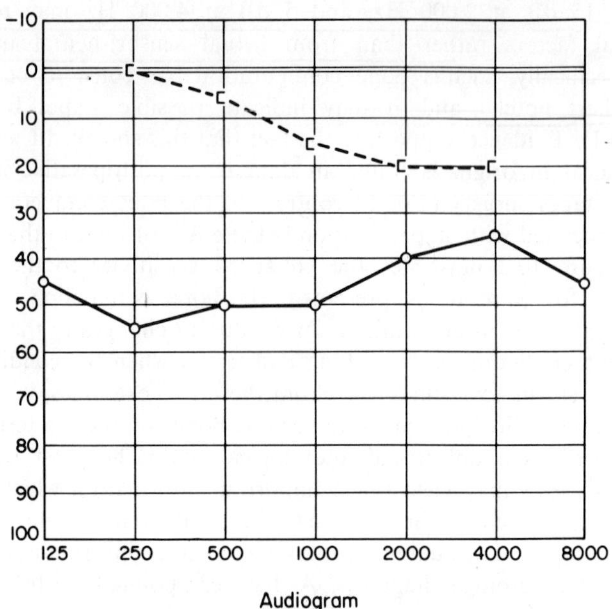

FIGURE 10.2 An audiogram for the right ear of a youngster having otitis media. Note the configuration of the bone-conduction thresholds reflecting better sensitivity for the low test frequencies.

clinician" (p. 254). However, two points must be stressed: First, as mentioned previously, the "diagnosis" of the auditory disorder is the responsibility of the physician, not the audiologist; thus, caution must be exercised when analyzing audiometric records. Second, a widely held generalization which has little validity in many instances is that sensori-neural hearing impairments result in high-frequency deficits, while conductive hearing losses are characterized by flat air-conduction curves. An analysis of clinical records quickly reveals that the differentiation of conductive and sensori-neural impairments on the basis of only the air-conduction audiogram is naive. Even though results from routine pure-tone audiometry may contain important clues beyond the usual consideration of the air to bone relationship, there are real dangers in overgeneralizing on the basis of such subtle indicators.

Another routine test which may further serve to differentiate conductive from sensori-neural disorders is the measurement of auditory discrimination for speech materials. However, as has been pointed out by Carhart (7), such variables as the difficulty of the test materials and the intensity level of presentation, as well as the site of dysfunction, determine in large part the score obtained for a given individual. As a generalization, persons with conductive hearing losses achieve higher scores on speech discrimination tests than do persons with sensori-neural deficits. However, many persons with sensori-neural hearing impairments have little difficulty in understanding speech in the quiet environment of the test chamber. Therefore, a high speech discrimination score (90 to 100 per cent) does not necessarily indicate a conductive hearing impairment. However, a score of 80 per cent or lower probably does suggest a sensori-neural involvement, provided that test materials of good quality are presented at sufficient intensity levels. Even though speech discrimination tests may be of some assistance for highlighting the presence of a sensori-neural deficit, the degree of such a loss cannot be predicted accurately on the basis of an auditory discrimination score for speech. The converse is also true, since one cannot anticipate with any degree of certainty the speech discrimination ability of a patient from his pure-tone audiogram.

Audiologists have recognized the importance of accurately establishing sensori-neural reserve when differentiating conductive from sensori-neural impairments, and yet have realized the problems in administering conventional bone-conduction tests. They have therefore developed alternate techniques for assessing the sensori-neural acuity level. These alternate techniques are discussed below and include the SAL test, brief-tone audiometry, the DL difference test, and acoustic impedance measurements.

In 1960, Jerger and Tillman published an article entitled "A New Method for the Clinical Determination of Sensori-neural Acuity Level (SAL)." The SAL technique they described as a substitute for bone-conduction audiometry was a modification of an approach reported by Rainville (33). Briefly, the methodology consists of delivering a masking noise via bone-conduction and establishing air-conduction thresholds in the presence of the noise stimulus. These masked air-conduction thresholds are then compared with the patient's air-conduction thresholds determined in quiet. The difference between these two sets of air-conduction thresholds is inversely proportional to the degree of sensori-neural involvement. In other words, a person with a conductive hearing loss will manifest a major shift with bone-conducted masking, while the effectiveness of the same masking signal is decreased when directed to the cochlea of an individual with a sensori-neural impairment. This approach elicited a good deal of interest in audiology and led to further research. Some of these investigations culminated in further modifications of the Rainville approach, and also suggested precautions which must be observed when employing this technique for the assessment of sensori-neural reserve. The major shortcoming of the SAL approach is related to the occlusion effect (40). Covering the external auditory meatus of a person with a normal middle-ear mechanism with a device such as an earphone enhances the signal level of the low-frequency components which reach the inner ear. This enhancement has been labeled the *occlusion effect*. This effect is not operative in patients with conductive hearing impairments. As a result, the sensori-neural acuity level for the conductive hearing loss case is underestimated with the SAL technique. This error occurs because an inequitable comparison is made. In the conductive patient, the occlusion effect is not operative, yet his response is compared to persons with normal hearing where the occlusion effect does play a role. Of course, it is in instances of middle-ear involvement that an accurate estimate of the status of the sensori-neural mechanism is most critical in the selection of candidates for middle-ear surgery. As a consequence, the SAL approach cannot be considered as a substitute for conventional bone-conduction testing. Instead, the SAL test should be considered as an alternate means for obtaining corroborative data from patients in whom the findings from bone-conduction audiometry are equivocal due to problems in masking and the like (40).

Another audiometric technique designed to determine the status of the sensori-neural mechanism is brief-tone audiometry as discussed by Miskolczy-Fodor (29). This approach takes advantage of the difference in thresholds obtained when the duration of the acoustic stimuli, either pure-tone or noise, is varied. It is well known that the auditory system integrates acoustic power over time, hence sensitivity for a stimulus of approximately 200 msec or longer is better than for signals of lesser durations. In other words, less intensity is required for a threshold response to a 200-msec tone than for one of perhaps 20 msec.

In the normal ear and the conductively impaired ear, the difference between thresholds for a 20 versus a 200 msec stimulus is approximately 8 dB. In sharp contrast, the listener with cochlear dysfunction shows a smaller difference in thresholds for stimuli differing in length by a factor of 10, i.e., 20/200 msec (34, 42). Thus, on the basis of a patient's response to brief tones, information may be gained as to whether a lesion exists in the middle ear or in the cochlea.

A third alternate technique for establishing sensori-neural acuity is the DL difference test as described by Jerger (20). In this procedure the difference limen for intensity at the octave test frequencies is established at two sensation levels, one near threshold and one at a higher sensation level. In the most recent work utilizing this technique, sensation levels of 10 and 40 dB were employed. In brief, normal or conductive listeners demonstrate a rather large difference in DL magnitude at these two sensation levels. Patients with known cochlear involvement, on the other hand, do not reflect such a large difference. In other words, their DL difference score is relatively small. In general, this procedure has not been adopted in clinical practice, even though findings from the DL difference test and from conventional bone-conduction audiometry were highly correlated, in that the smaller the difference scores, the more depressed was the bone-conduction threshold (20).

An entirely different approach for differentiating peripheral lesions is through acoustic impedance measurements of the impaired ear. This approach is feasible since it is known that only a portion of an air-conducted signal directed into the external auditory canal sets the tympanic membrane and the middle ear mechanism into vibration. A measureable amount of energy is reflected outward from the tympanic membrane due to the opposition (impedance) encountered by the sound wave in setting the conductive system into motion. The impedance of the middle ear mechanism is composed of such factors as friction (mechanical resistance), compliance (elasticity), and mass (inertia) (47). Commercial devices, called acoustic impedance bridges, have been developed for the measurement of this acoustic impedance of the ear at the eardrum.

The magnitude of the reflected energy measured with an acoustic impedance bridge is dependent upon the mobility of the middle-ear apparatus. Thus, intuitively, one would expect that the amount of the signal reflected at the eardrum would be abnormal in the presence of middle-ear pathologies. Research has shown that averaged data for samples of persons with various types of middle-ear lesions not only differ from each other but also from normals (11). In other words, on the average, different impedance values are obtained for persons with stapes fixation, as compared to individuals with ossicular chain interruption, while normals yield still different values. Unfortunately, the delineation among *individual* cases is not clear cut in that there is a great deal of variability in the absolute impedance values obtained for normals as well as for pathological cases. (1, 12, 41). Consequently, at present, measurements of absolute impedance are not widely undertaken in clinical settings.

Another type of impedance measurement, widely used in Europe, is referred to as the *relative* acoustic impedance method. With this technique, attention is focused upon the change in acoustic impedance that occurs upon eliciting a contraction of the middle-ear musculature. Unlike the absolute impedance method in which the quantification of impedance values is established, the relative impedance approach is directed toward detecting a change in the signal reflected from the eardrum due to the middle-ear reflex. In the normal ear, this reflex has been found to occur at sensation levels of 70 to 90 dB in the mid-test frequencies (17). It should be pointed out that this reflex can also be elicited by nonauditory stimuli such as electrical stimulation of the skin in the external auditory meatus, head movements, facial grimaces, air-jet stimulation of the orbital region of the eye, tactile stimulation of the ear, and caloric testing (17).

In general, the differentiation of a conductive from a cochlear lesion is made on the basis of the presence or absence of the acoustic reflex as observed from relative acoustic impedance testing. With many impairments of the middle-ear mechanism, the activity of the stapedius muscle cannot be demonstrated. Thus, the absence of the reflex to acoustic or nonacoustic stimulation is taken as one indication of a conductive impairment. Caution must be exercised in the interpretation of test findings, since dysfunction of the facial nerve, which innervates the stapedius muscle, may obliterate the reflex. In contrast to conductive hearing loss cases, the reflex is often obtained in patients with cochlear lesions at sensation levels less than 70 dB (17). Elicitation of this reflex at reduced sensation levels in such cases has been attributed to the abnormal growth of loudness (recruitment) frequently associated with lesions of the inner ear. Recent developments in commercial devices are stimulating renewed interest and research in relative impedance audiometry.

A variety of audiological approaches has been discussed for the differentiation of conductive and cochlear hearing disorders in the preceding section. These tests include conventional air- and bone-conduction audiometry, speech audiometry, the SAL technique, brief tone audiometry, the DL difference test, and aural acoustic impedance measurements. In the opinion of the writers, Tillman (40) has best summarized the present state of affairs in the following statement: "Recognizing the limitations of bone-conduction audiometry, an attempt must be made to develop more precise methods for quantifying sensori-neural acuity. In the meantime, however, one should continue to apply bone-conduction tests, following the best procedures available and utilizing all additional means at one's disposal ... to gain qualitative information which will aid in the interpretation of the results" (p. 220).

Sensory versus Neural Lesions

The problems of differentiating cochlear dysfunctions from eighth nerve lesions have received major emphasis during the past decade. In fact this area has been emphasized to the extent that some clinicians have limited their concept of differential audiology primarily to those tests that assist in localizing the deficit within the sensori-neural mechanism. Important as this aspect of differential audiology may be, it should receive no greater attention than other areas.

A large number of referrals for differential audiological evaluation consists of persons manifesting unilateral sensori-neural hearing loss. The primary reason that many such consultations are requested by the managing physician is that tests may assist in ruling out the presence of an eighth nerve tumor. While many referrals are made for this reason, it must be emphasized again that even the more sophisticated special auditory tests *cannot* determine the specific pathology underlying the disorder. Such tests may, however, highlight patterns of auditory behavior which have come to be associated with cochlear or neural involvement. Robertson (106) has discussed this issue with good insight.

Routine pure-tone and speech testing can yield valuable information on the site of lesion during the initial phase of the differential audiological study.

For example, a pure-tone configuration, which is often seen in cases with a medical diagnosis of Meniere's disease, is a unilateral hearing loss most pronounced in the low frequencies. In sharp contrast, patients with eighth nerve lesions frequently present a hearing impairment most evident in the high test frequencies in one ear. While such generalizations may describe a substantial number of cases falling into these two categories, there are numerous exceptions encountered with either a cochlear or a neural pathology (86).

In auditory discrimination for monosyllabic test words, there appears to be some differentiation of scores achieved by persons with cochlear involvements as compared to individuals with neural dysfunction. The general pattern appears to be best explained by the bottleneck principle (76). In other words, the most severe deficits in speech understanding are experienced by persons with eighth nerve pathology. This inability to discriminate speech far exceeds the difficulty that would be predicted on the basis of the pure-tone audiogram. In fact, it is not unusual for these patients to manifest great difficulty in repeating even spondaic words presented to the impaired ear. In contrast, it is rare for persons with cochlear involvements to exhibit deficits of this severity in auditory discrimination for speech, even though as a group their speech discrimination ability is not as good as the conductive hearing loss group. Again exceptions to the above generalization are encountered with some regularity (86, 88).

Recognition of the limitations of routine audiometric techniques as differential measures has led to the development of a more sophisticated battery of auditory tests.

LOUDNESS BALANCE TESTS

Historically, the father of differential audiology is Edmund Prince Fowler, Sr. (60, 61, 62). He first described the alternate binaural loudness balance (ABLB) test for the detection of abnormal loudness growth in a pathological ear. In this test, the task of the patient is to compare the loudness of a tone heard in his impaired ear to the loudness experienced when the same signal is alternately heard in his normal ear. Adjustments of the stimulus intensity presented to one ear are made until equal loudness is reported for the tone alternating between the two ears. Figure 10.3 illustrates a comparable loudness growth in both the normal and impaired ear, while Figure 10.4 indicates an abnormally rapid growth of loudness in the pathological ear. Specific recommendations for the administration and interpretation of this test have been given by Jerger (78).

A modification of Fowler's test was suggested by Reger (104) since the ABLB test cannot be appropriately administered to persons with bilateral hearing impairments. Reger's procedure is a monaural bi-frequency loudness balance (MBFLB) test during which the patient makes an equal loudness

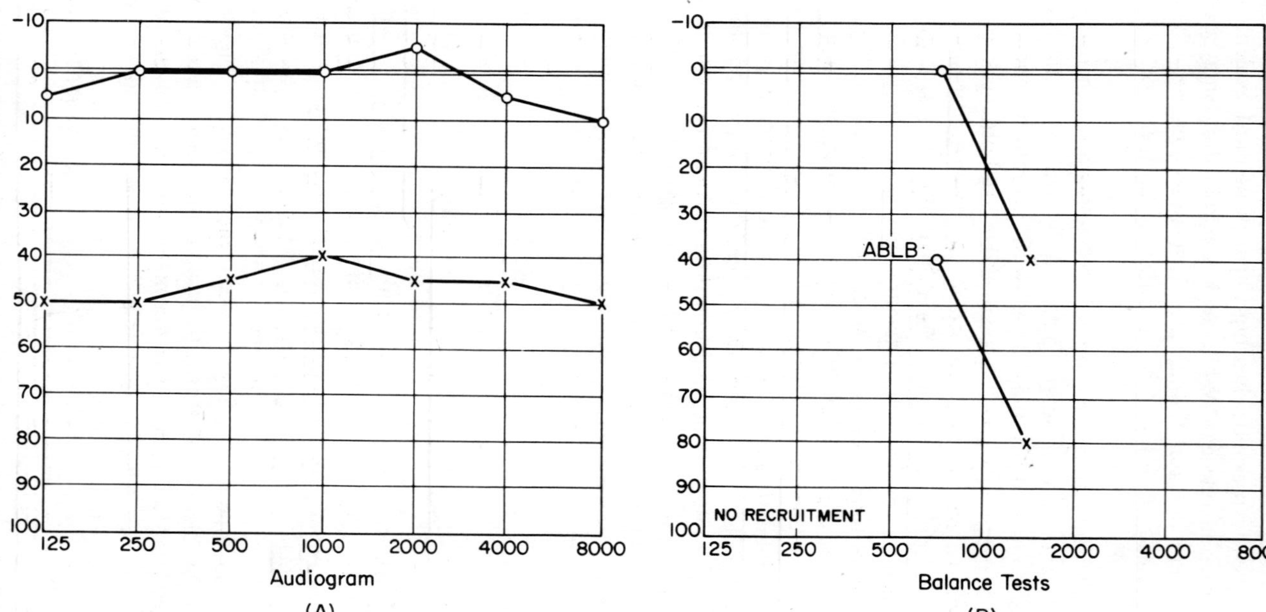

FIGURE 10.3 Air-conduction audiogram (A) and results from ABLB testing (B) indicating equivalent loudness growth in the two ears, i.e., no recruitment. Equal loudness is reported with a 40-dB SL signal in each ear.

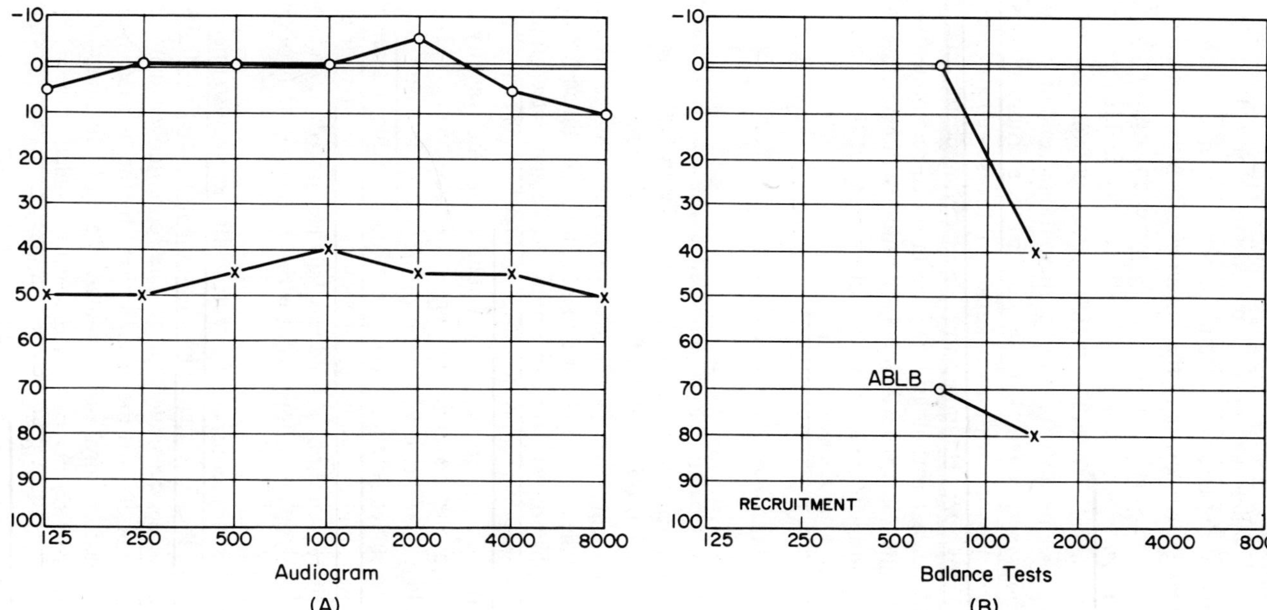

FIGURE 10.4 Air-conduction audiogram (A) and results from ABLB testing (B) indicating the presence of loudness recruitment, as reflected by unequal loudness growth in the two ears. Note that the patient reports equal loudness with a 40-dB SL signal in the left ear and a 70-dB tone in the right ear.

balance between two test frequencies in an ear having normal hearing at one or more frequencies. Thus, the loudness balance is made between two frequencies in the same ear, one for which hearing sensitivity is normal and the second for which hearing is impaired (*see* Figure 10.5). In many cases, at least one of these tests can be used to demonstrate whether or not abnormal loudness growth exists in the impaired ear. When an abnormally rapid growth of loudness is observed, the phenomenon is generally referred to as *loudness recruitment*. During the early years the loudness balance tests were used clinically to differentiate conductive from sensori-neural losses since it had been noted that cases with confirmed middle-ear involvement did not show recruitment. On the other hand, recruitment was often observed in many persons with a diagnosis of the so-called "perceptive hearing loss." Later Dix, Hallpike, and Hood (59) reported that it was the patient with cochlear pathology who demonstrated recruitment whereas their sample of individuals with eighth nerve tumors did not. As a result of this report, recruitment came to be viewed by many as the distinguishing feature of an ear with a cochlear lesion.

INTENSITY DL TESTS

Since the loudness balance tests described above could not be validly used in cases with hearing loss across all frequencies in both ears, research was initiated to develop other means for detecting the presence or absence of loudness recruitment. These investigations led to clinical tests for the measurement of the hearing-impaired patient's difference limen for intensity (58, 91). The supposition was that recruiting ears could detect abnormally small intensity changes at suprathreshold levels. However, the work of Hirsh, Palva, and Goodman (73) cast doubt upon the validity of this assumption. Subsequent research by Jerger and associates (82), which ultimately culminated in the development of the Short Increment Sensitivity Index (SISI) test, indicated that recruitment and a reduced intensity DL may represent two different auditory phenomena associated with cochlear damage. For this reason, both a loudness balance procedure and the SISI test are considered to be important tools for the differential study of auditory disorders.

Basically the SISI test consists of twenty 1-dB increments superimposed on a carrier tone of the same frequency at an intensity level of 20 dB above the threshold of the person under study. The score derived from this test reflects the percentage of 1-dB increments heard by the listener. Numerous reports in the literature have substantiated the early findings of Jerger, Shedd, and Harford (82) in that persons with cochlear lesions generally achieve a positive score on this test (70 to 100 per cent) at the higher test frequencies whether or not recruitment has been demonstrated during loudness balance testing (69, 98, 119, 122). In contrast, negative scores of 20 per cent

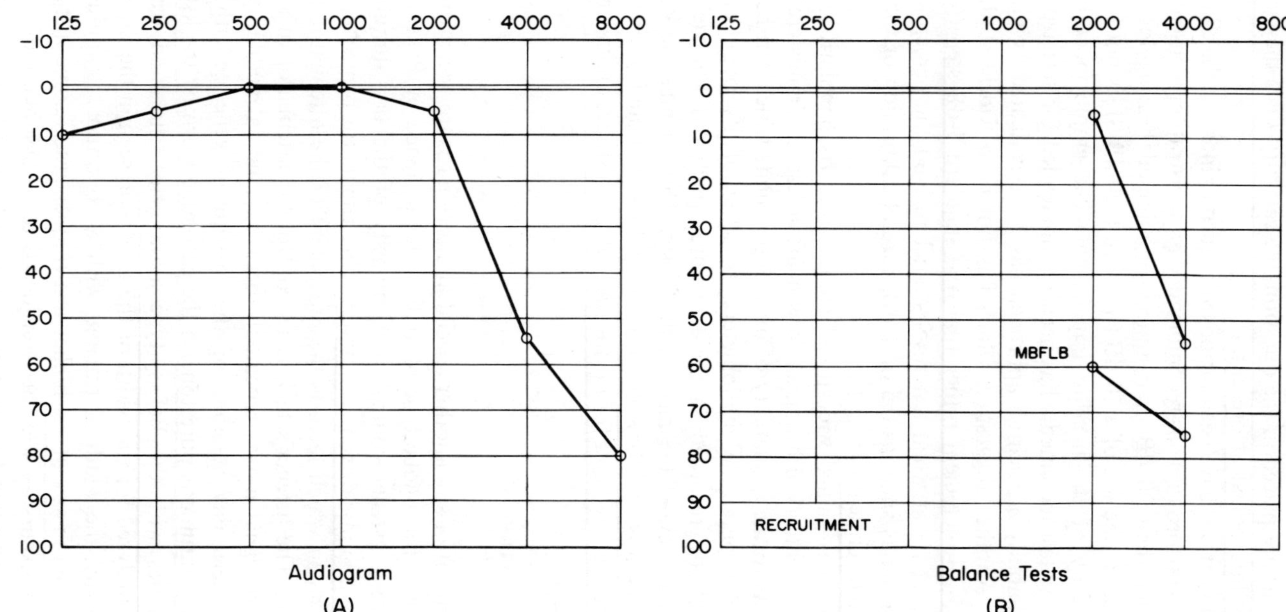

FIGURE 10.5 Air-conduction audiogram (A) and results from MBFLB (B) indicating the presence of recruitment. Note that 20-dB SL signal at 4,000 Hz and a 55-dB SL tone at 2,000 Hz were judged to be of equal loudness.

or less are often recorded for persons who subsequently are found through surgery to have eighth nerve lesions. Scores falling in the intermediate range (25 to 65 per cent) are placed in the questionable category since they cannot be meaningfully interpreted at present.

Several modifications have been proposed to further increase the efficiency of the SISI test. Harford (69) has recommended administration at a sensation level (SL) greater than 20 dB in instances of minimal hearing losses. In contrast, he suggests the use of a 10-dB SL when a 20-dB SL is not feasible due to the severity of the hearing impairment. The employment of ten rather than twenty test increments has been recommended for selected cases (69) and the reliability of such an approach has been evaluated by Griffing and Tuck (64). Another suggestion which has not been widely studied is to employ a 0.5-dB increment rather than the standard 1-dB step (67). It must be emphasized that when test results are based on the perception of intensity increments as small as 0.5 or 1 dB, careful calibration of the SISI apparatus becomes critical.

The SISI test has gained widespread clinical use. Its popularity is due in part to the straightforward manner in which the test is administered and scored, as well as to the availability of inexpensive units which can be used with conventional pure-tone audiometers. In spite of its popularity, a number of cases are recorded in the literature which did not yield the expected results in view of the medical diagnosis. Thus, it must be kept in mind that, as with any auditory measure, the SISI test should not be considered to be a perfect predictor for the location of the dysfunction underlying the hearing loss.

BEKESY AUDIOMETRY

The development of still another special auditory measure was prompted by the availability of a unique type of audiometer designed by Békésy (48). With this device a listener controls the intensity of the test stimulus by manually keying a motor-driven attenuator. This attenuator is mechanically linked to an ink pen which records the movement of the attenuator on an audiogram form. The listener's task is to control the attenuator in such a way that the test signal moves repeatedly between minimal audibility and inaudibility. Modern day versions of the instrument generate either an interrupted or a continuous pure tone in the earphone worn by the listener.

In early studies with the Bekesy-type audiometer, threshold tracings were primarily analyzed for the width of the excursion seen in the threshold tracing. Specifically, the width of tracings with a continuous stimulus was noted to be reduced in size at the higher test frequencies in some instances. This reduction in excursion size was considered to be a subtle indicator of a reduced difference limen for intensity. Consequently Bekesy audiometry was viewed as an indirect measure of recruitment. The reader may recall that it was during this early period that recruitment and a reduced DL size were considered to be a manifestation of the same phenomenon.

An entirely different observation was made by Reger and Kos (105) who described highly unusual auditory behavior during Bekesy audiometry in a patient later found to have an eighth nerve tumor. The individual exhibited pronounced threshold shift (auditory adaptation) while the examinee traced his threshold for a continuous tone. After further study, Lierle and Reger (89) suggested that the Bekesy threshold tracing may yield important differential audiological information.

Later observations by the research group at Northwestern University on patients with established medical diagnosis indicated that a fruitful approach for the interpretation of Bekesy audiograms was to make a comparison of threshold tracings obtained with interrupted and with continuous stimuli (77). On this basis, Bekesy audiograms were classified into four distinct types. After a correlation of the tracing patterns and the physician's otologic diagnosis was undertaken, the following generalizations were formulated:

A. Tracings were interwoven for both interrupted and continuous tones across the frequency range of 100 to 10,000 Hz for persons with pathologies of the middle ear. Such audiograms were arbitrarily labeled as Type I (*see* Figure 10.6).

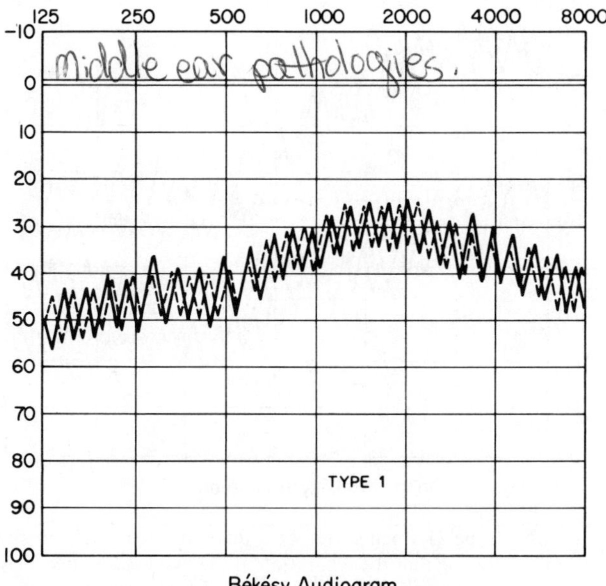

FIGURE 10.6 A Békésy audiogram reflecting interweaving tracings for the interrupted tone (dashed lines) and continuous tone (solid lines), i.e., Type I.

B. A Type II classification was assigned in those instances where the tracing for the continuous tone not only separated from the tracing for the interrupted tone but also showed a reduction of tracing amplitude above 1,000 Hz. The separation of the two did not exceed 20 dB with the continuous tone tracing always showing the greater loss (*see* Figure 10.7). These Type II audiograms were correlated with cochlear involvements.

C. The extreme adaptation to the continuous tone, first reported by Reger and Kos, was reflected in maximal separation of the two tracings and occurred even at the low test frequencies. This finding was seen in cases with subsequently confirmed eighth nerve tumors and was called a Type III audiogram (*see* Figure 10.8).

D. Another type of tracing was also encountered in some cases of eighth nerve lesion and was referred to as a Type IV Bekesy audiogram. Here the separation of the two tracings also occurred at the low test frequencies but the degree of adaptation was not pronounced since the continuous tone was perceived across the frequency range. However, the separation was greater than 20 dB and in this respect was differentiated from the Type II Bekesy audiogram (*see* Figure 10.9).

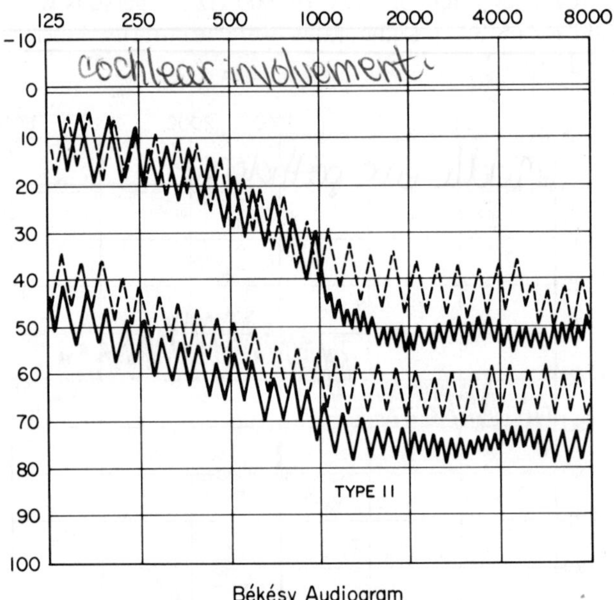

FIGURE 10.7 Type II tracings for two different ears. Note in the top tracing that the separation of the two tracings becomes very distinct above 1,000 Hz. The lower tracing is "atypical" in that the separation of the tracings occurs below 1,000 Hz and the narrowing of the continuous tracing occurs only for a segment of the higher test frequencies.

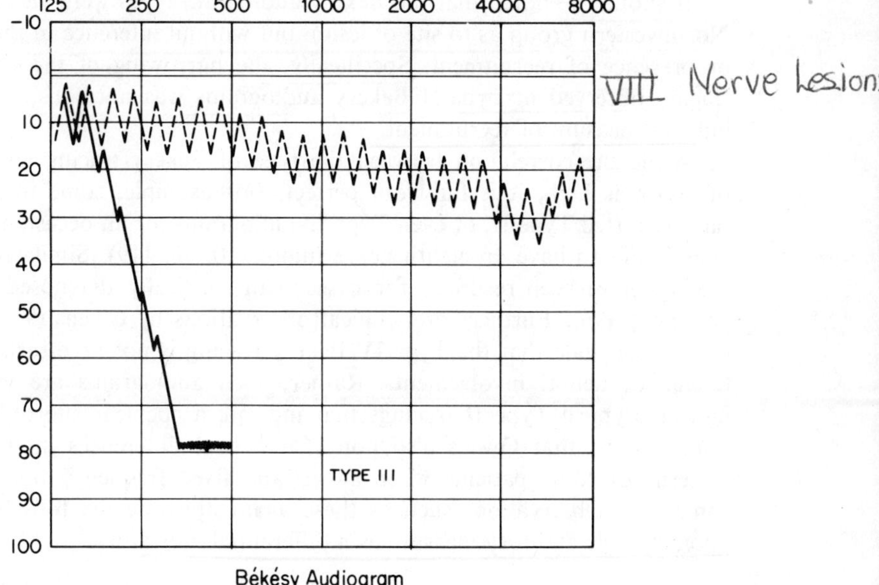

FIGURE 10.8 A Type III audiogram reflecting extreme adaptation in that the patient was unable to maintain perception of the continuous tone at the low test frequencies.

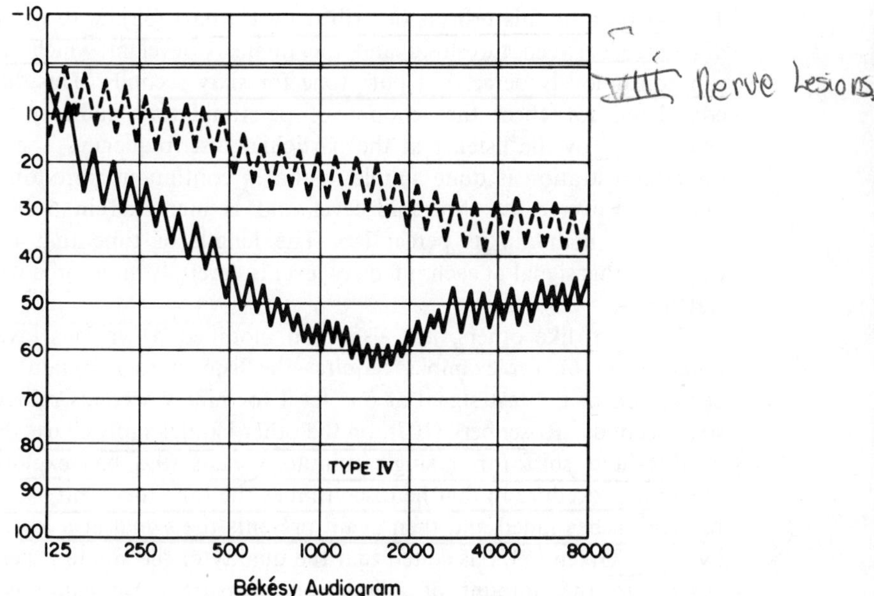

FIGURE 10.9 An audiogram classified as Type IV. Note the separation of the two tracings across frequency in excess of 20 dB.

It should be noted that the Bekesy audiogram types were viewed by the Northwestern group as to site of lesion but without inference to the absence or presence of recruitment. Specifically, the narrowing of the continuous tracing observed in Type II Bekesy audiograms was not considered as an indirect measure of recruitment.

While the correlation between the type of Bekesy tracing and the site of lesion is high, it is far from perfect. For example, some investigators have reported Type II, or even Type I, audiograms for an occasional person later found to have an eighth nerve tumor (50, 86, 119). Similarly, Type I tracings have been recorded for cases with medically diagnosed cochlear pathology (96). Furthermore, clinical observations by Owens (97) have led him to conclude that the Type IV Bekesy tracing is not necessarily characteristic of neural involvements. Rather, such audiograms are viewed by him as atypical Type II tracings that indicate a cochlear site of lesion. It is of interest that Owens also noted significant differences in the tracing patterns of some patients when sweep and fixed frequency tracings were compared. Observations such as these again illustrate the folly of relying upon a single auditory measure as a differential indicator.

THRESHOLD TONE DECAY TEST

A fourth differential auditory measure and one which requires only the use of a conventional pure-tone audiometer is the threshold tone decay test. The purpose of this test, as described by Carhart (52), is to determine the difference between threshold and the intensity level at which the patient can continuously perceive a pure tone for sixty seconds. This difference is considered to reflect the amount of perstimulatory auditory adaptation experienced by the listener at the particular test frequency. The procedure for administration is quite simple in that a continuous pure-tone signal is initially delivered at threshold level and is increased in 5-dB steps, as needed, to maintain its perception. The length of time that the patient perceives this signal at each intensity level is carefully monitored with a stopwatch.

This test, like others, has also been modified by various investigators. Sorenson (116), for example, requires the listener to maintain continuous perception of the test signal at one level for ninety seconds rather than for sixty seconds. Rosenberg (107), on the other hand, simply charts the amount of threshold shift for a single minute. Owens (99) has explored a still different procedure in that he discontinues the tone for twenty seconds after perception has faded and then again presents the signal at a level increased by 5 dB. Green (63) has stated that the quality of the stimulus perception is critical to the amount of adaptation measured. He cautions that the instructions to the listener should specify a response to tonal sensation rather than to the presence of just any type of sound.

Regardless of the procedure used, the aim of threshold tone decay testing remains the same, namely, to determine the amount of adaptation that occurs in the auditory system. With the procedure described by Carhart, tone decay of 30 dB or less is considered to reflect a cochlear lesion (119). In contrast, rapid adaptation in excess of 30 dB is most frequently encountered among patients with eighth nerve involvement. In fact, with an active eighth nerve pathology, it is not unusual to encounter such extreme tone decay that perception of the tone for the full sixty seconds is never maintained at any single intensity level even at the audiometer's maximum output. Simple as this test is, it is probably one of the most reliable differentiators between cochlear and neural pathologies (119).

PERIPHERAL AUDITORY TEST BATTERY

The four differential measures of auditory behavior which have been briefly discussed in the preceding section have come to constitute the standard battery of auditory tests used by numerous audiologists for isolating different peripheral sites of lesion. As has been pointed out, not one of these tests, be it the loudness balance procedures, the SISI test, Bekesy audiometry, or threshold tone decay testing, is infallible in pinpointing the site of lesion underlying the auditory abnormality under study. A perusal of various clinical studies suggests to these writers that any one of these tests may correctly localize the site of involvement in approximately 50 to 70 per cent of the cases reported. According to data of Tillman (119), it appears that Bekesy audiometry and tone decay testing are somewhat more sensitive to sensory versus neural lesions. However, there is good evidence that using a profile of results yielded by these four tests provides the investigator with a more accurate assessment of the various divisions in the auditory mechanism. That is to say, the probability of correctly identifying the site of lesion underlying a particular sensori-neural hearing disorder is greatly enhanced when the full array of test results is analyzed, rather than when one bases the audiological impression on the test finding from any particular special auditory measure.

A major problem in the interpretation of the results yielded by this peripheral auditory test battery occurs when an individual's profile of findings is equivocal. There clearly are instances in which some test results suggest a cochlear pathology while other test results for the same person indicate a neural lesion. However, there is the possibility that the patient's seemingly bizarre auditory behavior reflects a dual site of involvement. To date there has been no comprehensive study of such hearing-impaired individuals; therefore, a profile of contradictory test findings is poorly understood. Preliminary reports of patients with known dual sites of lesion (Meniere's patients with partial surgical section of the eighth nerve) have shown that an acute neural pathology may override cochlear test patterns, although a cochlear pattern may again predominate in some instances after an extended period of post surgical recovery (93).

Clearly, there is a need for detailed analysis of equivocal test results and their relationship to observations gleaned from postmortem temporal bone studies. Such studies would also make it feasible to test the following controversial hypothesis formulated by Carhart (51): "... there probably are lesions of the central auditory system which, when tested audiologically, mimic cochlear lesions in many respects and which, in consequence, are commonly misjudged to be peripheral hearing impairments" (p. 229). Carhart points out that positive SISI scores and a Type II Bekesy audiogram, as well as evidence of recruitment from loudness balance tests, that is, those findings which traditionally have come to be expected for an impairment of the inner ear, may also be seen in cases with a normal cochlea but with damage to lower brain stem structures. He bases this speculation primarily on test results obtained in young patients with hearing loss due to Rh incompatibility. Numerous histopathological studies have disclosed damage to the central auditory system in such cases, yet the special auditory test findings typify those seen in patients with known cochlear lesions (49, 92). Issues such as those discussed above clearly reveal the need for more research with the existing differential audiological tests as well as the need for further development of other auditory measures to facilitate neurological and otological diagnosis (53).

ADDITIONAL AUDITORY TESTS

Examples of other existing auditory procedures which have not been widely employed to assist in the differentiation of cochlear and neural hearing disorders are: brief-tone audiometry, acoustic impedance measures, and recordings of cochlear and neural electrical activity.

Reports by Miskolczy-Fodor (95) indicate that it may be possible to categorize the patient as having a cochlear or neural involvement through the comparison of results from brief-tone audiometry and from bone-conduction tests. Specifically, if air- and bone-conduction thresholds are equivalent while the difference between brief-tone thresholds for 20 and 200 msec stimuli is significantly less than 8 dB, the listener is considered to have an involvement of the inner ear. In the instance where the expected threshold shift (8 dB) for stimuli differing in duration by a factor of ten is seen, along with interweaving air- and bone-conduction curves, the lesion responsible for the hearing loss is thought to be neural in origin. In contrast, when an air bone gap exists this latter finding would be interpreted as confirmation of a conductive hearing loss. The validity of differentiating cochlear and neural lesions on the basis of brief-tone audiometry is open to question until a sufficient number of patients with cochlear dysfunction and with surgically confirmed eighth nerve lesions has been evaluated.

As was mentioned earlier, the significance of relative acoustic impedance measurements as a diagnostic indicator is being studied anew. The reader will recall that the acoustic reflex may be detected at sensation levels of less than 70 dB in instances of cochlear pathology. In contrast, it has been demonstrated that the reflex cannot be elicited at reduced sensation levels in the presence of a neural involvement. Thus, it has been suggested that relative impedance measure may represent an additional differential tool for locating the site of lesion in the peripheral auditory mechanism (94). However, the precautions mentioned earlier in conjunction with impedance audiometry as a differential tool must be kept in mind.

An entirely different experimental approach has been undertaken by Ruben (108, 109, 110). His technique involves the measurement and comparison of the electrical activity of the cochlea and the acoustic nerve. By surgically entering the middle ear and by placing electrodes on the round window, it is possible to measure the cochlear microphonic and the action potential of the peripheral auditory system. According to Ruben, the absence or reduction of the cochlear microphonic results from damage to the cochlea. In contrast, normal cochlear microphonics with aberrant neural activity, i.e., the absence of action potentials, are seen with eighth nerve damage (109, 111). Of course, such a procedure can only be initiated in a medical setting with the patient under some form of anesthesia. This technique has not gained widespread use since surgery is required. The subjection of human listeners to exploratory surgery for the recording of cochlear and eighth nerve potentials is open to criticism. However, recent work by Yoshie (123, 124) and by Sohmer (115) has demonstrated that it is possible to record eighth nerve potentials without surgery by placing pickup electrodes at the external ear. Again, little research is available on which to evaluate the merits of these procedures as additional differential tools.

The interest in recruitment tests laid the foundation for differential audiology. With the development of additional audiological tests, recruitment has come to be recognized as only one of several auditory phenomena which may be associated with a particular site of lesion. As a consequence the presence or absence of recruitment has been placed in its proper perspective, in that it is now considered as only one of several differential audiological findings of importance.

To be sure, different patterns of audiological test results emerge from the peripheral auditory test battery with different sites of lesion. While Bekesy audiometry, loudness balance measures, the SISI test, and threshold tone decay measurements constitute the battery of tests most widely employed, a number of additional techniques appear to offer promise in providing information as to the site of lesion underlying the hearing loss. Some of these techniques are relative acoustic impedance measure, brief-tone audiometry, and the recording of electrical activity from the cochlea and eighth cranial nerve. It is emphasized that the pattern of audiological test results, from a battery of measures rather than the findings from any single procedure, must be considered for differential purposes. Finally, it is apparent that a great deal of further exploration and research must be undertaken before test patterns are understood in the instance of a dual site of lesion. Similarly, the controversy of brain stem lesions "mimicking" cochlear pathology is yet to be resolved. Thus, it should be apparent that differential audiology, in and of itself, can only be considered as one source of important information upon which the final medical diagnosis of the auditory pathology can be made.

Detection of Central Auditory Disorders

The detection and description of central auditory lesions with differential techniques is still in the exploratory stage of development. There are a number of reasons why the study of central auditory disorders is largely an unexplored area, and these factors must be kept in mind when considering hearing tests for the study of central dysfunction. In the first place, few patients with central lesions are referred for audiological study. Consequently, most available research is based upon the evaluation of a relatively small sample of patients. Even in those cases whose auditory function has been assessed, the referring physician often has been unable to state the precise site and extent of the lesion in the central nervous system. Furthermore, the extreme neurological complexity of both the auditory tracts in the brain stem and the auditory centers in the cortical region would indicate that it is naive to expect a particular profile of test results when damage may occur at any one of many levels within the central auditory system.

As would be anticipated, lesions within the higher auditory system are difficult to detect. In fact, it is now recognized that many central auditory dysfunctions will not be demonstrated through the utilization of conventional audiological measurements (127). For this reason, a number of special auditory tests have been developed for evaluating patients with suspected lesions at the level of the brain stem and temporal cortex.

These patients, in the past, often have been categorized as cases of "central deafness." Such a label appears to be inappropriate since it has been demonstrated clearly that individuals with known lesions in the central auditory tracts do not manifest any significant hearing loss when tested by conventional pure-tone audiometry (127, 143). In fact, total removal of one hemisphere of the brain in human subjects has not resulted in any marked change of auditory sensitivity in either ear (131, 155).

Further, conventional speech audiometry for hemispherectomized patients has not shown any significant decrement in auditory understanding of speech in either ear (137, 138, 140).

Research by Jerger and Mier, on the other hand, reported differences in speech discrimination scores for PB–50 word lists of approximately 20 per cent between ears, with the poorer score obtained in the ear contralateral to the central auditory lesion (143). Interestingly, this difference was observed for patients with brain stem lesions as well as for persons with damage in the temporal lobe.

Observations with pure-tone and speech audiometry, such as those mentioned above, led to the formulation of the so-called "subtlety principle." This dictum states that the more central the lesion the more subtle is its manifestation (142). While lesions in the peripheral auditory mechanism may be detected with conventional auditory tests, a dysfunction of the central auditory system is quite elusive in its manifestation.

A possible exception to the preceding comment may be in the instance of a deficit at the level of the first auditory center in the brain stem, i.e., the cochlear nuclei. According to Carhart's postulation, such a lesion may in fact be exhibited through the use of both routine audiometry and the peripheral auditory test battery described in the previous section of this chapter (133, 134).

It is well known that the cochlear nuclei are quite unique in that they constitute the only way station in the central auditory system where one does not find a representation of neural coding from both ears (146). As a consequence, lesions at this level may be manifested in a far less subtle manner. At higher auditory levels, however, there is dual representation of both ears through numerous interconnections (136). Thus, a lesion above the cochlear nuclei or even a hemispherectomy does not prevent information presented to either ear from reaching one of the interpretive centers.

Despite the possible exception postulated by Carhart, the limitations of routine audiometry, as well as of the peripheral auditory test battery, in detecting central auditory damage is recognized.

Thus, a major thrust has been toward the development of tests that are sensitive to central lesions. One approach has used distorted speech stimuli. The rationale for such an approach is based upon the concept that a lesion within the central auditory system reduces the number of neural channels available for processing speech. Such a reduction in internal redundancy does not affect to any substantial degree the ability of the listener to understand speech of good fidelity. Bocca and Calearo (127) attribute this finding to the ability of the patient to compensate for a disturbance in the central auditory pathways by capitalizing upon the large number of redundant cues in speech stimuli. They theorize that by reducing the redundancy contained within a sample of speech, the presence of a central dysfunction may be highlighted. Consequently, a number of tests for the detection of central auditory disorders have utilized speech in which the redundancy has been reduced by distorting it in any number of ways, e.g., low-pass filtering, acceleration, low sensation level presentation, and periodic interruption[1] (126, 132, 147, 150).

The end result in such a reduction of speech redundancy is to increase the probability that even the normal listener may misinterpret some acoustic phonemes contained within the message. In contrast, it is expected that a lesion in the central auditory tracts will result in a significant increase in the number of errors made while decoding a distorted speech signal. The increased difficulty encountered by these latter subjects is probably due to a dual reduction in redundancy: that in the speech stimuli and in the number of intact central auditory tracts available for processing a message. Some writers have succinctly stated this premise in terms of a reduction of both external and internal redundancies. The reader is reminded that this discussion is based, in large part, on a theoretical construct which needs a great deal of additional study.

FILTERED SPEECH TESTS

The most widely studied technique for the detection of central auditory disorders has employed some form of filtered speech. For example, one test discussed by Jerger consists of speech test materials which have been low-pass filtered (below 500 Hz) (142, 143). These materials are presented monaurally at a sensation level of 40 dB. A second phase of this test is the monaural presentation of the same list of monosyllabic words without filtering at a very faint level (5-dB SL). Here it is readily apparent that the redundancy in the speech stimuli available to the listener has been reduced in two distinctly different ways. The anticipated result is that scores achieved on either test will be substantially poorer for the ear contralateral to the side of the lesion. (The reader will recall that the majority of the central auditory tracts for the right ear traverse the left side of the central system after leaving the cochlear nuclei. As a consequence, one would anticipate the result of a lesion in the left central auditory system to be reflected in the scores obtained on auditory tests presented to the right ear.) The efficiency of such testing was found to be increased by also assessing the listener's ability to centrally integrate information when the same test words with the two different redundancy reductions, as discussed above, were presented simultaneously. That is, low-pass filtered speech was fed to one ear and low sensation level unfiltered speech was delivered to the other ear. The normal listener takes advantage of both signals and, by synthesizing them, achieves

[1] Another technique used by Bocca was to increase the message length; however, it should be pointed out that such an approach does not appear to reduce the redundancy contained within speech but is a task which assesses a listener's auditory memory span.

a high score. In contrast, the patient with a central dysfunction achieves a similar score for both the monaural and binaural tasks due to a disruption of central processing (131, 141, 143). In other words, this test was designed to tax the central auditory system in two ways: the processing of redundancy reduced materials and the synthesis of two trains of neural events.

The test as described above has been useful in some instances; however, it has its inherent limitations. A critical variable is the accuracy with which threshold is determined, since in one phase of the testing the speech message is delivered at a sensation level of only 5 dB. An error in the estimated threshold will significantly affect the score achieved at such a low sensation level. A second and more serious limitation appears to be related to the fact that not all cases with auditory dysfunction in the central nervous system are highlighted with this approach, even though intuitively this test would appear to be very sound. Such an observation is not surprising when the extreme complexity of the neurological organization of the central auditory system is considered. Finally, as is the case with this test and others described below, it is the difference in test scores for the two ears which must be considered, since normative data are not available. In other words, the ear homolateral to the suspected lesion must serve as the reference.

A more recent application of filtered speech material with patients having a central nervous system lesion, as well as with persons having various peripheral hearing impairments, is reported by Tillman, Bucy, and Carhart (155). The impetus for this research was the report of Groen and Hellema (139), which suggested that binaural articulation functions for monosyllabic words among cases with CNS damage were equivalent to functions obtained with a monaural presentation. They interpreted this finding as reflecting an absence of binaural integration due to central damage, since their control group of normal listeners yielded steeper binaural articulation functions. Tillman and coworkers, however, found the performance of patients with CNS lesions to be quite similar to that recorded for the normal hearing and peripheral hearing loss groups. That is, articulation gain functions obtained for monaural presentations of low-pass and of high-pass filtered speech (monosyllabic words) were not equivalent to binaural slopes for any of their groups. These binaural functions were recorded when the same low-pass filtered and high-pass filtered words were presented to the two ears simultaneously. For all groups, the binaural articulation function was always steeper than either monaural slope. On the basis of these observations, the procedure in which binaural and monaural articulation functions are compared does not appear to be particularly sensitive to the presence of central auditory disorders.

Other investigators have also used filtered speech materials in tests for central lesions, and their approach has also been to deliver the same signal filtered in different ways to the two ears (147, 149). A breakdown on such test is thought to reflect disruption in the binaural integration ability of the listener, an auditory process that is thought to be mediated at the level of the brain stem (147).

With the exception of Italian investigators, little research has been reported on the alternate means of reduction in redundancy in the speech message through such ways as acceleration in the rate of the speech signal and interruption of the speech message. Consequently, there is little basis on which to evaluate the merit of these methods as tests for the detection of central auditory dysfunction. For further information regarding preliminary findings with such tests, the reader is referred to the discussion by Bocca and Calearo (127), and also Quiros (150).

COMPETING MESSAGE TESTS

Another promising method for the evaluation of central auditory disorders in which speech is presented to both ears is the competing message test (143). Here, a primary speech message (monosyllabic words) is presented to one ear while a secondary or competing message (sentences) is delivered simultaneously to the opposite side. Persons with normal auditory function can successfully attend to the primary message while ignoring the presence of the competing message. In like manner, persons with unilateral lesions at the level of the auditory cortex are not affected by the competing signal when it is delivered to the ear contralateral to the side of the lesion, and the primary message is heard in the other ear. However, when the signal presentations to the two ears are reversed, a marked breakdown in performance is observed. At present it is not certain what is to be expected with the competing message procedure in the instance of unilateral brain stem involvement. Returning to the data of Jerger, such subjects did not show any greater difference in scores for the two ears on competing message tasks than on conventional speech tests. Here again research with larger samples of persons having well documented lesions in either the brain stem or the auditory cortex is needed before a definitive interpretation of the findings from this test is possible.

Another manner in which competing signals are utilized is the staggered spondaic word test (SSW) described by Katz (145). With his technique a different bisyllabic word is presented to each ear. The timing of the presentation of these words is such that the second syllable of the word heard in one ear overlaps in time the first syllable of a different spondee presented in the opposite ear. According to Katz (145): "... this test appears to be both a practical and valid measure of central auditory dysfunction" (p. 144). In our opinion, the shortcomings of the SSW test in its present form that limit its immediate clinical application include the complicated method of scoring and the complex interpretation scheme. Here, too, sufficient investigation with patients having various types of central damage at known levels is lacking.

SPECIAL PURE-TONE MEASURES

Approaches using means other than speech stimuli for the detection of central lesions include the Alternate Binaural Loudness Balance (ABLB) test and the Simultaneous Binaural Median Plane Localization (SBMPL) test.[2] A comparison that has received little attention is the performance of a patient with suspected central auditory lesion on the ABLB and SBMPL tests. Jerger (141, 142), and more recently Davis and Goodman (135), have both reported cases for which an equal loudness experience at the two ears was achieved only with substantially greater stimulus intensity presented to the ear contralateral to the central lesion. This phenomenon has been referred to as decruitment and is suspected to reflect dysfunction at the cortical rather than at the brain stem level. In contrast, those patients who are unable to adjust the stimulus intensity of the signal delivered to one ear during the SBMPL test, so that an auditory image is perceived in the center of the head are suspected of having brain stem involvement (142). It has been theorized that equal loudness judgements are mediated at the cortical level, while the median plane localization task is subserved by an auditory mechanism at the subcortical level. At the present time, too little data are available for these writers to fairly evaluate the significance of such comparative testing to differentiate brain stem and cortical involvements.

Localization tasks which use stimuli other than pure tones, such as clicks or complex noise, have been reported by Walsh (156). In some instances, the signal has been presented via earphones with attention directed to interaural localization, since either the intensity or the time of arrival of the signal has been varied in the two earphones (147). Other investigators have presented similar sounds during sound-field listening conditions (152, 153). Although there is some suggestion that such tests may reflect aberrant auditory behavior in patients with central dysfunction, once again there is very limited information in current literature on the utility of these tests in a clinical setting.

From the preceding review, it is quite apparent that audiology has yet to develop definitive tests for the detection of central auditory lesions. The manifestation of these lesions is extremely subtle and consequently is not highlighted through the use of conventional pure-tone and speech audiometric measures. While distorted speech tests, as well as loudness balance and localization tasks, have been explored as differential tools, there is a lack of

2 In contrast to the alternate binaural loudness balance test, during which the signal is presented alternately to the two ears, the stimuli during the Simultaneous Binaural Median Plane Localization task are presented simultaneously in phase to the two ears. The intensity level of the signal is fixed in one ear and adjusted on the other ear until an intracranial median plane localization is reported. That is, the experience is one of hearing a single tone in the center of the head, not separate signals at the two ears.

research with patients having central auditory dysfunctions with confirmed lesions at a specific locus. Thus, this aspect of differential audiology must still be considered as being in its formative stage.

Detection of Nonorganic Hearing Problems (Pseudohypocusis)

The first difficulty encountered when discussing nonorganic hearing problems is the variety of terms used to describe this entity. For example, "pseudohypocusis," "nonorganic hearing loss," "functional hearing impairment," "hysterical deafness," "psychogenic hearing disorder," "simulated hearing problems," and "malingering" are some of the descriptive names that one finds in a review of the literature. In the following discussion "pseudohypocusis" is employed primarily, since it is a term which is descriptive and yet does not imply a categorization of the underlying causal factor. However, the term "nonorganic" is also used as a synonym. Some writers try to differentiate nonorganic hearing problems into psychogenic disorders or malingering. Implicit in such a differentiation is the assumption that some pseudohypocusics are individuals who willfully feign hearing impairment for monetary or other immediate gains (malingering), while the hearing loss may be based on subconscious motivational factors (psychogenic) in other instances. For an excellent review of the literature with specific emphasis on categorization and terminology, the reader is referred to Goldstein (185).

Regardless of the terminology used, it must be understood that the various special auditory tests for the detection of pseudohypocusis were never meant to identify causal factors. Although the clinician may believe that a particular patient is clearly a malingerer, it is not in the province of the audiologist to so label a patient. Such cases often involve medico-legal problems which are best handled by the referring physician. Thus, the audiologist's responsibility as a consultant is to detect the presence of pseudohypocusis and to estimate auditory thresholds on the basis of findings from selected hearing tests.

While the bulk of the literature dealing with pseudohypocusis is concerned with adults, the problem is also encountered among children. There is no firm estimate on the frequency of such problems among pediatric cases, yet there are ample reports of nonorganic hearing loss during childhood to forewarn astute clinicians of this possibility (157, 158, 204, 205). As was learned from the adult population in Veterans' Administration clinics, nonorganic hearing problems can easily go undetected unless the clinician is fully aware that pseudohypocusis does occur. This observation should serve as a warning to all clinicians, including those who work primarily with children.

Pseudohypocusis may take one of several forms. That is, the nonorganic loss may be either unilateral or bilateral. Furthermore, the degree of impairment reflected by various conventional auditory measures may range from mild to profound. Finally, some persons may have an organic hearing impairment upon which is superimposed a nonorganic component. Fournier (178) has referred to this latter group as "exaggerators." The particular auditory tests used to detect pseudohypocusis depend in part upon the type of loss observed during conventional pure-tone audiometry.

As is the case in all audiological evaluations, pure-tone audiometry serves as the point of departure for further audiological study. One of the first indications of the possible presence of pseudohypocusis is an inconsistent threshold response. Difficulty may be encountered in establishing reliable pure-tone thresholds using a conventional technique such as the one described by Carhart and Jerger (167). A suggestion made by Harris (192) in such cases is to plot an audiogram utilizing only ascending threshold explorations and then a second audiogram using the descending approach. If there is a marked discrepancy between the two audiograms, one has reason to suspect pseudohypocusis. Other subtle indications which should alert the tester are (1) a sensori-neural impairment with a saucer-shaped audiogram which may follow an equal loudness contour (166, 199), and (2) the absence of a shadow curve for either bone-conduction or air-conduction stimuli when masking has not been employed, even though a marked difference in thresholds was noted between the two ears.

Nonorganic hearing loss can be further confirmed by comparing the pure-tone average and the speech reception threshold (SRT). In the European literature this comparison is often called the "Carhart test" (178). It appears that at the same hearing level the loudness of a speech stimulus is substantially greater than that of a pure tone. As a consequence, the pseudohypocusic, who apparently bases his response on a loudness criterion, will repeat spondees at hearing levels substantially lower (better) than he voluntarily responded to tonal stimuli.

Having observed a marked discrepancy between the SRT and the pure-tone average, one can further substantiate the presence of a nonorganic impairment by using speech discrimination testing. One technique found particularly revealing by the present writers is to present lists of monosyllabic words at a level equivalent to the speech reception threshold, or even slightly lower. In contrast to the person with an organic hearing loss or to the normal listener who understands only a few words at these levels, the pseudohypocusic with encouragement often achieves a high score. This has been true for both adult subjects and children.

BEKESY AUDIOMETRY

An unexpected dividend from Bekesy audiometry has been the finding of another audiogram pattern which appears to characterize pseudohypocusis

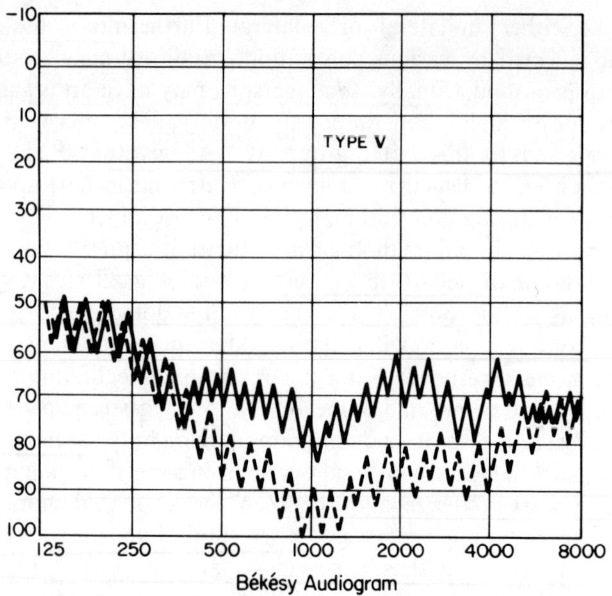

FIGURE 10.10 The Békésy audiogram for a patient later found to have essentially normal hearing. Note that tracing would suggest the presence of substantial hearing impairment; however, the fact that the interrupted tracing was poorer than the continuous tracing heightened the suspicion of pseudohypocusis. This audiogram was classified as Type V.

(198, 215, 218, 226). This particular type of Bekesy audiogram is labeled as a Type V tracing. Specifically, it has been noted that the tracings across frequency are unique in that the listener tracks his "threshold" at lesser intensity levels with the continuous tone than with the interrupted stimulus (*see* Figure 10.10). In all other categories of Bekesy audiograms, the continuous tracing is at the same or greater intensity levels than is the interrupted tracing.

One might speculate that the loudness experience at suprathreshold levels for a continuous tonal stimulus is greater than that for an interrupted signal at the same intensity. Hence, a Type V audiogram is recorded (194, 213, 218). Even though Bekesy audiometry may aid in the detection of pseudohypocusis, it must be emphasized that the individual's tracing for a continuous tone still does not represent a valid estimate of his actual hearing sensitivity.

SAL TEST

A report by Rintelmann and Harford (218) suggested that the SAL technique is not only useful for estimating sensori-neural reserve but also could be employed to aid in the identification of pseudohypocusis. These investigators noted in cases of nonorganic hearing impairment that the estimates of sensori-neural acuity by conventional bone-conduction audiometry and by the SAL technique were markedly discrepant. The SAL test indicates substantially less hearing loss. It would appear that the masking noise effectively disrupted the loudness criterion used by the listener as a gauge for his response to pure-tone stimuli. While the above findings suggest that the SAL method may be useful as another test for the detection of pseudohypocusis, these writers are unaware of any further reports on this application of SAL.

STENGER TEST

Unlike the preceding measures, the Stenger test is designed not only to detect pseudohypocusis but to estimate the auditory status in suspected *unilateral* nonorganic "hearing loss" (227). For this reason, it is one of the best techniques for evaluating pseudohypocusics. The basis for this test is the observation that a listener will perceive a diotic signal only in the ear in which it is loudest. The Stenger approach is administered by presenting the stimuli, which must be identical in both frequency and phase, simultaneously to the two ears. The level of the signal in the admittedly good ear is delivered at a low sensation level, while the tone of the "poor" ear is presented at a level below the threshold obtained during conventional audiometry. One of two responses should be anticipated: (1) if the tone is in fact not perceived in the "poor" ear, the patient will immediately respond to the low-level signal being simultaneously presented to the good ear and nonorganic causes can be ruled out, or (2) if the tone is in fact perceived in the "poor" ear, the patient will not respond since he will not admit to hearing a signal in that ear. He is unaware that the same stimulus is being presented at audible levels in his better ear. A lack of response under such test conditions is tantamount to admitting that the test signal is being heard in the "poor" ear. In the latter instance, one must suspect pseudohypocusis and try to estimate the actual threshold in the poorer ear by using the same technique.

To illustrate, assume that the thresholds obtained during routine testing show normal hearing (e.g., 10-dB HL) in the right ear and a moderate loss (e.g., 50-dB HL) in the left ear which is suspect. During the initial phase of the Stenger test, a signal of 20-dB HL, i.e., 10-dB SL, is fed to the better ear and simultaneously a tone identical in frequency and phase at 40-dB HL is delivered to the left ear. The listener fails to respond and thereby heightens the suspicion of a nonorganic involvement. An estimate of the threshold in the left ear is obtained by successively decreasing the signal to the poor ear in 5-dB steps until a response is obtained. At this point, perception of the stimulus is based on hearing in the good ear, and one would estimate that the actual threshold in the other ear is *approximated* by subtracting the sensation level for the good ear (10 dB) from the attenuator dial reading for the left ear.

A study by Peck (214) has disclosed that threshold could be predicted within 10 dB approximately 70 per cent of the time by utilizing the technique described above which was recommended by Fournier (178). Further, with thirty-five subjects the largest error in threshold prediction for the "impaired" ear was 20 dB. These data support the earlier comment that the Stenger test may serve as a technique for threshold estimation, as well as a test for detection of unilateral pseudohypocusis.

Another feature of this test which makes it appealing is the fact that speech, as well as pure tones, may serve as the test stimulus (228). Unlike some other measures in the nonorganic test battery, the Stenger test is virtually infallible. One possible exception is the case where the listener has diplacusis and feigns some degree of hearing loss in one ear, since he can detect the presence of a diotic tone which no longer sounds at the same pitch in the two ears. However, the speech Stenger test usually can be used with success even in these cases.

DELAYED AUDITORY FEEDBACK TESTS

Another way in which the audiologist can employ either speech or pure tones to aid in the identification of pseudohypocusis is the delayed auditory feedback approach (187, 188, 222, 223). A delay in the auditory feedback of speech disrupts the ability of a talker to self-monitor both the fluency and intensity of his verbal output, since one normally hears oneself without a perceptible lag. Thus, it becomes feasible to determine when a talker is aware of a delay in his auditory feedback by noting changes in his speech production.

To achieve the delay in auditory feedback, the subject's speech is picked up by a microphone and returned to his ears via earphones after an optimal delay of approximately 200 msec. The instrumentation necessary to effect such a lag is a tape recorder on which the record and playback modes can be activated simultaneously. In this way, the patient's speech is recorded on magnetic tape by the record head and almost immediately (200 msec later) is reproduced by the playback head whose output ultimately activates the earphones being worn by the patient. It should be noted that the delay comes about as a result of the physical separation between the two tape recorder heads. In other words, a particular segment of magnetic tape passes over the playback head 200 milliseconds after having passed over the record head. This is available on many commercial tape recorders.

When administering a delayed auditory feedback test, the patient with suspected pseudohypocusis is directed to read aloud a selected passage of printed material several times. In this way, the tester can determine what constitutes the individual's normal speech production according to rate, intensity, and fluency. The patient continues to read the same passage while the tester activates the delayed auditory feedback system whose intensity output is at levels less than admitted speech thresholds. In a unilateral hearing loss, the good ear must be masked during the test. With a bilateral impairment, the speech is fed to both ears. If an organic loss is present, the delayed signal will not alter his speech patterns while reading aloud. However, if the reader becomes nonfluent, increases the intensity of his vocalizations, or changes his reading rate, it is apparent that the delayed auditory feedback is being perceived. Again, the probable presence of pseudohypocusis must be investigated further.

Unfortunately, the tester cannot objectively quantify with ease subtle changes in the speech output which may occur. Furthermore, one cannot estimate with any degree of accuracy the patient's threshold levels for speech (191). Thus, this procedure can only be viewed as a method for detecting a nonorganic hearing disorder.

A recent modification of the delayed auditory feedback procedure uses pure tones and a key-tapping motor task (170, 171, 223). In this approach the listener is instructed to tap a particular pattern on a telegrapher's key. The tapping of the key activates an electronic apparatus which emits pure tones of short duration having the same temporal pattern as the tapping pattern. These pure-tone stimuli are fed to the ear of the subject first without delay, and then with a 200-msec delay. If the delayed feedback is audible, the subject's key tapping pattern becomes erratic, thus indicating auditory perception of the delayed signal.

In contrast to speech auditory feedback testing, it appears that the key-tapping approach with delayed pure-tone feedback not only serves as a test for uncovering nonorganicity but can also be used to estimate the actual threshold of hearing. Research indicates threshold estimates to be within approximately 5 dB of true auditory sensitivity (222).

DOERFLER-STEWART TEST

One of the earliest tests devised specifically for the detection of *bilateral* pseudohypocusis was the Doerfler-Stewart (D–S) test (175). With this method, an attempt is made to disrupt the loudness criterion set by the patient as the level for responding. In brief, this disruption is effected by introducing masking noise into the test situation while the listener is attempting to repeat spondaic words. Observations are recorded on the two SRT's in quiet, the level at which the masking noise interfered with the perception of spondaic words being presented at a 5-dB sensation level (NIL), and, finally, the intensity level at which the subject first acknowledges the awareness of the masking noise (NDT). The interpretation is rather complex in that it is based upon the relationship of the several findings.

Comparisons are made of: (1) SRT_1 versus SRT_2, (2) NDT versus SRT_1, and also versus SRT_2, and (3) SRT_1 plus 5 dB minus the noise interference level (NIL) and (4) NDT minus NIL. It is realistic to state that a difference greater than 5 dB between the two speech reception thresholds is suspect. However, it is not possible to set specific criteria for the interpretation of the three other comparisons, since the results obtained during the D–S test are dependent upon the specific type of noise stimulus used as the masker. The clinician should develop his own criteria for interpretation based upon the particular masking signal he plans to employ during clinical measurements.

While the Doerfler-Stewart test is one of the oldest measures in the audiologist's armamentarium, it may not be as sensitive to pseudohypocusis as was initially thought. In fact Ventry and Chaiklin (231, 232) have reported that with their particular sample of subjects taken from the Veterans' Administration population, the D–S measure was not as efficient in detecting nonorganic components as was the pure-tone average versus SRT comparison. Moreover, a significant number of patients with organic impairments also yielded positive results on this test.

LOMBARD TEST

An ancillary observation to any of the tests in which relatively intense masking signals are presented is the Lombard effect (194). This effect refers to the marked increase in the intensity of a subject's speech in the presence of noise. If the Lombard effect is elicited as "subliminal" masking intensity levels, one has subjective confirmation of nonorganic causes. Unfortunately, such observations are quite subjective and the sophisticated listener can often maintain a consistent vocal output even in the presence of intense noise.

IMPEDANCE AUDIOMETRY

Acoustic impedance measurements can also be used for the detection of pseudohypocusis in instances where voluntary responses to pure-tone stimuli are not obtained, or admitted thresholds suggest a profound hearing impairment. Obviously if acoustic reflexes are observed during impedance audiometry at hearing levels less intense than admitted thresholds, then a nonorganic component must be suspected. However, if acoustic reflexes are elicited at any sensation level relative to thresholds obtained during conventional audiometry, the examiner cannot make any interpretation on the presence or absence of nonorganic hearing impairment. Of course, the absence of acoustic reflex does not rule out pseudohypocusis in suspected cases either.

In other words, detection of pseudohypocusis with impedance audiometry is limited to those instances in which the acoustic reflex is elicited at hearing levels less intense than the admitted threshold, and even then the examiner cannot make any judgment as to actual threshold sensitivity.

ELECTROPHYSIOLOGICAL MEASUREMENTS

While it is apparent from the preceding discussion that a number of tests exist for the detection of nonorganic hearing loss, relatively few of the measures can establish precise auditory thresholds. For this reason, such electrophysiological techniques as electrodermal audiometry (EDA) and evoked response audiometry (ERA) play an important role in the assessment of the patient with a suspected nonorganic hearing involvement (184). EDA has sometimes been likened to a "lie detector" test and has been reportedly used with success in both civilian and Veterans' Administration hearing clinics. With this approach, the response consists of a change in the electrical resistance of the skin recorded from electrodes attached to an area rich in sweat glands, usually the pads of fingers. An audible tone is paired with a minimal electric shock which is usually delivered to the fingers of the other hand. Initially, the change in recorded skin resistance results from the presentation of the shock stimulus. However, after a number of paired presentations (tone-shock), conditioning occurs and electrodermal responses are then obtained for tone alone. Throughout the procedure, extinction of the responses to the pure-tone stimuli is prevented by periodically reintroducing pairs of tone-shock combinations.

The use of this technique with speech stimuli (spondaic words) has been discussed by Ruhm and Carhart (221). Here, the shock is paired with one "key" word. The electrodermal response is sought as this key word is presented within a group of various spondees. These stimuli are presented at various hearing levels until the speech threshold is established. Although there is some difficulty in objectively interpreting electrodermal response records, the skilled clinician can effectively estimate threshold with this technique.

A recent report by McCandless and Lentz (211) suggests that evoked response audiometry can also effectively obtain threshold information from cases with pseudohypocusis. Chapter 12 is devoted to a detailed discussion of this evoked response technique.

A number of tests which are useful for the identification of pseudohypocusis have been discussed. It should be quite apparent that the majority of such measures serve only to detect nonorganic hearing impairment. Only the Stenger test, delayed pure-tone feedback coupled with key-tapping, and the electrophysiologic measures (EDA and ERA) can be employed to approximate actual threshold sensitivity. Moreover, none of the auditory procedures discussed in this section can establish the basis for a nonorganic hearing disorder.

Differential audiology has been discussed by the different groups of auditory measures. Specifically, the various measures have been categorized as: (1) those tests most useful for differentiating conductive from sensori-neural hearing loss, (2) audiological procedures for localizing the site of lesion in sensori-neural deficits to either the cochlea or the eighth cranial nerve, (3) techniques for the detection of dysfunction in the central auditory nervous system, and (4) methods for the identification of pseudohypocusis. Throughout the various sections of this chapter, it has been repeatedly emphasized that it is necessary to employ a battery of audiological tests for the adequate assessment of the particular hearing disorder under study. Furthermore, overinterpretation on the basis of any single test has been discouraged. It has been pointed out that the auditory tests do not in any instance establish the causal factor underlying the hearing impairment. Rather, the profile of findings should be viewed as audiology's contribution to the differential diagnosis of hearing loss which must be based upon a multidisciplinary approach. Finally, while much progress has been made in the area of differential audiology for the study of auditory disorders, there is a good deal of ambiguity in the interpretation of test results. Such uncertainty suggests that much research is required before this phase of audiological testing can be considered as having reached any degree of maturity. 2-29-76

Bibliography

ASSESSMENT OF CONDUCTIVE HEARING IMPAIRMENT

1. Barry, S. J. "Some measurements of absolute aural acoustic impedance in normal hearing subjects." Unpublished Ph.D. Dissertation. Evanston, Ill.: Northwestern University, 1966.
2. Carhart, R. "Assessment of sensorineural response in otosclerotics." *Archives of Otolaryngology*, **71**: 141–49, 1960.
3. Carhart, R. "Audiometry in diagnosis." *Laryngoscope*, **68**: 253–77, 1958.
4. Carhart, R. "Audiometric manifestation of preclinical otosclerosis." *Annals of Otology, Rhinology and Laryngology*, **73**: 740–55, 1964.
5. Carhart, R. "Effects of stapes fixation on bone-conduction response." In H. Schuknecht, ed., *Otosclerosis*. Boston: Little, Brown and Company, 1962. Pp. 175–97.
6. Carhart, R. "Labyrinthine otosclerosis." *Archives of Otolaryngology*, **78**: 477–508, 1963.
7. Carhart, R. "Problems in the measurement of speech discrimination." *Archives of Otolaryngology*, **82**: 253–60, 1965.
8. Carhart, R. "The clinical application of bone-conduction audiometry." *Archives of Otolaryngology*, **51**: 798–807, 1950.
9. Dirks, D. "Factors related to bone-conduction reliability." *Archives of Otolaryngology*, **79**: 551–58, 1964.

10. Feldman, A. "Acoustic impedance measurement as a clinical procedure." *Journal of International Audiology*, **3**: 1–11, 1964.
11. Feldman, A. "Impedance measurements at the eardrum as an aid to diagnosis." *Journal of Speech and Hearing Research*, **6**: 315–27, 1963.
12. Feldman, A. S. "Acoustic impedance studies of the normal ear." *Journal of Speech and Hearing Research*, **10**: 165–76, 1967.
13. Feldman, A. and J. Zwislocki. "Effect of the acoustic reflex on the impedance at the eardrum." *Journal of Speech and Hearing Research*, **8**: 213–22, 1965.
14. Goldstein, D. P. and C. S. Hayes. "The occlusion effect in bone-conduction hearing." *Journal of Speech and Hearing Research*, **8**: 137–48, 1965.
15. Goldstein, D. P., C. S. Hayes, and J. L. Peterson. "A comparison of bone-conduction thresholds by conventional and Rainville methods." *Journal of Speech and Hearing Research*, **5**: 244–55, 1962.
16. Hood, J. D. "The principles and practice of bone-conduction audiometry." *Laryngoscope*, **70**: 1211–28, 1960.
17. Jepsen, O. "Middle-ear muscle reflexes in man." In J. Jerger, ed., *Modern Developments in Audiology*. New York: Academic Press, Inc., 1963. Pp. 193–239.
18. Jerger, J. F. "A new test for cochlear reserve in the selection of patients for fenestration surgery." *Annals of Otology, Rhinology and Laryngology*, **62**: 724–34, 1953.
19. Jerger, J. "A difference limen recruitment test and its diagnostic significance." *Laryngoscope*, **62**: 1316–32, 1952.
20. Jerger, J. "DL Difference Test." *Archives of Otolaryngology*, **57**: 490–500, 1953.
21. Jerger, J. and Susan Jerger. "Critical evaluation of SAL audiometry." *Journal of Speech and Hearing Research*, **8**: 103–28, 1965.
22. Jerger, J. and T. Tillman. "A new method for clinical determination of sensori-neural acuity level (SAL)." *Archives of Otolaryngology*, **71**: 948–55, 1960.
23. Keys, J. W. and B. Milburn. "The sensorineural acuity level (SAL) technique—an experiment with some observations." *Archives of Otolaryngology*, **73**: 710–16, 1961.
24. Kryter, K. D., C. Williams, and D. M. Green. "Auditory acuity and the perception of speech." *Journal of the Acoustical Society of America*, **34**: 1217–23, 1962.
25. Lightfoot, C. "The M-R test of bone-conduction hearing." *Laryngoscope*, **70**: 1552–59, 1960.
26. Lynn, G. E. and W. P. Pirkey. "Measurement of the sensorineural acuity level (SAL) in conductive hearing loss cases." *Journal of Auditory Research*, **2**: 323–26, 1962.
27. Martin, F. N. and H. A. T. Bailey, Jr. "Clinical comment on the sensorineural level (SAL) test." *Journal of Speech and Hearing Disorders*, **29**: 326–28, 1964.
28. Metz, O. "The acoustic impedance measured on normal and pathological ears." *Acta Oto-Laryngologica*, Supplement 63, 1946.
29. Miskolczy-Fodor, F. "The relation between hearing loss and recruitment and its practical employment in the determination of receptive hearing loss." *Acta Oto-Laryngologica*, **46**: 409–15, 1956.

30. Møller, A. "Intra-aural muscle contraction in man, examined by measuring acoustic impedance of the ear." *Laryngoscope*, **68**: 48–62, 1958.
31. Møller, A. "Bilateral contraction of the tympanic muscles in man, examined by measuring acoustic impedance change." *Annals of Otology, Rhinology and Laryngology*, **70**: 735–53, 1961.
32. Naunton, R. F. "The masking dilemma in bilateral conduction deafness." *Archives of Otolaryngology*, **72**: 753–57, 1962.
33. Rainville, M. J. "New method of masking for determination of bone-conduction curves." *Beltone Translation* No. 11, (1959). Translated from "Nouvelle méthode d' assourdissement pour le releve des courbes de conduction osseuse." *Journal France Otolaryngology*, **4**: 851–58, 1955.
34. Sanders, J. W. and E. A. Honig. "Brief-tone audiometry." *Archives of Otolaryngology*, **85**: 640–47, 1967.
35. Sanders, J. W. and W. F. Rintelmann. "Masking in audiometry—a clinical evaluation of three methods." *Archives of Otolaryngology*, **80**: 541–56, 1964.
36. Shambaugh, G. E., Jr. *Surgery of the Ear*. 2nd ed. Philadelphia: W. B. Saunders Co., 1967.
37. Studebaker, G. A. "On masking in bone-conduction testing." *Journal of Speech and Hearing Research*, **5**: 215–27, 1962.
38. Thompson, G. and R. Hoel. " 'Flat' sensorineural hearing loss and PB scores." *Journal of Speech and Hearing Disorders*, **27**: 284–85, 1962.
39. Tillman, T. W. "Clinical applicability of the SAL test." *Archives of Otolaryngology*, **78**: 20–32, 1963.
40. Tillman, T. W. "The assessment of sensorineural hearing acuity." In A. B. Graham, ed., *Sensorineural Hearing Processes and Disorders*. Boston: Little, Brown and Company, 1967. Pp. 211–21.
41. Tillman, T. W., P. J. Dallos, and T. Kuruvilla. "Reliability of measures obtained with the Zwislocki acoustic bridge." *Journal of the Acoustical Society of America*, **36**: 582–88, 1964.
42. Wright, H. N. "Clinical measurement of temporal auditory summation." *Journal of Speech and Hearing Research*, **11**: 109–27, 1968.
43. Zwislocki, J. "Acoustic measurement of the middle-ear function." *Annals of Otology, Rhinology and Laryngology*, **70**: 599–606, 1961.
44. Zwislocki, J. "An acoustic method for clinical examination of the ear." *Journal of Speech and Hearing Research*, **6**: 303–14, 1963.
45. Zwislocki, J. "Analysis of the middle ear function. Part I: Input impedance." *Journal of the Acoustical Society of America*, **34**: 1514–23, 1962.
46. Zwislocki, J. "Some impedance measurements on normal and pathological ears." *Journal of the Acoustical Society of America*, **29**: 1312–17, 1957.
47. Zwislocki, J. and A. Feldman. "Post-mortem acoustic impedance of human ears." *Journal of the Acoustical Society of America*, **35**: 104–07, 1963.

SENSORY VERSUS NEURAL LESIONS

48. Bekesy, George V. "A new audiometer." *Acta Oto-Laryngologica*, **35**: 411–22, 1947.
49. Blakeley, R. "Erythroblastosis and perceptive hearing loss: Responses of

athetoids to tests of cochlear function." *Journal of Speech and Hearing Research*, **2**: 5–15, 1959.

50. Brand, S. and P. Rosenberg. "Problems in auditory evaluation for neurosurgical diagnosis." *Journal of Speech and Hearing Disorders*, **28**: 355–61, 1963.
51. Carhart, R. "Audiologic tests: Questions and speculations." In F. McConnell and D. Ward, eds., *Proceedings of the Conference on Deafness in Childhood*. Nashville: Vanderbilt University Press, 1967. Pp. 229–51.
52. Carhart, R. "Clinical determination of abnormal auditory adaptation." *Archives of Otolaryngology*, **65**: 32–40, 1957.
53. Carhart, R. "Future horizons in audiological diagnosis." *Annals of Otology, Rhinology and Laryngology*, **77**: 706–16, 1968.
54. Carhart, R. "Labyrinthine otosclerosis." *Archives of Otolaryngology*, **78**: 477–89, 1963.
55. Carhart, R. "Probable mechanisms underlying kernicteric hearing loss." *Acta Oto-Laryngologica*, Supplement 221, 1–41, 1967.
56. Corso, J. and J. F. Wilson. "Additional variables on the Bekesy-type audiometer." *Archives of Otolaryngology*, **66**: 719–28, 1957.
57. Dallos, P. and T. Tillman. "The effects of parameter variations in audiometry in a patient with acoustic neurinoma." *Journal of Speech and Hearing Research*, **9**: 557–72, 1966.
58. Denes, P. and R. F. Naunton. "The clinical detection of auditory recruitment." *Journal of Laryngology*, **64**: 375–98, 1950.
59. Dix, M. R., C. S. Hallpike, and J. D. Hood. "Observations upon the loudness recruitment phenomenon with especial reference to the differential diagnosis of disorders of the internal ear and eighth nerve." *Journal of Laryngology and Otology*, **62**: 671–86, 1948.
60. Fowler, E. P. "A method for the early detection of otosclerosis: A study of sounds well above thresholds." *Archives of Otolaryngology*, **24**: 731–41, 1936.
61. Fowler, E. P. "Marked deafened areas in normal ears." *Archives of Otolaryngology*, **8**: 151–56, 1928.
62. Fowler, E. P. "Measuring the sensation of loudness." *Archives of Otolaryngology*, **26**: 514–21, 1937.
63. Green, D. S. "The modified tone decay test (MTDT) as a screening procedure for eighth nerve lesions." *Journal of Speech and Hearing Disorders*, **28**: 31–36, 1963.
64. Griffing, T. A. and G. A. Tuck. "Split-half reliability of the SISI." *Journal of Auditory Research*, **3**: 159–64, 1963.
65. Hallpike, C. S. and J. D. Hood. "Observations upon the neurological mechanism of loudness recruitment phenomenon." *Acta Oto-Laryngologica*, **50**: 472–86, 1959.
66. Hallpike, C. S. and J. D. Hood. "Some recent work on auditory adaptation and its relationship to the loudness recruitment phenomenon." *Journal of the Acoustical Society of America*, **23**: 270–74, 1951.
67. Hanley, C. N. and J. F. Utting. "An examination of the normal hearer's response to the SISI." *Journal of Speech and Hearing Disorders*, **30**: 58–65, 1965.
68. Harbert, F. and I. Young. "Threshold auditory adaptation measured by tone

decay test and Bekesy audiometry." *Annals of Otology, Rhinology and Laryngology*, **73**: 48–60, 1964.

69. Harford, E. R. "Clinical application and significance of the SISI test." In A. B. Graham, ed., *Sensorineural Hearing Progresses and Disorders*. Boston: Little, Brown and Co., 1967. Pp. 223–34.
70. Harris, J. D. "A brief critical review of loudness recruitment." *Psychology Bulletin*, **50**: 190–203, 1953.
71. Harris, J. D., H. L. Haines, and C. K. Myers. "Brief-tone audiometry." *Archives of Otolaryngology*, **67**: 699–713, 1958.
72. Harris, J. D., et al. "Loudness perception for pure tones and for speech." *Archives of Otolaryngology*, **55**: 107–34, 1952.
73. Hirsh, I. J., T. Palva, and A. Goodman. "Difference limen and recruitment." *Archives of Otolaryngology*, **60**: 525–40, 1954.
74. Hirsh, I. J. "Loudness and recruitment." In *The Measurement of Hearing*. New York: McGraw-Hill Book Company, 1952. Pp. 203–30.
75. Hopkinson, Norma. "Modifications of the four types of Bekesy audiograms." *Journal of Speech and Hearing Disorders*, **31**: 79–82, 1966.
76. Jerger, J. "Audiological manifestations of lesions in the auditory nervous system." *Laryngoscope*, **70**: 417–25, 1960.
77. Jerger, J. "Bekesy audiometry in the analysis of auditory disorders." *Journal of Speech and Hearing Research*, **3**: 275–87, 1960.
78. Jerger, J. "A difference limen recruitment test and its diagnostic significance." *Laryngoscope*, **62**: 1316–32, 1952.
79. Jerger, J. "Hearing tests in otologic diagnosis." *ASHA*, **4**: 139–45, 1962.
80. Jerger, J. and P. Bucy. "Audiologic findings in an unusual case of eighth nerve lesion." *Journal of Auditory Research*, **1**: 26–35, 1960.
81. Jerger, J., R. Carhart, and J. Lassman. "Clinical observations on excessive threshold adaptation." *Archives of Otolaryngology*, **68**: 617–23, 1958.
82. Jerger, J., J. L. Shedd, and E. Harford. "On the detection of extremely small changes in sound intensity." *Archives of Otolaryngology*, **69**: 200–11, 1959.
83. Jerger, J. "DL difference test." *Archives of Otolaryngology*, **57**: 490–501, 1953.
84. Jerger, J. "Recruitment and allied phenomena in differential diagnosis." *Journal of Auditory Research*, **1**: 145–51, 1960.
85. Jerger, J. and E. R. Harford. "Alternate and simultaneous binaural balancing of pure tones." *Journal of Speech and Hearing Research*, **3**: 15–30, 1960.
86. Johnson, E. W. "Auditory test results in 110 surgically confirmed retrocochlear lesions." *Journal of Speech and Hearing Disorders*, **30**: 307–17, 1965.
87. Johnson, E. W. and J. Sheehy. "Audiological aspects of the diagnosis of acoustic neuromas." *Journal of Neurosurgery*, **24**: 621–28, 1966.
88. Johnson, E. W. and W. P. House. "Auditory findings in fifty-three cases of acoustic neuromas." *Archives of Otolaryngology*, **80**: 667–77, 1964.
89. Lierle, D. M. and S. N. Reger. "Experimentally induced temporary threshold shifts in ears with impaired hearing." *Annals of Otology, Rhinology and Laryngology*, **64**: 263–77, 1955.
90. Lundborg, T. "Diagnostic problems concerning acoustic tumors: A study of 300 verified cases and the Bekesy audiogram in the differential diagnosis." *Acta Oto-Laryngologica*, Supplement 99, 1–111, 1951.

91. Luscher, E. and J. Zwislocki. "Comparison of the various methods employed in the determination of the recruitment phenomenon." *Journal of Laryngology*, **65**: 187–95, 1951.
92. Matkin, N. D. and R. Carhart. "Auditory profiles associated with Rh incompatibility." *Archives of Otolaryngology*, **84**: 502–13, 1966.
93. Matkin, N. D., W. R. Hodgson, R. Carhart, and T. W. Tillman. "Audiological manifestations of acute neural lesions in cases with Meniere's disease." *Journal of Speech and Hearing Disorders*, **30**: 370–75, 1965.
94. Metz, O. "Threshold of reflex contraction of muscles of middle ear and recruitment of loudness." *Archives of Otolaryngology*, **55**: 536–43, 1952.
95. Miskolczy-Fodor, F. "The relationship between hearing loss and recruitment and its practical employment in the determination of perceptive hearing loss." *Acta Oto-Laryngologica*, **46**: 409–15, 1956.
96. Owens, E. "Bekesy tracings and site of lesion." *Journal of Speech and Hearing Disorders*, **29**: 456–68, 1964.
97. Owens, E. "Bekesy tracings, tone decay, and recruitment." *Journal of Speech and Hearing Disorders*, **30**: 50–57, 1965.
98. Owens, E. "The SISI test and eighth nerve versus cochlear involvement." *Journal of Speech and Hearing Disorders*, **30**: 252–62, 1965.
99. Owens, E. "Tone decay in eighth nerve and cochlear lesions." *Journal of Speech and Hearing Disorders*, **29**: 14–22, 1964.
100. Pestalozza, G. and C. Cioce. "Measuring auditory adaptation." *Laryngoscope*, **72**: 240–61, 1962.
101. Price, L. "Threshold testing with Bekesy audiometer." *Journal of Speech and Hearing Research*, **6**: 64–69, 1963.
102. Price, L., D. C. Shepard, and R. Goldstein. "Abnormal Bekesy tracings in normal ears." *Journal of Speech and Hearing Disorders*, **30**: 139–44, 1965.
103. Reger, S. N. "A clinical and research version of the Bekesy audiometer." *Laryngoscope*, **62**: 1333–58, 1952.
104. Reger, S. N. "Differences in loudness response of the normal and hard-of-hearing ear at intensity levels slightly above the threshold." *Annals of Otology, Rhinology and Laryngology*, **45**: 1029–39, 1936.
105. Reger, S. N. and C. M. Kos. "Clinical measurements and implications of recruitment." *Annals of Otology, Rhinology and Laryngology*, **61**: 810–20, 1952.
106. Robertson, D. "Use of Bekesy findings in auditory diagnosis." *Journal of Speech and Hearing Disorders*, **30**: 367–68, 1965.
107. Rosenberg, P. E. "Rapid clinical measurements of tone decay." Presented at the convention of the American Speech and Hearing Association. November, 1958.
108. Ruben, R. J. "Cochlear potentials as a diagnostic test in deafness." In A. B. Graham, ed., *Sensorineural Hearing Processes and Disorders*. Boston: Little, Brown and Company, 1967. Pp. 313–37.
109. Ruben, R. J. "Physiological techniques in the differential diagnosis of non-conductive deafness." In *Report of the Proceedings of the International Congress on Education of the Deaf*, 1963. Pp. 368–77.
110. Ruben, R. J., J. E. Bordley, G. Nager, J. Sekula, G. G. Knickerlocker, and H. Fisch. "Human cochlear response to sound stimuli." *Annals of Otology, Rhinology and Laryngology*, **69**: 459–72, 1960.

111. Ruben, R. J., A. T. Lieberman, and J. E. Bordley. "Some observations on cochlear potentials and nerve action potentials of children." *Laryngoscope*, **72**: 545–54, 1962.
112. Sanders, J. W. and E. A. Honig. "Brief-tone audiometry." *Archives of Otolaryngology*, **85**: 640–47, 1967.
113. Shambaugh, G. "Team approach to early diagnosis and removal of acoustic neuromas." *Archives of Otolaryngology*, **83**: 570–73, 1966.
114. Simmons, R. B. and R. F. Dixon. "Clinical implications of loudness balancing." *Archives of Otolaryngology*, **83**: 449–53, 1966.
115. Sohmer, H. and M. Feinmesser. "Cochlear action potentials recorded from the external ear in man." *Annals of Otology, Rhinology and Laryngology*, **76**: 427–35, 1967.
116. Sorensen, H. "A threshold tone decay test." *Acta Oto-Laryngologica*, Supplement 158, 356–60, 1960.
117. Thompson, G. "A modified SISI technique for selected cases of suspected acoustic neurinoma." *Journal of Speech and Hearing Disorders*, **28**: 299–302, 1963.
118. Tillman, T. W. "Audiologic diagnosis of acoustic tumors." *Archives of Otolaryngology*, **83**: 574–81, 1966.
119. Tillman, T. W. "Special hearing tests in otoneurologic diagnosis." *Archives of Otolaryngology*, **89**: 51–56, 1969.
120. Yantis, P. A. "Clinical applications of the temporary threshold shift." *Archives of Otolaryngology*, **70**: 779–87, 1959.
121. Yantis, P. A. "Locus of the lesion in recruiting ears." *Archives of Otolaryngology*, **62**: 625–31, 1955.
122. Yantis, P. A. and R. L. Decker. "On the short increment sensitivity index (SISI Test)." *Journal of Speech and Hearing Disorders*, **29**: 231–46, 1964.
123. Yoshie, N. "Auditory nerve action potential responses to clicks in man." *Laryngoscope*, **78**: 198–215, 1968.
124. Yoshie, N., T. Ohashi, and T. Suzuki. "Nonsurgical recordings of auditory nerve action potentials in man." *Laryngoscope*, **77**: 76–85, 1967.

DETECTION OF CENTRAL AUDITORY DISORDERS

125. Bocca, E. "Binaural hearing: Another approach." *Laryngoscope*, **65**: 1164–71, 1955.
126. Bocca, E. "Clinical aspects of cortical deafness." *Laryngoscope*, **68**: 301–9, 1958.
127. Bocca, E. and C. Calearo. "Central hearing processes." In J. Jerger, ed., *Modern Developments in Audiology*. New York: Academic Press, Inc., 1963. Pp. 337–70.
128. Bocca, E., C. Calearo, and V. Cassinari. "A new method for testing hearing in temporal lobe tumors." *Acta Oto-Laryngologica*, **44**: 219–21, 1954.
129. Bocca, E., C. Calearo, V. Cassinari, and F. Migliavocca. "Testing 'cortical' hearing in temporal lobe tumors." *Acta Oto-Laryngologica*, **45**: 289–304, 1955.
130. Bunch, C. C. "Auditory acuity after removal of the entire right cerebral hemisphere." *Journal of the American Medical Association*, **90**: 2102, 1928.

131. Calearo, C. "Binaural summation in lesions of the temporal lobes." *Acta Oto-Laryngologica*, **47**: 392–95, 1957.
132. Calearo, C. and A. Lazzaroni. "Speech intelligibility in relation to speed of the message." *Laryngoscope*, **67**: 410–19, 1957.
133. Carhart, R. "Audiologic tests: Questions and speculations." In F. McConnell and D. Ward, eds., *Proceedings of the Conference on Deafness in Childhood.* Nashville: Vanderbilt University Press, 1967. Pp. 229–51.
134. Carhart, R. "Probable mechanisms underlying kernicteric hearing loss." *Acta Oto-Laryngologica*, Supplement 221, 1–41, 1967.
135. Davis, H. and A. C. Goodman. "Subtractive hearing loss, loudness recruitment, and decruitment." *Annals of Otology, Rhinology and Laryngology*, **75**: 87–94, 1966.
136. Galambos, R. "Neural Mechanisms in Audition." *Laryngoscope*, **68**: 378–401, 1958.
137. Goldstein, R. "Hearing and speech in follow-up of left hemispherectomy." *Journal of Speech and Hearing Disorders*, **26**: 126–29, 1961.
138. Goldstein, R., A. Goodman, and R. King. "Hearing and speech in infantile hemiplegia before and after left hemispherectomy." *Neurology*, **6**: 869–75, 1956.
139. Groen, J. J. and A. C. M. Hellema. "Binaural speech audiometry." *Acta Oto-Laryngologica*, **52**: 397–414, 1960.
140. Hodgson, W. R. "Audiological report of a patient with left hemispherectomy." *Journal of Speech and Hearing Disorders*, **32**: 39–45, 1967.
141. Jerger, J. "Audiological manifestations of lesions in the auditory nervous system." *Laryngoscope*, **70**: 417–25, 1960.
142. Jerger, J. "Observations in auditory behavior in lesions of the central auditory pathways." *Archives of Otolaryngology*, **71**: 797–806, 1960.
143. Jerger, J. "Auditory tests for disorders of the central auditory mechanism." In W. S. Fields and B. R. Alford, eds., *Neurological Aspects of Auditory and Vestibular Disorders.* Springfield: Charles C Thomas, Publisher, 1964. Pp. 77–86.
144. Jungert, S. "Auditory pathways in the brain stem." *Acta Oto-Laryngologica*, Supplement 138, 1958.
145. Katz, J. "The SSW test: An interim report." *Journal of Speech and Hearing Disorders*, **33**: 132–46, 1968.
146. Lorente de No., R. "Anatomy of the Eighth Nerve III—General Plan of Structure of the Primary Cochlear Nuclei." *Laryngoscope*, **43**: 327–50, 1933.
147. Matzker, J. "Two new methods for the assessment of central auditory function in cases of brain disease." *Annals of Otology, Rhinology and Laryngology*, **68**: 1185–96, 1959.
148. Neff, W. D. and I. T. Diamond. "The neural basis of auditory discrimination." In H. F. Harlow and C. N. Woolsey, eds., *Biological and Biochemical Basis of Behavior.* Madison: University of Wisconsin Press, 1958. Pp. 101–26.
149. Portman, N. and C. Portman. *Clinical Audiometry.* Trans. B. Proctor and S. Wevers. Springfield: Charles C Thomas, Publisher, 1961.
150. Quiros, J. B. "Accelerated speech audiometry." *Translations of Beltone Institute for Hearing Research*, **17**: 5–40, 1964.
151. Roberts, L. "The cerebral cortex and hearing." *Annals of Otology, Rhinology and Laryngology*, **69**: 830–46, 1960.

152. Sanchez Longo, L., F. Forster, and F. Auth. "A clinical test for sound localization and its applications." *Neurology*, **7**: 655–63, 1957.
153. Sanchez Longo, L. and F. Forster. "Clinical significance of impairment of sound localization." *Neurology*, **8**: 119–26, 1958.
154. Stein, L. "Auditory behavior in hemispherectomy and infantile spastic hemiplegia." Unpublished Ph.D. dissertation. Evanston, Ill.: Northwestern University, 1963.
155. Tillman, T. W., P. C. Bucy, and R. Carhart. "Monaural versus binaural discrimination for filtered CNC materials: The impaired auditory mechanism SAM-TR-66-64." July, 1966.
156. Walsh, E. G. "An investigation of sound localization in patients with neurological abnormalities." *Brain*, **80**: 222–50, 1957.

DETECTION OF NONORGANIC HEARING PROBLEMS (PSEUDOHYPOCUSIS)

157. Barr, B. "Nonorganic hearing loss in children." *Acta Oto-Laryngologica*, **52**: 337–46, 1960.
158. Berger, K. "Nonorganic hearing loss in children." *Laryngoscope*, **75**: 447–57, 1965.
159. Berk, R. L. and A. S. Feldman. "Functional hearing loss in children." *New England Journal of Medicine*, **259**: 214–16, 1958.
160. Blegvad, N. R. "Psychogenic deafness (emotional deafness)." *Acta Oto-Laryngologica*, **40**: 283–96, 1951.
161. Brockman, S. J. and Gloria H. Hoversten. "Pseudo neural hypoacusis in children." *Laryngoscope*, **70**: 825–39, 1960.
162. Butler, R. A. and F. T. Galloway. "Performances of normal-hearing and hard-of-hearing persons on the delayed feedback task." *Journal of Speech and Hearing Research*, **2**: 84–90, 1959.
163. Calearo, C. "Detection of malingering by periodically switched speech." *Laryngoscope*, **67**: 130–36, 1957.
164. Campanelli, P. A. "Simulated hearing losses in school children following identification audiometry." *Journal of Auditory Research*, **3**: 91–108, 1963.
165. Carhart, R. "The determination of hearing loss." *Audiology Information Bulletin*, Veterans' Administration. Washington, D.C.: U.S. Government Printing Office, 1960.
166. Carhart, R. "Tests for malingering." *Transactions of the American Academy of Ophthalmology and Otolaryngology*, **65**: 437, 1961.
167. Carhart, R. and J. Jerger. "Preferred method for clinical determination of pure-tone thresholds." *Journal of Speech and Hearing Disorders*, **24**: 330–45, 1959.
168. Chaiklin, J. B. and I. M. Ventry. "Functional hearing loss." In J. Jerger, ed., *Modern Developments in Audiology*. New York: Academic Press, Inc., 1963. Pp. 76–125.
169. Chaiklin, J. B., I. M. Ventry, L. S. Barrett, and Gretchen A. Skalbeck. "Pure-tone threshold patterns observed in functional hearing loss." *Laryngoscope*, **69**: 1165–79, 1959.

170. Chase, R. A., S. Harvey, Susan Standfast, Isabelle Rapin, and S. Sutton. "Comparison of the effects of delayed auditory feedback on speech and keytapping." *Science*, **129**: 903–4, 1959.
171. Chase, R. A., S. Sutton, E. P. Fowler, Jr., T. H. Fay, Jr., and H. B. Ruhm. "Low sensation level delayed clicks and keytapping." *Journal of Speech and Hearing Research*, **4**: 73–78, 1961.
172. Cohen, M., S. M. Cohen, M. Levine, R. Maisel, H. Ruhm, and R. M. Wolfe. "Interdisciplinary pilot study of nonorganic hearing loss." *Annals of Otology, Rhinology and Laryngology*, **72**: 67–82, 1963.
173. Dixon, R. F. and H. A. Newby. "Children with nonorganic hearing problems." *Archives of Otolaryngology*, **70**: 619–23, 1959.
174. Doerfler, L. G. "Psychogenic deafness and its detection." *Annals of Otology, Rhinology and Laryngology*, **60**: 1045–48, 1951.
175. Doerfler, L. and K. Stewart. "Malingering and psychogenic deafness." *Journal of Speech and Hearing Disorders*, **11**: 181–86, 1946.
176. Ewertsen, H. W. "Delayed speech test." *Acta Oto-Laryngologica*, **45**: 383–87, 1955.
177. Feldman, A. S. "Impedance measurements at the eardrum as an aid to diagnosis." *Journal of Speech and Hearing Research*, **6**: 315–27, 1963.
178. Fournier, J. E. "The detection of auditory malingering." *Translations of the Beltone Institute for Hearing Research*, No. 8. February, 1958.
179. Galloway, F. T. and R. A. Butler. "Conditioned eyelid response to tone as an objective test of hearing." *Journal of Speech and Hearing Disorders*, **21**: 47–55, 1956.
180. Getz, S. B. "A note on voice quality in emotional deafness." *Journal of Speech and Hearing Disorders*, **23**: 52–53, 1958.
181. Gibbons, E. W. and H. M. Boyd. "A delayed sidetone test to detect unilateral nonorganic deafness: Its clinical application." *Transactions of the American Academy of Ophthalmology and Otolaryngology*, **63**: 769–77, 1959.
182. Gibbons, E. W. and R. A. Winchester. "A delayed sidetone test for detecting uniaural functional deafness." *Archives of Otolaryngology*, **66**: 70–78, 1957.
183. Goldstein, R. "Effectiveness of conditioned electrodermal responses (EDR) in measuring pure-tone thresholds in cases of nonorganic hearing loss." *Laryngoscope*, **66**: 119–30, 1956.
184. Goldstein, R. "Electrophysiologic Audiometry." In J. Jerger, ed., *Modern Developments in Audiology*. New York: Academic Press, Inc., 1963. Pp. 167–92.
185. Goldstein, R. "Pseudohypocusis." *Journal of Speech and Hearing Disorders*, **31**: 341–52, 1966.
186. Graham, J. T. "Evaluation of methods for predicting speech reception threshold." *Archives of Otolaryngology*, **72**: 347–50, 1960.
187. Hanley, C. N. and W. R. Tiffany. "Auditory malingering and psychogenic deafness: Comments on new test and some case reports." *Archives of Otolaryngology*, **60**: 197–201, 1954.
188. Hanley, C. N. and W. R. Tiffany. "An investigation into the use of electromechanically delayed side tone in auditory testing." *Journal of Speech and Hearing Disorders*, **19**: 367–74, 1954.
189. Hanley, C. N., W. R. Tiffany, and Jacqueline M. Brungard. "Skin resistance

changes accompanying the sidetone test for auditory malingering." *Journal of Speech and Hearing Research*, **1**: 286–93, 1958.

190. Hardy, W. G. "Special techniques for the diagnosis and treatment of psychogenic deafness." *Annals of Otology, Rhinology and Laryngology*, **57**: 65–95, 1948.
191. Harford, E. R. and J. F. Jerger. "Effect of loudness recruitment on delayed speech feedback." *Journal of Speech and Hearing Research*, **2**: 361–68, 1959.
192. Harris, D. A. "A rapid and simple technique for the detection of nonorganic hearing loss." *Archives of Otolaryngology*, **68**: 758–60, 1958.
193. Hattler, K. W. "The Type V Bekesy pattern: The effects of loudness memory." *Journal of Speech and Hearing Research*, **11**: 567–74, 1968.
194. Heller, M. F. and P. Lindenberg. "Evaluation of deafness of nonorganic origin." *Archives of Otolaryngology*, **58**: 575–81, 1953.
195. Hood, J. D. "Modern masking techniques and their application to the diagnosis of functional deafness." *Journal of Laryngology and Otology*, **73**: 536–43, 1959.
196. Hood, W. H., R. A. Campbell, and C. L. Hutton. "An evaluation of the Bekesy ascending descending gap." *Journal of Speech and Hearing Research*, **7**: 123–32, 1964.
197. Jepsen, O. "Intratympanic muscle reflexes in psychogenic deafness (impedance measurements)." *Acta Oto-Laryngologica*, Supplement 109, 61–69, 1953.
198. Jerger, J. and G. Herer. "Unexpected dividend in Bekesy audiometry." *Journal of Speech and Hearing Disorders*, **26**: 390–91, 1961.
199. Johnson, K. O., W. P. Work, and G. McCoy. "Functional deafness." *Annals of Otology, Rhinology and Laryngology*, **65**: 154–70, 1956.
200. Juers, A. L. "Pure-tone threshold and hearing for speech—diagnostic significance of inconsistencies." *Laryngoscope*, **66**: 402–09, 1956.
201. Klotz, R. E., A. W. Koch, and T. P. Hackett. "Psychogenic hearing loss in children." *Annals of Otology, Rhinology and Laryngology*, **69**: 199–205, 1960.
202. Lamb, L. E. and J. L. Peterson. "Middle-ear muscle reflex measurements in pseudohypoacusis." *Journal of Speech and Hearing Disorders*, **32**: 46–50, 1967.
203. Larr, A. L. and B. V. Leamer. "Problems in the identification of nonorganic hearing loss." *Annals of Otology, Rhinology and Laryngology*, **66**: 182–86, 1957.
204. Lehrer, Nancy D., S. Hirschenfang, M. H. Miller, and Shokri Radpour. "Nonorganic hearing problems in adolescents." *Laryngoscope*, **74**: 64–69, 1964.
205. Leshin, G. J. "Childhood nonorganic hearing loss." *Journal of Speech and Hearing Disorders*, **25**: 290–92, 1960.
206. Lewis, A. N. and V. Sipr. "A simplified instrument for pure-tone delayed auditory feedback." *Journal of Speech and Hearing Research*, **10**: 93–98, 1967.
207. Livingood, W. C. "Extraauditory hypoacusis." *Annals of Otology, Rhinology and Laryngology*, **73**: 72–81, 1964.
208. Marean, C. E., Sr. "The nonorganic component as manifested in predominantly unilateral aural impairment." *Journal of Auditory Research*, **3**: 241–47, 1963.

209. Martin, F. N. and R. R. Hawkins. "A modification of the Doerfler-Stewart test for the detection of nonorganic hearing loss." *Journal of Auditory Research*, **3**: 147–50, 1963.
210. Martin, N. A. "Psychogenic deafness." *Annals of Otology, Rhinology and Laryngology*, **55**: 81–89, 1946.
211. McCandless, G. A. and W. E. Lentz. "Evoked response audiometry in non-organic hearing loss." *Archives of Otolaryngology*, **87**: 123–28, 1968.
212. Melnick, W. "Comfort levels and loudness matching for continuous and interrupted signals." *Journal of Speech and Hearing Research*, **10**: 99–109, 1967.
213. Miller, A. L. "The use of masked bone-conducted speech as an aid in the detection of feigned unilateral hearing losses." *Journal of Speech and Hearing Disorders*, **29**: 333–35, 1964.
214. Peck, J. "A comparison of the ascending and descending methods for administering the pure-tone Stenger test." Unpublished Master's Thesis. Storrs, Conn.: University of Connecticut, 1967.
215. Peterson, J. L. "Nonorganic hearing loss in children and Bekesy audiometry." *Journal of Speech and Hearing Disorders*, **28**: 153–58, 1963.
216. Resnick, D. M. and K. S. Burke. "Bekesy audiometry in nonorganic auditory problems." *Archives of Otolaryngology*, **76**: 38–41, 1962.
217. Rintelmann, W. F. and R. Carhart. "Loudness tracking by normal hearers via Bekesy audiometer." *Journal of Speech and Hearing Research*, **7**: 79–93, 1964.
218. Rintelmann, W. and E. Harford. "The detection and assessment of pseudo-hypocusis among school-age children." *Journal of Speech and Hearing Disorders*, **28**: 141–52, 1963.
219. Rintelmann, W. F. and E. Harford. "Type V Bekesy pattern: Interpretation and clinical utility." *Journal of Speech and Hearing Research*, **10**: 733–44, 1967.
220. Ross, M. "The variable intensity pulse count method (VIPCM) for the detection and measurement of the pure-tone thresholds of children with functional hearing losses." *Journal of Speech and Hearing Disorders*, **29**: 477–82, 1964.
221. Ruhm, H. B. and R. Carhart. "Objective speech audiometry: New method based on electrodermal response." *Journal of Speech and Hearing Research*, **1**: 169–78, 1958.
222. Ruhm, H. B. and W. A. Cooper, Jr. "Delayed feedback audiometry." *Journal of Speech and Hearing Disorders*, **29**: 448–55, 1964.
223. Ruhm, H. B. and W. A. Cooper, Jr. "Some factors that influence pure-tone delayed auditory feedback." *Journal of Speech and Hearing Research*, **6**: 223–37, 1963.
224. Ruhm, H. B. and O. J. Menzel. "Objective speech audiometry in cases of nonorganic hearing loss." *Archives of Otolaryngology*, **69**: 212–19, 1959.
225. Shepherd, D. C. "Nonorganic hearing loss and the consistency of behavioral auditory responses." *Journal of Speech and Hearing Research*, **8**: 149–63, 1965.
226. Stein, L. "Some observations on Type V Bekesy tracings." *Journal of Speech and Hearing Research*, **6**: 339–48, 1963.

227. Taylor, G. J. "An experimental study of tests for the detection of auditory malingering." *Journal of Speech and Hearing Disorders*, **14**: 119–30, 1949.
228. Thomsen, K. A. "Case of psychogenic deafness demonstrated by measuring of impedance." *Acta Oto-Laryngologica*, **45**: 82–85, 1955.
229. Ventry, I. M. and J. B. Chaiklin. "Functional hearing loss: A problem in terminology." *ASHA*, **4**: 251–54, 1962.
230. Ventry, I. M. and J. B. Chaiklin. "Reply." *ASHA*, **5**: 499, 1963.
231. Ventry, I. M. and J. B. Chaiklin. "Multidiscipline study of functional hearing loss." *Journal of Auditory Research*, **5**: 179–272, 1965.
232. Ventry, I. M. and J. B. Chaiklin. "Evaluation of pure-tone audiogram configurations used in identifying adults with functional hearing loss." *Journal of Auditory Research*, **5**: 212–18, 1965.
233. Ventry, I. M., J. B. Chaiklin, and W. F. Boyle. "Collapse of the ear canal during audiometry." *Archives of Otolaryngology*, **73**: 727–31, 1961.
234. Yates, A. J. "Delayed auditory feedback." *Psychology Bulletin*, **60**: 213–32, 1963.

11

The Mentally Retarded and Mentally Ill

Paul A. Rittmanic, Ph.D.

The receptive and expressive communication disorders of the mentally retarded are comparable in type and degree to those found among non-mentally retarded children and adults. Expressive disorders range from complete MUTISM and unintelligible vocalizations to mild articulation problems. Perusal of the literature shows that the incidence of the various speech and hearing disorders is much greater for the institutionalized mentally retarded in all age groups than would typically be found in the noninstitutionalized populations of similar ages (50).

Speech pathologists and audiologists who work with this type of patient spend a great deal of the time upon standard diagnostic and treatment procedures which are, in many instances, inadequate for the task of evaluating and modifying the *receptive* and *expressive* language behavior of these handicapped individuals. In spite of the multiple communication problems so often encountered among the mentally retarded and mentally ill, there is much that has been done and can be done to adequately identify and treat these communication problems.

The objectives of this chapter are: (1) to discuss the problem of evaluation of auditory disorders among the mentally retarded and emotionally disturbed; (2) to review and evaluate audiological techniques and tests that have been used or can be used to assess auditory function; (3) to provide treatment program guidelines.

The recent increase of national interest in problems of mental retardation and mental illness has tended to center the attention of both the professional worker and private citizen on the needs of these populations. As a result, a concerted effort is being made to assist the mentally retarded and mentally ill by using a multidisciplinary evaluation and treatment approach aimed at the HABILITATION and REHABILITATION of as many patients as possible. This shift of emphasis from the traditional custodial to active institutional programming to community programming has far-reaching implications for all professions and certainly for the field of speech pathology and audiology. The role of the hearing and speech specialist in multidisciplinary team evaluation and treatment has assumed increasing importance.

Mental Retardation

DEFINITIONS

The term MENTAL RETARDATION may be considered as a condition that originates during the developmental period and is characterized by significantly subnormal intellectual functioning, with the result of a varying degree of social inadequacy (Rothstein, 71).

As might be expected, there is considerable variation in the terminology describing this condition in the United States and in other countries. The World Health Organization recommended that the problem of mental retardation be referred to as mental subnormality with two major subdivisions according to causative factors. These would include:

1. Mental deficiency caused by biological factors resulting in dysfunction of the central nervous system.
2. Mental retardation resulting from social, economic, cultural, and psychological factors.

However, the American Association on Mental Deficiency has not followed this terminology recommendation and has advocated the overall use of the term "mental retardation."

The difficulty of proper classification and identification is not just an individual matter but also is related to the condition itself. Traditionally, mental retardation was thought of as a mental health concern only. However, contemporary thinking based on more comprehensive knowledge has emphasized that such identification is most misleading and is apt to hinder program development. This is obvious when one considers that there are nearly one hundred causative factors which have been identified as being associated with mental retardation and which represent a large number of

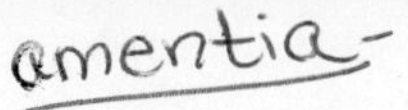

medical, psychological, psychiatric, and other conditions. To make it even more difficult, it must be remembered that several causative factors are usually operative in any one individual and thus require diagnostic and treatment procedures from different fields.

It is extremely difficult to secure any really accurate numerical evaluation of the incidence of mental retardation. However, the most authoritative sources do agree that the present number of mental retardates may be estimated at approximately five million individuals or nearly thirty per thousand population (Rothstein). Approximately one in thirty is severely retarded and the remainder ranges from the moderate to the mildly impaired intellectually and socially. These are some representative definitions of mental retardation based on a specific frame of reference:

1. The mentally deficient person is (1) socially incompetent, that is, socially inadequate, occupationally incompetent, and unable to manage his own affairs; (2) mentally subnormal; (3) retarded intellectually from birth or early age; (4) retarded at maturity; (5) mentally deficient as a result of constitutional origin, through heredity or disease, and (6) essentially incurable (Doll, 15).
2. Mental deficiency or amentia, then, is a condition in which the mind has failed to reach complete or normal development (Tredgold, 86).
3. Mental deficiency may be defined, from a medical point of view, as a condition of arrested or incomplete mental development induced by disease or injury before adolescence or arising from GENETIC causes (Jervis, 35).
4. Mental retardation may be viewed as a deficit of intellectual function that results from varied intrapersonal or extrapersonal determinants, but has as a common proximate cause a diminished efficiency of the nervous system, and thus entails a lessened general capacity for growth in perceptual and conceptual integration and consequently in environment adjustment (Benoit, 5).

EVALUATION AND CLASSIFICATION

Any diagnostic or evaluation process assumes efficient and reliable methods of testing. This is critical because classification follows these evaluation and diagnostic activities, and furnishes essential guidance in formulating programs for prevention, training, education, and research. Because of the multiphasic nature of mental retardation, it is quite important that the analysis and interpretation of all data and the subsequent PROGNOSTIC determinations be done in a multidisciplinary setting.

Fortunately, it is not necessary to examine great numbers of retarded children in special diagnostic or institutional outpatient clinics. The largest percentage of these mentally retarded children are classified as EDUCABLE

RETARDED and are thus adequately identified and diagnosed by the public school personnel. The Illinois State Department of Public Instruction has developed specific procedures for school psychologists to use in selecting and placing retarded children in special classes (62).

The physician is the professional worker who has the major responsibility for the supervision and for the health of the whole child. This responsibility requires periodic examinations and evaluations administered longitudinally in order to give more information than could possibly be obtained from a single evaluation. Abnormal factors that cannot be explained by the history require more special studies, i.e., laboratory, psychometric, x-ray, and audiologic.

CAUSES

Mental retardation has been associated with approximately one hundred different diseases, SYNDROMES, and ETIOLOGIES. However, most of these are rarely found and only about 20 per cent are encountered with sufficient frequency to be of practical importance.

These can be classified etiologically into three large groups: (1) prenatal, (2) natal, and (3) postnatal.

Most admissions to institutions for the mentally retarded are classified as either GENETICALLY or PRENATALLY determined. Pregnancy studies on abnormal children, including the mentally retarded, have shown a high incidence of maternal bleeding, TOXEMIAS of pregnancy, prematurity, and RUBELLA.

Another significant group factor associated with mental retardation includes those involving NATAL and PERINATAL processes. These include cerebral birth injury and ASPHYXIA. A high incidence of neurological abnormalities such as convulsive disorders and cerebral palsy has been associated with this category.

Postnatal conditions that are most common include inflammations of the central nervous system such as MENINGITIS and ENCEPHALITIS. The next most common cause is cerebral trauma occurring during infancy.

COMMUNICATION PROBLEMS

There is a high incidence of both receptive and expressive communication disorders among the mentally retarded. The occurrence of expressive disorders in speech has been reported to range as high as 90 per cent, depending on the type of population, whether it was institutional or non-institutional, and the criteria used to evaluate speech and language (50).

The literature on hearing testing of the mentally retarded has a number of reports of hearing surveys (1, 6, 7, 20, 26, 34, 36, 43, 44, 48, 54, 55, 57, 63, 67, 68, 72, 73, 74, 75, 77, 78, 79, 81, 89, 91, 92). These show considerable variance (ranging from 8 to 56 per cent) on the incidence of hearing impairment reported for mentally retarded populations. These variations in incidence have resulted from a number of factors such as test validity, test reliability, pass or fail criteria, test environment, intelligence quotient, and chronological age. In addition, several studies presented a rather substantial number of patients who were classified as untestable or difficult to test.

Notwithstanding these differences in incidence studies reported for the mentally retarded, there is no question that there is a higher incidence of auditory dysfunction among the mentally retarded than in comparable nonmentally retarded populations. It may be well to point out that there is a greater number of studies on the incidence of hearing impairment among the institutionalized mentally retarded than among comparable samples of mentally retarded subjects tested in the community.

Auditory Assessment of the Mentally Retarded

It has been the common experience of state school and state hospital speech and hearing staff members that hearing loss often goes undetected unless it is moderately severe. Other handicaps such as character disorders, DYSPHASIA, and cerebral damage so often found among the mentally retarded frequently confuse and obscure the diagnosis. However, the application of careful differential testing will often separate those with PERIPHERAL hearing impairment from those with a central auditory pathology.

The findings of these incidence studies emphasize that audiometric testing should be included in the routine examination of all mentally retarded and brain-injured patients. This information is vital, not only to the speech and hearing specialist, but to the psychologist who relies mainly on functional tests; to the special education personnel who must plan programs for these patients; to the ward attendants who must communicate daily with the patients; to the physician who is concerned with the general health, care, and management of the patient; and to all staff members who are equally concerned about social communication as it affects patient management. In general, the superintendents and clinical directors of the various state schools, state hospitals, and zone centers as well as administrative and special education personnel in the public school system have been quite cooperative with speech and hearing personnel and are generally eager to obtain specialized services. Nevertheless, the responsibility of the hearing and speech specialist includes the education and instruction of other professional personnel regarding the audiologist's activities and responsibilities, since audiology is a relatively recent entry into the multidisciplinary institutional and noninstitutional programs for the mentally retarded.

The profession of speech pathology and audiology is just beginning to turn its attention to the problems of differential diagnosis and treatment of mentally retarded and brain-injured children with communicative disorders (69). Traditionally, speech pathologists and audiologists have tended to look upon the mentally retarded as a last choice in the selection of handicapped persons who will receive the benefit of their professional skills. This is most unfortunate because many of these mentally retarded and perceptually impaired individuals have been prevented from returning to any useful socioeconomic function because of a receptive or expressive communication disorder that was far more handicapping than their basic problem of mental retardation or emotional disturbance.

AUDIOLOGIC ORIENTATION

A major problem for the clinical audiologist is the development of RELIABLE and VALID test techniques for testing the mentally retarded child. Most formal auditory tests were developed for adults and have often been assumed to be equally useful for infants and young children. In recent years, this assumption has been increasingly questioned. The accumulation of research and clinical data strongly indicates that the problem of assessing the auditory capabilities of the mature adult is considerably different from the task of determining the auditory capacity of young children. Consequently, it is mandatory that clinical audiologists who assess the hearing of children be aware of whether their tests and procedures are developmentally appropriate, or whether their methods are beyond the mental and physical maturity of the child.

Equally important is the need for the clinician to be aware that no response to sound is not a sure indication of auditory dysfunction. In fact, the younger the child or the more severe the developmental delay, the greater is the likelihood of no response. Therefore, the audiologist has the problem of determining whether an impairment of auditory acuity is responsible for the lack of response, or whether there are other complicating factors.

In the older child who should have developed normal speech but has not, the common presumption is that his speech delay is due to peripheral deafness. This has resulted in many incorrect diagnoses and in much inappropriate programming. There is little doubt that when children do not develop speech normally, problems of impaired auditory acuity are the most common cause. However, it is the responsibility of the examining audiologist to differentiate among problems such as mental deficiency, emotional disturbance, and auditory dysfunction associated with central nervous problems.

An evaluation of the auditory capacity must take into account the general mental and emotional development of the child. Auditory dysfunction may include impairment of acuity or the inability to interpret sound meaningfully or both. Auditory problems may be caused by physical and psychological factors.

The clinical audiologist engaged in pediatric audiology will encounter several types of response behavior. Some children will make no apparent response to sound, despite the fact that they have normal hearing acuity. Other infants and children will respond to certain sounds consistently even though they have a hearing loss which will affect speech and language development. Still other children will give intermittent or inconsistent responses. Therefore, the clinical audiologist must always be prepared to evaluate the variable responses in children. The child's overall behavior in the presence of various auditory stimuli must be related very carefully to all other SYMPTOMATOLOGIES before a clinical opinion or diagnosis is offered.

These considerations are especially important when we consider that a large number of children may have one or more conditions causing the apparent and inconsistent auditory response. The problem of multiple handicaps often requires the evaluation of several specialists for both differential diagnostic purposes as well as for program planning.

LANGUAGE CONSIDERATIONS

Every clinical audiologist should have broad training in speech and language development and in speech and language disorders. Commonly, children are referred to the clinical audiologist when it has been observed by parents or other professional workers that the child is not developing speech and language commensurate with his age. Therefore, it is necessary to assess not only the auditory capability of the child but also the type and the degree of the expressive problem.

Myklebust (60) cautions that neither speech nor hearing should be viewed as the totality of language, although both are essential for normal language development. He further states that before a child can speak, he must be able to hear, then to interpret, and lastly, to relate the interpreted verbal symbols to the speech motor system. He further categorizes language into the three areas—inner, receptive, and expressive.

DIAGNOSTIC PROCEDURE

In order to arrive at a diagnostic determination, there are certain essential elements that must be considered. Doll (15) has emphasized that four basic factors need to be considered in the diagnostic process. These include the previous condition; that is, the determination of the onset and early development of the problem. The second factor includes obtaining information on the present status of the child. The third determination is the future status or prognosis. The final consideration is to determine the cause. Since the four basic factors are closely related, it follows that the diagnostic procedure calls for both analysis and SYNTHESIS in order to prevent an incorrect etiological determination.

Doll (15) also stresses another factor that is significant in making any differential diagnosis in young children who have auditory dysfunction. This is the determination of the age of onset of the condition, since it is directly related to finding the etiology. That is, the child's present behavioral symptoms should be fairly consistent with expectations according to the age at which the auditory dysfunction was incurred.

Myklebust (60) suggests that the differential diagnosis of auditory problems in young children emphasize these three steps. First, the examiner must obtain a DIFFERENTIAL HISTORY; second, he must make careful clinical observation of the child; and third, he must make a clinical examination that uses informal as well as formal tests. Myklebust further emphasizes that these steps are not separated but are often accomplished simultaneously. A thorough discussion of the essential factors to be considered and of differential history-taking is presented in his textbook.

It has been this writer's experience that otherwise well-trained clinical audiologists often neglect or minimize the differential history-taking and its subsequent interpretation and evaluation. This is most unfortunate since a considerable amount of time could be saved in the clinical examination phase of the differential diagnostic procedure. Also, it would alert the audiologist to watch for certain types of responses during the clinical observation.

The etiological factors responsible for the auditory dysfunction are often revealed in the examination of the case history. Such factors as type of birth, perinatal behavior, RH INCOMPATIBILITY, prenatal disease, health history, emotional disturbances, ages of rolling over, crawling, sitting, standing, walking, *babbling*, and responding to sound are only a few of the essential factors which must be considered in any etiological determination.

CLINICAL OBSERVATION

One of the most challenging tasks for the clinical audiologist is to determine whether apparent auditory dysfunction is only a manifestation of general developmental delay, or whether a true organic hearing problem exists. This problem is encountered quite frequently by clinical audiologists who work in multidisciplinary mental health, public health, and medical center programs. Due to the nature of their patient population, clinicians in these agencies typically see a large number of suspected mentally retarded children as well as infants and children with central nervous system impairments and emotional disturbances.

It is a well known fact that language acquisition is related to the level of intelligence. The majority of mentally deficient children who are referred to audiology clinics for suspected auditory dysfunction in infancy and early life manifest very limited speech and language development. Since speech is acquired when mental development reaches approximately twelve to eighteen months, it is not unusual to have nonverbal children referred for auditory testing due to their lack of language development. However, when the mentally deficient child is compared to the peripherally deaf child, it is apparent that the retarded child does not use vision and tactile sensory avenues in a compensatory manner. He does understand sounds and words on his mental level. Karlin and Strazulla (41) reported data that showed the differences among severe, moderate, and mildly retarded children in relation to their age of word acquisition as compared to their ages of sitting and walking. They found that speech was more retarded than motor development, although motor development was also delayed in comparison to the nonmentally retarded child.

The majority of mentally retarded children do develop speech but at a later chronological age, since they need more time to achieve the necessary intellectual capability. Therefore, the speech sound acquisition as well as the language development is delayed. The child is also delayed in nearly all other aspects of his genetic development. This developmental delay is the most significant symptom in differentiating auditory dysfunction from problems of mental retardation, peripheral hearing impairment, and auditory dysfunction associated with central nervous system damage or psychological disturbances.

The mentally retarded individual does use his hearing projectively to maintain contact with his surroundings, to explore his auditory environment, and to relate to others. However, it is necessary for the clinician to remember that the retarded child responds primarily to sounds that are meaningful to him. Several of the authors whose papers are reported by Lloyd and Frisina (50) indicate that a great deal of inaccurate hearing testing and diagnoses could be prevented if the child were evaluated using sounds that are meaningful to him rather than using the more complicated and inappropriate test materials of pure-tone and speech audiometry evaluation.

In summary, it can be said that most mentally retarded children with normal hearing demonstrate normal vocal tone quality, use vocalizations for pleasure, utilize gesture language at their mental level, can respond to simple meaningful sounds, exhibit emotional behavior commensurate with their mental age, and respond auditorily to *meaningful* acoustic signals. Especially important is the factor of delayed motor development and reduced social awareness commensurate with the child's delayed development. These factors are much easier to observe in the severely and moderately retarded child than in the child with a mild degree of retardation. Fortunately, although the degree of genetic developmental delay is less pronounced with the more mildly retarded, it also follows that these subjects are easier to assess by standard techniques and usually present a less complicated evaluation problem.

AUDITORY TESTING

The majority of infants and children who have auditory dysfunction are also children who manifest nonverbal behavior. Since they lack the ability for verbal communication or for reception and comprehension of spoken language, they are especially difficult to test with the standard tests. Therefore, the clinical audiologist must be discerning in the choice and interpretation of tests as well as creative in modifying and developing new test techniques.

No matter what informal or formal tests are used and whether or not they are standardized or not standardized, certain factors must be taken into consideration when testing the nonverbal child. First, the audiologic tests must be suitable to the developmental level of the child. If they are not appropriate to the genetic level of the child and he does not respond, no useful information has been secured. The second factor that must be considered is whether the clinician is obtaining the maximum response from the child. The maximum response is assumed to be a threshold response, unless stated otherwise. This determination is particularly difficult to make, since very young or very impaired children are unable to give appropriate responses. Third, the clinician must know if the test is aimed at assessing listening acuity or comprehension ability.

Although there are a rather large number of standardized psychological tests for young children, many of the auditory tests have not been standardized to the extent that many of the tests of mental ability have been. Consequently, the clinician using such tests must make a comparison with the normal that is based to a great extent on his clinical experience. The elicitation of responses which can be evaluated and compared with the responses of others is an important and necessary aspect of auditory testing. The audiologic tests should provide the clinician with a systematic observation of the child's behavior that can be repeated by other examiners or by the same examiner. It is also important to relate the audiologic test information to data obtained on intellectual ability, adaptive behavior, and emotional status.

IDENTIFICATION TESTING

Considerations. Frisina (21) emphasizes that there is no single audiologic definition for children. That is, whether a procedure is appropriate for a specific subject depends upon the way in which the procedure has been standardized. Generally, it is not so important what the specific classification of the subject or patient is, but whether he can be reliably and validly tested.

This type of rationale also applies to the auditory evaluation of the mentally retarded. There is no question that many of the mentally retarded infants and children can be assessed reliably and validly with existing audiological tests. However, it is essential in all audiologic testing to specify and control the various stimulus-response criteria carefully. This basic principle holds true especially in the testing of mentally retarded children. Unless the clinical audiologist is rigorous in his establishment of stimulus and response criteria, there will be a serious question as to whether he has really measured the absolute threshold. It would be well to point out that a number of tests involving reflexes such as the MORO, STARTLE, AUROPALPEBRAL, and STAPEDIAL REFLEX tests are not strict measurements of hearing.

The auditory measurements which are usually of the most concern to the clinical audiologist are the absolute threshold for pure-tone air-conduction and bone-conduction tests, speech reception, and speech sound discrimination ability.

Auditory assessment of neonates. Audiologic evaluation of NEONATES has been studied by several researchers: Buhler (8), Ewing and Ewing (17), Gesell and Armatruda (27), Downs and Sterritt (16), Price and Goldstein (64), Cody and Bickford (10), Froeschels and Beebe (23), Green and Richard (31), Nelson (61), and Waldon (87). The earlier work consisted of systematic testing and observation of responses such as the startle reflex, crying responses, attentional modifications, change of activity, and similar types of responses. However, these tests were very gross in that the spectrum of the sounds presented was extremely wide, and it was also necessary to employ relatively high-intensity sounds in order to produce observable responses.

On the other hand, the later work of investigators employing electrophysiological techniques indicated that more specific frequency information could be obtained and that these could be obtained at lower intensity levels. However, ELECTROPHYSIOLOGIC AUDIOMETRY has not provided definite baseline data on the limits of absolute threshold pure-tone and noise measurements for neonates. Nevertheless, a substantial amount of systematic observation and testing by such investigators as Wedenberg (90), Froding (22), Hardy and Pauls (33), Ewing (19), and others point out that there are definite observable responses to various stimuli at certain intensity levels to which neonates will respond. This type of auditory testing can be applied successfully to the mentally retarded child as well as to the nonmentally retarded child.

Infant testing (two to twenty-four months). Several investigators who have pursued longitudinal studies of behavioral responses during the infancy period have reported a number of observable behavioral changes in response to certain sounds. Gesell and Armatruda (27) indicate that after two to three months, the infant is no longer as responsive to very loud sounds and seems to assume a listening or attentional posture in the presence of loud sounds. As maturation continues into the fourth or fifth month, the infant may respond to sounds with a change in facial expression, and within a few weeks an attempt to localize is evident. At approximately seven months of age, the ability to localize is achieved. At about eight and one-half to nine months of age, the infant begins to engage in sound imitation, and comprehension begins to occur at sometime around one year of age.

Ewing (19) used a number of different auditory stimuli when testing infants and established a clinical set of norms that can be expected with the average hearing infant. Subsequently, Hardy and Pauls (33) used some of Ewing's findings in a screening study of infants. In 1961, DiCarlo and Bradley (13) reported that when children fail localization tests at the age where it is typically observed, it is quite suggestive of some auditory dysfunction.

It should be emphasized that the clinical audiologists should be familiar with and definitely utilize the normative data that has been reported by the various investigators. No adequate sample of properly diagnosed mentally retarded children with such pathologies as MONGOLISM, PKU SYNDROME, and other identifiable pathologies has been tested to discover if the various types of auditory reflexive responses are delayed or present at comparable chronological ages in nonmentally retarded subjects. Therefore, extreme caution must be exercised in the interpretation of any results that are positive, since a true auditory dysfunction may not be present, but the maturational delay may cause the lack of response and thus mislead the audiologist. Ideally, ELECTROPHYSIOLOGIC TECHNIQUES such as AUDITORY EVOKED POTENTIAL testing should be attempted whenever there is any suggestion of a condition commonly associated with mental retardation and other positive audiologic findings.

Hearing assessment of young children (two to five years). A number of writers, Lowell et al. (52), Barr (3), Dix and Hallpike (14), Denmark (11), Shimizu and Nakamura (80), Statten and Wishart (85), Guilford and Haug (32), Keaster (42), DiCarlo and Bradley (13), and Geyer and Yankauer (29) have reported on the various facets of both IDENTIFICATION AUDIOMETRY and threshold audiometry with very young children. In general, their findings show that play audiometry is undoubtedly the most useful technique when attempting to evaluate the auditory capabilities of preschool children. There seems to be little doubt that with the careful application of modified pure-tone and speech reception test techniques, reliable and valid identification of hearing-impaired preschool children can be achieved.

These techniques have also been found to be quite applicable for use with the mentally retarded. A number of investigators, Lloyd and Frisina (50), Schlanger (75), Webb et al. (89), Rigrodsky et al. (67), Rittmanic (69), Siegenthaler and Krzwicki (81), and others have reported achieving reliable and valid test results.

FACTORS RELATED TO HEARING LOSS AMONG THE MENTALLY RETARDED

The clinical audiologist engaged in testing mentally retarded subjects should keep in mind that there are a number of factors that contribute to the problem of test reliability with this type of patient. The first of these would include the reliability and validity of the audiometric tests that are being used. As mentioned previously, extreme care must be exercised not only to stimulus control but especially to the observation of responses and their interpretation. Secondly, the mentally retarded, and especially the institutionalized retarded, have poor listening habits. This limitation often results in the partial or total lack of understanding of directions for a proper test response. Thirdly, there is a much higher incidence of sensori-neural hearing impairment coexisting with other central nervous system dysfunction. This undoubtedly results in more frequent breakdown of auditory comprehension. Fourth, it has been reported that there is a greater incidence of CENTRAL AUDITORY DYSFUNCTION in the mentally retarded than would be found in comparable samples of nonmentally retarded subjects. However, due to the problems inherent in diagnosing a central auditory dysfunction with nonmentally retarded brain-injured children, it still remains to be demonstrated whether this is true. Because of the not uncommon occurrence of multiple handicaps and their complications, a substantial number of these mentally retarded children have been classified as untestable. Fifth, there is a relatively high incidence of emotional disturbance with the mentally retarded. This is especially true at the time of the admission to an institution and when the diagnostic tests are being administered. This further complicates the evaluation process and has been the cause of much spurious diagnostic information. Finally, the incidence of NONORGANIC HEARING IMPAIRMENT is relatively high with the higher IQ children and must be considered by the audiologist.

BEHAVIORAL AUDIOMETRY

Behavioral audiologic tests and measurements presume the subject's ability to respond voluntarily in a certain manner to a specific stimulus. This technique is generally used with adults and children who are capable of understanding instructions and responding correctly.

With very young children and with a large number of mentally retarded subjects, it is not possible to obtain reliable responses at threshold or suprathreshold levels. Therefore, it becomes necessary to modify the responses and employ conditioned response or play audiometry. This type of activity may include placing a ring on a peg, dropping a block in a box, or some social reward such as a pat on the back or a vocal approval. Further modifications of this include the well-known puppet show technique, which involves a voluntary pressing of a button with the reward of a picture. These types of play audiometric techniques have been successful with children with chronological ages as low as twenty-four months.

Reflex tests. The auditory assessment of the very young child still remains one of the major challenges in audiological diagnosis. Obviously, the more conventional tests are not applicable to this age group, and it is necessary for the examiner to depend on other means for obtaining information on auditory function.

It is often necessary for the clinical audiologist to depend on the observation of gross responses in an effort to determine if there is a serious hearing impairment, and if the child needs further comprehensive audiologic evaluation. It is common practice to use reflexive movements for determining the presence or absence of hearing. The acoustical-palpebral reflex is one of the first tests utilized. This reflex action consists of a quick closing and opening of the eyelids immediately after a loud acoustic stimulation. The audiologist must be very careful to see that the eyelids and the facial muscles of the child are relaxed before this type of reflex test is attempted. It is well to remember that the palpebral reflex can be elicited only at very intense levels (approximately 110 dB-SPL) and is not designed to assess threshold. It is only used to obtain an indication of whether hearing is present or absent.

It must be cautioned that the audiologist is not to automatically infer that there is a profound hearing loss if no response is elicited by this type of test but to consider it only an indication of possible auditory dysfunction. There are a number of other reflexes that are useful to the audiologist in determining if hearing is present. These include the eye blink test (acoustical palpebral reflex), eye rolling (orientation reflex), head turning, Moro reflex, and the startle reflex. Several authors, Nelson (61), Green and Richard (31), Ewing (19), Froeschels and Beebe (23), Gesell et al. (28), and Hardy and Pauls (33), are among those who have done extensive testing utilizing reflex observational techniques.

In general, it was found that eye movement was the predominant response at the one-month level with a gradual rolling of the eyes towards the sound stimulus beginning to occur in the second and third months. The Moro reflex was also evident during the first two to four months. This reflex is characterized by an extension of the arms with the spreading, adduction, and half-flexion of the fingers and an extension of the legs and toes. This reflex usually consists of symmetrical and consecutive outward, upward, and inward grasp motions of the arms with crying often accompanying them.

The startle reflex can be described as a general startle reaction when a very loud noise is presented to the child. He may begin to throw up his hands and feet and he often begins crying. Closing of the eyes and thrusting forward of the head, forward movement of the trunk, and contraction of the abdomen and neck may also be evident.

The Moro reflex begins to disappear by about the fourth month, but the other reflexes such as eye opening, eye rolling, startle reflex, and head turning remain throughout the first year with the development of learned responses occurring in the second year of life. The pediatrician and the neurologist have traditionally observed reflex behavior in their assessment of the auditory as well as other sensory and motor functions. This has not been true of clinical audiologists in general, and many of the common observational techniques are not used to their fullest extent by clinical audiologists. However, there is still a considerable uncertainty about the hearing level for infants when using the various reflexes. Waldon (87) points out that such reflexes as eye blinks, eye rolling, head turning, and the Moro reflex can be utilized in the reliable determination of threshold but states that the startle reflex is not useful for obtaining threshold levels because of the high level of sound intensity needed to excite the reflex.

There is ample experimental and clinical evidence to show that children are capable of responding to auditory signals at an extremely early age, and that the responses depend upon the infant's age and the type of signal presented. As the child matures, these responses become more definite, and learned responses begin to replace the generalized body movements.

These observational techniques and criteria should be used in the auditory assessment of suspected or known mentally retarded children. Data presented by Lloyd and Melrose (49) shows that reliable audiometric testing can be achieved with older mentally retarded children when certain precautions are taken. Therefore, if reliable pure-tone and speech audiometric testing can be done with mentally retarded children of moderate to relatively high levels of intelligence, it follows that careful observation of their early reflex behavior toward loud sounds should give us gross information on the auditory system. However, no study has conclusively shown whether the reflex behavior of the severe, moderate, and mildly retarded child is significantly delayed when compared to the nonmentally retarded child of comparable chronological age. It may be that there is very little if any difference in reflex behavior, or that definite differences for comparable chronological ages may be evident.

Pure-tone and speech audiometry. Few studies have been reported on the reliability of pure-tone and speech audiometry measurements for the normal hearing mentally retarded child as well as on the hearing-impaired mentally retarded child. This is somewhat surprising since incidence data mentioned earlier in this chapter reported that hearing loss among the mentally retarded ranges from 8 to 56 per cent. As mentioned previously, these significant variations in incidence have led many to question the inter- and intratest reliability of the measures used.

Kopatic (45) tested forty-seven adult females in the mildly retarded IQ range binaurally for eleven frequencies four times at periodic intervals. He reported correlations of 0.62 for the right ear and 0.63 for the left ear and thus concluded that the reliability coefficients on the thresholds for these patients cast considerable doubt on the applicability of pure-tone testing with the mentally retarded. Unfortunately, Kopatic did not furnish otologic and audiologic information for his subjects; there was no description of the test environment, no description of the audiometric procedure or instructions utilized, the type of threshold criterion, or the qualifications of the audiometrist administering these tests.

In 1964, Fulton and Graham (25) reported on the results of a study investigating pure tone-test reliability with the mentally retarded of four functioning levels: borderline—dull normal, mild, moderate, and severe. The study results indicated that the standard plus or minus 5-dB test-retest reliability criteria employing standard pure-tone stimuli could be obtained with the dull-normal and mild groups, but that the test-retest step difference increased with the more severely retarded children.

Lloyd and Melrose (49) published the results of a study that investigated the intramethod agreement of pure-tone and speech audiometry with forty mentally retarded patients with specific levels of retardation. Pure-tone thresholds for the 500 to 2,000 cps pure-tone average were obtained using four methods (standard, modified ear-choice, play, and slide-show audiometry). Measurements of the speech reception threshold were also obtained using the standard and picture method. The data reported from their investigation indicated that all six methods demonstrated high reliability. Most of the actual differences for each subject were within plus or minus 5 dB, with high intraclass correlations. The highest intraclass correlations reported showed that the play audiometry method was the most reliable of the four pure-tone techniques. They also reported that the two methods measuring speech reception threshold yielded slightly higher reliability than any of the four pure-tone methods.

Rittmanic (69) presented data which indicated that when qualified clinical audiologists administered pure-tone and speech audiometric tests, it was not necessary to provide immediate routine repeat testing of all mentally retarded subjects. This finding is contrary to other reports in the literature (78, 45).

A note of caution is in order when considering the relationship of the 500 to 2,000 cps pure tone average with the speech reception threshold. The pure-tone test is intended primarily to obtain information specifically about a determination of the integrity of the peripheral mechanism, and it will not provide full information on the functional hearing of mentally retarded and brain-injured children for oral language comprehension. In all cases where auditory dysfunction is suspected (not withstanding a normal pure-tone measurement), speech audiometry should be administered.

Watkins et al. (88) utilized an experimental test (the Animal Sound Test) consisting of vowel-consonant combinations presented by live voice and matched to specific picture cards of animals. This new test was devised for measuring hearing acuity in mentally retarded subjects with mental ages of less than four years and was compared with two conventional methods of hearing testing (pure tone and speech reception). They reported that the Animal Sound Test yielded lower thresholds with more subjects who had been untestable by the standard methods, but who were able to be tested with this special test.

Operant conditioning audiometry. Skinner defines operant behavior as that which operates on the environment with the behavior being controlled by its consequences. These consequences have been called *reinforcers,* and they may be either positive or negative. A positive reinforcer may be a class of events which increases the probability of the reoccurrence of the response that reduces or terminates it.

Examples of positive reinforcers for test subjects may be food, candy, social approbation, and the like. Examples of negative reinforcers are shock, unpleasant noise, and heat or cold. Spradlin (83) discussed four possible applications of operant principles to audiometry when testing the profoundly retarded subjects.

The clinical audiologist usually does not have much difficulty in accomplishing a reliable audiologic evaluation of the majority of mentally retarded subjects. The major difficulty arises when the mentally retarded person does not respond or is substantially inconsistent in his responses or is unable to follow verbal directions. Naturally, with the more retarded and multiply handicapped child, there is a greater likelihood of unreliable test results.

Spradlin (83) points out that the audiologist's verbal responses are actually a reinforcement in conventional behavior audiometry, but that this is not very effective with a profoundly retarded child. Dix and Hallpike (14) described the "peep show" technique for testing young children. This technique has been successful with testing children from approximately twenty months of age and older and is a form of operant or instrumental testing procedure. In this case, the reinforcement of the response is the presentation of an interesting picture. Lloyd (51) has modified the peep show technique and applied it with some success to the hearing evaluation of severely retarded children.

It would be well for the clinical audiologist to remember that operant conditioning audiometry is merely a variation of behavioral audiometry with the major emphasis on the use of reinforcers. Furthermore, this type of instrumental testing has several limitations and we still must seek a more objective and reliable method to assess retarded, brain-injured, and other multiply handicapped children. The next section will deal with the quest to evolve this type of test.

ELECTROPHYSIOLOGICAL TESTS

Goldstein (30) differentiates very clearly between behavioral audiometry and electrophysiologic audiometry. He states, "Electrophysiologic audiometry differs from behavioral audiometry in that the response of the acoustic stimulation manifests itself by some change in the observed electrical properties of the person under test, while in behavioral audiometry, the response is some overt bodily reaction." Furthermore, in behavioral audiometry overt responses may be voluntary or involuntary.

This apparent objectivity of electrophysiologic audiometry must be carefully qualified, since the technique may be called objective but the interpretation of the graphic recordings, meter variations, or other signals are still open to subjective error.

Goldstein's (30) review of electrodermal response audiometry (EDA) or psychogalvanic skin response audiometry (PGSR) and electroencephalographic audiometry (EEA) is very thorough and comprehensive and will not be reviewed in detail at this time but is discussed in Chapters 10 and 12. It must be stated, however, that these two techniques along with auditory evoked potential audiometry have been of considerable assistance in the identification of threshold hearing levels in otherwise untestable subjects.

In general, it has been found that EDA and EEA hearing threshold levels will be essentially equivalent. Also, reliable behavioral audiometric thresholds tend to agree rather closely with thresholds obtained by EDA and EEA techniques.

Although EDA and EEA tests may reveal essentially normal thresholds, there may be a real or apparent auditory disorder in any given mentally retarded or emotionally disturbed subject. Even if the hearing threshold level has been determined reliably by electrophysiologic audiometry, we are still aware of only the acuity factor in the overall auditory dysfunction.

There is still a critical need to obtain baseline data on a large number of neurologically identifiable cases of an impaired central nervous system. Electrophysiologic audiometry data is needed on large numbers of mentally retarded and emotionally disturbed children and adolescents who manifest "delayed speech development" or apparent receptive and expressive aphasic syndromes. Until this is done, it will continue to be quite hazardous to make any general diagnostic statements about individual electrophysiologic test results.

Electrodermal audiometry with the mentally retarded has been studied by very few investigators. Irwin et al. (34), Kodman et al. (43), Moss et al. (58), Webb et al. (89), and Fulton (24) have reported on the results of research done with mentally retarded subjects. The results of these experimenters were not in agreement concerning the validity and reliability of GSR audiometry with the mentally retarded. Webb, Fulton, Irwin, and Kodman were able to achieve conditioning with the severely retarded and to secure some threshold measurements. In general, the results of GSR testing have not been shown to be as reliable as previously mentioned methods using operant or play audiometry test techniques. Obviously, the research data does point up the lack of standardized information on GSR techniques with the mentally retarded and suggests the definite need for systematic and long-term research.

Recently, Price and Goldstein (64) reported on the use of auditory evoked potential audiometry with various types of brain-injured and mentally retarded subjects. Some success was achieved in securing auditory threshold values using the auditory evoked potential technique but once again, the apparent lack of large samples of matched subjects placed the findings in serious question. Yet, the major contribution of this beginning work is that hearing threshold levels were obtained from some of these subjects and were also verified by other electrophysiologic techniques as well as by behavioral audiometry.

DIFFERENTIAL DIAGNOSIS

Audiologically, a differential diagnosis of auditory dysfunction implies the location of the site of lesion in the auditory system. There is a rather large and growing battery of audiologic procedures to assist the clinical audiologist in arriving at this determination (*see* Chapters 9 and 10). However, when we are considering the auditory evaluation of mentally retarded, brain-injured, and emotionally disturbed children, it is implied that we are going to assist in the differential diagnosis of oral language delay. Frisina (21) has serious reservations on whether the present observational and measurement techniques used by audiologists are sufficient at this time to permit the audiologist to make a differential diagnosis of language disorder.

There is little doubt that that reservation is a legitimate one, but this diagnostic job should not fall solely within the province of the audiologist. Mentally retarded and brain-injured children who manifest receptive and expressive communicative disorders require a multidisciplinary evaluation. Therefore, the audiologist frequently will furnish very important information to the physician, psychiatrist, psychologist, neurologist, and other specialists for a diagnosis of the site of lesion and the possible etiology of the language delay. Moreover, he can immediately provide the educational specialist with a very good estimate of the patient's present functional level, whatever the eventual etiological classification and the direction of habilitative and rehabilitative programs.

MULTIDISCIPLINARY EVALUATION AND PLANNING

Evaluation and treatment of the mentally retarded and brain-injured child is a multidisciplinary task. Youngsters should receive a routine medical evaluation, psychological and social evaluation, speech and hearing evaluation, educational evaluation, and possible specialized examinations such as neurological, psychiatric, serological, x-ray, and otological. Due to the high incidence of hearing impairment reported for both the institutionalized and the noninstitutionalized mentally retarded child, it is most important to develop a sound otoaudiological screening and evaluation program.

Otoaudiological programming. If a mentally retarded subject fails the audiological screening examination, a retest should be scheduled and a second screening examination administered. If the patient performs reliably and fails the screening examination a second time, a pure-tone air-conduction and bone-conduction test must be administered along with tests for speech reception threshold and speech discrimination. Following these diagnostic tests, the patient should be scheduled for an ear, nose, and throat examination to be administered by an otolaryngologist.

The otolaryngological examination may result in several types of follow-up services. First, the examining physician may find no evidence of ear pathology and may recommend only periodic threshold testing to check whether the hearing loss is progressive in nature. If the loss is a psychosocially handicapping, a recommendation may be made for hearing-aid evaluation and possible hearing-aid selection, depending on the overall status of the patient's behavior. A second course of action may require short-term or long-term medication with subsequent oto-audiologic evaluations throughout the period of treatment. A third possibility is the recommendation for surgical correction of certain conditions such as otosclerosis, cholesteatoma removal, myringotomy, and tympanectomy.

Obviously, the clinical audiologist is intimately involved in the oto-audiologic evaluation and treatment program. However, another major aspect of the audiologic evaluation of the hard-of-hearing or deaf mentally retarded patient includes hearing evaluation, selection of a hearing aid, and intensive aural rehabilitation programming.

Two Illinois Department of Mental Health institutions (Dixon State School and Lincoln State School) have developed what can be classified as a diagnostic hearing-aid therapy program. If a resident's hearing loss is serious enough to warrant amplification, and the ENT examination indicates that medication or surgery will not help in correcting the impairment, a period of diagnostic therapy is arranged to determine whether or not a resident can utilize amplification adequately. During this period of approximately one to three months, the resident is exposed to auditory amplification with a portable auditory training unit or wearable amplification. An attempt is made to determine whether or not the resident can profit from wearable amplification, if he has a desire to do so and if the desire can be developed. The ward or cottage living situation is also evaluated to determine whether or not a resident can use a hearing aid in this environment and take care of it adequately. The child's social adequacy, intellectual capacity, emotional stability, and other related factors are reviewed to determine if further audiologic rehabilitative services are indicated.

Assuming that the period of evaluation indicates that a hearing-aid evaluation is in order, the examination is scheduled and conducted at the audiologic clinic located in the institution. A full stock of hearing aids is kept at the clinic, and it is available for testing on the residents. The hearing-aid evaluation is a further attempt to obtain refined information on the appropriateness of wearable amplification for the specific patient. At this time, a specific aid is selected and immediately fitted on the patient.

The next step in rehabilitation involves a three- to six-month hearing-aid orientation and aural rehabilitation program geared to the specific needs of the patient. The wearable instrument is kept at the clinic during the initial phases of the program and eventually the patient is permitted to wear the aid not only at the therapy sessions but at his work assignment, school classes, and on the wards. At the end of this period, a final determination is made as to whether he can adequately use his hearing aid.

When patients are discharged and placed in the community on regular work assignments, in sheltered care homes, or in nursing homes, they are still periodically evaluated by the speech and hearing department for the effectiveness of wearable amplification.

Large numbers of patients who require hearing-aid evaluations and a program of aural rehabilitation also usually need intensive speech and language work as well. A number of patients are involved in a broad program of speech and language therapy as well as in the aural rehabilitation program.

It is common for the speech and language diagnostic team to discover related perceptual, neuromuscular, dental, neurologic, and other conditions that affect the communicative ability of the patient. The services of specialists in pediatric neurology, aural surgery, radiology, and other specialities are available for further evaluation and treatment. All referrals from the speech and hearing staff for other services are coordinated through the chief of the medical staff.

This program is described in detail in order to furnish the reader with what the author has observed to be both an effective habilitative or rehabilitative approach that can be established for the mentally retarded and brain-injured child who has a receptive or expressive disorder related to auditory impairment, and who needs an intensive and comprehensive otoaudiologic program.

Over thirty studies have been reported on the incidence of hearing impairment and have suggested tests for audiologic diagnosis of the mentally retarded. However, very few authors (68, 76) discuss the important postevaluation activities that any good diagnostic program implies. This is not only a deficiency of a great number of audiologic programs for the

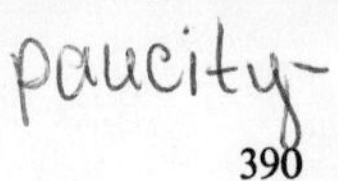

mentally retarded, but is also an unfortunate trend in many university and medical center audiology settings. The emphasis continues to be strong on the evaluation, diagnosis, and classification of disorders, but the habilitative and rehabilitative aspects of auditory dysfunction have been neglected. Not only has there been a general failure to apply what is known about auditory training, lip reading, hearing-aid orientation, and related activities, but also there has not been a long-term systematic evaluation of these techniques with the mentally retarded and brain injured. A number of institutions and programs are now becoming interested in this type of clinical research, and it is anticipated that there will be a strong research effort directed to this aspect of rehabilitative audiology.

Audiologic Assessment of the Mentally Ill and Emotionally Disturbed

The recent national emphasis on mental health problems has resulted in the development of interest not only of average citizens but of professional workers in a number of related fields. The profession of speech pathology and audiology has begun to display some interest toward the psychiatric patient, and in some states nonpsychiatric services, including speech and hearing, are now being developed. One state, Illinois, has begun to provide state-wide speech and hearing services for the mentally ill as well as for the mentally retarded (69, 70).

AUDIOLOGIC SURVEY

There is a paucity of literature on hearing testing of psychiatric hospital patients. Lamb and Graham (47) reported a study designed to evaluate the validity, reliability, and efficiency of certain auditory screening tests when used with patients in a psychiatric hospital. They classified the patients not according to a psychiatric diagnosis but according to "least disturbed," "moderately disturbed," and "severely disturbed." They used a one-frequency 4,000 Hz technique and a standard audiometric sweep frequency screening test for the frequencies 250 through 8,000 Hz. The best method of testing used the sweep frequency technique, which obtained the least false positives. They reported that the sample tested (110 patients, 53 females and 57 males) did not have a significantly higher incidence of hearing impairment than would be found in the general population.

Barker (2) reported a pilot study of hearing-impaired psychotic patients at the Rochester State Hospital in Rochester, Minnesota. This study reported only on patients who were considered to be deaf on the basis of ward personnel reports and who were thought to be physically and mentally able to cooperate in testing. This study concluded that otoaudiological services should be an integral part of the treatment program provided for mentally ill and emotionally disturbed patients.

Sprinkle et al. (84) did an otolaryngologic and audiologic assessment of 170 consecutive admissions to the Western State Hospital in Stanton, Virginia. Alcoholics and drug addicts were not reported in this study, only patients who had specific psychiatric classifications. The results indicated that approximately five (3 per cent) could not be tested because of their severe disturbance; 154 (97 per cent) patients were able to complete the testing. Those with handicapped hearing in the speech range was 5.1 per cent (a loss greater than 30 decibels ASA in the better ear). Approximately 7.7 per cent of the patients were also found to have otolaryngologic pathology. Their conclusion was that hearing loss does not appear to be a statistically significant variable with the mentally ill. However, they too, recommended the provision of otolaryngologic and audiologic rehabilitation.

The most comprehensive hearing survey was done by McCoy and Plotkin (53) at the Elgin State Hospital, Elgin, Illinois. This institution has approximately 5,000 patients, and of these, over 4,000 were assessed with the audiometric screening technique advocated by Lamb and Graham (47). The intention was to study several variables: (1) the hearing loss patterns of a large state psychiatric hospital population; (2) the possible relationship between hearing loss and residency in a state mental hospital; (3) the appropriateness of sweep frequency audiometry with large psychiatric programs (because of its reliability and efficiency); and (4) the development of effective speech, hearing, and otologic services in a large state hospital program.

The incidence of hearing loss in the various age groups as shown in Table 11.1 indicates that there is a higher than average incidence of hearing

TABLE 11.1. INCIDENCE OF HEARING LOSS IN A LARGE STATE PSYCHIATRIC HOSPITAL*

Unit	*Total Population*	*Not Present*	*Total Screened***	*Passed*	*Failed*	*Difficult to Test*
1	780	135	645	297 (46%)	290 (45%)	58 (9%)
2	758	69	689	154 (22%)	272 (40%)	263 (38%)
3	524	62	462	134 (29%)	219 (47%)	109 (24%)
4	607	0	607	22 (2%)	62 (11%)	523 (87%)
5	126	0	126	90 (71%)	21 (16%)	15 (13%)
6	975	65	910	181 (20%)	488 (54%)	241 (26%)
7	746	59	687	203 (29%)	363 (53%)	121 (18%)
8	107	27	80	44 (55%)	33 (41%)	3 (4%)
9	114	53	61	22 (36%)	38 (62%)	1 (2%)
10	Cannot be done on a screening basis.					
Totals	4,737	470	4,267	1,147 (27%)	1,786 (42%)	1,334 (31%)

* The table shows the total population of each Unit, the number of patients on each Unit that were not present when screening was conducted, the total number of patients that were screened, as well as the number and percentage of patients in each of the three groups—Passed, Failed and Difficult to Test.

** *Percentages based upon total screened.*

impairment in a large state psychiatric hospital than would be found in nonpsychiatric samples from the community.

AUDITORY DYSFUNCTIONS IN MENTALLY ILL AND EMOTIONALLY DISTURBED CHILDREN

Ramsdell (66) emphasized that the auditory system is one of the primary sensory avenues that the individual utilizes in order to maintain contact with the environment. In previous discussions, it has been stressed that normal auditory capacity, acuity, and comprehension are needed in order for a child to develop normal language. However, in addition to the need for a normal sensory and integrative auditory pathway, it is also essential that the emotional status of the child not be severely impaired. A number of investigators have pointed out adequate auditory functioning cannot be separated from the overall affective behavior of the child. Kanner (37) points out that when a severe emotional conflict is present in the child, it can result in the loss of part or all of the normal auditory sensory behavior. If the affective disturbance occurs at an early enough age, it can result in the delay of oral language development (28, 38, 40, 56, 59). These authors suggest that certain psychological factors may have a critical effect upon speech development in the age range between six months and twenty-four months of age. Mowrer (59) suggests that the child does not associate sound in general with well being, and that this could impair the normal use of the auditory system and, in turn, affect oral language development.

CASE HISTORY AND CLINICAL OBSERVATION INFORMATION

Case history information obtained on adolescents agrees with much of the information reported on children who manifest psychological hearing impairments. It appears that all psychologically induced auditory disorders are primarily a defensive measure on the part of the child or adolescent to avoid threatening or punishing stimuli. Psychiatric opinion emphasizes that this type of psychologic reaction is an unconscious one and not volitional. These are some of the psychodynamic factors of the children and adolescents who have been examined at state hospital, mental health center, and state school programs and who were referred primarily because of an observable breakdown in auditory or expressive behavior.

Children and adolescents who have an auditory dysfunction due to emotional or mental disturbances do display certain patterns of behavior. Some individuals are very aggressive and domineering and oftentimes are also hyperactive. Conversely, large numbers of young children and adolescent patients are withdrawn and dissociated. Furthermore, certain types of emotional disorders are associated with psychologically induced hearing impairment more than others.

Kanner (37) described a severe emotional problem that appears in infancy and named it "*infantile autism.*" Mahler (56) reported in more detail on the behavior of the autistic child. He stated that infantile autism is often confused with peripheral deafness, since one of the outstanding symptoms of the autistic child is his absence of vocalization and his inattention to auditory stimuli. It would be well for the reader to also review some of the behavioral characteristics of the severely mentally retarded child. It will be apparent that it is easy to confuse infantile autism with the mental retardation syndrome.

Whatever the etiological factors are that produce autism, the audiologist should note certain salient developmental characteristics observed in these cases. The autistic child presents a history of involvement from the preverbal period but usually does not have any behavioral symptomology of identified central nervous system damage. Also important is the fact that verbal language is absent. Admittedly, there are some writers who feel that infantile autism cannot in most instances be explained on a psychological or psychiatric basis, but is due to an organic lesion of the central nervous system that is subclinical in nature.

Another major mental illness identified primarily with children and adults is childhood schizophrenia. Bender (4) has described the nature and cause of this emotional disturbance in young children. He mentions that this type of mentally disturbed child usually has had a fear of sound during infancy. Furthermore, since the child with schizophrenia may be unable to respond correctly to the usual standard audiometric tests, he is often labeled as having peripheral hearing impairment.

As in the case of the autistic child, the clinical audiologist is not primarily concerned with the psychodynamics that underly aberrant auditory behavior shown by the schizophrenic child. It is important that the clinician be aware of certain behavior of these children. Frequently, the history of this type of child will reveal that he has used hearing in a normal manner and that he has developed normal or near-normal oral language; but he has then become gradually or precipitously disturbed affectively with concomitant disturbances in expressive and receptive behavior. Childhood schizophrenia is often diagnosed between the ages of eighteen and thirty-six months, since the disturbance of speech, language, and hearing are often reported at this time and deafness and mental deficiency are suspected.

The examining audiologist must be aware that the schizophrenic child and adolescent may manifest what seems to be AUDITORY HALLUCINATIONS, although this is very difficult to determine and can only be inferred from some of the child's bizarre verbal and nonverbal behavior. The child's verbalizations are usually quite limited, but he may have had a history of normal language development during the first year or two of life. As the severity of the affective disorder increases, the child may demonstrate complete muteness. This is quite different from the mentally deficient, peripherally hard-of-hearing, and aphasic child who is rarely without some kind of vocalization or verbalization. Careful long-term observation of these children often reveals essentially normal auditory acuity and even normal oral language development.

Typically, the schizophrenic child does not attempt to speak and will not respond to the wide range of motivational techniques that the hearing and speech specialist usually employs with the nonverbal child. This resistance or inability to respond to a wide range of multisensory stimulation is strikingly different from the behavior of the mentally retarded, peripherally impaired, and brain-injured child. The schizophrenic child does not respond to sound in a consistent manner and does not use his hearing projectively. These children also do not use gesture like the mentally retarded and peripherally impaired child. He also does not use his voice to call his parents or siblings, but when he does vocalize, the acoustic characteristics of his voice are essentially normal. Basic emotional responses such as crying, laughing, and smiling are bizarre. These children may weep without tears and respond to apparent fantasy activity with inappropriate laughing and smiling.

It is not unusual for children to cry when brought to the clinic for a speech and hearing evaluation, since this is a somewhat threatening situation to many. The child with a severe affective disorder rarely, if ever, cries when he is brought into a strange situation. Furthermore, these children may not even cry in appropriate circumstances when they have been injured or hurt. These behavioral responses and characteristics must be carefully observed and noted by the examining clinician during the evaluation process.

Another outstanding behavioral characteristic of schizophrenic children is their lack of interest in face-to-face contact. There are some who will look at the face of the examining clinician but without apparent awareness. There is a manifest lack of eye contact. Generally, these schizophrenic individuals do not respond to tactile sensations. This contrasts sharply with the response of peripherally hard-of-hearing, mentally retarded, and aphasic children who do tend to respond in a compensatory manner. However, it would be well to note that some children with affective disorders do respond to tactile stimulation.

The child with affective disorders appears to have a reasonably good motor ability. The majority of the patients this author has examined and observed appear to be relatively healthy. Inspection of the child's case history often shows that motor development was within the normal range during the first year or two of life, and observation of current behavior shows that they are capable of doing many of the common self-care tasks, such as eating, drinking, and dressing, with no apparent difficulty. This is in contrast to the mentally deficient child who shows a delay commensurate with the amount of overall retardation.

Socially, the child diagnosed as autistic or schizophrenic exhibits consistently aberrant social perception and response. They tend to behave as though other people are not present. These children also play in a manner that is not normal for their ages. Kanner (38) states that they are likely to prefer plain blocks, which they use to construct complicated designs and patterns. They often will play with these blocks for long periods of time without interruption.

AUDITORY TESTING

Repeatable responses to standard audiometric tests (pure-tone and speech) are difficult to obtain from these emotionally disturbed children. The examining audiologist must be very observant, since the subject often gives only one response or indication of having heard the sound stimuli. In general, it is very difficult to place earphones on this type of child or adolescent and to obtain reliable responses to pure-tone or speech stimuli. The best test procedure employs various types of sound field stimuli (noise, tapes, or phonograph records of animal sounds, whispered speech, and noise-makers). Significant responses are often observed when stimuli are presented at very low intensity levels. As a matter of procedure, it is far better to begin formal testing in a sound field environment presenting stimuli by an ascending method rather than by the typical descending method that is used when testing the peripherally deafened and the mentally retarded child. Whereas play-conditioned audiometry is very effective with the mentally retarded and peripherally deafened, it is consistently not effective with this type of emotionally disturbed person.

Whenever the clinical audiologist has obtained reliable information on the auditory system for acuity or comprehension, he must be extremely careful not to inform the patient directly that he is aware that the patient has normal hearing. This is especially true with the adult psychiatric patient who seems to have a hearing loss and firmly believes that he does have a hearing problem. This information must be conveyed to the psychiatrist or medical staff member who has overall responsibility for the management and treatment of the psychiatric patient. This information can then be combined with other multidisciplinary evaluation and treatment findings.

In summary, it can be stated that the primary responsibility of the clinical audiologist with the emotionally disturbed patient is to find out if any organic hearing impairment is present and then to identify the type and degree. Proper referrals should then be made to the psychiatrist with appropriate recommendations for possible aural rehabilitation programming, if the overall status of the patient permits this type of treatment.

PROGRAM CONSIDERATIONS

Complete audiological facilities and a full clinical audiology staff are available at a few large psychiatric institutes, as well as some mental health centers, to provide the necessary evaluation and treatment. A number of mentally ill and emotionally disturbed patients have been found to have marked hearing impairment (otosclerosis, sensori-neural losses, and all other types of hearing impairment) who can and have profited from an intensive otoaudiologic program and from intensive aural rehabilitation services.

Psychiatric and medical personnel have reported to this author some remarkable changes in the affective behavior of a number of patients who heretofore had been unreachable by counseling and psychotherapy. In fact, one twenty-eight-year-old depressive woman, who had been reporting head noises and was very withdrawn and confused, was found to have a maximum conductive hearing loss due to advanced otosclerosis. After audiometric screening, air- and bone-conduction threshold testing, and speech audiometry, she was scheduled for corrective surgery. As a result of successful middle-ear surgery, the air-bone gap was closed to the point where she had a 15-decibel 500 to 2,000 average hearing level. The ward psychiatrist pointed out there was a marked change in behavior, that the patient became more outgoing and no longer reported the awareness of ear ringing and certain other head noises, which the psychiatrist had incorrectly attributed to auditory hallucinations.

This anecdote along with the high incidence of communicative disorders among the mentally ill should convince the hearing and speech specialist that here is a relatively untapped area for the development of extensive rehabilitation programming. Traditionally, speech pathologists and audiologists have tended to avoid or neglect the mentally ill and emotionally disturbed except in a few programs. This is most unfortunate. Many of these patients are prevented from returning to useful socioeconomic function and from experiencing possible recovery from their psychiatric disorders because their receptive or expressive disorder may be far more handicapping than their basic problem. This is especially evident in the adolescent and young adult psychiatric populations who need every asset in order to reenter society as adjusted and contributing members.

Therefore, the speech pathologist and audiologist should give serious thought to the development of quality clinical programs for the evaluation and treatment of the mentally ill and mentally disturbed patient with communication disorders. Furthermore, university training programs should include the availability of clinical practicum experience with these types of patients. Lastly, the research on auditory problems of this population must be greatly expanded.

There are a relatively small number of state hospitals and mental health clinics that have an available speech pathology and audiology resident staff. However, only one state, Illinois (Rittmanic, 69), have provided a statewide speech and hearing program which has the responsibility for providing clinical training, and research programs in speech pathology and audiology.

Therefore, it would seem that state departments of public health and mental health should give serious consideration to the initiation and development of statewide speech and hearing programs to serve their psychiatric population. Although there is a limited amount of information available at present on the extent of communication disorders among this population, it is still sufficient to furnish administrators and program staff with the backup information they need to justify the recruitment of qualified personnel, the purchase of necessary equipment, and the provision of space. The contribution of the hearing and speech specialists to the multidisciplinary evaluation and treatment team of the psychiatric hospital or mental health clinic has been found to be a meaningful and important one.

The minimum level of preparation for a person hired to organize and supervise a speech and hearing service for a mental health state hospital or state school program should be a Master's degree in speech pathology or audiology, and at least four years' clinical experience. This recommendation is based on the author's first-hand experience with staff who have had lesser academic training and experience. The type of cases encountered, the need for advanced theoretical information and professional experience, the requirement for working with other highly trained staff, and the inherent difficulty of diagnosing and treating the cases have shown that a staff trained only on the undergraduate level and with minimum or no experience is not adequate. This results in a disservice to the patient, to the multidisciplinary team, and to the speech and hearing specialist himself.

Adequate equipment and facilities for speech therapy activities should be provided at any mental health facility. There should also be audiometric test suites with equipment that will provide for both sound field and earphone testing by pure-tone and speech stimuli. This is especially important for the pre- and postotological testing and also for the differential diagnosis of organic and nonorganic hearing impairments that are found among the psychiatrically disturbed.

Glossary

ADAPTIVE BEHAVIOR Problem-solving behavior.

APHASIC SYNDROME Language disturbances resulting from brain damage. Symbolic functioning (speech comprehension and oral language usage) may be impaired.

ASPHYXIA Suffocation; also, suspended animation from suffocation.

AUDITORY EVOKED POTENTIAL A detectable acoustically stimulated electrical change, recorded from a part of the brain.

AUDITORY HALLUCINATIONS Subjective auditory sensations, such as hearing voices and responding as if the voices were real.

AUROPALPEBRAL REFLEX (APR) The eyeblink response characterized by either a slight or a very marked drawing of the eyelids together.

CENTRAL AUDITORY DYSFUNCTION Auditory dysfunction caused by a lesion in the auditory pathways to the brain, i.e., cochlear nucleus to the temporal lobe.

CHOLESTEATOMA A cystic mass with a lining of stratified squamous epithelium, usually of keratinizing type, filled with desquamating debris frequently including cholesterol. Steatomas occur in the meninges, the central nervous system, and in the bones of the skull, but are most common in the middle-ear and mastoid region.

DIFFERENTIAL HISTORY The collation and interpretation of specific case history information obtained by each specialist involved in the evaluation of a particular patient.

DYSPHASIA Impairment of speech, consisting in lack of coordination and failure to arrange words in their proper order.

EDUCABLE RETARDED Many state education codes define educable mentally retarded children as those incapable of doing normal class work. Also, the IQ range of 50 to 75 may often be used as a classification criterion.

ELECTROPHYSIOLOGIC AUDIOMETRY A means of measuring hearing that uses observed bodily changes in electrical reactions which result from acoustic stimulation.

ELECTROPHYSIOLOGIC TECHNIQUES Electrodermal audiometry, electroencephalographic audiometry, and auditory evoked potential.

ENCEPHALITIS Inflammation of the brain.

ETIOLOGY The study or theory of the causation of any disease; the sum of knowledge regarding causes.

GENETIC Mode of development.

HABILITATION The development of capabilities or skills not previously possessed.

HEREDITY Organic resemblance based on descent.

IDENTIFICATION AUDIOMETRY The utilization of audiometric screening tests to discover hearing loss.

INFANTILE AUTISM Infants who appear severely dissociated from interpersonal relationships.

MENINGITIS Inflammation of the meninges.

MONGOLISM A condition characterized by a small, anteroposteriorly flattened skull; a short, flat-bridged nose; epicanthus; short phalanges; and a widened space between the first and second digits of hands and feet, with moderate to severe mental retardation, and associated with a chromosomal abnormality.

MORO REFLEX This reaction is characterized by symmetrical movements. The arms are extended, spread, and then adducted with the fingers spread and half-flexed. The legs are extended and the toes bent. This embracing motion of the arms and general muscle tension is usually accompanied by a cry.

MUTISM Inability or refusal to speak.

MYRINGOTOMY Surgical incision of the membrana tympani.

NATAL Pertaining to birth.

NEONATE A newborn infant.

NONORGANIC HEARING IMPAIRMENT Any auditory disturbance with no apparent anatomical or physiological causation.

OTOAUDIOLOGICAL SCREENING The use of otological screening tests and audiometric screening tests to discover hearing loss.

OTOSCLEROSIS The formation of spongy bone in the capsule of the labyrinth of the ear.

PERINATAL Pertaining to or occurring in the period shortly before and after birth; in medical statistics, this period is generally considered to begin with completion of twenty-eight weeks of gestation and is variously defined as ending one to four weeks after birth.

PERIPHERAL Pertaining to or situated at or near the periphery (the outward part or surface).

PHENYLKETONURIA (PKU) A congenital faulty metabolism of phenylalanine, because of which phenylpyruvic acid appears in the urine. This condition will result in severe mental retardation if not detected and corrected very early in life.

PRENATAL Existing or occurring before birth.

PROGNOSTIC Affording an indication as to prognosis (a forecast of the probable result of an attack of disease; the prospect of recovery from a disease as indicated by the nature and symptoms of the case).

PSYCHODYNAMICS The science of mental processes.

PSYCHOSOCIAL HANDICAPPING LOSS A degree of hearing loss which is severe enough to adversely affect the individual's personal and social behavior.

REHABILITATION Assistance in restoring a person to a former capacity. It may involve diagnostic and treatment services.

RELIABLE Self-consistent.

RH INCOMPATIBILITY Serologic incompatibility between the fetus and the mother.

RUBELLA An acute exanthematous febrile virus disease with an eruption not unlike that of measles.

SCHIZOPHRENIA Bleuler's term for dementia praecox which, according to his interpretation, represents a cleavage or fissuration of the mental functions.

STAPEDIAL REFLEX Loud acoustic stimulation causes the stapedius muscle to contract. Indirect observations include movements of the malleus or drum membrane, air pressure changes in the middle ear cavity, fluid changes in the labyrinth, and changes in ear impedance.

STARTLE REFLEX This reaction is evoked by a loud sound. It is characterized by throwing of the hands and feet, eye closing, forward movement of the trunk, forward head thrust, contraction of the abdomen and neck, and promotion of the lower arms.

SYMPTOMATOLOGY The systematic discussion of symptoms.

SYNDROME A set of symptoms which occur together; the sum of signs of any morbid state; a symptom complex.

SYNTHESIS The combination of separate elements into a whole.

TOXEMIA A general intoxication due to the absorption of bacterial products (toxins) formed at a local source of infection.

TYMPANECTOMY Excision of the tympanic membrane.

VALID Basically a test is valid when it measures what it is presumed to measure.

Bibliography

1. Atkinson, C. J. "Perceptual and responsive abilities of mentally retarded children as measured by several auditory threshold tests." *Perceptual and Response Abilities of Mentally Retarded Children.* U.S. Office of Education, Cooperative Research Project No. 176 (6471), Southern Illinois University, Carbondale, Illinois, 1–47, 1960.
2. Barker, F. B. "Impaired hearing in psychotic patients: A pilot study." Mental Hospital of Rochester State Hospital, Rochester, Minnesota, **15**: 434–35, 1964.
3. Barr, B. "Pure tone audiometry for pre-school children: A preliminary report." *Acta Oto-Laryngologica,* Supplement 110: 89–92, 1954.
4. Bender, L. "Childhood schizophrenia." *American Journal of Orthopsychiatry,* **17**: 40–44, 1947.
5. Benoit, E. P. "Toward a new definition of mental retardation." *American Journal of Mental Deficiency,* **63**: 559–65, 1959.
6. Birch, J. W. and J. Mathews. "The hearing of mental defectives: Its measurement and characteristics." *American Journal of Mental Deficiency,* **55**: 384–93, 1951.
7. Bradley, E., W. E. Evans, and A. M. Worthington. "The relationship between administration time for audiometric testing and the mental ability of mentally deficient children." *American Journal of Mental Deficiency,* **60**: 346–53, 1955.
8. Buhler, C. *The First Year of Life.* New York: John Day Publishing Company, 1930.
9. Bzoch, K. *An Investigation of the Speech of Pre-school Cleft Palate Children.* Ph.D. Thesis, Northwestern University, 1956.
10. Cody, D. T. R. and R. Bickford. "Cortical audiometry: An objective method of evaluating auditory acuity in man." *Mayo Clinic Proceedings,* **40**: 273–87, 1965.
11. Denmark, F. G. W. "A development of the peep-show audiometer." *Journal of Laryngology and Otology,* **64**: 357–60, 1950.
12. Despert, L. "Psychotherapy in childhood schizophrenia." *American Journal of Psychiatry,* **104**: 36–40, 1947.
13. DiCarlo, L. M. and W. H. Bradley. "A simplified auditory test for infants and young children." *Laryngoscope,* **71**: 628–33, 1961.
14. Dix, M. R. and C. S. Hallpike. "Peep-show: new technique for pure-tone audiometry in young children." *British Medical Journal,* **2**: 719–24, 1947.
15. Doll, E. A. "The essentials of an inclusive concept of mental deficiency." *American Journal of Mental Deficiency,* **46**: 214–19, 1941.
16. Downs, M. P. and G. Sterritt. "Identification audiometry for neonates: A preliminary report." *Journal of Audiological Research,* **4**: 69–80, 1964.
17. Ewing, I. R. and A. W. G. Ewing. "The ascertainment of Deafness in infancy and early childhood." *Journal of Laryngology and Otology,* **59**: 309–14, 1944.
18. Ewing, I. and A. Ewing. *Opportunity and the Deaf Child.* University of London Press, London, England, 1947.
19. Ewing, I. *Educational Guidance and the Deaf Child.* A. W. G. Ewing, ed., Manchester University Press, Manchester, England, 1958.

20. Foale, M. and J. Paterson. "The hearing of mental defectives." *American Journal of Mental Deficiency*, **59**: 254–58, 1954.
21. Frisina, D. R. "Measurement of hearing in children." J. Jerger, ed., *Modern Developments in Audiology*, New York and London: Academic Press, 126–66, 1963.
22. Froding, C. "Acoustic investigation of newborn infants." *Acta Oto-Laryngologica*, **52**: 31–46, 1960.
23. Froeschels, E. and H. Beebe. "Testing hearing of newborn infants." *Archives of Otolaryngology*, **44**: 710–15, 1946.
24. Fulton, R. T. *Psychogalvanic Skin Response and Conditioned Orientation Reflex Audiometry with Mentally Retarded Children*, Ph.D. Thesis, Purdue University, 1962.
25. Fulton, R. T. and J. T. Graham. "Pure tone reliability with the mentally retarded." *American Journal of Mental Deficiency*, **69**: 256–68, 1964.
26. Gaines, J. A. L. *A Comparison of Two Audiometric Tests Administered to a Group of Mentally Retarded Children.* M. A. Thesis, University of Nebraska, 1961.
27. Gesell, A. and C. Armatruda. *Developmental Diagnosis*, New York: Harper and Row, Publishers (Hoeber), 1947.
28. Gesell, A., Halverson, H. M., Thompson, H., Frances, L., Burton, M. C., Ames, L. B., and Amatruda, C. S. *The First Five Years of Life*, New York: Harper and Row, Publishers, 1940.
29. Geyer, M. and A. Yankauer. *Journal of Exceptional Children*, **72**: 723–26, 1957.
30. Goldstein, R. "Electrophysiologic audiometry." J. Jerger, ed., *Modern Developments in Audiology*, Academic Press: New York, London, 168–90, 1963.
31. Green, M. and J. B. Richard. *Pediatric Diagnosis*, Philadelphia and London: W. B. Saunders Company, 1954.
32. Guilford, F. and O. Haug. "Diagnosis of deafness in the very young child." *American Medical Association Archives of Otolaryngology*, **55**: 101–6, 1952.
33. Hardy, W. and M. Pauls. "Significance of problems of conditioning in GSR audiometry." *Journal of Speech and Hearing Disorders*, **24**: 123–26, 1959.
34. Irwin, J. B., J. E. Hind, and A. E. Aronson. "Experience with conditioned GSR audiometry in a group of mentally deficient individuals." *Training School Bulletin*, Training School at Vineland, New Jersey, **54**: 26–31, 1957.
35. Jervis, G. S. "Medical aspects of mental deficiency." *American Journal of Mental Deficiency*, **57**: 175–88, 1952.
36. Johnston, P. W. and M. J. Farrell. "Auditory Impairment among resident school children at the Walter E. Fernald State School." *American Journal of Mental Deficiency*, **58**: 640–43, 1954.
37. Kanner, L. "Autistic disturbances of affective content." *Nervous Child*, **2**: 217–21, 1943.
38. Kanner, L. "Early infantile autism." *Journal of Pediatrics*, **25**: 211–17, 1944.
39. Kanner, L. *Child Psychiatry*, Springfield, Illinois: Charles C. Thomas, 1948.
40. Kanner, L. "A discussion of early infantile autism." *Digest of Neurology and Psychiatry*, **29**: 158–62, 1951.
41. Karlin, I. W. and M. Strazzula. "Speech and language problems of mentally deficient children." *Journal of Speech and Hearing Disorders*, **17**: 286–94, 1952.
42. Keaster, J. "A quantitative method of testing the hearing of young children." *Journal of Speech and Hearing Disorders*, **12**: 159–60, 1947.

43. Kodman, F., Jr., A. Fein, and A. Mixson. "Psychogalvanic skin response audiometry with severe mentally retarded children." *American Journal of Mental Deficiency*, **64**: 131–36, 1959.
44. Kodman, F., Jr., T. R. Powers, P. P. Philip, and G. M. Weller. "An investigation of hearing loss in mentally retarded children and adults." *American Journal of Mental Deficiency*, **63**: 460–63, 1958.
45. Kopatic, N. J. "The reliability of pure-tone audiometry with the mentally retarded: Some practical and theoretical considerations." *Training School Bulletin*, Training School at Vineland, New Jersey, **60**: 130–36, 1963.
46. LaCrosse, E. L. and H. Bidlake. "A method to test the hearing of mentally retarded children." *Volta Review*, **66**: 27–30, 1964.
47. Lamb, L. E. and J. T. Graham. "Audiometric screening in a psychiatric hospital." *Journal of Auditory Research*, **3**: 338–49, 1963.
48. Lloyd, L. L. and M. Reid. *The Percent of Hearing Impaired and Difficult to test Patients at Parsons State Hospital and Training Center*. A special report presented at the March Audiology Conference, 1965. (More complete data is scheduled for analysis and subsequent reporting later as Parsons Demonstration Project Report No. 47.)
49. Lloyd, L. L. and J. Melrose. "Inter-method comparisons of selected audiometric measures used with normal hearing mentally retarded children." *Journal of Audiological Research*, **6**: 205–17 (a), 1966.
50. Lloyd, L. L. and E. R. Frisina. *Audiologic Assessment of the Mentally Retarded: Proceedings of a National Conference*. University of Kansas, Bureau of Child Research and the Parsons State Hospital and Training Center, 1965.
51. Lloyd, L. L. "Behavioral audiometry viewed as an operant procedure." *Journal of Speech and Hearing Disorders*, **31**: 128–36, 1966.
52. Lowell, E., G. Rushford, G. Hoverston, and M. Stoner. "Evaluation of pure-tone audiometry with pre-school age children." *Journal of Speech and Hearing Disorders*, **21**: 292–302, 1956.
53. McCoy, D. F. and W. H. Plotkin. "Audiometric screening of a psychiatric population in a large state hospital." *Journal of Auditory Research*, **7**: 327–34, 1967.
54. McIntire, M. S., F. J. Menolascino, and J. H. Wiley. "Mongolism—some clinical aspects." *American Journal of Mental Deficiency*, **69**: 794–800, 1965.
55. MacPherson, J. B. *The Evaluation and Development of Techniques for Testing the Auditory Acuity of Trainable Mentally Retarded Children*. Ph.D. Thesis, University of Texas, 1960.
56. Mahler, M. S. "On child psychosis in schizophrenia; autistic and symbiotic infantile psychosis." *Psychoanalytic Study of the Child*, New York, International Universities Press, 7, 1952.
57. Melmer, P. E. *The Speech Characteristics of a Selected Group of Institutionalized Mentally Retarded Children of School Age*. M. A. Thesis, University of Nebraska, 1958.
58. Moss, J. W., M. Moss, and J. Tizard. "Electrodermal response audiometry with mentally defective children." *Journal of Speech and Hearing Research*, **4**: 41–47, 1961.
59. Mowrer, O. H. *Learning Theory and Personality Dynamics*, New York: The Ronald Press, 1950.

60. Myklebust, H. *Auditory Disorders in Children*, New York, Grune and Stratton, Inc., 1954.
61. Nelson, W. E. *Textbook of Pediatrics*, Philadelphia and London: W. B. Saunders Company, 1964.
62. Page, R. Superintendent, Illinois Office of the Superintendent of Public Instruction. *Rules and Regulations to Govern the Administration and Operation of Special Education*, 1964.
63. Pantelakos, C. G. "Audiometric and otolaryngologic survey of retarded students." *North Carolina Medical Journal*, **24**: 238–42, 1963.
64. Price, L. L. and R. Goldstein. "Averaged evoked responses for measuring auditory sensitivity in children." *Journal of Speech and Hearing Disorders*, **31**: 248–56, 1966.
65. Price, L. L., B. Rosenblut, R. Goldstein, and D. C. Shepherd. "The averaged evoked response to auditory stimulation." *Journal of Speech and Hearing Research*, **9**: 361–70, 1966.
66. Ramsdell, D. A. "The psychology of the hard of hearing and the deafened adult." H. Davis, ed., *Hearing and Deafness*, New York: Murray Hill Books, 1947.
67. Rigrodski, S., F. Prunty, and L. Glovsky. "A study of the incidence, types and associated etiologies of hearing loss in an institutionalized mentally retarded population." *Training School Bulletin*, Training School at Vineland, New Jersey, **58**: 30–44, 1961.
68. Rittmanic, P. A. "Hearing rehabilitation for the institutionalized mentally retarded." *American Journal of Mental Deficiency*, **63**: 778–83, 1959.
69. Rittmanic, P. A. "A state-wide speech and hearing program for the mentally retarded and mentally ill." *Journal of the American Speech and Hearing Association*, **8**: 182–87, 1966.
70. Rittmanic, P. A. *Audiological Aspects of Mental Retardation*, presented at the Illinois Speech and Hearing Association Annual Convention, 1966.
71. Rothstein, J. H., ed., *Mental Retardation*, New York: Holt, Rinehart and Winston, 1962.
72. Roy, R. *Incidence and Severity of Hearing Loss of Institutionalized Mentally Retarded Adults of Various Intelligence Levels.* M.A. Thesis, University of Nebraska, 1959.
73. Schlanger, B. B. "Speech examination of a group of institutionalized mentally handicapped children." *Journal of Speech and Hearing Disorders*, **18**: 339–50, 1953.
74. Schlanger, B. B. *Speech Therapy With Slow Learning Children.* Unpublished report: Division of Mental Hygiene, State Department of Public Welfare, Wisconsin, 1953 (b).
75. Schlanger, B. B. and R. Gottsleben. "Testing the hearing of the mentally retarded." *Journal of Speech and Hearing Disorders*, **21**: 487–93, 1956.
76. Schlanger, B. B. "The speech and hearing program at the training school." *Training School Bulletin*, Training School at Vineland, New Jersey, **53**: 262–72 (10), 1957.
77. Schlanger, B. B. and R. Gottsleben. "Testing the hearing of the mentally retarded." *Training School Bulletin*, Training School at Vineland, New Jersey, **54**: 21–25 (8), 1957.
78. Schlanger, B. B. "Effects of listening training on auditory thresholds of

mentally retarded children." *Journal of the American Speech and Hearing Association*, **8**: 273–75, 1962.

79. Schlanger, B. B. and N. J. Christensen. "Effects of training upon audiometry with the mentally retarded." *American Journal of Mental Deficiency*, **68**: 469–75, 1964.
80. Shimizu, H. and F. Nakamura. "Pure-tone audiometry in children; lantern-slide test." *Annals of Otology, Rhinology and Laryngology*, **66**: 392–98, 1957.
81. Siegenthaler, B. and Doris Krzwicki. "Incidence and patterns of hearing loss among an adult mentally retarded population." *American Journal of Mental Deficiency*, **64**: 444–49, 1959.
82. Skinner, B. F. *Science and Human Behavior*, New York: Appleton-Century-Crofts, 1953.
83. Spradlin, J. E. "Operant principles applied to audiometry with severely retarded children." Lloyd and Frisina, eds., *The Audiologic Assessment of the Mentally Retarded, Proceedings of a National Conference*, University of Kansas Bureau of Child Research and Parsons State Hospital and Training Center, 1965.
84. Sprinkle, P., G. S. Fitz-Hugh, G. Harden, and D. Waldren. "Incidence of hearing loss and otolaryngologic disorders in consecutive admissions to a state mental hospital." *Virginia Medical Monthly*, **92**: 124–29, 1965.
85. Statten, P. and D. E. S. Wishart. "Pure-tone audiometry in young children; psychogalvanic skin resistance and peep show." *Annals of Otology, Rhinology and Laryngology*, **65**: 511–34, 1956.
86. Tredgold, A. F. *A Textbook of Mental Deficiency*, 7th edition, Williams and Wilkins, Baltimore, Maryland, 1947.
87. Waldon, E. F. "The baby cry test: A new audiometric technique for testing very young children." B. Prowrie, ed., *Proceedings of International Congress on Education of the Deaf, and the 41st Meeting of the Convention of American Instructors of the Deaf*, 1963. U.S. Government Printing Office, No. 106, Gallaudet College, Washington, D.C., 1964.
88. Watkins, E. O., J. H. Steward, and M. D. Ryan. "A novel hearing test for retardates with mental ages below four years." *American Journal of Mental Deficiency*, **71**: 396–400, 1966.
89. Webb, C., S. Kinde, B. Weber, and R. Beedle. *Procedures for Evaluating the Hearing of the Mentally Retarded*, U.S. Office of Education, Cooperative Research Project No. 1731, Central Michigan University, Mt. Pleasant, Michigan, 1964.
90. Wedenberg, E. "Auditory tests on newborn infants." *Acta Oto-Laryngologica*, **46**: 446–49, 1956.
91. Wiley, J. H. and G. Jacobs. "The incidence and characteristics of hearing loss in an institutionalized, mildly retarded population." L. L. Lloyd and D. R. Frisina, *The Audiologic Assessment of the Mentally Retarded: The Proceedings of a National Conference*. Parsons, Kansas: Speech and Hearing Department at Parsons State Hospital and Training Center, 1965. (This study is not reported in Appendix C but it was cited as the source of the studies reported as No. 12 and No. 17.)
92. Wolfe, W. G. and J. R. MacPherson. *The Evaluation and Development of Techniques for Testing the Auditory Acuity of Trainable Mentally Retarded Children*. U.S. Office of Education, Cooperative Research Project No. 172, University of Texas, Austin, Texas, 1959.

12

Electroencephalic Audiometry

Geary A. McCandless, Ph.D.

Electroencephalic Audiometry

Numerous attempts have been made to utilize physiological measures for assessing hearing sensitivity in those humans who, because of age or other factors, fail to respond to conventional audiometric tests. Some of the so-called "objective" tests have monitored changes in heart rate (42), blood pressure, pupillary dilation, and cochlear potentials (39), to determine hearing sensitivity. However, none of these tests has received general acceptance in clinical use. The most widely used test that relies on autonomic responses is electrodermal audiometry described in 1947 (29, 14). Since these initial reports, much has been written on the potential use of electrodermal audiometry (16). A main drawback to this test is the disturbing effect it may have on children, since its administration is dependent upon the introduction of a noxious shock stimulus for conditioning.

Recently much attention has been directed toward various measures of electrical activity within the central nervous system as a possible means of assessing hearing function. Such tests are based on the observation that small changes appear in the ongoing electrical activity of the brain when a sensory stimulus is introduced to an intact auditory system. Compared with other physiological measures, the recording of brain potentials is a relatively recent development. The first electroencephalographic recordings (EEG) from human brains were made in Germany by Hans Berger in 1924 and were published in 1929 (2). Since that time the technique has been widely used clinically in the diagnosis of epilepsy and brain damage.

More recently, physiologists have attempted to "decode" the EEG recording in an attempt to evaluate the possible relationship of the electrical activity of the brain to behavioral, subjective experiences in man. One way this relationship can be studied is to examine how the brain responds to the presentation of controlled sensory stimuli such as flashes of light, tactile stimuli, or sound. The resulting electrical potentials from the brain are commonly referred to as *cortically evoked responses* and can be measured from many recording sites on the head. In applying these measures to audiometry, hearing sensitivity is determined by eliciting an auditory electroencephalic response (ER) from the subject without depending on his subjective response.

The evoked cortical response in man was first described by P. A. Davis (10), who used auditory, visual, and tactile stimuli, and labeled the response the "K Complex." Because the electroencephalic response was seen to arise principally from an area at or near the vertex of the head, it was later called the "vertex" or "V potential" (1). In fact, this response is quite diffuse and can be measured over most of the head. It may be described as "non-sensory specific" since it can be elicited by any sensory modality, visual, tactile, auditory, or olfactory (17, 22). The response waveform is similar in general pattern for all types of stimuli, but there are some minor waveform and latency differences for specific modalities. The actual central pathways and structures which mediate a response to auditory stimuli are not known at present, but because of the long latencies this response may be represented by associative structures in addition to the primary auditory projections areas of the temporal lobe.

Characteristics of the Electroencephalic Auditory Response

An idealized response is characterized by a polyphasic wave having fairly consistent latencies (Figure 12.1), but any single response may contain only a portion of the characteristic peaks. The negative and positive peaks and valleys have been labeled P_1, N_1, P_2, and N_2. Typical latencies of the specific peaks in the response for a 2,000-Hz tone at 60-dB sensation level are $P_1 = 50$ msec, $N_1 = 100$ msec, $P_2 = 175$ msec, $N_2 = 300$ msec (12, 32, 8). The amplitude of individual responses rarely exceeds 20 microvolts. Components earlier than 75 msec are sometimes seen but are very small and difficult to visualize. Some investigators report the early response components that appear 10 to 75 msec following stimulus onset may reflect myogenic activity from muscles attached to the skull (3). More recently Ruhm and his associates (40) indicate that the early components do indeed reflect cortical activity.

Electroencephalic responses to auditory stimuli appear generally similar in waveform for all subjects. There are, however, subtle individual differences which are highly reproducible over long periods of time—even years.

An important characteristic of the evoked potential is that it can be initiated by any sudden change in the sensory environment. This fact suggests that the associated underlying mechanism is a "change detector." Its function is to alter or orient the brain to abrupt change in the sensory input. For example, an evoked off-response can be seen at the termination of a stimulus that lasts longer than about 500 msec (10, 36). Likewise, an evoked response can be produced when a tone of 1,000 Hz is suddenly changed to a 2,000 Hz tone of the same loudness. Similar evoked responses can be obtained by changes in sound intensity (28).

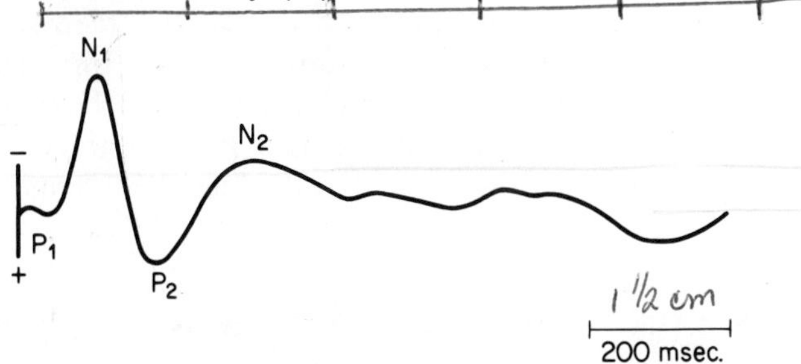

FIGURE 12.1 A typical electroencephalic response in an adult to a 2,000 Hz tone at 60-dB sensation level.

Early Electroencephalic Response Tests of Auditory Function

Since presentations of sound stimuli to the ear were found to produce predictable changes in the EEG tracing, this technique was naturally evolved to be used for testing hearing acuity on subjects unable or unwilling to respond to conventional hearing tests. This technique lay unused for over twenty-five years following its discovery. During this period the use of the EEG as a diagnostic clinical tool had become well established in the detection of brain tumors, epilepsy, or other pathological changes which alter the on-going rhythms of electrical brain activity. Marcus (22) reported using the raw EEG technique to determine hearing function in a group of seventy-one young children suspected of having hearing disorders or abnormal speech and language development. By comparing the "arousal response" on the EEG tracing with the intensity of a sound stimulus, Marcus was able to determine when a child did or did not hear. The stimuli he used to elicit responses were uncalibrated, i.e., the mother's voice, a drum, police whistle, cow bell, and pitch pipes. These gross stimuli did not permit a fine determination of auditory acuity; nonetheless valuable diagnostic information was provided which might have otherwise been unattainable in very young children.

Later Derbyshire and McDermott (13) refined the technique of EEG audiometry by presenting pure tones of known intensity to subjects. Successive presentations were lowered in intensity, and later the recordings were read and a threshold assigned as being the lowest level at which a response could be visualized on the conventional EEG recording. Further, these authors described four distinct changes in the ER which could be observed when a sound was presented to the ear: (1) an "on" effect; (2) an "off" effect; (3) an increase or reduction in voltage; and (4) late effects that are reflected by a change in the overall sleep level.

In spite of early successes, the EEG-audiometric technique was not widely used. One reason was undoubtedly the fact that the ER to auditory stimuli were highly variable and not readily apparent from one stimulus to the next, using conventional EEG recordings (Figure 12.2). In addition, it was difficult to separate the response from the background of ongoing cortical activity, since the response becomes smaller in amplitude as the test stimulus is decreased to near threshold.

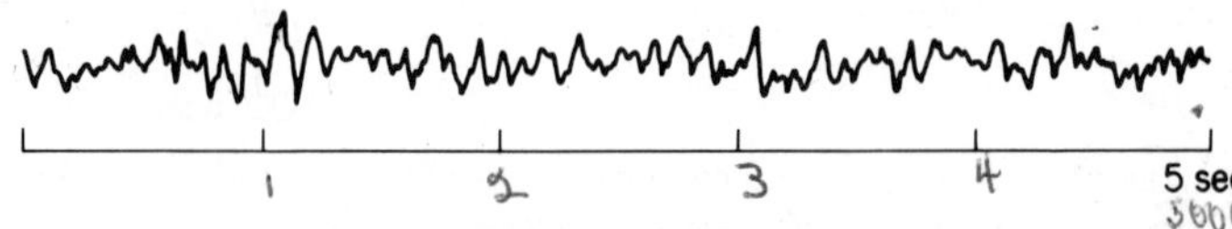

FIGURE 12.2 A series of electroencephalic responses as seen in a conventional EEG recording. Five auditory clicks were presented at an 80-dB sensation level at one-second intervals as shown on the time base marker.

Extracting the Electroencephalic Response to Sensory Stimuli from Background Activity

AVERAGED ELECTROENCEPHALIC RESPONSES (AER)

Certain neurophysiological data often appear to be unpredictable and quite random. However, when proper techniques are used, these events that at first appear to be disorganized or unrelated begin to assume a degree of order. Sometimes when single events seem to have little meaning, we say that *on the average* certain things occur. Applying this "average" principle to the avoked response phenomenon, we find that a response cannot always be seen in raw EEG recordings each time a sensory stimulus is introduced. At one moment it may be clearly observable, while at another only a portion or none of the response can be seen. Subtle changes in the ongoing activity of the brain often appear to be random and unrelated to any specific sensory event such as the hearing of a sound. This fact made the clinical use of raw EEG recordings difficult because the response representing a change in cortical activity was frequently lost in the biological noise that is part of the normal active brain.

Dawson reported using a method of photographic superimposition to enhance a time-locked response when somatosensory stimuli were used (11). This technique is illustrated in Figure 12.3. The characteristic ER with its rather definitive features can be seen clearly in contrast to the random brain activity. Only those changes related to the click are reproduced in a consistent time relationship to the stimulus onset. The portions of the spontaneous EEG activity unrelated to the stimulus are minimized. The constant time relationship of the evoked potential to the onset of the stimulus makes an averaging or summing process feasible.

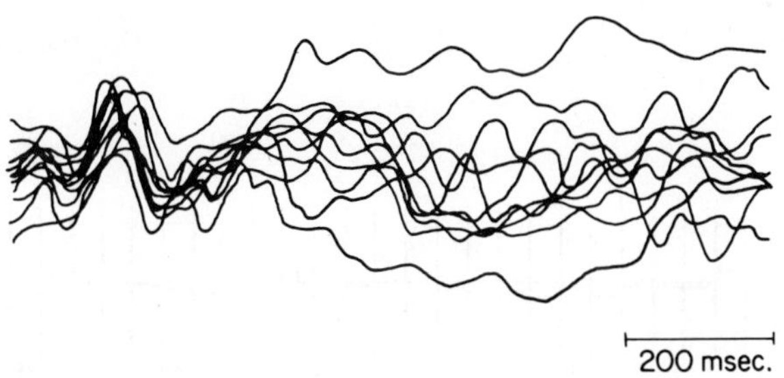

FIGURE 12.3 A superimposition of ten individual responses. The characteristics of the responses emerge as a dark envelope during the first 300 msec following the stimulus. The later EEG activity is clearly more random.

SUMMING COMPUTERS

The recent advent of high-speed electronic computers has made possible the electronic averaging or summing of ER from background electrical activity. Geisler et al. (15) first studied the evoked response to clicks by using a computer. They were able to see the summed responses at as low a level as 5-dB SL, thus pointing up the possible use of the computer as a method of testing auditory function.

Technically, most computers do not "average" the electroencephalic response, since the term "average" denotes first summing the responses then dividing them by the number of stimuli. Rather, most computers in use today are summing devices which, through a process of algebraic addition, extract the time-related cortical events and diminish the amplitude of the more random ongoing electrical activity. As each stimulus is presented to the ear, the computer is programmed to sort or add into a series of separate bins or channels the voltage at any moment for a specified time following the stimulus onset. Each bin represents a specific time period after the onset of the stimulus. The computer "remembers" or stores the instantaneous voltage of the signals in its memory bank. The memory bank is composed of the entire collection of time bins, i.e., each bin of the computer is time-locked to a specific poststimulus time. Electrical activity from the brain that is unrelated to the stimuli will cancel out, since one can expect approximately the same number of positive and negative potentials for each bin. Figure 12.4 illustrates the bin concept of the

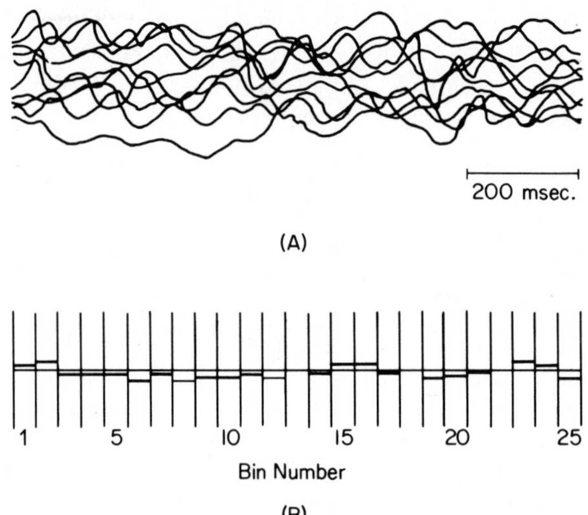

FIGURE 12.4 Part (A) of this figure is an overlay of a series of ten bursts of one-second EEG activity where no stimulus is presented to the ear. Being somewhat random, this background activity averages near zero for each of the computer bins (B).

computer and what might be visualized in a series of twenty-five bins when random electroencephalic activity is presented ten times. No characteristic response is seen because the ongoing activity nearly equals zero for each bin. In theory, the assumption is that at any given point in time the voltage will equal zero with an infinite number of runs. Figure 12.5 illustrates what might be visualized for ten sweeps in the computer bins when responses to stimuli occur. With each succeeding algebraic addition of the stimulus-response sequence, the electroencephalic response appears to grow in amplitude as the background noise is diminished.

Most computers today have 50 to 1,000 or even more bins. This number allows for excellent resolution of the summed electroencephalic response over a scan of one or even two seconds, when a sufficient number of time-locked stimulus presentations is algebraically added.

After a predetermined number of stimuli have been summed, the voltage from each of the bins is visually displayed on an oscilloscope or read out on a graphic recorder for a permanent record.

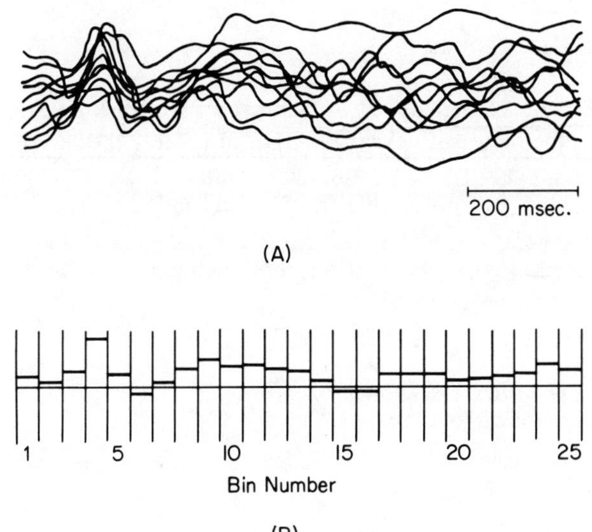

FIGURE 12.5 Part (A) of this figure is an overlay of a series of ten one-second segments of EEG activity immediately following stimulation of the ear with a tone. Part (B) illustrates how this series of single responses are algebraically added in the computer memory, yielding a summed electroencephalic response.

Computer Use in Testing Auditory Function

Lowell et al. (20, 21) used a specially built summing device to detect responses to auditory stimuli in order to develop the technique as a potential tool in diagnostic audiology. He obtained clear responses from the intact scalps of humans which demonstrated that at least the earlier components of the ER resulting from a click could be seen at levels that approached voluntary threshold.

Since 1960 several special summing or averaging devices have been built specifically for the study of audition (5, 21, 26). Presently there is a variety of commercial summing computers available for clinical and experimental use.

Tests of auditory function using averaged electroencephalic audiometry (AEA) undoubtedly require the most elaborate equipment of any auditory test presently available. A further complication of AEA is the fact that considerable training is required to administer the tests and interpret the results. Because of the complexity of the test, it is essential to understand some of the ramifications of the testing procedures as well as those factors which influence the evoked response itself.

RECORDING PROCEDURE

After the scalp of the subject is cleaned, a silver disk or other electrode is attached to the scalp with electrode paste at or near the vertex of the head. A reference electrode is placed on the mastoid or earlobe, and a ground lead is placed on the opposite ear, the forehead, or the nasion. During the test, raw electroencephalic activity is amplified and monitored on a recorder or oscilloscope. It is also simultaneously fed into the summing device for online data processing.

Effects of Stimulus Variables on the Electroencephalic Response

TYPES OF AUDITORY STIMULI

Good responses can be elicited from a variety of stimuli. Earlier, it was thought an ER could be produced only when a very brief intense sound was presented, such as a click. Because of its rapid onset, a click produces a good response but may not be particularly well adapted for tests of auditory sensitivity, since the response to a click, even when filtered, adds limited information about the auditory system's ability to respond at various frequencies.

Pure tones can also be used as stimuli and have the advantage of being produced and calibrated according to standard audiometric reference levels (25). Speech, bands of noise, or other auditory stimuli may also be used to elicit an ER, but procedures using these stimuli have not as yet been thoroughly investigated.

NUMBER OF STIMULI

The relative success of the encephalographic response technique depends upon the efficiency with which the evoked potential can be visualized or "read" from the background EEG. The averaging process depends on the concept that the time-locked stimuli will grow in direct proportion to the total number of stimuli (N). The signal-to-noise ratio is improved by the square root of N in averaging N samples. Thus the amplitude of the noise is reduced with each averaging of the signal. The signal which is time locked adds each time and as such increases with each signal. Approximately fifty stimuli appear to be sufficient to produce a visible response in most subjects, even when the stimulus is near threshold. Adding twenty-five or fifty more does not significantly improve visualization of the response. At suprathreshold levels, fewer sweeps may be adequate.

STIMULUS REPETITION RATE

The ER from a population of neurons follows many of the same physiological principles common to all neural tissue. When stimulated at an increasing rate, single nerves and groups of nerves may reach a point at which they have insufficient time between stimuli to recover or to permit continued firing. The neural tissue responsible for the slow components of ER behaves in somewhat the same fashion; that is, if stimuli are presented at sufficiently fast repetition rates, the response tends to be reduced in amplitude. This effect of one response on the next begins to be noticeable at repetition rates as slow as one every ten seconds. Stimulus repetition rates faster than about one per second reduce the ER amplitude markedly, and make response identification difficult (8, 24). There is a question as to whether this is truly a refractory function or just an interaction of response peaks; nonetheless, when stimuli are presented in close time approximation, they certainly have a limiting effect on the successive responses, even though each of the stimuli may be heard as equally loud by the subject.

RISE TIME AND DURATION

A critical stimulus parameter affecting the ER is the rise time of the stimulating sound. Differences in response latency can, indeed, be seen between a click having almost instantaneous rise time and a tone of similar intensity having a rise-decay time of 25 to 30 msec (26). Lamb and Graham (18) found shifts in latency with changes of up to 95 msec in the rise time. There is, however, some question as to whether the latency shift was entirely due to rise time and not, at least partially, due to a problem of instrumentation.

Onishi and Davis (31), using a linear on and off ramp to control stimulus rise and decay, found that the response latency of the N_1 component increased as rise time increased from 3 to 300 msec. Interestingly, with tonal durations of 30 msec or longer, only a very slight decline in response amplitude was found as a function of longer stimulus rise times. When the duration of the stimulus plateau is less than 30 msec, the response amplitude is greater with a fast rise time (3 msec) than with a slower rise time (30 msec).

Rose et al. (38) report that at 40-dB SL the stimulus duration makes no significant difference in the response amplitude. At threshold levels, however, increasing stimulus durations from 10 to 100 msec produce an increase in the response amplitude, corresponding to a subjective increase in loudness (9).

Responses can be elicited by stimuli lasting many seconds. The evoked response is not seen past about 500 msec even though the tone continues, demonstrating that the response is to the initiation of the tone rather than to factors of duration. The response is produced not by the total on time of the tone, but by the initial on effect, which reflects a change in the sensory state.

FREQUENCY

In the cochlea there are more sensory units responsive to low frequencies than to the higher frequencies. This is because the areas in the cochlea responsible for transmitting low tones involve a wide area along the apical and middle turn. Higher frequencies are represented by a rather restricted area on the basal portion of the cochlea.

At the cortex, therefore, one might predict a greater response amplitude for low-frequency stimuli based on the normal neural population for certain frequencies. There appears to be only a slight difference in the response amplitude of the mid-frequencies, 500, 1,000, and 2,000 Hz (25, 36). When comparing the very low frequencies (100 to 500 Hz) with those above 2,000 Hz, however, the low tones do indeed produce responses of greater amplitude (19). The response amplitude of the very low tones may be twice as large as that of the high frequencies.

INTENSITY

The stimulus parameter exerting greatest influence on the response waveform is intensity. As the loudness of the test stimulus is increased, the amplitude of the ER generally becomes greater. Simultaneously, the latency of the characteristic peaks is shortened. Davis and Zerlin (9) point out that the input (stimulus)–output (ER voltage) relationship is not a linear function; that is, the sensation of subjective loudness grows at a much faster rate than does the amplitude of the ER. Loudness sensation is doubled by an increase of only 10 dB, whereas approximately a 25-dB increment is needed for a similar growth of the electroencephalic potential voltage. Moore and Rose (30) have shown that the amplitude of the evoked response does not increase at levels above 70 to 90-dB SL.

Studies by Rapin (33), McCandless and Best (24), Rose and Ruhm (37), and McCandless and Lentz (27) suggest that the latency of the evoked response components undergo a systematic prolongation as the sensation level is lowered. Rapin, for example, noted a shift in latency of approximately 43 msec between the 5-dB and 50-dB sensation level for component N_1 of the ER. Significant shifts in latency for all of the characteristic peaks of the ER were observed by McCandless and Lentz (27) as the stimulus presentation level was lowered to threshold. However, all the peaks do not appear to shift equally with a stimulus intensity change (37).

Clinically, the effects on the response of the stimulus sensation level are of utmost importance. Deciding whether an ER is present or absent near threshold level is contingent on understanding how the stimulus sensation level alters the response amplitude and latency as a function of the sensation level.

Figure 12.6 shows a series of summed responses from an adult subject

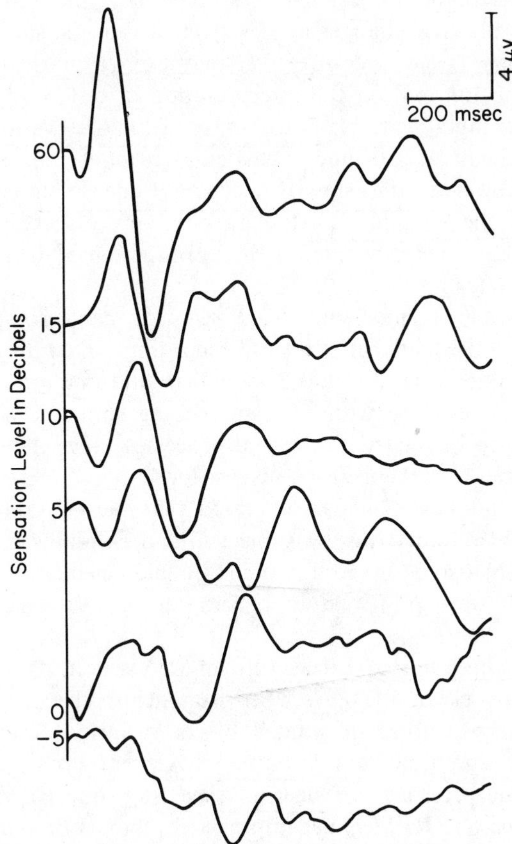

FIGURE 12.6 A series of summed responses to tones obtained from an adult. The response amplitude is very large at 60-dB SL. As the stimulus level is lowered to threshold, the response amplitude tends to decrease and the latency of the peaks becomes longer. The response is still clearly identifiable at 5-dB SL but becomes more obscure at 0 dB SL. At −5-dB SL, the characteristic peaks are not seen.

at 60-dB, 15-dB, 10-dB, 5-dB, 0-dB, and −5-dB sensation levels. The response is smaller in amplitude near threshold but can still be readily seen at 0-dB SL.

Effects of the Psychophysiological State on the Auditory Electroencephalic Response

Of clinical importance in ER audiometry are variables which may influence or alter the response waveform in some manner during a test. The source of variables outside the subject such as frequency and intensity can be carefully controlled. Any changes arising from within the subject, however, are difficult or impossible to control, yet may exert a marked influence on the pattern of the ER and on the interpretation of test results.

Because of the highly variable nature of the state of arousal in individual subjects, it is difficult to attribute a particular response characteristic to a specific state. However, the slow wave amplitude is enhanced by the improbability of the stimulus, by the novelty, or by increased attention. The state of arousal, the sleep state, or the introduction of drugs also modify the response waveform.

In some subjects a sufficiently loud stimulus can produce responses that can be seen consistently in raw EEG recordings. Even in these subjects there is considerable variation of the waveform and amplitude of the slow component of the response with each succeeding stimulus. These changes must be assumed to be related to internal processes, since the sound stimuli and the environment are kept at a constant level.

McCandless and Best (24) demonstrated that the ER amplitude could be increased slightly by having the subject attend carefully to the auditory stimulus. Davis (6) also observed that the ER could be enhanced significantly when the stimuli were presented in relation to a task which required a decision.

The greatest alteration of ER waveform is observed as a subject goes to sleep. Williams et al. (41) described significant changes in the total auditory response waveform in adult subjects at various levels of natural sleep. The most significant alteration of waveform does not appear in adults until the deeper stages of sleep or in a stage-one REM (Rapid Eye Movement). Stage-one REM is accompanied by bursts of rapid eye movements, which may be associated with dreaming. The behavioral alerting and ER thresholds are highly variable in this state.

In young children and infants, the psychophysiological state changes very rapidly, sometimes from second to second, causing considerable test-retest variability. Even when the child appears to be in a steady sleeping state, there is sufficient alteration of the state to produce significant changes in the response waveform. If the ER waveform is altered markedly by the state of the subject, considerable difficulty is encountered in interpreting the presence or absence of a response, especially when testing at low sensation levels. Rapin (33) used AER audiometry with click stimuli on a group of children with communicative disorders. The earlier response components decreased and the amplitude of the later portion of the response increased when the children were drowsy. In the alert state, however, the earlier components appeared to be more stable.

Figure 12.7 illustrates the kind of test-retest variability seen in young subjects. This figure shows a change in the ER pattern of a normal child, eight weeks of age, throughout a normal sleep state, from drowsiness to alertness. Fifty presentations of a 2,000 Hz tone at 60-dB HL were used as stimuli for each response measure and were averaged with a computer. All tests were made at ten-minute intervals over a one-hour period. Definite alteration in waveform can be seen resulting from changes in the alert state. The possibility of rather large, momentary changes in responsivity must be considered when interpreting the presence or absence of a response in tests of auditory acuity.

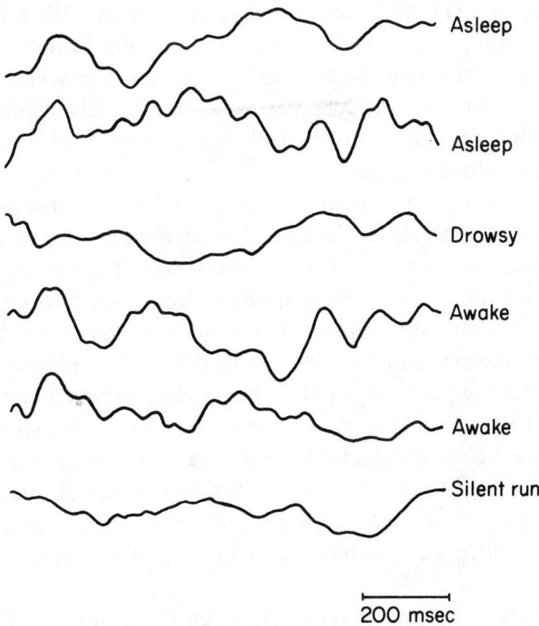

FIGURE 12.7 This illustrates changes in the electroencephalic response caused by shifts in the alerting state in an eight-week-old normal child. The tests were taken at ten-minute intervals for one hour, keeping the stimulus intensity constant. The alteration of the response waveform reflects the changes in the psychophysiological state of the subject.

Attempts have been made to modify the waveform of the ER by hypnotic suggestion. However, even under a deep hypnotic state, the ER persists and is altered little, if at all, by suggestions that a loud tone cannot be heard, or that a soft stimulus is very loud.

Clinical Testing

THRESHOLD DETERMINATION

Since the ER amplitude seems to relate closely to the sensation of loudness, it has a natural application as an objective testing device for auditory sensitivity in uncooperative patients. It should be stressed that the ER reflects only the fact that the auditory impulses have reached the brain. At the present time we are unable to draw absolute inferences as to whether or not the patient "hears." In other words, it is safe to assume that the appearance of a response indicates that a sound has alerted the cortex, but in no way does it imply that the patient can use auditory information meaningfully. The absence of a response on the other hand may not mean the child cannot hear, since some children with brain damage respond overtly to sound, but give inconsistent or no electroencephalic responses. In practice, however, there does seem to be a relationship between the behavioral indication of hearing and the presence of electroencephalic responses to pure-tone stimuli.

At present no criterion has been established for determining or reading the presence or absence of an averaged electroencephalic response. As the stimulus intensity is decreased toward threshold, it becomes more difficult to subjectively differentiate the responses from the background activity, even though the responses represent a sum of as many as fifty individual stimuli. Some investigators have chosen to define the presence of a response by requiring that the peaks of a particular latency exceed a certain amplitude (21, 37). The ER threshold has also been described as the stimulus intensity that produces a visually detectable response, when an intensity decrement of 5 or 10 dB does not produce a waveform which is similar (33). This technique allows each subject to be his own response control, and has considerable value since each subject's responses, in general, have their own peculiarities.

A positive response at a relatively high sensation level is sometimes obtained at the beginning of the test in order to serve as a reference for the recognition of similar patterns at lower sensation levels. It should be remembered, however, that the latencies are prolonged at lower SL's, so a direct comparison of response latencies to very intense stimuli to responses at near-threshold stimuli cannot be used.

The determination of an ER near threshold may also be accomplished by the use of a template and is derived by drawing the averaged response of a group of subjects for varying sensation levels.

McCandless and Lentz (27) reported that for older children and adults one can expect to visualize an evoked response in one of two runs 91 per cent of the time at a 5-dB sensation level. At 0 dB sensation level, one is able to visualize a response approximately 50 per cent of the time. In younger children, however, a readable response is seen much less frequently. Rapin and Graziani (34) reported that even at a high-intensity level there was a 10 per cent chance of obtaining a false response where none exists for an individual "averaged" run.

RELATIONSHIP OF AVERAGED ENCEPHALOGRAPHIC RESPONSE THRESHOLDS TO VOLUNTARY THRESHOLDS

The first application of a special computer to detect the auditory threshold was reported by Lowell et al. (21). Looking only at the early components of the evoked response, he found that responses could be detected at +5-dB SL 24 per cent of the time and 82 per cent at +30-dB SL in normally hearing adults.

Cody and Bickford (4) reported testing twenty normal ears with AEA. They found that of sixty individual test tones tabulated, 43 per cent gave identical thresholds on both the AEA and conventional audiograms; 40 per cent differed by 5 dB, 12 per cent differed by 10 dB, and only 5 per cent differed by 15 dB. These results show good agreement between conventional procedures and AEA. These investigators compared the voluntary threshold responses with the ER thresholds of adults who had sensori-neural deafness and found that the difference in the method of testing rarely exceeded 10 dB. McCandless and Lentz (27) reported that in normal hearing adults the mean difference between the voluntary and the ER threshold did not exceed 5 dB. Roeser and Rose (35) reported that the ER thresholds for individuals with cochlear pathology was nearer behavioral audiometric thresholds than the ER thresholds for a group of individuals with no pathology of the ear.

In children, the relationship between voluntary and AEA thresholds are somewhat difficult to evaluate since behavioral tests are not easily obtained in this group. Studies have indicated that AEA thresholds in children older than four years approximate the voluntary audiometric thresholds within 0 to 15 dB (7). Care must be taken in assuming that the ER thresholds and voluntary thresholds are equivalent. The electroencephalic potential is an electrophysiological measure while behavioral audiometry is a psychophysiological measure. The two measures may be compared, but an inherent relationship need not necessarily exist.

In children younger than eighteen months, there appears to be a greater separation of the behavioral threshold from the ER measure. These greater differences may be due to the extreme variability in state and the increased difficulty in interpreting the presence of an evoked response.

TESTING CHILDREN

Even in normally hearing children, the ER to auditory stimuli can be observed shortly after birth, but it is highly variable. It begins to stabilize with age and seems to be related to the change in the sleep-awake ratio in the child. There is considerable difficulty in eliciting unequivocal responses at levels below 40-dB HL on children three months and younger. By age six months, the ER at hearing levels less than 40 dB may be obtained with much greater consistency. Children may be tested either awake, in natural sleep, or under sedation, but subtle differences may be expected in the waveform of the response in these various states. Children can be tested while awake and held in their mother's arms, or in a crib or bassinet.

Older children and adults are tested while seated in a chair and are asked to remain quiet or to read. It is inadvisable to test infants when they are sucking a pacifier, feeding, or in a transitional period (i.e., from alertness to drowsiness or from drowsiness to sleep), since these conditions produce extreme variations in the response. More response stability can be expected when the child is either awake and alert or in quiet, deep, flaccid sleep. Tests may be administered under sedation, but certain response variations may still be seen depending upon the depth of sleep and the type of sedation used.

The interpretation of AEA with children having brain damage is most difficult. Those with emotional disorders are not as difficult to test. The presence of a clear ER suggests that the sound is being heard, but the absence of a response does not necessarily imply the reverse. In these cases, replication is necessary to interpret the data, and all ancillary information available must be used to obtain meaningful test results.

The ER audiometric technique appears to be an important adjunct to conventional and other behavioral tests of auditory sensitivity. With this technique it is possible to gain information on the auditory system that cannot always be obtained by other techniques. In addition, children showing autistic behavior, brain damage, or other organic or behavioral anomalies may be assessed for their residual hearing, where other techniques prove inadequate. In this regard AEA adds significantly to the armamentarium of clinical tests.

4-12-76.

Bibliography

1. Bancaud, J., V. Bloch, and J. Paippard. "Contribution EEG á l'étude des potentials évoques chez l'homme au niveau du vertex." *Review of Neurology*, **89**: 399–418, 1953.
2. Berger, H. "Uber das elektrenkephalogramm des menschen." *Archives of Psychiatry Nervenker*, **87**: 527–70, 1929.

3. Bickford, R. G., J. L. Jacobson, and D. T. R. Cody. "Nature of averaged evoked potentials to sound and other stimuli in man." *Annals of the New York Academy of Science*, **112**: 204–23, 1964.
4. Cody, D. T. R. and R. G. Bickford. "Cortical audiometry: An objective method of evaluating auditory acuity in man." *Mayo Clinic Proceedings*, **40**: 273–87, 1965.
5. Cox, R. R. and E. V. Evarts. "An evoked response detector." *Electroencephalography and Clinical Neurophysiology*, **13**: 487–90, 1960.
6. Davis, H. "Enhancement of evoked cortical potentials in humans related to a task requiring a decision." *Science*, **145**: 182–83, 1964.
7. Davis, H. "Validation of evoked response audiometry." *International Audiology–Audiologie Internationale*, **2**: 77–81, 1966.
8. Davis, H., T. Mast, N. Yoshie, and S. Zerlin. "The slow response of the human cortex to auditory stimuli: Recovery process." *Electroencephalography and Clinical Neurophysiology*, **21**: 105–13, 1966.
9. Davis, H. and S. Zerlin. "Acoustic relations of the human vertex potential." *Journal of the Acoustical Society of America*, **39**: 109–16, 1966.
10. Davis, P. A. "Effects of acoustic stimuli on the waking brain." *Journal of Neurophysiology*, **2**: 494–99, 1939.
11. Dawson, G. D. "A summation technique for the detection of small evoked potentials." *Electroencephalography and Clinical Neurophysiology*, **6**: 65–84, 1954.
12. Derbyshire, A. J. and G. A. McCandless. "Template for the EEG response to sound." *Journal of Speech and Hearing Research*, **7**: 96–98, 1964.
13. Derbyshire, A. J. and M. McDermott. "Further contributions to the EEG method of evaluating auditory function." *Laryngoscope*, **68**: 558–70, 1958.
14. Doerfler, L. G. "Neurophysiological clues to auditory acuity." *Journal of Speech and Hearing Disorders*, **13**: 227–32, 1948.
15. Geisler, C. D., L. S. Frishkopf, and W. A. Rosenblith. "Extracranial responses to acoustic clicks in man." *Science*, **128**: 1210–11, 1958.
16. Goldstein, R. "Electrophysiologic audiometry." In J. Jerger, ed., *Modern Developments in Audiology. Academic Press*, New York and London: Academic Press, Inc., 1963. Pp. 167–92.
17. Katzman, R. "Sensory evoked response in man." *Annals of the New York Academy of Science*, **112**: 1–546, 1964.
18. Lamb, L. E and J. T. Graham. "Influence of signal variables on evoked response to sound." *Journal of Speech and Hearing Research*, **10**: 257–67, 1967.
19. Lowell, E. L. *Research in Sensory Threshold Measurement*. Final report to the Physiological Psychology Branch, Physiological Science Division (450). Washington, D.C.: Office of Naval Research, 1967.
20. Lowell, E. L., C. I. Troffer, E. A. Warburton, and A. M. Rushford. "Temporal evannation: A new approach in diagnostic audiology." *Journal of Speech and Hearing Disorders*, **25**: 340–45, 1960.
21. Lowell, E. L., C. I. Williams, R. M. Ballenger, and P. P. Alvig. "Measurement of auditory threshold with a special purpose analog computer." *Journal of Speech and Hearing Research*, **4**: 105–12, 1961.
22. Marcus, R. E. "Hearing and speech problems in children: Observation and use of electroencephalography." *Archives of Otolaryngology*, **53**: 134–46, 1951.

23. McCandless, G. A. "Clinical application of evoked response audiometry." *Journal of Speech and Hearing Research*, **10**: 468–78, 1967.
24. McCandless, G. A. and L. G. Best. "Evoked responses to auditory stimuli in man using a summing computer." *Journal of Speech and Hearing Research*, **7**: 193–202, 1964.
25. McCandless, G. A. and L. G. Best. "Summed evoked responses using pure-tone stimuli." *Journal of Speech and Hearing Research*, **9**: 266–72, 1966.
26. McCandless, G. A., L. G. Best, and J. H. Larkins. "A summing computer for measuring evoked responses in man." *Journal of Medical Electronics*, **4**: 78–81, 1965.
27. McCandless, G. A. and W. E. Lentz. "Evoked response (EEG) audiometry in nonorganic hearing loss." *Archives of Otolaryngology*, **87**: 123–28, 1968.
28. McCandless, G. A. and D. E. Rose. "Evoked cortical responses to stimulus change." *Journal of Speech and Hearing Research*, In Press.
29. Michels, M. W. and C. T. Randt. "Galvanic skin response in differential diagnosis of deafness." *Archives of Otolaryngology*, **45**: 302–11, 1947.
30. Moore, E. J. and D. E. Rose. "Acoustically evoked responses in man to high-intensity pure-tone stimuli." *International Audiology*, **8**: 172–81, 1969.
31. Onishi, S. and H. Davis. "Effects of duration and rise time of tone bursts on evoked V potentials." *Journal of the Acoustical Society of America*, **44**: 582–91, 1968.
32. Price, L. L., B. Rosenblut, R. Goldstein, and D. C. Shepherd. "The averaged evoked response to auditory stimulation." *Journal of Speech and Hearing Research*, **9**: 361–70, 1966.
33. Rapin, I. "Evoked responses to clicks in a group of children with communication disorders." *Annals of the New York Academy of Science*, **112**: 183–203, 1964.
34. Rapin, I. and L. J. Graziani. "Auditory evoked responses in normal, brain damaged, and deaf infants." *Neurology*, **17**: 881–94, 1967.
35. Roeser, R. and D. E. Rose. "Electroencephalic audiometry in the determination of cochlear pathology." *Journal of Auditory Research*, **8**: 135–41, 1968.
36. Rose, D. E. and J. C. Malone. "Some aspects of the acoustically evoked response to the cessation of stimulus." *Journal of Auditory Research*, **5**: 27–40, 1965.
37. Rose, D. E. and H. B. Ruhm. "Some characteristics of the peak latency and amplitude of the evoked response." *Journal of Speech and Hearing Research*, **9**: 412–22, 1966.
38. Rose, D. E., D. Teter, and E. Curtiss. "Effects of duration on the acoustically produced evoked response." *Journal of Auditors Research*. In Press.
39. Ruben, R. J., J. E. Bordley, and A. T. Lieberman. "Cochlear potentials in man." *Laryngoscope*, **71**: 1141–64, 1961.
40. Ruhm, H., E. Walker, and H. Flanigin. "Acoustically evoked potentials in man: Mediation of early components." *Laryngoscope*, **127**: 806–22, 1967.
41. Williams, H. L., H. C. Morlock, J. V. Morlock, and A. Labin. "Auditory evoked responses and the EEG stages of sleep." *Annals of the New York Academy of Science*, **112**: 172–79, 1964.
42. Zeaman, D. and N. Wegner. "Cardiac reflex to tones of threshold intensity." *Journal of Speech and Hearing Disorders*, **21**: 71–75, 1956.

13

Industrial and Military Audiology

Gerald A. Studebaker, Ph.D.
William T. Brandy, Ph.D.

Audiologists have a vital role today in the evaluation of people with suspected hearing losses who are referred to clinics for extensive hearing tests, hearing-aid evaluations, and rehabilitative training in speech-reading and listening. However, the problems of noise and hearing loss in industrial and military situations have received little attention from audiologists. This chapter reflects an expectation and a hope that in the future, audiologists will become increasingly involved in the prevention as well as in the evaluation of hearing losses caused by noise.

The effective prevention of hearing loss from noise requires the coordination of a number of professional specialities. Because of the audiologist's training in anatomy and physiology, physics of sound, psychology, statistics, hearing testing, and hearing rehabilitation, he is in a unique position to make significant contributions to industrial and military hearing conservation programs. The audiologist has the potentially important role of bridging the gap between the medical and engineering approaches to noise and noise-induced hearing disorders. Finally, the audiologist has a potential role as a consultant to, or as a director of, personnel engaged in hearing conservation programs.

Noise Parameters

DEFINITION OF NOISE

Noise may be defined in any one of several ways depending upon the intent of the writer. To an acoustician, noise may be defined as erratic, inharmonic, meaningless, or statistically random variations in sound pressure. To an audiologist, noise may be defined as a useful acoustic signal used to elevate the hearing threshold or to reduce the intelligibility of speech. To a communications specialist, noise may be any signal (acoustic or nonacoustic) which reduces the efficiency of communication. To a noise-control engineer, noise may be defined as any undesirable acoustic signal. To those interested in hearing conservation, noise may be any acoustic signal, meaningful or not, which is injurious to the hearing mechanism. Most of the preceding definitions, except those applied to noise used for experimental or clinical purposes, include the concept of "undesirability." For example, the neighbor's "hi-fi" set may be desirable sound under some circumstances; under others it may be undesirable. It may be music for the owner of the set and noise for the neighbor.

Noise, like all acoustic events, can be described physically according to frequency, intensity, and time parameters. More specific descriptions may include spectrum (intensity by frequency), phase, on-off ratio, rise and decay times, and frequency bandwidth of the noise. Tompkins, in Chapter 1 of this text, presents the basic principles of the physical description of sound. There are a number of factors discussed here, however, which are particularly relevant to the description of noise.

LEVEL

Sound level is customarily expressed in decibels according to the reference sound pressure of 0.0002 microbar. Sound pressure level is equal to 20 log P_1/P_0 where P_1 is equal to the observed sound pressure and P_0 is equal to the reference sound pressure. The word "level" means that the physical magnitude of the observed sound is expressed in decibels. The absence of the word "level" indicates that the sound magnitude is expressed directly in units of some physical quantity (for example, dynes or watts).

Other references and scales are used for certain purposes. For example, many sound-level calculations are more conveniently performed by using a sound intensity scale. The usual sound intensity reference is 10^{-12} watt per square meter or 10^{-16} watt per square centimeter (these two values are equal). Sound intensity level is equal to 10 $\log_{10} I_1/I_0$, where I_1 is equal to the observed sound intensity and I_0 is equal to the reference sound intensity.

The formulas 20 $\log_{10} P_1/P_0$ and 10 $\log_{10} I_1/I_0$ yield the same number of decibels for a given observation, because intensity is proportional to pressure squared (*see* Chapter 1). However, the reference sound pressure (0.0002 microbar) and the reference sound intensity (10^{-12} watt per square meter) are only approximately equal. Actual equality between the two is observed only under specific conditions of atmospheric pressure and temperature. For practical purposes, it may be assumed that the two references are equal under ordinary ground level atmospheric conditions with the error seldom greater than ± 0.5 dB (78).

Another sound magnitude scale which is used frequently in the study of noise is sound power level. Sound power is measured in watts, with the area unspecified. Sound power level is equal to ten times the logarithm of the ratio of the observed sound power to the reference sound power. The usual sound power reference is 10^{-12} watt, although 10^{-13} watt has been used. A sound magnitude scale that is not used in the measurement of airborne sound is sound force level. This scale is used in expressing the output of bone-conduction vibrators. The reference sound force is one dyne. Both sound force and sound power are expressed with the area unspecified because they are expressions of the total force or power while pressure and intensity are force and power per unit area. Decibel values are related to sound force and sound power in the same way as are sound pressure and sound intensity, respectively.

WORKING WITH THE DECIBEL

A number of procedures associated with noise measurement computations illustrate the importance of a thorough knowledge of decibel notation. Often it is desirable to estimate the spectrum level (the level per cycle) of a noise on the basis of measurements that must be made in bandwidths considerably wider than 1 Hz. Or, it is sometimes necessary to calculate the effect of adding or subtracting sound sources upon the overall sound level. In order to accomplish these tasks, it is essential, first, to convert sound levels into sound intensity; second, to perform the arithmetic operation desired; and third, to convert the answer back to sound level.

Tables 13.1 and 13.2 present information which can be used for various sound-level calculations. In Table 13.1, the first column records sound levels in 10-dB steps. The second column records the sound pressures in microbar and in 20-dB intervals. Column two illustrates that every ten-fold increase in sound pressure (or sound force) results in a 20-dB increase in sound level. Column three records the sound intensities associated with various sound levels expressed for the 10^{-16} watt per square centimeter reference, and column four gives the same information for the 10^{-12} watt per square meter reference. The scale in the fourth column also applies to sound power and illustrates that every ten-fold increase in intensity or

TABLE 13.1. PRESSURE, POWER, AND DECIBEL EQUIVALENTS

dB	*Pressure re:* 0 *dB* = 0.0002 *microbar*	*Intensity re:* 0 *dB* = 10^{-16} *watt/cm²*	*Intensity re:* 0 *dB* = 10^{-12} *watt/m²*
−20	0.00002 microbar	10^{-18} watt/cm²	10^{-14} watt/m²
−10		10^{-17} ,,	10^{-13} ,,
0	0.0002 ,,	10^{-16} ,,	10^{-12} ,,
10		10^{-15} ,,	10^{-11} ,,
20	0.002 ,,	10^{-14} ,,	10^{-10} ,,
30		10^{-13} ,,	10^{-9} ,,
40	0.02 ,,	10^{-12} ,,	10^{-8} ,,
50		10^{-11} ,,	10^{-7} ,,
60	0.2 ,,	10^{-10} ,,	10^{-6} ,,
70		10^{-9} ,,	10^{-5} ,,
80	2.0 ,,	10^{-8} ,,	10^{-4} ,,
90		10^{-7} ,,	10^{-3} ,,
100	20.0 ,,	10^{-6} ,,	10^{-2} ,,
110		10^{-5} ,,	10^{-1} ,,
120	200.0 ,,	10^{-4} ,,	10^{0} ,,
130		10^{-3} ,,	10^{1} watts/m²
140	2000.0 ,,	10^{-2} ,,	10^{2} ,,

TABLE 13.2. DECIBEL, POWER RATIO, AND PRESSURE RATIO EQUIVALENTS*

GIVEN: Decibels **TO FIND: Power and Pressure Ratios**

TO ACCOUNT FOR THE SIGN OF THE DECIBEL

For positive (+) values of the decibel—Both pressure and power ratios are greater than unity. Use the two right-hand columns.

For negative (−) values of the decibel—Both pressure and power ratios are less than unity. Use the two left-hand columns.

Example—*Given:* ± **9.1** dB. *Find:*

	Power Ratio	*Pressure Ratio*
+9.1 dB	8.128	2.851
−9.1 dB	0.1230	0.3508

← − *dB* + →

Pressure Ratio	*Power Ratio*	*dB*	*Pressure Ratio*	*Power Ratio*
1.0000	**1.0000**	**0**	**1.000**	**1.000**
.9886	.9772	.1	1.012	1.023
.9772	.9550	.2	1.023	1.047
.9661	.9333	.3	1.035	1.072
.9550	.9120	.4	1.047	1.096
.9441	.8913	.5	1.059	1.122
.9333	.8710	.6	1.072	1.148
.9226	.8511	.7	1.084	1.175
.9120	.8318	.8	1.096	1.202
.9016	.8128	.9	1.109	1.230

← − *dB* + →

Pressure Ratio	*Power Ratio*	*dB*	*Pressure Ratio*	*Power Ratio*
.7079	**.5012**	**3.0**	**1.413**	**1.995**
.6998	.4898	3.1	1.429	2.042
.6918	.4786	3.2	1.445	2.089
.6839	.4677	3.3	1.462	2.138
.6761	.4571	3.4	1.479	2.188
.6683	.4467	3.5	1.496	2.239
.6607	.4365	3.6	1.514	2.291
.6531	.4266	3.7	1.531	2.344
.6457	.4169	3.8	1.549	2.399
.6383	.4074	3.9	1.567	2.455

* Table One of Peterson, A. P. G. and E. E. Gross, Jr., *Handbook of Noise Measurement* (6th ed.). West Concord, Mass.: General Radio Company, 1967. Pp. 204, 205.

TABLE 13.2—*continued*

Pressure Ratio (− dB)	Power Ratio (− dB)	dB	Pressure Ratio (+ dB)	Power Ratio (+ dB)
.8913	**.7943**	**1.0**	**1.122**	**1.259**
.8810	.7762	1.1	1.135	1.288
.8710	.7586	1.2	1.148	1.318
.8610	.7413	1.3	1.161	1.349
.8511	.7244	1.4	1.175	1.380
.8414	.7079	1.5	1.189	1.413
.8318	.6918	1.6	1.202	1.445
.8222	.6761	1.7	1.216	1.479
.8128	.6607	1.8	1.230	1.514
.8035	.6457	1.9	1.245	1.549
.7943	**.6310**	**2.0**	**1.259**	**1.585**
.7852	.6166	2.1	1.274	1.622
.7762	.6026	2.2	1.288	1.660
.7674	.5888	2.3	1.303	1.698
.7586	.5754	2.4	1.318	1.738
.7499	.5623	2.5	1.334	1.778
.7413	.5495	2.6	1.349	1.820
.7328	.5370	2.7	1.365	1.862
.7244	.5248	2.8	1.380	1.905
.7161	.5129	2.9	1.396	1.950
.5012	**.2512**	**6.0**	**1.995**	**3.981**
.4955	.2455	6.1	2.018	4.074
.4898	.2399	6.2	2.042	4.169
.4842	.2344	6.3	2.065	4.266
.4786	.2291	6.4	2.089	4.365
.4732	.2239	6.5	2.113	4.467
.4677	.2188	6.6	2.138	4.571
.4624	.2138	6.7	2.163	4.677
.4571	.2089	6.8	2.188	4.786
.4519	.2042	6.9	2.213	4.898
.4467	**.1995**	**7.0**	**2.239**	**5.012**
.4416	.1950	7.1	2.265	5.129
.4365	.1905	7.2	2.291	5.248
.4315	.1862	7.3	2.317	5.370
.4266	.1820	7.4	2.344	5.495
.4217	.1778	7.5	2.371	5.623
.4169	.1738	7.6	2.399	5.754
.4121	.1698	7.7	2.427	5.888
.4074	.1660	7.8	2.455	6.026
.4027	.1622	7.9	2.483	6.166
.3981	**.1585**	**8.0**	**2.512**	**6.310**
.3936	.1549	8.1	2.541	6.457
.3890	.1514	8.2	2.570	6.607
.3846	.1479	8.3	2.600	6.761
.3802	.1445	8.4	2.630	6.918
.3758	.1413	8.5	2.661	7.079
.3715	.1380	8.6	2.692	7.244
.3673	.1349	8.7	2.723	7.413
.3631	.1318	8.8	2.754	7.586
.3589	.1288	8.9	2.786	7.762

Pressure Ratio (− dB)	Power Ratio (− dB)	dB	Pressure Ratio (+ dB)	Power Ratio (+ dB)
.6310	**.3981**	**4.0**	**1.585**	**2.512**
.6237	.3890	4.1	1.603	2.570
.6166	.3802	4.2	1.622	2.630
.6095	.3715	4.3	1.641	2.692
.6026	.3631	4.4	1.660	2.754
.5957	.3548	4.5	1.679	2.818
.5888	.3467	4.6	1.698	2.884
.5821	.3388	4.7	1.718	2.951
.5754	.3311	4.8	1.738	3.020
.5689	.3236	4.9	1.758	3.090
.5623	**.3162**	**5.0**	**1.778**	**3.162**
.5559	.3090	5.1	1.799	3.236
.5495	.3020	5.2	1.820	3.311
.5433	.2951	5.3	1.841	3.388
.5370	.2884	5.4	1.862	3.467
.5309	.2818	5.5	1.884	3.548
.5248	.2754	5.6	1.905	3.631
.5188	.2692	5.7	1.928	3.715
.5129	.2630	5.8	1.950	3.802
.5070	.2570	5.9	1.972	3.890
.2818	**.07943**	**11.0**	**3.548**	**12.59**
.2786	.07762	11.1	3.589	12.88
.2754	.07586	11.2	3.631	13.18
.2723	.07413	11.3	3.673	13.49
.2692	.07244	11.4	3.715	13.80
.2661	.07079	11.5	3.758	14.13
.2630	.06918	11.6	3.802	14.45
.2600	.06761	11.7	3.846	14.79
.2570	.06607	11.8	3.890	15.14
.2541	.06457	11.9	3.936	15.49
.2512	**.06310**	**12.0**	**3.981**	**15.85**
.2483	.06166	12.1	4.027	16.22
.2455	.06026	12.2	4.074	16.60
.2427	.05888	12.3	4.121	16.98
.2399	.05754	12.4	4.169	17.38
.2371	.05623	12.5	4.217	17.78
.2344	.05495	12.6	4.266	18.20
.2317	.05370	12.7	4.315	18.62
.2291	.05248	12.8	4.365	19.05
.2265	.05129	12.9	4.416	19.50
.2239	**.05012**	**13.0**	**4.467**	**19.95**
.2213	.04898	13.1	4.519	20.42
.2188	.04786	13.2	4.571	20.89
.2163	.04677	13.3	4.624	21.38
.2138	.04571	13.4	4.677	21.88
.2113	.04467	13.5	4.732	22.39
.2089	.04365	13.6	4.786	22.91
.2065	.04266	13.7	4.842	23.44
.2042	.04169	13.8	4.898	23.99
.2018	.04074	13.9	4.955	24.55

TABLE 13.2—*continued*

Pressure Ratio (− dB)	Power Ratio (− dB)	dB	Pressure Ratio (+ dB)	Power Ratio (+ dB)
.3548	**.1259**	**9.0**	**2.818**	**7.943**
.3508	.1230	9.1	2.851	8.128
.3467	.1202	9.2	2.884	8.318
.3428	.1175	9.3	2.917	8.511
.3388	.1148	9.4	2.951	8.710
.3350	.1122	9.5	2.985	8.913
.3311	.1096	9.6	3.020	9.120
.3273	.1072	9.7	3.055	9.333
.3236	.1047	9.8	3.090	9.550
.3199	.1023	9.9	3.126	9.772
.3162	**.1000**	**10.0**	**3.162**	**10.000**
.3126	.09772	10.1	3.199	10.23
.3090	.09550	10.2	3.236	10.47
.3055	.09333	10.3	3.273	10.72
.3020	.09120	10.4	3.311	10.96
.2985	.08913	10.5	3.350	11.22
.2951	.08710	10.6	3.388	11.48
.2917	.08511	10.7	3.428	11.75
.2884	.08318	10.8	3.467	12.02
.2851	.08128	10.9	3.508	12.30
.1585	**.02512**	**16.0**	**6.310**	**39.81**
.1567	.02455	16.1	6.383	40.74
.1549	.02399	16.2	6.457	41.69
.1531	.02344	16.3	6.531	42.66
.1514	.02291	16.4	6.607	43.65
.1496	.02239	16.5	6.683	44.67
.1479	.02188	16.6	6.761	45.71
.1462	.02138	16.7	6.839	46.77
.1445	.02089	16.8	6.918	47.86
.1429	.02042	16.9	6.998	48.98
.1413	**.01995**	**17.0**	**7.079**	**50.12**
.1396	.01950	17.1	7.161	51.29
.1380	.01905	17.2	7.244	52.48
.1365	.01862	17.3	7.328	53.70
.1349	.01820	17.4	7.413	54.95
.1334	.01778	17.5	7.499	56.23
.1318	.01738	17.6	7.586	57.54
.1303	.01698	17.7	7.674	58.88
.1288	.01660	17.8	7.762	60.26
.1274	.01622	17.9	7.852	61.66
.1259	**.01585**	**18.0**	**7.943**	**63.10**
.1245	.01549	18.1	8.035	64.57
.1230	.01514	18.2	8.128	66.07
.1216	.01479	18.3	8.222	67.61
.1202	.01445	18.4	8.318	69.18
.1189	.01413	18.5	8.414	70.79
.1175	.01380	18.6	8.511	72.44
.1161	.01349	18.7	8.610	74.13
.1148	.01318	18.8	8.710	75.86
.1135	.01288	18.9	8.811	77.62

Pressure Ratio (− dB)	Power Ratio (− dB)	dB	Pressure Ratio (+ dB)	Power Ratio (+ dB)
.1995	**.03981**	**14.0**	**5.012**	**25.12**
.1972	.03890	14.1	5.070	25.70
.1950	.03802	14.2	5.129	26.30
.1928	.03715	14.3	5.188	26.92
.1905	.03631	14.4	5.248	27.54
.1884	.03548	14.5	5.309	28.18
.1862	.03467	14.6	5.370	28.84
.1841	.03388	14.7	5.433	29.51
.1820	.03311	14.8	5.495	30.20
.1799	.03236	14.9	5.559	30.90
.1778	**.03162**	**15.0**	**5.623**	**31.62**
.1758	.03090	15.1	5.689	32.36
.1738	.03020	15.2	5.754	33.11
.1718	.02951	15.3	5.821	33.88
.1698	.02884	15.4	5.888	34.67
.1679	.02818	15.5	5.957	35.48
.1660	.02754	15.6	6.026	36.31
.1641	.02692	15.7	6.095	37.15
.1622	.02630	15.8	6.166	38.02
.1603	.02570	15.9	6.237	38.90
.1122	**.01259**	**19.0**	**8.913**	**79.43**
.1109	.01230	19.1	9.016	81.28
.1096	.01202	19.2	9.120	83.18
.1084	.01175	19.3	9.226	85.11
.1072	.01148	19.4	9.333	87.10
.1059	.01122	19.5	9.441	89.13
.1047	.01096	19.6	9.550	91.20
.1035	.01072	19.7	9.661	93.33
.1023	.01047	19.8	9.772	95.50
.1012	.01023	19.9	9.886	97.72
.1000	**.01000**	**20.0**	**10.000**	**100.00**

Pressure Ratio (− dB)	Power Ratio (− dB)	dB	Pressure Ratio (+ dB)	Power Ratio (+ dB)
3.162×10^{-1}	**10^{-1}**	**10**	**3.162**	**10**
10^{-1}	10^{-2}	20	10	10^{2}
3.162×10^{-2}	10^{-3}	30	3.162×10	10^{3}
10^{-2}	10^{-4}	40	10^{2}	10^{4}
3.162×10^{-3}	10^{-5}	50	3.162×10^{2}	10^{5}
10^{-3}	10^{-6}	60	10^{3}	10^{6}
3.162×10^{-4}	10^{-7}	70	3.162×10^{3}	10^{7}
10^{-4}	10^{-8}	80	10^{4}	10^{8}
3.162×10^{-5}	10^{-9}	90	3.162×10^{4}	10^{9}
10^{-5}	**10^{-10}**	**100**	**10^{5}**	**10^{10}**

power results in a 10-dB increase in sound level. Again, it should be noted that the values in column two are seldom exactly interchangeable with the values in columns three and four because of atmospheric effects. These differences are sufficiently small, however, so that the values in columns two, three, and four are considered equivalent for usual noise computation purposes.

It is possible to construct a table of decibel, dyne, and watt equivalents at any time. First, it should be remembered that doubling intensity results in approximately a 3-dB increase and that doubling pressure results in approximately a 6-dB increase. More precisely, the increases are 3.0103 dB and 6.0206 dB for intensity and pressure, respectively. It should also be recalled from basic mathematics that $10^{-2} = 0.01$; $10^{-3} = 0.001$; $3 \times 10^{-2} = 0.03$; $4.5 \times 10^{-5} = 0.000045$.

Considering the intensity scale, if 90 dB = 0.001 watt/m^2 (which is 10^{-3} watt/m^2), then 93 dB $\simeq$ 0.002 watt/m^2, 96 dB $\simeq$ 0.004 watt/m^2, and 99 dB $\simeq$ 0.008 watt/m^2. Further, 102 dB $\simeq$ 0.016 watt/m^2 and, thus, 92 dB $\simeq$ 0.0016 watt/m^2. Finally, 95 dB $\simeq$ 0.0032 watt/m^2, 98 dB $\simeq$ 0.0064 watt/m^2, 101 dB $\simeq$ 0.0128 watt/m^2, and 91 dB $\simeq$ 0.00128 watt/m^2. Hence, with a knowledge of the effects of doubling and multiplying by 10, one can construct the entire scale for whole-number decibel steps. It should be pointed out that because doubling does not result in an exact 3-dB increase, a cumulative error develops. In order to reduce this factor to a minimum, all of the doublings should be done in one or two decade ranges, moving to other decade ranges in multiples of ten.

A similar procedure can be followed with sound pressure. On this scale, however, only the even whole-number decibel steps can be found. Consequently, if 80 dB $\simeq$ 2 dynes/cm^2, then 86 dB $\simeq$ 4 dynes/cm^2, 92 dB $\simeq$ 8 dynes/cm^2, 98 dB $\simeq$ 16 dynes/cm^2, 104 dB $\simeq$ 32 dynes/cm^2, 84 dB $\simeq$ 3.2 dynes/cm^2, etc. In order to obtain levels for other values of pressure or intensity ratios, it is necessary to consult tables prepared for this purpose or to utilize a table of common logarithms. Both the *Handbook of Noise Control* (29) and the *Handbook of Noise Measurement* (53) (from which Table 13.2 is drawn) contain tables specifically designed for decibel work and do not require a thorough knowledge of logarithms in order to be used effectively.

Common problems using decibel calculations involve the combining or subtracting of sound sources, the calculation of spectrum level from a knowledge of overall level and bandwidth, and the calculation of the overall level from spectrum level for a given bandwidth. In each instance, the computation is figured on an energy basis, that is, on the intensity or power scale. When two identical sound sources are presented at the same time, the overall level of the combined sources is 3 dB higher than either source presented alone, because the sound from the two sources combines on an energy basis. Thus, 90 dB + 90 dB $\simeq$ 93 dB. But what is the overall level when a second source of say 87 dB (when sounded alone) is added to a room where the level is 90 dB before the second source is added? Converting to watt/m^2: 90 dB = 0.001 watt/m^2 and 87 dB $\simeq$ 0.0005 watt/m^2. The sum of the two is equal to about 0.0015 watt/m^2. Because 0.0015 is 1.5 times as large as 0.001, and because this ratio represents a decibel increase of approximately 1.8 dB over 90 dB, the overall level of the combined sources is calculated to be 91.8 dB. The 1.8 dB is obtained by consulting a decibel table (such as Table 13.2) or a table of common logarithms.

Subtraction is handled similarly. If the overall level in a room is 90 dB and a source of 87 dB (when sounded alone) is removed, what will be the resulting overall level? Ninety dB = 0.001 watt/m^2 and 87 dB $\simeq$ 0.0005 watt/m^2. Subtraction results in an answer of 0.0005 watt/m^2 or 87 dB. Hence, by removing a source which alone is 3 dB below the overall level, the overall level is reduced by 3 dB. A second problem further illustrating the manner of reduction is 90 dB minus 84 dB. Converting to the intensity values and subtracting, 0.001 watt/m^2 − 0.00025 watt/m^2 = 0.00075 watt/m^2. Converting back to intensity level, 0.00075 watt/m^2 equals approximately 1.25 dB. Therefore, the overall level is reduced to 88.75 dB through the removal of the 84-dB source. It should be noted that if the level of the source removed (when sounded alone) is within 3 dB of the overall level of all the sources combined, then this single source is producing the majority of the sound energy, and its removal results in a greater than 3-dB decrease in overall level. If the level of the source removed (when sounded alone) is more than 3 dB below the overall level of combined sources, it is a minor source of the total sound energy and its removal results in less than a 3-dB decrease in the overall level. Figure 13.1, which is from the *Handbook of Noise Measurement*, presents a graphic method of adding and subtracting decibels without calculation.

In spectrum level calculations, it is assumed that the noise in question is reasonably flat across frequencies within the band being studied. In actual practice, however, the spectrum level across the band is seldom flat except for intentionally produced "white" noises, and even these noises are shaped by the frequency response of the electroacoustic system being used. Nevertheless, when the bands are sufficiently narrow, the degree of error introduced through this assumption is small unless the noise contains strong narrow-band or pure-tone components.

In order to find the average spectrum intensity (watts per square meter) within a given bandwidth of a noise with a known intensity, it is necessary only to divide the intensity of the band by the width of the band in Hz. This procedure is analogous to dividing a total weight by the number of items included in the total in order to find the average weight of the individual items. However, since sound magnitude normally is expressed in decibels rather than in watts, it is first necessary to convert the sound levels to intensity, then divide, and then convert back to decibels. An alternative

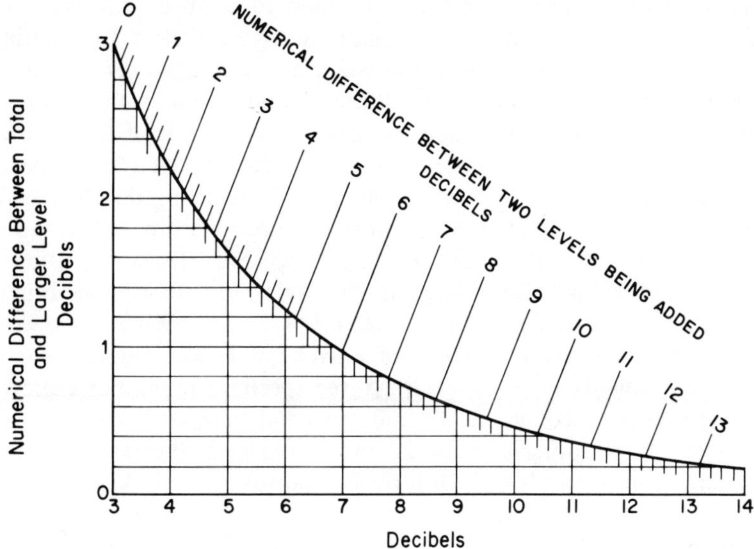

FIGURE 13.1 Combining levels of uncorrelated noise signals.

TO ADD LEVELS

Enter the graph with the NUMERICAL DIFFERENCE BETWEEN TWO LEVELS BEING ADDED. Follow the line corresponding to this value to its intersection with the curved line, then left to read the NUMERICAL DIFFERENCE BETWEEN TOTAL AND LARGER LEVEL. Add this value to the larger level to determine the total.

Example: Combine 75 dB and 80 dB. The difference is 5 dB. The 5-dB line intersects the curved line at 1.2 dB on the vertical scale. Thus the total value is 80 + 1.2 or 81.2 dB.

TO SUBTRACT LEVELS

Enter the graph with the NUMERICAL DIFFERENCE BETWEEN TOTAL AND LARGER LEVELS if this value is less than 3dB. Enter the chart with the NUMERICAL DIFFERENCE BETWEEN TOTAL AND SMALLER LEVELS if this value is between 3 and 14 dB. Follow the line corresponding to this value to its intersection with the curved line, then either left or down to read the NUMERICAL DIFFERENCE BETWEEN TOTAL AND LARGER (SMALLER) LEVELS. Subtract this value from the total level to determine the unknown level.

Example: Subtract 81 dB from 90 dB. The difference is 9 dB. The 9-dB vertical line intersects the curved line at 0.6 dB on the vertical scale. Thus the unknown level is 90-0.6 or 89.4 dB.

(This graph is based on one developed by R. Musa.)

Source: Peterson, A. P. G., and E. E. Gross, Jr. Appendix II, *Handbook of Noise Measurement* (6th ed.), West Concord, Mass.: General Radio Company, 1967.

method, which requires only one conversion to decibels, is based on the fact that adding and subtracting logarithms is equivalent to multiplying and dividing the antilogarithms (the watts per square meter). In this procedure, find 10 $\log_{10}$ of the bandwidth in Hz, and subtract this result from the band level to obtain the spectrum level. For example, if the bandwidth is 10,000 Hz and the overall level of the band is 100 dB, the average spectrum level is 60 dB (10 $\log_{10}$ of 10,000 = 40 dB; 100 dB minus 40 dB = 60 dB). A somewhat more complicated example is a bandwidth of 200 Hz and an overall level of 100 dB. Since 10 $\log_{10}$ of 200 $\simeq$ 23 (because 10 $\log_{10}$ of 100 = 20 and 200 is twice as large as 100, giving 23 dB), the spectrum level equals about 77 dB (100 dB minus 23 dB = 77 dB). When the spectrum level is known and the overall level of a given band is desired, the procedure is to add 10 $\log_{10}$ of the bandwidth to the spectrum level. For example, if the spectrum level equals 20 dB and the bandwidth is 400 Hz, the band level is 46 dB (10 $\log_{10}$ of 100 = 20 and 10 $\log_{10}$ of 400/100 $\simeq$ 6; thus the 20-dB spectrum level plus 26 dB for the bandwidth equals 46 dB).

FREQUENCY

Most noises are complex broad band acoustic signals. For many applications, a knowledge of the distribution of sound energy along the frequency scale is required. Frequency is normally plotted on a natural logarithmic scale (log to the base two: $\log_2$). That is, each successively higher octave has a bandwidth which is double that of the one below. In music, the successive octaves are given the natural logarithmic labels of C_1, C_2, C_3, etc. In acoustics, logarithmic labels generally are not used except for the one-third octave bands.

It is well known that a two-to-one ratio represents a one-octave interval. Among audiologists, however, it is not generally recognized that 1,500 Hz, 3,000 Hz, etc., do not represent the mid-octave points between 1,000 and 2,000 Hz, and 2,000 and 4,000 Hz. These values are used on audiometers, apparently, because they are arithmetically convenient. In order to find the actual mid-octave intervals, third-octave intervals, or other fractional octave intervals, use the following procedure: because frequencies are on a $\log_2$ scale, raise 2 to the fractional power desired (1/2, 1/3, 1/4) and multiply the base frequency (the lowest frequency of the band) by the answer. For example, in order to find the mid-octave interval of the 1,000 to 2,000 Hz octave, first find $2^{1/2}$ (this is equivalent to the square root of two), which is 1.4142, and multiply that by 1,000 to get an answer of 1,414.2 Hz. One-third octaves are found by multiplying $2^{1/3}$, which is 1.259921 and is equivalent to the cube root of two, by the base frequency. For the 1,000 to 2,000 Hz octave, the one-third octave intervals are 1,000.0 to 1,259.9 Hz, 1,259.9 to 1,587.2 Hz, and 1,587.2 to 2,000.0 Hz. Normally, it is unnecessary to find smaller fractional intervals, but narrower intervals can be found similarly or by finding the $\log_{10}$ of 2 (which is 0.30103), dividing this value by the number of divisions desired (4, 5, 6, etc.), and then finding the antilogarithm of the quotient. This number is then used as the value by which each successive base frequency is multiplied. For example, 0.30103 divided by 3 = 0.10034, the antilogarithm of which is about 1.2599. This antilogarithm value is then multiplied by the base frequency to give the upper limit of the third-octave band in question.

In psychoacoustics, bandwidth is sometimes expressed in decibels. Bandwidth in dB equals 10 $\log_{10}$ of the bandwidth in Hz. For example, a bandwidth of 20 dB equals a bandwidth of 100 Hz, and a bandwidth of 2,000 Hz equals a bandwidth of 33 dB. Thus, bandwidth expressed in dB can be converted to Hz and, at the same time, can indicate the difference between the overall band level and the spectrum level (band level minus bandwidth in dB equals spectrum level).

DURATION

The duration of exposure to noise is an important parameter, but exposure durations are normally expressed in intervals that require no discussion (minutes, hours, days, and years). Exceptions are noises of less than 0.2 seconds in duration, which will be discussed in a subsequent section of this chapter.

Instrumentation for Noise Measurement

SOUND LEVEL INSTRUMENTS

The general-purpose sound-level meter is the basic instrument for the measurement of noise level. The fundamental characteristics of this instrument are set forth in standard number S1.4–1961 ("Specification for General-Purpose Sound-Level Meters") of the United States of America Standards Institute (USASI) (67). The general-purpose sound-level meters consist principally of a calibrated microphone, suitable amplifiers, a frequency weighting network, a calibrated attenuator, an indicating meter, and an output connection to accomodate additional measuring equipment. The unit must have a means of calibrating the electrical circuitry. The microphone can be calibrated only by some external means such as by free field substitution, by reciprocity calibration, by using a pure-tone signal source produced by manufacturers specifically for calibration purposes, or by a pistonphone. Sound-survey meters are essentially the same as the general-purpose sound-level meters, except that they are smaller, lighter in weight, and less expensive. These advantages are achieved by limiting the versatility of the instrument and by manufacturing the instrument to somewhat larger tolerances.

Sound-survey meters do not meet all of the requirements of USASI S1.4–1961.

Of particular significance are the three weighting networks A, B, and C found on all sound-level meters. The weightings of the three networks are shown in Figure 13.2. Each is designed to approximate a Phon or loudness level curve. The A setting approximates the 40-Phon curve, B the 70-Phon curve, and C the 100-Phon curve. These meters may also include a "20–KC" setting where the frequency response is flat up to 20,000 Hz within the limits imposed by the microphone at a particular angle of incidence. The USASI. S1.4–1961 standard specifies the limits within which the actual response of the instrument must fall. A precision sound-level meter is one which meets the tolerance requirements of the IEC 179 "Precision Sound-Level Meters–1965 Standard" (55). This standard is more stringent in the high frequencies but less so in the low frequencies than S1.4–1961. In 1967 and 1968, there were references found to N and D weighting networks. Following the suggestion of Technical Committee 29 of the International Electrotechnical Commission (IEC/TC29), technicians must now refer to the inverse NOY curve passing through 1,000 Hz at the same level as A, B, and C as the D weighting curve. This curve was formerly called N. The letter N is now reserved for a curve parallel to D but 7-dB higher (3).

It should be noted that the name of this device is "sound-level meter" rather than "sound-pressure-level meter" even though the basic reference pressure is 0.0002 microbar. The reason for this is that with the device on

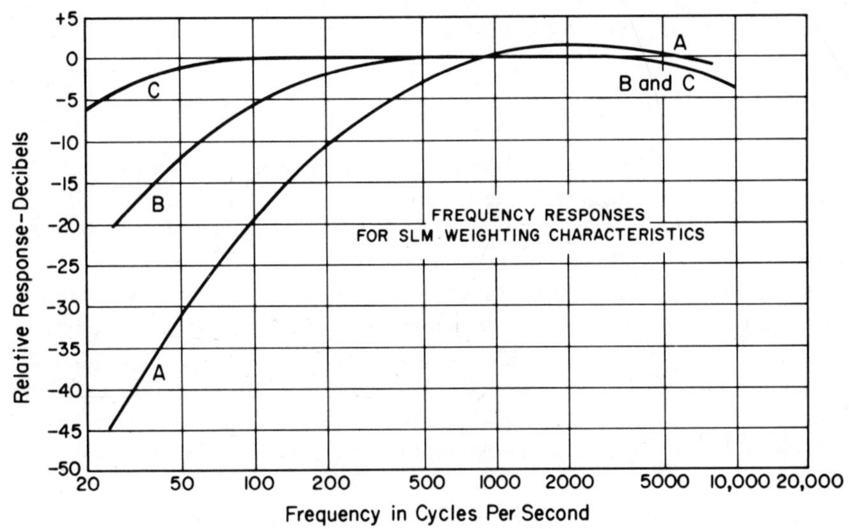

FIGURE 13.2 Frequency-response characteristics of the USASI S1.4-1961 "Standard for General Purpose Sound-Level Meters."

Source: American Standard Specification for General Purpose Sound Level Meters (S1.4-1960), Figure 2, p. 8.

the A, B, or C settings, the meter indication may not represent dB above 0.0002 microbar because the filtering characteristics of the weighting networks reduce the meter indication. Sound level is simply defined as the level measured by a sound-level meter meeting the specifications of USASI S1.4–1961 with the weighting network specified.

Sound levels are obtained by adding the meter reading to the attenuator value indicated, when the latter is set at a position necessary to obtain an onscale meter deflection. The choice of the weighting network depends upon the application. In the past, in order to obtain readings which approximate the manner in which human beings perceive sound at various intensity levels, it was recommended that the A scale be used for levels below 55 dB, the B scale for levels in the 55 to 85-dB range, and the C scale for levels above 85 dB (52). In the latest edition of the *Handbook of Noise Measurement* (53), Peterson and Gross reflect the current practice of using the A scale for most sound-level readings. This practice is based upon observations that the A-weighting scale readings correlate well with subjective judgments of noise loudness and annoyance (53, 32, 79). In 1967, Botsford (5) presented evidence that A scale readings are as good as more complicated methods for evaluating the hearing damage risk potential of a noise. Further, Webster (76) has concluded that speech interference levels are estimated very well by A scale readings. However, when making a frequency analysis of noise with associated equipment, measurements should be made on the C scale or the "20–KC" setting in order to deliver a relatively flat signal to the analysis or recording equipment.

The weighting networks also may be used to approximate the distribution of noise energy across frequency. If the readings on the A setting are much lower than on the C setting, then the A-filtering network has prevented a significant portion of the noise from reaching the meter. It may be concluded that such a noise has relatively strong low-frequency components because the A network filters primarily the low frequencies.

FREQUENCY-BAND ANALYZERS

The most widely used instrument for the frequency analysis of noise is the octave-band analyzer. This instrument consists of a microphone, amplifiers, calibrated attenuators, filter circuits, an indicating meter, and an output jack. Also included are provisions for the input of signals from sound-level meters or other appropriate equipment. The analyzer usually includes "C" and "20–KC" weighting networks.

Octave-band analyzers are available with either one of two sets of bands. One set is based on the USASI Z24.10–1953 standard ("Specification for an Octave-Band Filter Set for Analysis of Noise and Other Sounds") (65) and is labeled according to the nominal cut-off frequencies of the bands; 150 to 300 Hz, 300 to 600 Hz, 600 to 1,200 Hz, etc. The other set is based on the USASI S1.6–1960 standard ("Preferred Frequencies for Acoustical Measurements") (56) and is designated by the center frequency of the bands; 250 Hz, 500 Hz, 1,000 Hz, etc. The nominal cutoff frequencies of these bands are given in Table 13.4. It should be pointed out that the nominal cutoff frequencies for octave-band analyzers are the 3-dB down points. Also the cutoff frequencies presented in Table 13.4 do not correspond to the 1953 values. The "preferred frequencies" have come into increasingly common use in recent years and are gradually replacing the older values.

TABLE 13.3. THE PREFERRED OCTAVE-BAND SERIES FROM USASI S1. 6–1960

The preferred octave band series:

Center Frequency Hertz	*Effective Band Hertz*	*Band No.*
31.5	22.1 to 44.2	15
63	44.2 to 88.4	18
125	88.4 to 177	21
250	177 to 354	24
500	354 to 707	27
1,000	707 to 1,414	30
2,000	1,414 to 2,828	33
4,000	2,828 to 5,657	36
8,000	5,657 to 11,314	39

The preferred center frequencies in one-third-octave steps are:

No.	*Hertz*	*No.*	*Hertz*	*No.*	*Hertz*
10	10	20	100	30	1,000
11	12.5	21	125	31	1,250
12	16	22	160	32	1,600
13	20	23	200	33	2,000
14	25	24	250	34	2,500
15	31.5	25	315	35	3,150
16	40	26	400	36	4,000
17	50	27	500	37	5,000
18	63	28	630	38	6,300
19	80	29	800	39	8,000

The octave-band analyzer is calibrated in the same manner as the sound-level meter. In order to check the calibration of the individual bands, the levels observed in each band may be summed on an energy basis (as explained earlier) and compared with the overall levels in the presence of a reasonably flat broad band noise. The sum of the bands should be within one or two dB of the overall level. When high-quality white noise is presented to the analyzer (bypassing the microphone), each higher octave band reads 3 dB greater than the one below. This occurs because each successively higher band is twice as wide and, thereby, contains twice the energy of the band immediately below. This is yet another way to check filter networks.

Equipment employing band widths narrower than octave bands are less frequently used than octave-band analyzers because of greater cost and complexity. In addition, such detailed information is usually unnecessary in industrial and military noise measurement applications. Some special noise problems, particularly those in which narrow-band or pure-tone components are suspected, may require this more sophisticated instrumentation.

Narrow-band analyzers are of the constant-ratio type (including octave-band analyzers) or the constant bandwidth type. A common constant ratio type is the one-third octave-band analyzer. The bands are based on $10^{1/10}$ (or 1.2589) times the base frequency rather than $2^{1/3}$ (or 1.2599) times the base frequency, and are numbered according to 10 $\log_{10}$ of the center frequency. That is, the band centered at 1,000 Hz is labeled band number 30, the band centered at 2,000 Hz is labeled number 33, etc. The ratio $10^{1/10}$ is used instead of $2^{1/3}$ in the construction of one-third octave-band analyzers so that the system can be extended conveniently into the infrasonic and ultrasonic regions (USASI S1.6–1960). The resulting error is very small. As with the octave-band analyzer, a flat spectrum input results in higher readings in each successively higher band. The rate of increase is one dB per one-third octave-band step. Other constant ratio analyzers are one-tenth octave and constant percentage types. Bandwidths as narrow as 3 per cent of the nominal center frequency are available.

Constant bandwidth analyzers are available with nominal bandwidths as narrow as 3 Hz. The constant bandwidth types have the distinct advantage of providing observed levels which are always the same number of dB above the spectrum level. With the constant ratio types, the difference between the observed level and the spectrum level varies with frequency, complicating the calculation of spectrum level. However, constant bandwidth analyzers are generally more costly than constant ratio analyzers.

IMPACT ANALYZERS

Some noises encountered in industrial and military establishments, such as punch presses or gunfire, are characterized by short durations and fast rise times. When a sound-level meter is presented with such brief inputs (less than about 0.2 second), the mass of the movement of the indicating meter prevents the meter from reaching full deflection before the cessation of the input. The meter thereby underestimates the level of the noise. This underestimation is substantial for very brief pulses.

The level of short duration signals is measured more accurately with impact meters or oscilloscopes. An impact meter such as General Radio, Type 1556–B, is a device which stores the input signal in a capacitor for a period of time which is sufficient for the meter to reach full deflection. Such a device produces accurate level indications for impulse durations as short as 50 microseconds. The meter remains within one dB of the peak value for about 10 seconds. Impact meters also measure time-averaged noise levels which are averaged over a selection of intervals from about 0.002 to 0.2 second. The difference between peak values and time-averaged values is used to estimate the duration of the sound pulse. Shorter sound pulses produce greater differences between the peak level and the time-average level when averaged over a duration significantly longer than the pulse duration. Necessary information for making these estimates is provided in the manufacturer's instruction manuals (Operating instructions, General Radio, Type 1556–B, Impact-Noise Analyzer, 1962) (49).

Oscilloscopes are also used for impact noise measurements. The electron beam reacts essentially instantaneously to the input, because the beam is virtually without mass. However, these devices are quite expensive, and they are relatively inconvenient to use outside of the laboratory.

TAPE RECORDERS

Tape recorders are used to bring noises into the laboratory, or to store noises for future reference. Although a complete discussion of tape recorders is beyond the scope of this chapter, it should be noted that the instrument imposes limitations upon the analysis. One requirement of a tape recorder used for noise analysis is a frequency response equal to or exceeding that of a sound-level meter. This, in turn, requires a tape speed of at least seven and one-half inches per second. In addition, the signal-to-noise ratio must be at least 45 dB (63). Since sound-level meters generally have a moderately high output impedance, the bridging input should be used on the recorder. It is important not to overload the recorder or the tape, particularly when dealing with sounds of short duration. Because of these and other problems, the analysis of signals recorded on tape should not be attempted without a thorough understanding of the characteristics of the individual tape recorder in use. Peterson (51) presents a thorough discussion of the features of a tape recorder designed specifically for noise measurements.

The Noise Survey

The proper choice of noise measurement positions requires a thorough understanding of temporal and spatial work patterns. Each environment has its own peculiar set of circumstances which should be studied thoroughly by the surveyor. For such a study, he must have a complete knowledge of his equipment, including the effects of humidity, temperature, angle of incidence, observer position, as well as the effects of cables and microphones. A noise hazard should be measured with the microphone at the position of the employee's most exposed ear. The microphone should be oriented at several angles of incidence. When these several obtained levels are within 2 or 3 dB of each other, an average is used as the sound level at that position. If the sound source is close and it is clear that sound arriving directly from the source is stronger than the reflected sound, the microphone may be oriented at any angle to the source for which the free field calibration of the microphone is known. The sound can be assumed to be arriving directly from the source when it is observed that moving the microphone away from the source results in a significant reduction in level.

Of particular importance are the records of noise measurements. These must include floor plans with machinery locations, indications of machinery elevations from the floor, locations of measurement positions, and the noise levels obtained. In addition, all measurement conditions must be noted, including the date and time of day; the temperature; the location and number of workers, the operating conditions for the machinery; a description of walls, floors, and ceilings; and the position of the surveyor. A complete description of the measuring equipment, including type and serial number, weighting network used, microphone sensitivity and serial number, meter speed, extent of meter fluctuation, any correction factors applied, position and orientation of the microphone, as well as the results of calibration checks are recorded. For further details of survey techniques, consult Williams (77), Peterson and Gross (53), and the instructions accompanying the noise measuring equipment.

It is necessary to measure the noise levels within the audiometric test space in order to determine whether the observed noise levels are sufficient to influence hearing test results obtained in this space. While the desired degree of quiet depends upon whether the room is used for research work, clinical work, or hearing survey work, the procedures are essentially the same. Measurements are made with the microphone at the position normally occupied by the subject's head and at the same time of day the hearing tests are to be conducted. Levels should be obtained in bands not wider than one octave. USASI standard S3.1–1960 ("Criteria for Background Noise in Audiometer Rooms") (7) gives octave-band levels, one-third octave-band levels, and spectrum levels which can not be exceeded in order to measure hearing thresholds down to the level of 0 dB, according to the USASI standard Z24.5–1951 ("Specifications for Audiometers for General Diagnostic Purposes") (66). This standard assumes that thresholds are measured with audiometers meeting USASI standard Z24.5–1951 and Z24.12–1952 ("Specifications for Pure-Tone Audiometers for Screening Purposes") (68). If for each test tone frequency, the octave-band level of the background noise is less than the value given in the standard, the room is usable under the conditions given in the standard. In order to obtain accurate thresholds at test tone levels below 0 dB according to USASI Z24.5–1951, lesser ambient noise levels are required. The stringency of the criteria is increased by the difference between the USASI Z24.5–1951 levels and the proposed

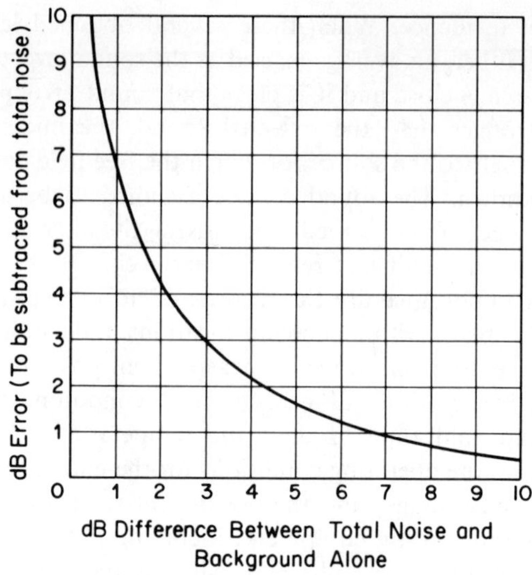

FIGURE 13.3 Background noise correction for sound-level measurements.

test tone levels. When unoccluded thresholds are obtained, the attenuation provided by the MX/41/AR cushion should be subtracted from the criteria, also. If other earphone cushions are used, the criteria are changed by the amount of difference in the attenuation provided by that cushion relative to the amount provided by the MX/41/AR. The criteria for background noise in audiometer rooms expressed in octave bands, one-third octave bands, and spectrum levels from USASI S3.1–1960, are reproduced in Tables 13.4 and 13.5. In 1968 a USASI committee approved by the Acoustical Society of America began work on updating this standard.

Because of the low levels measured, circuit noise in the measuring equipment may confound the measurements. The manufacturers' instructions for the measurement of circuit noise should be carried out, and if the measured noise level is less than 10 dB above the circuit noise, a correction for summation should be made according to Figure 13.3 (53). If the measured level is less than 3 dB above the circuit noise, it is apparent that the circuit noise is the major contributor to the meter indication, and a valid estimate of the room noise cannot be made in that band.

Hearing Loss from Noise

KIND AND DEGREE

Of particular interest to the audiologist are the nature and the extent of hearing losses resulting from exposure to noise. Reviews of the early

TABLE 13.4. MAXIMUM ALLOWABLE SOUND PRESSURE LEVELS FOR NO MASKING ABOVE THE ZERO HEARING-LOSS SETTING OF A STANDARD AUDIOMETER

(*Decibels ref* 0.0002 *Microbar*)

Audiometric test frequency (cps)	125	250	500	750	1,000	1,500	2,000	3,000	4,000	6,000	8,000
$\frac{1}{3}$ *octave band center frequency (cps)*	125	250	500	800	1,000	1,600	2,000	3,200	4,000	6,400	8,000
Sound pressure level (dB)	35	35	35	35	35	37	42	47	52	57	62
$\frac{1}{2}$ *octave band cut-off frequencies (cps)*	106–150	212–300	425–600	600–850	850–1,200	1,200–1,700	1,700–2,400	2,400–3,400	3,400–4,800	4,800–6,800	6,800–9.600
Sound pressure level (dB)	37	37	37	37	37	39	44	49	54	59	68
Octave band cut-off frequencies (cps)	75–150	150–300	300–600	600–1,200	600–1,200	1,200–2,400	1,200–2,400	2,400–4,800	2,400–4,800	4,800–10,000	4,800–10,000
Sound pressure level (dB)	40	40	40	40	40	42	47	52	57	62	67

Source: Table One of USASI S3.1–1960 ("Background Noise in Audiometer Rooms"), p. 9.

TABLE 13.5. MAXIMUM ALLOWABLE SPECTRUM LEVELS FOR NO MASKING ABOVE THE ZERO HEARING-LOSS SETTING OF A STANDARD AUDIOMETER

(*Decibels ref* 0.0002 *Microbar for* 1-*cps band*)

Audiometric test frequency (cps)	125	250	500	750	1,000	1,500	2,000	3,000	4,000	6,000	8,000
Spectrum level of narrow-band sound whose center frequency is nearly that of the test tone	21	18	15	12	12	11	16	18	23	25	30

Source: Table Two of USASI S3.1–1960 ("Background Noise in Audiometer Rooms"), p. 9.

literature by Kryter (36) and Glorig (18) suggest that while there was some awareness of hearing loss due to noise for a century or more, it was not until the 1930's and the 1940's that the problem was widely studied. Following World War II, the Subcommittee on Noise in Industry was established by the Committee on Conservation of Hearing of the American Academy of Ophthalmology and Otolaryngology. The American Standards Association Committee Z24–X–2 was established in 1952, and shortly thereafter the Committee on Hearing and Bioacoustics (CHABA) of the National Academy of Science was established. Kryter's 1950 study provided considerable impetus toward the establishment of the latter two committees. The purposes of these committees were to study noise and its effect on hearing, to attempt to set forth guidelines for acceptable levels of noise, and to establish hearing conservation methods in industry.

The major characteristics of hearing loss due to noise were recognized early, and they have become increasingly well defined over the years. Hearing losses due to noise exposure are divided into two broad categories; acoustic trauma and noise-induced hearing loss. Lawrence (40) describes acoustic trauma as damage to the ear resulting from a sharply rising wavefront, such as an intense blast. Lawrence states that in true acoustic trauma, the auditory insult occurs usually only once and the damage is produced at that time. His studies demonstrate that acoustic trauma often results in a rupture of the eardrum with resultant bleeding and a conductive loss of hearing. In addition, there may be damage to the inner ear such as the dislodgement of a part of the organ of Corti from the basilar membrane. Noise trauma, then, can produce both conductive losses, which may be only temporary, and sensori-neural losses, which are often permanent.

The second type, noise-induced hearing loss, constitutes the vast majority of hearing losses observed in industrial and military situations. Noise-induced hearing loss is caused by daily exposure to intense sound over a long period of time (months or years). Such noises are not sufficiently intense to produce acoustic trauma. Nevertheless, the noise is injurious and gradually, over time, slight insult is added to slight insult until a permanent hearing loss is produced. Lawrence (40) explains the pathophysiology of this process by noting that the organ of Corti does not have a direct blood supply. This condition prevents a rapid exchange of nutrients and waste products at the cellular level during auditory stimulation. Lawrence believes that continued stimulation depletes the energy resources of the cells and produces a temporary threshold shift. If auditory stimulation is removed, the ear usually recovers, but if the cellular changes are sufficiently extensive, they may produce a permanent loss of hearing.

The earliest physical changes in the cell are difficult to detect visually and may be confined to the supporting cell structures (45). As injury level increases, however, Deiter's cells become difficult to distinguish, the tunnel of Corti becomes filled with debris, and the nuclei of the outer hair cells begin to disappear. Intense stimulation causes a disappearance of the organ of Corti, disruptions in Reissner's membrane, and other destruction. As time passes, the organ of Corti is replaced by a layer of simple epithelial cells (40, 45). Both Lawrence (40) and Schuknecht and Tonndorf (62) observed that although the end result of acoustic trauma and noise-induced hearing loss appear audiometrically similar, the former is the result of an immediate mechanical destruction of the organ of Corti, while the latter results from cumulative depletion of the cells' ability to perform their function.

Ward, Fleer, and Glorig (74) demonstrated that exposure to repeated small arms fire produced hearing losses not significantly different from those produced by exposure to continuous noise. Lindquist, Neff, and Schuknecht (41) demonstrated that the histopathological appearance of the cochlear lesion is identical for animals exposed to gunfire and for those subjected to head blows. These studies indicate that the same inner-ear structures lose their function in the same order in most forms of traumatic injury, whether over a short or long duration.

The 4,000 Hz sensori-neural notch has, for many years, been recognized as the principal audiometric feature of a hearing loss resulting from excessive auditory stimulation. Other characteristics of noise-induced hearing loss have been identified by Ward, Glorig, and Fleer (74). These include the observations that the 4,000 Hz notch often includes 6,000 Hz with approximately the same degree of loss at both frequencies; that the degree of loss is less pronounced at 8,000 Hz than at the two lower frequencies; and that hearing sensitivity for sounds below 4,000 Hz is relatively unaffected, with greater resistance to injury at lower and lower frequencies. These authors also inspected the individual configurations and found that the steepness of the audiometric curve above the cutoff frequency (the highest frequency at which normal hearing is observed) is unrelated to the cutoff frequency. In addition, improved hearing sensitivity at the frequency region just below the cutoff frequency was noted. The authors speculate that this latter finding results from the loss of inhibitory fibers located just basalward from the area responsive to the cutoff frequency.

Another common observation is that noise-induced hearing losses do not usually exceed 50 to 60-dB HL (according to USASI Z24.5–1951). It is hypothesized that this level may represent the threshold of the inner hair cells which are more resistent to injury than the outer hair cells (10). A second possibility is that when the test tone level reaches 50 to 60 dB (USASI Z24.5–1951), the excitation pattern on the basilar membrane becomes sufficiently broad to stimulate relatively normal adjacent areas (74). Observations by Ward, Glorig, and Fleer reveal mild to moderate tone decay in some noise exposure losses but not in others. Their observations also show that loudness recruitment is almost always present and that it reaches complete recruitment at 100-dB SPL, regardless of the amount of hearing loss. This feature is similar to that described by Hallpike and

Hood (27) as a characteristic of Meniere's disease. Ward, Glorig, and Fleer found that speech discrimination is affected in noise-induced hearing losses to the extent that would be expected if the hearing loss functioned as a simple filter.

Schuknecht and Tonndorf (62) review various hypotheses to explain the reason for the 4,000 Hz notch. They conclude that there are basically two schools of thought. The first maintains that upon stimulation, strong mechanical forces develop in the area of the organ of Corti responsive to 4,000 Hz tones. The second maintains that the area of the organ of Corti responsive to 4,000 Hz is more susceptible to damage. As an example of the susceptibility point of view, Schuknecht and Tonndorf mention the work of Crowe, Guild, and Polvolgt (8) who suggested that the blood supply to the 4,000 Hz area of the organ of Corti is relatively poor. Today, most investigators, including Schuknecht and Tonndorf, support the mechanical approach. In 1946, Ruedi and Furrer (61) proposed the "dual-eddy theory," and in 1953 Hilding (31) proposed the "jet theory." Both of these theories follow the mechanistic approach and both maintain that the mechanics of cochlear action place excessive strains on the 4,000 Hz area of the organ of Corti. Schuknecht and Tonndorf agree that excessive strain is the probable cause. Furthermore, they believe that this strain is due to the acceleration of the basilar membrane during stimulation. They assume that stress is approximately proportional to acceleration, and that the acceleration of the basilar membrane depends upon the amplitude of the membrane and the position along the membrane.

Acceleration of the basilar membrane is greatest at the basal end, becoming progressively less toward the apical end. Schuknecht and Tonndorf reason that the higher frequencies areas are more susceptible to injury because the accelerative forces are greater and, therefore, the rise time is shorter at the basilar end. They state that acceleration in response to tones above 6,000 Hz is less because auditory sensitivity is less, and large displacement amplitudes are not possible in that region of the membrane. Therefore, according to Schuknecht and Tonndorf, the point of maximum stress on the membrane occurs at the region where the amplitude and the rise time of the traveling bulge combine to produce the greatest acceleration stress (the 4,000 to 6,000 Hz region).

Other factors may contribute to the greater loss in the 4,000 Hz region. High-frequency tones produce greater temporary threshold shifts (TTS) than low-frequency tones (73). This is true of permanent threshold shifts (PTS) as well (21, 39). The maximum TTS for moderate-level to high-level tones occurs from one-half to two octaves above the frequency of the fatiguing tone (73). If a band of noise is the fatiguer, the maximum TTS develops one-half to two octaves above the upper cutoff frequency of the noise band. If the upper cutoff frequency is above 3,000 Hz, the maximum effect is still produced in the 4,000 to 6,000 Hz region (73). Thus, fatiguers containing frequencies in the 1,000 Hz to 3,000 Hz region produce their greatest effect in the 2,000 Hz to 8,000 Hz region. Since the acoustic reflex does not attenuate inputs in this frequency region but does attenuate lower frequency inputs, the effect is to permit those frequencies which produce the greatest damage in the 4,000 Hz region to reach the inner ear unattenuated. Another contributing factor to this notch is the natural resonance of the ear canal which produces maximal enhancement of sound in the 2,000 to 3,000 Hz region (4, 54). Signals in this frequency range produce their greatest effect upon the ear in the 4,000 to 6,000 Hz region.

FACTORS INFLUENCING NOISE-INDUCED LOSS

A number of factors influence the extent of the hearing loss produced by noise. While there is a great deal of accumulated evidence on the influence of frequency, intensity, and duration upon TTS, relatively little is known about the influence of these parameters upon PTS. The basic problem is that PTS develops over periods of months or years, which makes it difficult or impossible to conduct longitudinal studies (i.e., studying different groups of individuals who have been exposed to the same noise for different durations).

Figure 13.4 from Glorig, Ward, and Nixon (21), illustrates the course

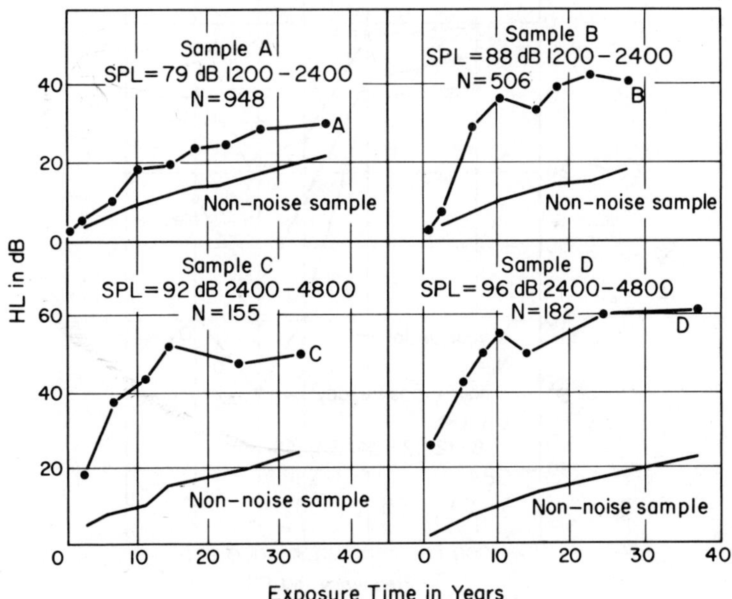

FIGURE 13.4 Median hearing levels at 4,000 Hz as a function of years of exposure.

Source: Glorig, A., W. D. Ward, and J. Nixon. "Damage risk criteria and noise-induced hearing loss." *Archives of Otolaryngology*, **74**: 419, 1961.

of PTS at 4,000 Hz as a function of exposure time and noise level. Although each data point is based upon different subjects, the results indicate that higher noise levels produce greater hearing loss. A difference is noted between those exposed to an octave-band sound level of 79 dB and those exposed to an octave-band sound level of 88 dB or more. The former group evidences only slightly more hearing loss than a nonnoise-exposed sample, whereas the latter group evidences considerably more hearing loss. In addition, the amount of hearing loss increases rapidly at first and then reaches a plateau in about ten years. After that, the rate of hearing loss increase is about equal to that observed for the nonnoise-exposed group. It must be remembered that these data are for 4,000 Hz only.

The next four figures are also taken from Glorig, Ward, and Nixon (21) and illustrate several additional features of noise-induced hearing loss. These figures record the first, second, and third quartile hearing losses (labeled Q_1, Q_2, and Q_3) for four different samples of subjects. Each sample was exposed to the same noise but for different durations. The average duration of exposure was four years for those subjects whose hearing thresholds are recorded in Figure 13.5. The 4,000 Hz notch is apparent in this figure.

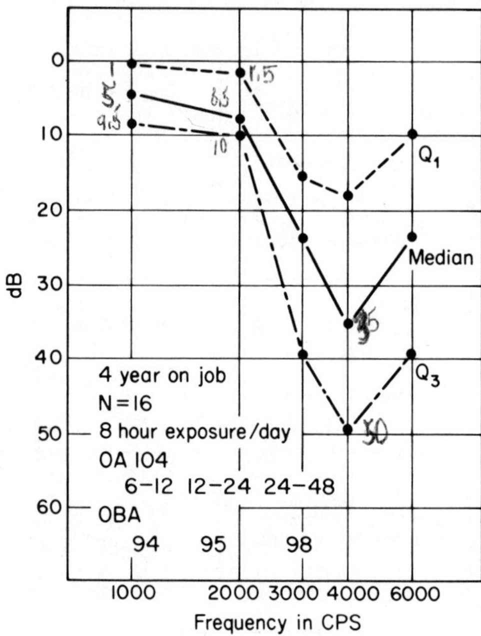

FIGURE 13.5 Noise-induced permanent threshold shift, at four years on the job.

Source: Glorig, A., W. D. Ward, and J. Nixon. "Damage risk criteria and noise-induced hearing loss." *Archives of Otolaryngology*, **74**: 419, 1961.

Of particular interest is the extent of the difference between Q_1 and Q_3. After only four years on the job, 25 per cent of the subjects evidenced losses in excess of 50 dB at 4,000 Hz, while 25 per cent of the subjects showed losses of less than 20 dB (both dB levels according to USASI Z24.5–1951). Obviously, substantial differences in susceptibility exist across individuals.

Figure 13.6 shows the results obtained on ninety-two subjects exposed

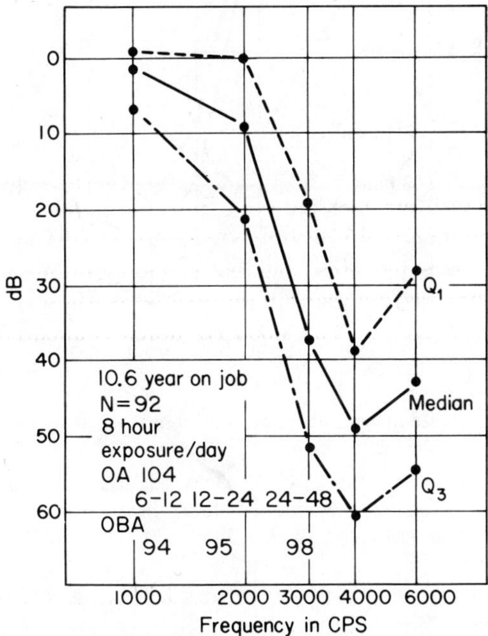

FIGURE 13.6 Noise-induced permanent threshold shift at ten years on the job.

Source: Glorig, A., W. D. Ward, and J. Nixon. "Damage risk criteria and noise-induced hearing loss." *Archives of Otolaryngology*, **74**: 419, 1961.

to the same noise levels for ten years. All quartiles are greater (increased hearing loss) but Q_1 has advanced more than Q_2 or Q_3, thus reducing the dispersion at both 4,000 and 6,000 Hz. At 2,000 Hz, however, the dispersion has increased with 25 per cent of the subjects showing significant hearing loss and 25 per cent of the subjects showing no hearing loss. Figure 13.7 illustrates that after twenty-one years on the job, 25 per cent of the subjects show very significant losses at 2,000 Hz, while 50 per cent of the subjects still evidence little or no hearing loss. The dispersion at 3,000 Hz, 4,000 Hz, and 6,000 Hz has decreased further, with Q_1 and Q_2 increasing more than Q_3; this reflects the previously discussed ceiling effect at 50 to 60 dB (according to USASI–1951 reference levels). At 1,000 Hz, 25 per cent of

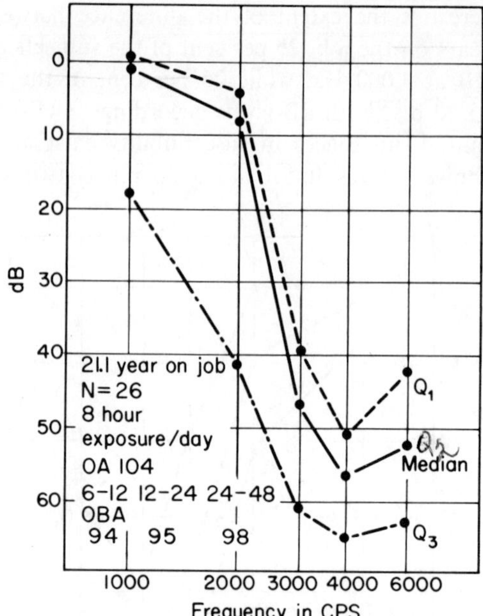

FIGURE 13.7 Noise-induced permanent threshold shift at twenty-one years on the job.

Source: Glorig, A., W. D. Ward, and J. Nixon. "Damage risk criteria and noise-induced hearing loss." *Archives of Otolaryngology*, **74**: 419, 1961.

the subjects revealed significant hearing loss following this twenty-one-year employment history. Finally, after thirty-three years, as shown in Figure 13.8, Q_3 for 1,000 Hz is substantially increased, while Q_1 and Q_2 show a slight increase. At 2,000 Hz all quartiles are depressed, while the interquartile ranges at all frequencies above 1,000 Hz are decreased further. The decreased steepness of the audiometric curve below 4,000 Hz indicates that the amount of increased loss is greater at the frequencies below 4,000 Hz than at 4,000 Hz. It is apparent that while sensitivity at 4,000 Hz reaches a plateau after ten years, sensitivity for the more important lower frequencies continues to decrease through the thirty-third year.

It must be remembered that all of the data for these four figures are based on different groups of subjects. However, an interfigure comparison suggests that the hearing sensitivity of susceptible ears at susceptible frequencies decreases sooner than that of less susceptible ears or at less susceptible frequencies. A plateau is then reached by the susceptible ears and susceptible frequencies. After a greater exposure time, the less susceptible ears and less susceptible frequencies "catch up," decreasing the interquartile range and decreasing the difference between hearing thresholds of adjacent test tone frequencies.

It is often assumed that noise-induced hearing loss and hearing loss due to presbycusis progress independently and are additive, although there is no definite evidence in support of this assumption at this time (35, 30, 6, 13). The average loss of hearing sensitivity as a function of age in a nonnoise-exposed population is now well established (13, 6), although there is wide variability in noise-induced and presbycusis hearing losses across individuals. At the present time, the relative contributions of the two etiologies to the total hearing loss of a given individual is impossible to determine (17).

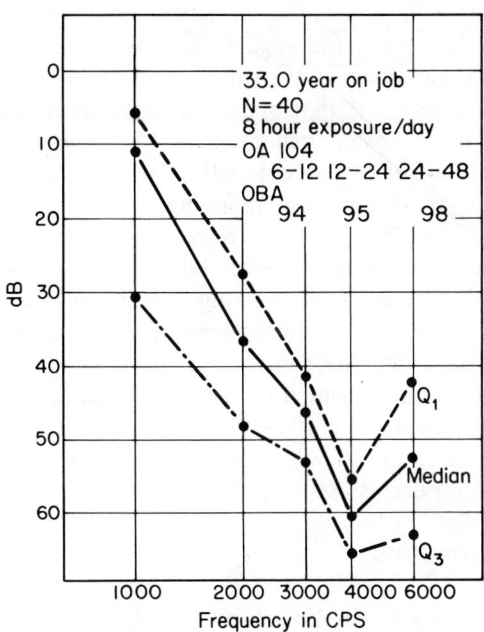

FIGURE 13.8 Noise-induced permanent threshold shift at thirty-three years on the job.

Source: Glorig, A., W. D. Ward, and J. Nixon. "Damage risk criteria and noise-induced hearing loss." *Archives of Otolaryngology*, **74**: 419, 1961.

Damage-Risk Criteria and Contours

EARLY DEVELOPMENTS

The term "damage-risk criteria" has generally referred to overall noise levels which are believed to represent the maximum levels to which an average human being could be exposed for eight hours a day over a working lifetime without acquiring a significant noise-induced hearing loss. Kryter

(36) pointed out that specifying noise in terms of overall level is inadequate, because overall level does not reveal the distribution of sound energy across the frequency range. He proposed the use of critical-band levels on the assumption that noise outside the critical band does not contribute to the deafening effect of the noise within the band. However, critical band levels have not been shown to be superior to octave or one-third octave-band levels as a basis for damage-risk criteria. The use of octave bands instead of critical bands avoids the additional step of calculating critical-band levels.

Since Kryter's 1950 publication, a number of damage-risk criteria have appeared in the literature. Eldredge (12) reviews these and evaluates the significance of each. Among the more important concepts developed during the 1950's were: (1) that a zone of hazardous noise levels, rather than a single noise level, delineates hazardous from nonhazardous levels (28); (2) that noises concentrated in narrow bands or noises with strong pure-tone components are more hazardous at a given level than broadband noises (36, 58); (3) that low-frequency noises are less hazardous than high-frequency noises (1, 36, 58); and (4) that reasonable damage-risk criteria do not protect everyone, making it necessary to accept significant hearing loss in some arbitarily chosen percentage of the people (13, 58, 59). AFR 160–3 (1) presented the concepts of recommended ear protection at one level of exposure and mandatory ear protection at a higher level. Also introduced in this document is a method for rating exposures of less than a full working day based on the assumption that the ear integrates successive exposures on a total energy basis.

RECENT DEVELOPMENTS

Continuous Exposure. In 1960 Jones and Church (34) reported a procedure based upon the work of Kryter (36), Hardy (28), and upon AFR 160–3 (1). Glorig, Ward, and Nixon (21) presented damage-risk criteria based upon the accumulated evidence of the Subcommittee on Noise in Industry. The committee stressed that all ears cannot be protected by any reasonable set of noise level criteria and, therefore, ongoing hearing testing must be included in a hearing conservation program in order to detect susceptible individuals. In addition, the authors stress that the damage-risk criteria should be established on the premise that hearing impairment is based upon the reduced ability to hear and understand speech.

A basic assumption underlying the Glorig, Ward, and Nixon work is that for a given noise, the amount of TTS developed over a short period of time by a group can be used to predict the amount of PTS developed by a group over a working lifetime of exposure. This is reasonably well demonstrated only at 4,000 Hz. Moreover, large intersubject variability makes this assumption inapplicable to individuals. On the basis of the TTS produced by various levels and durations of noise exposure, Glorig, Ward, and Nixon recommend the initiation of hearing conservation procedures if the noise level in any octave band exceeds the International Noise Rating Curve 85 (NR–85). This curve is presented in Table 13.6. The curve is

TABLE 13.6. HEARING DAMAGE RISK CRITERIA

Octave Band Levels for NR Curve 85

Octave Midfrequency	63	125	250	500	1,000	2,000	4,000	8,000
SPL (dB)	102	95	91	87	85	82	80	79

Source: Glorig, A., W. D. Ward, and J. Nixon, "Damage-Risk Criteria and Noise-Induced Hearing Loss." *Archives of Otolaryngology*, **74**; 421, 1961.

labeled according to the sound pressure level of the octave band on the curve which centers at 1,000 Hz. The other octave-band levels on the curve are levels which are believed to be equally damaging to hearing. The presence of higher permissible levels in the low frequencies reflects the observation that at a given level the low-frequency components of a noise are less injurious than the high-frequency components. The NR–85 curve was chosen as the criterion on the basis of evidence that octave-band levels at or below those of NR–85 will produce a TTS of 12 dB or less at 2,000 Hz (the most susceptible "speech frequency") in a workday of five hours or more. Therefore, an average PTS of 12 dB or less at 2,000 Hz is expected in a working lifetime.

In 1963 and 1965, Kryter (37, 38) redefined the term "damage-risk criteria" to refer to the extent of the acceptable hearing loss rather than to the maximum permissible sound levels. Since the maximum permissible sound levels are usually depicted as curves, he proposed labeling them "damage-risk contours." Kryter went on to propose damage-risk criterion hearing levels of not greater than 10 dB at 1,000 Hz, not more than 15 dB at 2,000 Hz, and not more than 20 dB at frequencies of 3,000 Hz or higher over a ten-year exposure period (all hearing levels according to USASI Z24.5–1951). On the basis of his review of the literature and his own investigations, Kryter concluded that the temporary threshold shift observed two minutes after a full day's exposure (TTS) can be used to predict PTS expected after ten or more years of exposure (PTS ten year). He cautioned against implying a causal relationship between TTS and PTS. Kryter also presented a set of damage-risk contours on the basis of TTS data for various exposure levels and daily durations, It should be noted that these contours, as previous contours, protect only 50 per cent of the employees from hearing losses in excess of the criterion. In order to protect nearly everyone, the noise-exposure levels must be lowered by 10 dB. If the latter is not possible, he recommends a program of monitoring audiometry to detect those employees who might develop a hearing loss.

In 1966 Kryter et al. (39) reported the results of deliberations by Working Group 46 of the Committee on Hearing and Bioacoustics (CHABA) of the National Academy of Science. This report principally reflects the work of Kryter and the Subcommittee on Noise in Industry. The definitions of damage-risk criteria and damage-risk contours follow those of Kryter (37, 38). Working Group 46 used TTS data to establish damage-risk contours for long-term daily exposures. The evidence available to them indicated that TTS_2 data underestimate the degree of hearing loss after ten years or more of noise exposure by about 3 dB at 4,000 Hz, overestimate it by about 5 dB at 2,000 Hz, and approximately estimate it at 1,000 Hz.

Figure 13.9, presented by Kryter in 1963 and 1965 and then again by Kryter et al. in 1966, shows damage-risk contours for various "one exposure per day" durations for noises measured in octave or one-third octave bands. The principal features of this figure are: (1) 135 dB should not be exceeded for any duration; (2) greater intensity is permitted in the lower and higher frequencies than in the 2,000 to 4,000 Hz frequency region; (3) greater exposure levels are permitted if the exposure duration is shortened; and (4) the permissible exposure levels are 5 dB lower for sound energy concentrated into a one-third octave band or less, or measured in one-third octave bands, than for wide-band noises measured in octave bands. Permissible levels for pure tones are presented in another figure and are approximately 5 dB less than for broad band noises in the high frequencies. The contours for low-frequency pure tones for the shorter exposure durations reflect the observation that pure tones are less effective than noises in eliciting and maintaining the acoustic reflex (72).

In 1969 the provisions of the Walsh-Healey Public Contracts Act of 1936 were revised by the U.S. Department of Labor to protect the hearing of employees of private firms doing more than $10,000 worth of business per year with the federal government. The corrected provisions provide that when employees are subjected to greater sound levels than those listed in Table 13.7 that "feasible administrative or engineering controls shall be

TABLE 13.7. PERMISSIBLE NOISE EXPOSURES UNDER THE WALSH-HEALEY ACT (AS REPORTED BY MAAS 1969)

Duration per day in hours	*Sound level dBA slow response*
8	90
6	92
4	95
3	97
2	100
1–1/2	102
1	105
1–1/2	110
1/2	115
1/4 or less	

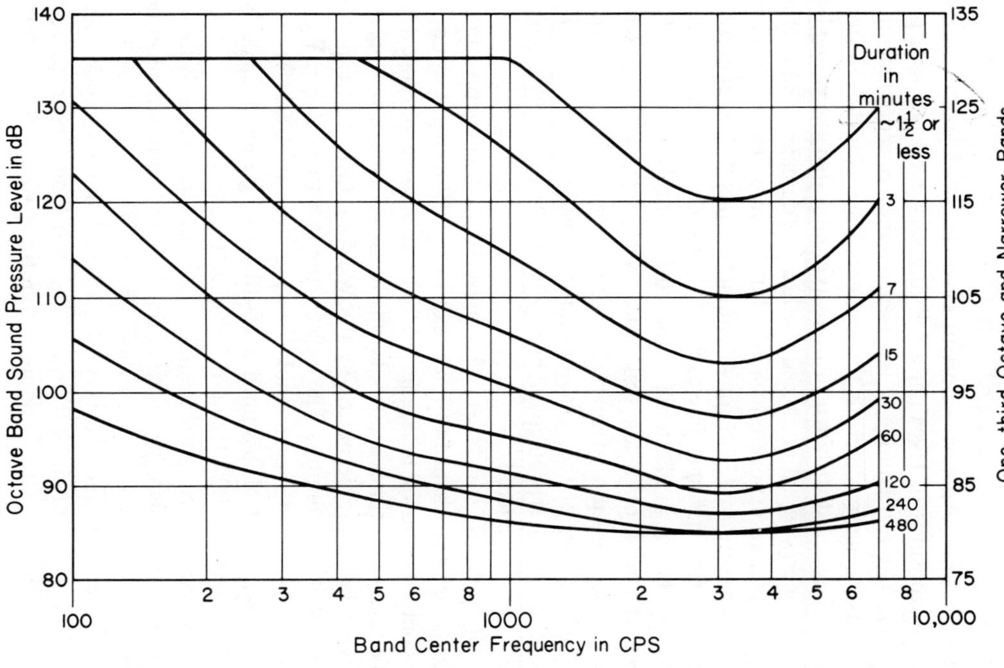

FIGURE 13.9 Damage-risk contours for one exposure per day to one-octave and one-third octave bands of noise.

Source: Kryter et al. "Hazardous exposure to intermittent and steady-state noise." *Journal of the Acoustical Society of America*, **39**: 456, 1966.

utilized" (Sect. 50–204.10 Walsh-Healey Public Contracts Act). If these fail to reduce the levels below those in Table 13.7, then personal protection must be provided and used.

Note that the levels in Table 13.7 are A scale readings using the slow sound-level meter response. Provision is also made to convert octave band readings into equivalent A-weighted sound levels. The report by Botsford (5) appears to have been instrumental in the basic measurement used in the Walsh-Healey Act.

Interrupted Exposure. An early effort to evaluate the degree of hazard of one or several exposures of less than a full day was published as a part of AFR 160–3 (1). The procedure "... is based on the concept that equal quantities of acoustic energy entering the ear canal are equally injurious, regardless of how they are distributed in time, assuming that the equivalent quantities of noise energy equal or exceed the hearing damage-risk criteria" (1, p. 6). For example, an exposure to 85 dB for 480 minutes is considered equivalent to an exposure to 95 dB for 48 minutes. Since 95 dB represents ten times as much energy per unit time as 85 dB, the same amount of energy will be absorbed by the ear in one-tenth of the time. On this basis, a trading relationship between time on a log scale and level (which is a log scale) was established. The duration of several separate periods of exposure is figured as the simple sum of the noise on-times. The AFR 160–3 (1) formulation proved to be overprotective, primarily because recovery during quiet intervals is not considered.

In 1961, Glorig, Ward, and Nixon (21) presented a formulation based upon TTS data for less than five-hour exposures. Working Group 46 presented the contours shown in Figure 13.9 for this same purpose (39). The permissible levels and times are similar in the two formulations, except that slightly higher levels are permitted by the Working Group at exposure durations in excess of ten minutes. This reflects the fact that Glorig, Ward, and Nixon assumed a 12-dB permissible hearing loss at 2,000 Hz as a criterion, whereas Kryter et al. assumed a 15-dB hearing loss at 2,000 Hz and 20-dB hearing loss at 3,000 Hz and above as a criterion.

Both Glorig, Ward, and Nixon (21) and Kryter et al. (39) present figures which can be used to calculate permissible on-time and required off-times for on-off exposures during a working day. These formulations are based primarily upon the growth and recovery of TTS and the assumption that TTS_2 at the end of a day predicts PTS_{10yr}. The Working Group presents separate graphs for noises with long-burst durations (over two minutes) and short-burst durations (less than two minutes). The latter are treated as a continuous exposure to a noise with a given on-fraction. Long-burst durations are treated as requiring certain off-times before reexposure is permissible.

The calculation of damage-risk contours for exposures to interrupted noise is more involved that for single exposure to continuous noise over a

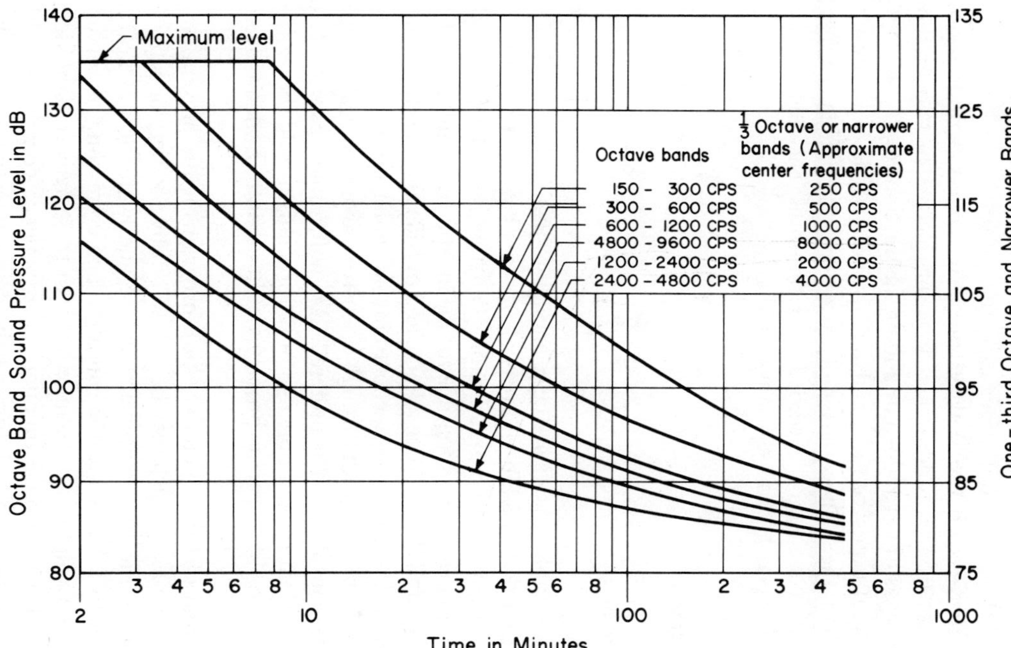

FIGURE 13.10 Damage-risk contours for one exposure per day to certain one-octave and certain one-third octave or narrower bands of noise.

Source: Kryter et al. "Hazardous exposure to intermittent and steady-state noise." *Journal of the Acoustical Society of America*, **39**: 456, 1966.

whole or a part of a working day. Considerations of growth and recovery rates of TTS, the acoustic reflex latencies and recovery, the type of signal eliciting the reflex, and the portion of the basilar membrane protected by the reflex are usually included. In addition, the question of whether the influence of these factors upon PTS is the same as their influence upon TTS must be considered. Kryter et al. (39) and Glorig, Ward, and Nixon (21) indicate considerably less confidence in the contours for interrupted exposures than in those for continuous exposures.

As shown in Table 13.7, the Walsh-Healey Act covers periods shorter than eight hours as well. In addition, if exposure occurs in two or more periods, then the exposures are added by adding the fractions $C_1/T_1 + C_2/T_2$, where C is the actual exposure time, and T is the permissible exposure time at that level. When the sum equals unity or more, then the permissible exposure has been equaled or exceeded. Relationships between on- and off-times and cycles per day are not considered.

Hearing Conservation

GENERAL CONCEPTS

Few industrial establishments are large enough to justify the employment of highly specialized personnel in all areas of working hazards (eye and skin irritants, air pollutants, atomic radiations, and noises). Typically, the physician and the engineer are responsible for the identification and correction of working hazards, and they use consultants and outside agencies to evaluate special problems. Military establishments follow a similar procedure, except that many problems are dealt with through extensive use of technical bulletins before an outside consultant is considered. An unfortunate aspect of the consultant system is that the full potential of the specialist is seldom realized, because he is asked to solve specific problems rather than to evaluate overall problem areas.

The primary goal of hearing conservation programs is the prevention of noise-induced hearing loss, which may be carried out by a variety of activities including the modification of equipment, the use and evaluation of hearing tests and ear protectors, as well as the education and counseling of administrative personnel and employees. Because many of these activities are highly technical, personnel with diverse training and experience contribute to the hearing conservation program. Unfortunately, communication among these personnel is often inadequate and the full potential of the program is not realized. This is particularly true between those who measure and control noise and those who medically evaluate the noise-induced hearing losses. As mentioned earlier, the audiologist could bridge this communication gap.

In 1948, the Court of Appeals of the State of New York decided that hearing loss resulting from long-term noise exposure is a condition for which an employee may collect compensation from his employer, even though a loss of time or wages is not evident (Matter of Slawinski vs. J. H. Williams & Co., 298 N.Y. 546). This decision and subsequent decisions in Wisconsin and Missouri prompted legislative action in these states as well as the initiation of hearing conservation programs in many industries (35). With the growing public awareness of noise problems in industrial and military settings, these programs will be expanded in the future.

NOISE CONTROL PROCEDURES

The first step in a hearing conservation program is the evaluation of the noise in question and a comparison of the results with the damage-risk contours. If the noise levels in any band exceed the contours, noise control procedures should be undertaken. These procedures include the following: (1) reducing the noise output of the equipment itself through modification in design or usage; (2) surrounding the equipment with sound-deadening materials; (3) moving the employees farther from the equipment and, if necessary, using remote control devices to operate the equipment; or (4) placing sound barriers between the noise source and the personnel. The application of noise control procedures are highly technical and are outside the scope of this chapter. Detailed discussions of noise source and noise pathway controls are contained in Harris (29) and Peterson and Gross (53).

EAR PROTECTION

If the sound levels at the employee's ears still exceed the damage-risk contours after the completion of noise control procedures, personal ear protection devices should be worn. Such devices are available in two basic forms, earplugs inserted into the ear canal and earmuffs covering the entire external ear. Figure 13.11 after Guild (26) records the attenuation provided by typical devices of each type, and by the two worn together. This figure illustrates that the attenuation provided by both types is greater at the higher frequencies, that the combination of the two types provides the greatest amount of attenuation, and that the total attenuation of the two together is far less than the simple addition of the attenuation provided by each.

Other sound transmission pathways limit the total amount of attenuation that can be achieved by simply covering and plugging the ears. When an individual wears an earplug, sound reaches his ear along several pathways. Sound energy may pass through the earplug material, it may move the earplug as a whole and set up pressure waves within the ear canal, or it may enter the ear canal through air leaks around the edge of the earplug. In order to reduce transmission through the earplug itself, it should be made

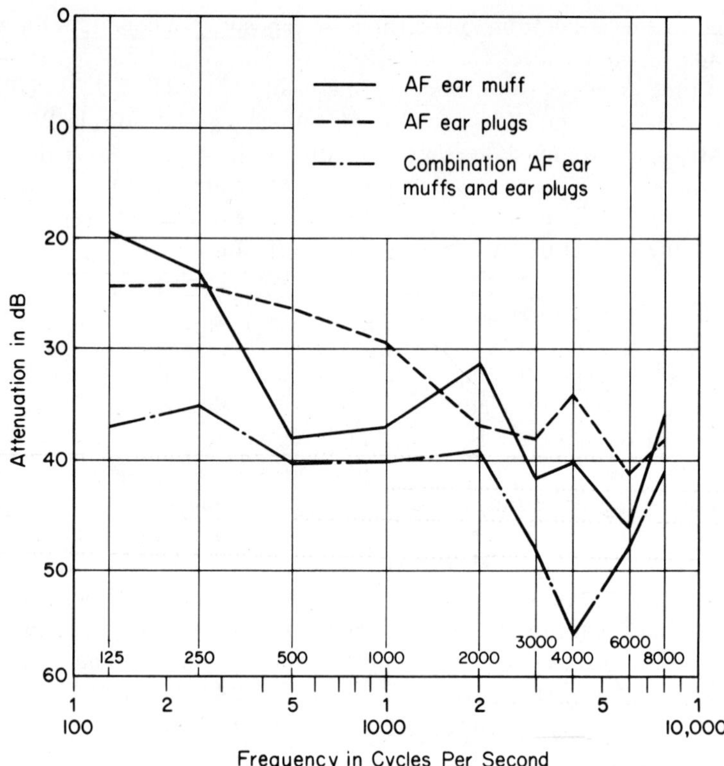

FIGURE 13.11 Attenuation characteristics of ear protectors.
Source: Guild, Elizabeth. "Ears can be protected." *Noise Control*, **4**: 35, 1958.

of material with low compliance and high mass. However, a compliant material is needed for good fit and comfort, this makes compromises in earplug construction necessary. A substantial increase in mass above that currently used is required in order to produce a significant effect. Furthermore, greater mass increases discomfort and creates a problem of keeping the devices in the ear. An air leak can cause a significant reduction in attenuation at all frequencies but, particularly, in the lower frequencies (80). For this reason, a flexible material that conforms to the shape of the individual ear canal, a good initial selection of earplug size, and the proper use of the earplug by the employee are all required.

Earmuffs offer the following advantages: they are relatively easy to put on and use; they do not cause discomfort in the ear canal; and they do not require much care in initial selection or in daily use. Earmuffs also offer some disadvantages. The weight of the earmuff is objectionable to some employees, the heat under the earmuff may be objectionable, and air leaks may occur where the cushion crosses the earpiece of eyeglasses (81, 42, 47).

The design of the cushion on the earmuff is dictated by two conflicting considerations. The first is that a flexible soft cushion is needed to provide maximum comfort and a tight air seal around the earmuff. The second is that a relatively stiff cushion is required to reduce the piston-like movement of the earmuff as a whole in response to sound waves (81). Zwislocki (81) proposed the use of "semi-plastic" cushions containing a substance which flows slowly and which is enclosed within a plastic covering. This material slowly conforms to the contours of the head but appears "stiff" in response to higher frequency vibrations. Other cushions are made of a plastic foam. These are flexible on the outer margin to allow for a good seal, but are relatively stiff deeper in the material and along the inner margin, in order to reduce the relative movement between the earmuff and the head.

The attenuation characteristics of an earmuff can be increased by enlarging the volume of air contained under the earmuff or by increasing its mass. The extent of the increase in size and weight is limited by considerations of comfort and wearability (81).

A good hearing conservation program includes checks on the actual amount of attenuation provided by the ear protectors. Because the devices are not always fitted or used properly, and because the aging of rubber or plastic may cause changes in the acoustical characteristics of the devices, the attenuation figures provided by manufacturers may be greater than the values actually achieved in practice. A standard method for measuring the amount of attenuation provided by ear protectors is covered in USASI Z24.22–1957 ("Method for the Measurement of the Real Ear Attenuation of Ear Protectors at Threshold"). This publication also discusses required ambient noise levels, frequencies to be tested, required equipment specifications, data recording, and number of subjects. The standard should be consulted in detail whenever attenuation measurements of ear protectors are made.

A hearing conservation program also should include some means of determining whether the employees actually use, and use correctly, the devices issued to them. Nonuse and misuse of ear protectors are common problems in hearing conservation programs. Employees complain that they hurt the ear or are hot, that they are too much trouble, that they have been lost or forgotten, or that failure to use them previously did not result in any hearing difficulty. Both individual and group attitudes influence the employees' resistance to wearing ear protectors. Certain individuals do not wish to appear afraid of risk or injury. Others yield to group pressure against abiding by safety rules. Still others fail to use these devices simply because it is required by authority figures. Maas (42) has discussed these employee reactions in relation to successful hearing conservation programs. Employees may be encouraged to wear ear protection through lectures, films, and posters (22, 23).

Fletcher (14) investigated the feasibility of using the acoustic reflex as a means of protecting the ear from injury due to impulsive sounds. In his procedure, a reflex-eliciting signal is presented 200 msec before the sound impulse. In this way the reflex reaches its maximum level by the time the impulse arrives, thus reducing the input to the cochlea. Fletcher demonstrated that the TTS exhibited by an ear protected in this way is less than that exhibited by an unprotected ear. However, he also showed that except for frequencies below 1,000 Hz where there is a slight advantage in favor of the reflex, a simple inexpensive earplug is superior to the reflex in protecting the ear from TTS. Because of the cost, complexity, and relative ineffectiveness of the acoustic reflex as a protective mechanism in most frequency regions, it appears unlikely that this procedure will be applied except under unusual circumstances.

THE HEARING TESTING PROGRAM

Each employee should receive a preemployment (often called "reference" or "entrance") hearing test. All employees working in environments where any octave-band level is greater than 10 dB below the damage-risk contour for the appropriate daily exposure duration should be monitored for changes in hearing sensitivity. The monitoring program should include these employees because noise levels within 10 dB of the contours will produce some hearing losses in excess of the criterion. Finally, all employees should receive hearing tests upon termination of their employment.

The reference audiogram should consist of pure-tone air-conduction thresholds for each ear at 500, 1,000, 2,000, 3,000, 4,000, and 6,000 Hz as given by the Guide for Conservation of Hearing in Noise (1964) (23). Frequencies below 500 Hz are not included because they contribute very little information for an industrial or military situation, and because it is difficult and expensive to provide an environment quiet enough in the low frequencies. Three thousand Hertz is included because hearing sensitivity at this frequency is sometimes used in the calculation of compensation (16). The use of 6,000 Hz rather than 8,000 Hz is recommended because relatively greater variability in test results is observed at the latter frequency (11). Any person showing an average loss in the speech frequencies of more than 15 dB (according to USASI Z24.5–1951) should be referred for otological evaluation and a "placement evaluation" (23).

Monitoring audiometry is accomplished in several ways and at varying time intervals, depending upon the equipment and methods used as well as the noise levels to which the workers are exposed. The testing procedures may range from a full pure-tone air-conduction threshold test to a simple screening test. Screening procedures often consist of the presentation of one frequency or two frequencies at one or several previously determined screening levels. The "Guide for Conservation of Hearing in Noise" (23) recommends that the first monitoring hearing test take place nine to twelve months after employment "unless an earlier test is indicated by long, continuous exposure to noise levels greater than 100-dB average OBL at 300 to 600, 600 to 1,200 and 1,200 to 2,400 cps ..." (23, p. 20). Other indications for earlier tests are reports of severe tinnitus or subjectively noticeable temporary threshold shifts. The Guide for Conservation of Hearing in Noise further recommends that if the individual's threshold appears to have increased by 10 dB or more at 2,000 Hz, or by 15 dB or more at 3,000 Hz or above, he should be given a complete threshold test. If this test confirms the screening results, measures to conserve the employee's hearing should be undertaken. All hearing tests should be given after a period of at least sixteen hours during which the employee has not been exposed to noise levels in excess of 85 dB in the octave bands (23, 75).

The termination or exit audiogram has the same requirements as the preemployment audiogram. If a significant increase in hearing loss is noted, the employee should be evaluated by an audiologist certified by the American Speech and Hearing Association. This is particularly true when compensation is involved.

All hearing tests should be carried out in an environment that is sufficiently quiet. Tables 13.4 and 13.5 give the maximum allowable background noise levels for testing to levels as low as 0 dB (according to USASI Z24.5–1951) as recommended in USASI S3.1–1960. These levels assume the use of well-fitted earphone cushions. The levels recommended by the Guide for Conservation of Hearing in Noise are taken from 1960 USASI standard. Commercially available prefabricated test booths have proved to be the most satisfactory way of achieving the desired degree of quiet (23, 15). There are three basic types of hearing testing equipment used in industrial and military settings: self-recording audiometers; manually operated threshold audiometers; and screening devices. Self-recording audiometers are discussed in detail by Rudmose (60), and manual audiometers are familiar to all audiologists. The typical screening device used in monitoring audiometry is a small, solid-state, battery-operated unit which produces one or two test tones (either 4,000 Hz or 4,000 and 2,000 Hz) at one, two, or three hearing levels.

It is essential that adequately trained and supervised personnel perform the hearing tests. In 1958, the American Speech and Hearing Association's Committee on Clinical Standards in Hearing formed a subcommittee to establish guidlines for the training of audiometric technicians. While recognizing the desirability of using fully qualified audiologists, the subcommittee realized that this is not feasible in most industrial and military situations. Therefore, it was recommended that technicians work under the supervision of an otologist or an audiologist. The subcommittee believed that the technicians should be limited to pure-tone air-conduction testing and that they should be excluded from performing bone-conduction tests, tests using masking, speech tests, as well as all procedures designed for the detection and measurement of nonorganic hearing disorders. Furthermore, it was recommended that decisions regarding all procedures used in the testing program should be made by the otologist or audiologist directing the program (57).

The subcommittee also suggested that the training program for the technicians should be of a few weeks', rather than a few days', duration. It was suggested that the technicians should have instruction in anatomy and physiology of the ear, physics of sound, the operation of test equipment, and the indications of equipment failure. The subcommittee further recommended that the training program include supervision in taking a minimum of ten complete pure-tone air-conduction threshold audiograms. The technicians also should be taught to make simple listening checks on the equipment before each day of testing (57).

In 1965 the American Speech and Hearing Association endorsed in principle a program of training for industrial audiometric technicians meeting the following minimum requirements:

1. The training program shall consist of a minimum of two and a half days with five days as an optimum,

2. The scope and nature of the course be as outlined in the second draft of Guide for Training of Industrial Audiometric Technicians, dated April 28, 1965,

3. The training program director hold certification in audiology by ASHA or in otolaryngology by the American Board of Otolaryngology,

4. That there be a minimum period of five hours of supervised practice as outlined in the Guide for Training,

5. That a final examination be given before satisfactory completion of the course ... (48).

It is important that the procedures taught to the technicians be highly standardized and explained in great detail. It is suggested that the technicians be taught to follow a check-list similar to that presented in Table 13.8. In order to insure accurate test results, technicians should be trained to follow a well-defined procedure without deviation. Several authors, among them Glorig and Harris (19), House and Glorig (20), and Fox (15), have suggested specific test methodologies and instructions for use by technicians. Suggestions for record-keeping forms can be found in the Guide for Conservation of Noise in Industry (23) and Glorig and Harris (19).

The calibration of the testing equipment is essential. In addition to the daily checks made by the technician (Table 13.8), all equipment should be calibrated electroacoustically at least once a month. Calibration units are available today that are both inexpensive and sufficiently easy to use. Such equipment provides calibration readings that are more precise and less time consuming than the "biological calibration" recommended by the Guide for Conservation of Hearing in Noise (23). The following alterations in output can be considered significant: (1) greater than ± 4 dB from dial readings at frequencies of 2,000 Hz and below; (2) greater than ±5 dB from dial readings at frequencies above 2,000 Hz (66, 68). Deviations up to ±10 dB may be permitted temporarily provided that mathematical corrections are made. If significant alterations in output cannot be corrected by supervisory or local repair personnel, the equipment should be returned to the manufacturer or his representative. A spare audiometer is extremely valuable when this occurs.

UTILIZATION OF HEARING TEST RESULTS

Preemployment audiograms have several uses. First of all, they are used as a reference against which later hearing tests can be compared. Secondly, in some states they are used to determine the amount of hearing loss for which a particular employer will not be responsible. That is, the employer may not have to pay for the amount of hearing loss that predated the individual's current employment. Finally, these audiograms are used to identify "tender" ears (ears which already exhibit PTS) or ears that exhibit a hearing disease that may be progressive. It is important for the employer to identify the latter group of hearing disorders because, potentially, he could become liable for hearing loss caused by disease which subsequently could not be differentiated from that caused by noise.

If the preemployment audiogram demonstrates the presence of a hearing loss, this justifies placing that individual in a relatively quiet working

TABLE 13.8. DAILY AUDIOMETER CHECK-LIST

Audiometer____________________
Date________________________

	500		1,000		2,000		4,000		6,000	
	R	*L*	*R*	*L*	*R*	*L*	*R*	*L*	*R*	*L*
Technician thresholds										
Linearity check of intensity dial (increase dial slowly from 0 to 80-dB)										
Stability check of tone (set intensity dial at 60-dB)										
Interrupter switch check (clicks and noises)										
Wire check (wiggle wire at one intensity and frequency and listen for variations in tone)										
Remarks										

Technician ____________________

environment. Unfortunately, such hearing losses may be used as sufficient reason to deny employment. Under United States Air Force regulations, any individual having a reference audiogram that shows Class C hearing (average thresholds of 20 dB or more according to USASI Z24.5–1951 at 500, 1,000, and 2,000 Hz "... will not be assigned to duty where hazardous noise exposure will occur" (2, p. 2).

The primary function of monitoring audiometry is the identification of those individuals who appear to be developing a hearing loss. United States Air Force civilian and military personnel are removed from hazardous noise areas (areas with octave-band levels greater than 85 dB) whenever an audiogram taken 40 hours after exposure shows a threshold shift of 10 dB or more at 2,000 and/or 3,000 Hz, and/or a threshold shift of 15 dB or more at 4,000 and/or 6,000 Hz. The Guide for Conservation of Hearing in Noise (23, p. 20) recommends that when monitoring audiometry indicates a change of 10 dB at 2,000 Hz or below, or a change of 15 dB at 3,000 Hz or above, "... appropriate steps should be taken to conserve the employee's hearing."

In 1963, Hermann presented the Early Loss Index (ELI) to systematize the application of the results of monitoring audiometry. After analyzing the distribution of the hearing sensitivity of noise-sheltered male and female subjects, he determined that at 4,000 Hz a hearing loss of more than 22 dB greater than the loss expected at the age of the individual or group in question is exceeded by only 2.5 per cent of the noise-sheltered group (a standard deviation of 1.96). Therefore, an employee exhibiting a hearing loss of this extent or greater is suspected of having a noise-induced hearing loss. In addition, he determined that for the same frequency, a hearing loss more than 29.6 dB greater than that expected for the age is exceeded by only 0.5 per cent of the noise-sheltered group (a standard deviation of 2.5). Therefore, a hearing loss of this extent probably is related to noise exposure, assuming other causes of hearing loss are ruled out. Table 13.9

TABLE 13.9. EARLY LOSS INDEX 4,000 CPS AUDIOMETRY

Age specific Presbycusis, dB			*ELI Scale*		
Age	*Women*	*Men*	*Grade*	*Exceeds ASPV by:*	*Remarks*
25	0	0	A	< 8 dB	Normal—excellent
30	2	3	B	8–14	Normal—good
35	3	7	C	15–22	Normal—within expected range
40	5	11	D	23–29	Suspect NIL
45	8	15	E	30 or more	Strong indication of NIL
50	12	20			
55	15	26			
60	17	32			
65	18	38			

Source: Table 11 of E. R. Hermann, "An audiometric approach to noise control." *American Industrial Hygiene Association Journal*, **24**; 349, 1963.

is a reproduction of the table given by Hermann. Included are the average amounts of hearing loss at 4,000 Hz expected in nonnoise exposed groups at various ages for men and women as well as the ELI scale. Any individual with an ELI of D or E should wear ear protection or be removed from the noise. Averages for groups exposed to noise which correspond to an ELI of D or E are sufficient cause for the initiation of noise-control procedures.

Several aspects of Hermann's report are particularly important. First, the extent of the hearing loss considered significant is put on a statistical basis. Second, the report illustrates how the average hearing loss due to presbycusis in each age group is subtracted from the observed hearing loss. Most important, however, it points out how hearing test results can be utilized in the evaluation of individual hearing problems as well as in the evaluation of the noise itself. Thus, the noxiousness of plant noise levels, together with individual susceptibility, can be monitored by a properly designed and utilized hearing testing program.

Exit audiograms are used to demonstrate that an individual does or does not have a hearing loss upon termination of employment. In addition, they can be used to protect the employer from claims for increased hearing loss which actually developed following termination. Finally, exit audiograms are used for the determination of compensation under existing Workman's Compensation laws or, in the case of federal civil service, under United States Department of Labor regulations.

COMPENSATION

A workman applying for compensation under Workman's Compensation laws must do so according to the regulations of the state in which he is employed. If he is a federal civil service employee he must apply through the United States Department of Labor. The regulations vary widely across the state. The laws of most states provide for the compensation of employees who have incurred hearing loss due to acoustic trauma. However, noise-induced hearing loss is not specifically mentioned as a compensable impairment in most states. A survey by Fox (16) indicated that compensation for noise-induced hearing loss can be obtained through general provisions of the compensation laws in many of these states. In New York, Wisconsin, and Missouri, specific laws governing compensation for acoustic trauma and noise-induced hearing loss have been passed. The various federal and state compensation laws are not discussed in detail in this chapter. More information can be obtained from Nelson (46), Newby (47), Fox (16), Kalmykow (35), and Symons (69).

In 1961, the American Medical Association (AMA) published the "Guides to the Evaluation of Permanent Impairment (for) Ear, Nose, Throat, and Related Structures" (25). This document contains several important definitions and it endorses the computational method for determining the degree of hearing impairment published by the American Academy of Ophthalmology and Otolaryngology (AAOO) in 1959 (24). This computational method has superseded the AMA formula of 1947, "Tentative Standard Procedure for Evaluating the Percentage Loss of Hearing in Medicolegal Cases" (70). In the 1961 AMA Guide, permanent impairment is defined as "... any anatomic or functional abnormality or loss after maximal medical rehabilitation has been achieved and which abnormality or loss the physician considers stable or nonprogressive at the time the evaluation is made." Permanent disability "... is not a purely medical condition ..." but a reduction in a person's "... actual or presumed ability to engage in gainful activity ... ." Impairment, then, represents loss of function while disability represents the extent to which this impairment disables the individual. Impairment is a medical evaluation while "evaluation of permanent disability is an appraisal of the patient's present and probable future ability to engage in gainful activity as it is affected by nonmedical factors such as age, sex, education, economic and social environment, and the medical factor—permanent impairment" (25).

According to Fox (16), ratings of hearing impairment in the various states are made in one of three ways: (1) by relying upon "expert medical testimony"; (2) by applying the AMA formula of 1947; or (3) by applying the AAOO formula of 1959. The AAOO (24), the AMA (25), and Fox (16) all urge the adoption of the AAOO method. This method is based upon the average of the pure-tone thresholds for 500, 1,000, and 2,000 Hz because these frequencies are the most important for the understanding of speech. This average is labeled the "estimated hearing level for speech." Speech reception thresholds are not used because speech materials are not standardized sufficiently and because of the confusion surrounding the thresholds for the various speech materials used in speech tests. The computations of AAOO (24) are based upon the reference levels specified in USASI Z24.5–1951. It is assumed that no impairment exists if the hearing level for speech is 15 dB or less ("low fence") and that total impairment exists if the hearing level for speech is in excess of 81.7 dB ("high fence"). Impairment increases at the rate of 1.5 per cent per dB between 15 and 81.7 dB. The good ear is given a weighted value which is five times that of the poor ear in the calculation of the per cent of binaural hearing impairment.

Workmen's Compensation laws designate the number of weeks' salary an individual may receive for a total impairment of hearing in either one or both ears. In order to arrive at the number of weeks' salary a workman will receive for a partial impairment, the number of weeks for total impairment is multiplied by the percentage of hearing impairment. Compensation payments made by the United States Veterans' Administration may be based upon pure-tone thresholds (voluntary or electrodermal results) or upon the results of speech audiometry, although the latter are preferred.

The classification of the hearing loss is based upon both the speech reception thresholds and the speech discrimination scores, by a procedure that is based on the Social Adequacy Index of Davis (9).

Bibliography

1. Air Force Regulation No. 160–3. "Hazardous noise exposure." Washington, D.C.: Department of the Air Force, 1956.
2. Air Force Regulation No. 160–3A. "Hazardous noise exposure." Washington, D.C.: Department of the Air Force, 1960.
3. Batchelder, L. Letter to readers of *Sound & Vibration*, **2**: 13, 1968.
4. Bekesy, G. von. "Uber den Einfluss der durch den Kopf und den Gehorgang bewirkten Schalifeldverzerrungen auf die Horschwelle." *Annalen der Physik*, **14**: 267–71, 1932. As translated in Bekesy, G. von., *Experiments in Hearing*. New York: McGraw-Hill Book Company, 1960.
5. Botsford, J. H. "Simple method for identifying acceptable noise exposures." *Journal of the Acoustical Society of America*, **42**: 810–19, 1967.
6. Corso, J. F. "Age and sex differences in pure-tone thresholds." *Archives of Otolaryngology*, **77**: 385–405, 1963.
7. "Criteria for background noise in audiometer rooms. (S3.1–1960)." New York: United States of America Standards Institute, 1960.
8. Crowe, S. J., S. R. Guild, and L. M. Polvolgt. "Observations on pathology of high-tone deafness." *Bulletin Johns Hopkins Hospital*, **54**: 315–79, 1934. Cited by H. F. Schuknecht and J. Tonndorf. *Laryngoscope*, **70**: 479–505, 1960.
9. Davis, H. "The articulation area and the social adequacy index for hearing." *Laryngoscope*, **58**: 761–78, 1948.
10. Davis, H. "A mechano-electrical theory of cochlear action." *Annals of Otology, Rhinology and Laryngology*, **67**: 789–801, 1958.
11. Davis, H., G. Hoople, and H. O. Parrack. "The medical principles of monitoring audiometry." *Archives of Industrial Hygiene and Occupational Medicine*, **17**: 1–20, 1958.
12. Eldredge, D. H. "The problems of criteria for noise exposure." Armed Forces-NRC Committee on Hearing and Bioacoustics, 1960. Quoted by C. D. Yaffee and H. H. Jones. *Noises and Hearing*. Public Health Service Publication No. 850. Washington, D.C.: U.S. Public Health Service, 1961.
13. Exploratory Subcommittee Z24–X–2. *The Relations of Hearing Loss to Noise Exposure*. New York: United States of America Standards Institute, 1954.
14. Fletcher, J. L. "Comparison of the attenuation characteristics of the acoustic reflex and the V51-R earplug." *Journal of Auditory Research*, **2**: 111–16, 1961.
15. Fox, M. S. "Industrial Audiometry." In A. Glorig, ed., *Audiometry, Principles and Practice*. Baltimore: Williams & Wilkins Company, 1965.
16. Fox, M. S. "Comparative provisions for occupational hearing loss." *Archives of Otolaryngology*, **81**: 257–60, 1965.
17. Gallo, R. and A. Glorig. "Permanent threshold shift changes produced by noise exposure and aging." *American Industrial Hygiene Association Journal*, **25**: 237–45, 1964.

18. Glorig, A. "The effects of noise on hearing." *Journal of Laryngology and Otology*, **75**: 447–78, 1961.
19. Glorig, A. and J. D. Harris. "Audiometric testing in industry." In C. M. Harris, ed., *Handbook of Noise Control.* New York: McGraw-Hill Book Company, 1957.
20. Glorig, A. and H. House. "A new concept in auditory screening." *Archives of Otolaryngology*, **66**: 228–32, 1957.
21. Glorig, A., W. D. Ward, and J. Nixon. "Damage-risk criteria and noise-induced hearing loss." *Archives of Otolaryngology*, **74**: 413–23, 1961.
22. Grzona, Alice. "An occupational health nurse's program." *Nursing Outlook*, **9**: 283–84, 1961.
23. "Guide for conservation of hearing in noise." (*Supplement of the*) *Transactions of the American Academy of Ophthalmology and Otolaryngology*, 1964.
24. "Guide for the evaluation of hearing impairment: A report of the Committee on Conservation of Hearing." *Transactions of the American Academy of Ophthalmology and Otolaryngology*, **63**: 236–38, 1959.
25. "Guides to the evaluation of permanent impairment (for) ear, nose, throat, and related structures." *Journal of the American Medical Association*, **177**: 489–501, 1961.
26. Guild, Elizabeth. "Ears can be protected." *Noise Control*, **4**: 33–35, 1958.
27. Hallpike, C. S. and J. D. Hood. "Observations upon the neurological mechanism of the loudness recruitment phenomenon." *Acta Oto-Laryngogica*, **50**: 472–86, 1959.
28. Hardy, H. C. "Tentative estimate of a hearing damage risk criterion for steady-state noise." *Journal of the Acoustical Society of America*, **24**: 756–61, 1952.
29. Harris, C. M., ed. *Handbook of Noise Control.* New York: McGraw-Hill Book Company, 1957.
30. Hermann, E. R. "An audiometric approach to noise control." *American Industrial Hygiene Association Journal*, **24**: 344–56, 1963.
31. Hilding, A. C. "Studies on otic labyrinth; anatomic explanation for hearing drip at 4096 characteristic of acoustic trauma and presbycusis." *Annals of Otology, Rhinology and Laryngology*, **62**: 950–56, 1953.
32. Hillquist, R. K. "Objective and subjective measurement of truck noise." *Sound and Vibration*, **1**: 8–13, 1967.
33. Industrial audiometric technician training guide for instructors." (Second draft, March 1, 1967).
34. Jones, A. R. and F. W. Church. "A criterion for evaluation of noise exposures." *American Industrial Hygiene Association Journal*, **21**: 481–85, 1960.
35. Kalmykow, A. "Legal developments concerning loss of hearing from noise in industry." *A.M.A. Archives of Industrial Hygiene*, **21**: 216–21, 1960.
36. Kryter, K. D. "The effects of noise on man." *Journal of Speech and Hearing Disorders*, Supplement No. 1, 1950.
37. Kryter, K. D. "Exposure to steady-state noise and impairment of hearing." *Journal of the Acoustical Society of America*, **35**: 1515–25, 1963.
38. Kryter, K. D. "Damage risk criterion and contours based on permanent and temporary hearing loss data." *American Industrial Hygiene Association Journal*, **26**: 34–44, 1965.

39. Kryter, K. D., W. D. Ward, J. D. Miller, and D. H. Eldredge. "Hazardous exposure to intermittent and steady-state noise." *Journal of the Acoustical Society of America*, **39**: 451–64, 1966.
40. Lawrence, M. "Current concepts of the mechanism of occupational hearing loss." *American Industrial and Hygiene Association Journal*, **25**: 269–73, 1964.
41. Lindquist, S. E., W. D. Neff, and H. F. Schuknecht. "Stimulation deafness: A study of hearing losses resulting from exposure to noise to blast impulses." *Journal of Comparative Physiology and Psychology*, **47**: 406–11, 1954.
42. Maas, R. B. "Hearing protection in industry." *Nursing Outlook*, **9**: 281–83, 1961.
43. Maas, R. B. "New industrial noise standards contained in Walsh-Healey Act Reviews." *ASHA*, **11**: 1969.
44. "Method for the measurement of the real-ear attenuation of ear protectors at threshold (Z24.22-1957)." New York: United States of America Standards Institute, 1957.
45. Miller, J. D., C. S. Watson, and W. P. Covell. "Deafening effects of noise on the cat." *Acta Oto-Laryngologica*, Supplement 176: 91, 1963.
46. Nelson, H. A. "Legal liability for loss of hearing." In C. M. Harris, ed., *Handbook of Noise Control.* New York: McGraw-Hill Book Company, 1957.
47. Newby, H. A. *Audiology*. 2nd ed. New York: Appleton-Century-Crofts, 1964.
48. "Official minutes of the convention, American Speech and Hearing Association, October 30–November 2, 1965." *ASHA*, **8**: 125, 1966.
49. *Operating instructions*, *General Radio Type* 1556-*B*, *Impact-Noise Analyzer*. West Concord, Mass.: General Radio Company, 1962.
50. Peterson, A. P. G. "Personal communication with authors." 1967.
51. Peterson, A. P. G. "The tape recorder in acoustical measurements." *Sound and Vibration*, **1**: 14–20, 1967.
52. Peterson, A. P. G. and E. E. Gross, Jr. *Handbook of Noise Measurement.* 5th ed. West Concord, Mass.: General Radio Company, 1963.
53. Peterson, A. P. G. and E. E. Gross, Jr. *Handbook of Noise Measurement.* 6th ed. West Concord, Mass.: General Radio Company, 1967.
54. Pollack, I. "Specification of sound pressure levels." *American Journal of Psychology*, **62**: 412–17, 1949.
55. *Precision Sound Level Meters IEC 179.* New York: International Electrotechnical Commission, 1965.
56. "Preferred frequencies for acoustical measurements (S1.6–1960)." New York: United States of America Standards Institute, 1960.
57. "Report of committee on short courses in audiometric techniques." *Transactions of the American Academy of Opthalmology and Otolaryngology*, **63**: 852–53, 1959.
58. Rosenblith, W. A. and K. N. Stevens. "Noise and man." *Handbook of Acoustic Noise Control.* Washington, D.C.: Vol. 11. U.S.A.F., W.A.D.C., Tech. Rep. No. 52–204 (1953).
59. Rudmose, W. "Hearing loss resulting from noise exposure." In C. M. Harris, ed., *Handbook of Noise Control.* New York: McGraw-Hill Book Company, 1957.
60. Rudmose, W. "Automatic audiometry." In J. Jerger, ed., *Modern Developments in Audiology.* New York: Academic Press, Inc., 1963.

61. Ruedi, L. and W. Furrer. "Das akustische trauma." *Pract. Oto-Rhino-Laryngol.*, **8**: 177–372, 1946. Cited by H. F. Schucknecht, and J. Tonndorf. *Laryngoscope*, **70**: 479–505, 1960.
62. Schuknecht, H. F. and J. Tonndorf. "Acoustic trauma of the cochlea from ear surgery." *Laryngoscope*, **70**: 479–505, 1960.
63. Scott, H. H. "Noise measuring techniques." In C. M. Harris, ed., *Handbook of Noise Control.* New York: McGraw-Hill Book Company, 1957.
64. "Slawinski *v.* J. H. Williams Company, 298 N. Y. 546." Cited by Symons, N. S., *Archives of Industrial Hygiene and Occupational Medicine*, **5**: 138–56, 1952.
65. "Specification for an octave-band filter set for analysis of noise and other sounds (Z24.10–1953)." New York: United States of America Standards Institute, 1953.
66. "Specification for audiometers for general diagnostic purposes (Z24.5–1951)." New York: United States of America Standards Institute, 1951.
67. "Specification for general-purpose sound-level meters (S1.4–1961)." New York: United States of America Standards Institute, 1961.
68. "Specification for pure-tone audiometers for screening purposes (Z24.12–1952)." New York: United States of America Standards Institute, 1952.
69. Symons, N. S. "The legal aspects of occupational deafness." *Archives of Industrial Hygiene and Occupational Medicine*, **5**: 138–56, 1952.
70. "Tentative standard procedure for evaluating the percentage loss of hearing in medicolegal cases: Report of the Council on Physical Medicine." *Journal of the American Medical Association*, **133**: 396–97, 1947.
71. "Walsh-Healey Public Contracts Act Section 50–204.10." Cited by Maas, R. B. *ASHA*, **11**: 1969.
72. Ward, W. D. "Damage-risk criteria for line spectra." *Journal of the Acoustical Society of America*, **34**: 1610–19, 1962.
73. Ward, W. D. "Auditory fatigue and masking." In J. Jerger, ed., *Modern Developments in Audiology*. New York: Academic Press, Inc., 1963.
74. Ward, W. D., R. E. Fleer, and A. Glorig. "Characteristics of hearing losses produced by gunfire and by steady noise." *Journal of Auditory Research*, **1**: 325–56, 1961.
75. Ward, W. D., A. Glorig, and D. L. Skiar. "Temporary threshold shift produced by intermittent exposure to noise." *Journal of the Acoustical Society of America*, **31**: 791–94, 1959.
76. Webster, J. C. "SIL—Past, Present, and Future." *Sound and Vibration*, **3**: 22–26, 1969.
77. Williams, C. R. "Principles of noise measurement." In J. Sataloff, ed., *Industrial Deafness.* New York: McGraw-Hill Book Company, 1957.
78. Young, R. W. "Physical properties of noise and their specification." In C. M. Harris, ed., *Handbook of Noise Control.* New York: McGraw-Hill Book Company, 1957.
79. Young, R. W. "Single-number criteria for room noise." *Journal of the Acoustical Society of America*, **36**: 289–95, 1964.
80. Zwislocki, J. "Acoustic filters as ear defenders." *Journal of the Acoustical Society of America*, **23**: 36–40, 1951.
81. Zwislocki, J. "Ear protectors." In C. M. Harris, ed., *Handbook of Noise Control.* New York: McGraw-Hill Book Company, 1957.

14

Hearing Aids

Kenneth W. Berger, Ph.D.
Joseph P. Millin, Ph.D.

After organic hearing loss has been identified and quantified, and attempts have been made to determine the anatomical location as well as the etiology of hearing dysfunction, it is the responsibility of the physician to administer medical or surgical treatment if indicated. Should significant, untreatable hearing loss remain after medical intervention, or should such intervention not be indicated, it usually becomes the responsibility of the audiologist to determine if the patient can benefit from amplification. In addition to determining amplification needs, the audiologist should assume responsibility for determining the approximate amplification requirements for an instrument. After the instrument has been purchased from the hearing aid dealer, the audiologist has the responsibility of helping the individual to learn the proper use of the aid. In addition to the hearing instrument, such therapy as speech-reading and auditory training may be recommended, and often vocational and educational guidance may be appropriate.

The roles of the otologist, audiologist, and hearing aid dealer should be clear, although these roles sometimes overlap (4, 11). The otologist is responsible for diagnosing the hearing impairment and the medical or surgical treatment of the ear. The audiologist makes available to the physician audiologic diagnostic test results for the overall medical diagnosis. The audiologist also evaluates the patient's need for amplification and, if indicated, determines the approximate instrument requirements for the individual (123). He also has the responsibility of directing the overall aural rehabilitation of the patient. The hearing aid dealer is responsible for the precise fitting of the aid and its earmold, selling it, servicing it, and for helping the individual to adjust to amplification when no great problems are encountered. The training of these specialists is designed to prepare each of them to best perform his function in meeting the needs of the patient. Within this framework the patient should be assured of adequate management of his hearing problem.

The Hearing Aid

Broadly conceived, a hearing aid can be described as any device that brings sound to the ear more effectively. In the narrower and more frequently used sense the modern hearing aid is a miniaturized amplifier circuit which, though it takes many forms, is designed specifically for improving human hearing.

The function of a hearing aid is to amplify sound energy and to present the amplified sound to the ear with as little undesirable distortion as possible. Since sound cannot be adequately amplified directly, it is necessary to change the acoustic energy to an electrical signal. This electrical signal is then amplified and reconverted to acoustic energy at the ear.

The amount of amplification is generally expressed as the difference, in decibels, between the input and the output of the hearing aid. This difference is called *gain.* To accomplish amplification, the transistor hearing aid is provided with three basic components:

1. Microphone. The microphone responds to the mechanical sound vibrations and converts them into an electrical equivalent of the acoustic signal.

2. Amplifier. This device amplifies (by means of a transistorized circuit) the electrical signal which comes from the microphone.

3. Earphone or receiver. The receiver reconverts the electrical signal (now amplified) into audible sound waves, which are then directed to the ear.

In addition to these basic components most hearing aids have an on-off switch, a volume control, an internal or external tone control, a battery compartment, a cord or tube, and an earmold. Many aids also include a telephone pickup coil and perhaps other circuitry designed to meet special hearing problems. While all modern hearing aids contain similar circuitry and operate on the same principle, they may be divided into two major kinds: the desk aid (or auditory trainer); and the wearable aid. The desk aid is primarily used for auditory training or in the deaf classroom and may be designed for a single listener or a group. (For a brief discussion of auditory trainers, see Chapter 7 in the book by Oyer [99].) Our principle interest will be the wearable, or individual, hearing aid.

Wearable aids are often classified as to where they are worn: body, ear-level, and in-the-ear styles. Until recently the most common type of aid was the body or conventional type available with either an air- or a bone-conduction receiver. The case is generally rectangular or box-like in shape and is carried in the pocket or clasped to the clothing. Occasionally smaller body aids can be worn in the hair, supported by a barrette.

A relatively recent development, available for all but severe hearing loss cases, the ear-level aid comes in two styles, the behind-the-ear model (called "post auricle" or "over-the-ear" by some manufacturers) and the aid built into eyeglass temples. Both of these styles most commonly provide sound by air conduction, but eyeglass models are available that provide hearing by bone conduction. More recently, in-the-ear aids have appeared, but most of them have too little power to be of much use to a person with significant hearing impairment. Future developments in design are likely to make the in-the-ear style of use to a greater number of persons.[1]

In hearing aid design and manufacture, there have been great strides in miniaturization within the past decade or so, frequently with little or no loss in power or fidelity. The sizes of the hearing aids may be illustrated by the following data from one representative manufacturer:

	Width	*Length*	*Thickness*	*Weight (no battery)*
Body aid	1.72 in.	2.64 in.	0.70 in.	2.3 oz.
Behind-ear aid	0.56 in.	1.60 in.	0.40 in.	0.24 oz.

It should be emphasized that difficulties of further miniaturization of hearing aids do not stem from any limitations of solid-state circuitry. Actually, transistors and integrated circuits are more durable and capable of better quality performance than the older vacuum-tube circuits. The major limitations are found in the microphone and receiver. First, if they are placed too close together, acoustic feedback will occur, even at low-gain levels. Second, the size of these transducers cannot be reduced without also drastically reducing their ability to respond to the signal with good fidelity. Until these problems have been overcome by some breakthrough in transducer design, further miniaturization of hearing aids is of doubtful value.

1 Statistics furnished by the Hearing Aid Industry Conference, Inc. for 1968 show that of the hearing-aid sales, 51.3 per cent were behind-the-ear styles, 25.7 per cent eyeglass aids, 14.8 per cent body aids, and 8.2 per cent in-the-ear models.

Electronic Amplification

Our treatment of the complex topic of amplifier electronics will be limited to describing some simple circuits. Exhaustive consideration of amplifier theory is beyond the scope of this chapter, and is readily available in numerous excellent works. Let us now look at several of the most important components and properties of amplifiers.

MICROPHONE

The exterior portion of the microphone consists of a case with a sealed lid, which is a very thin and flexible diaphragm. The diaphragm vibrates in response to the varying air pressure of the sound waves striking it and is light enough to enable it to follow the fine and rapid vibrations produced by speech and music.

The older vacuum-tube hearing aid usually employed a crystal microphone, which was compatible with the needs of a vacuum-tube circuit. Transistor circuits function better with magnetic microphones. In transistor hearing aids, the transduction of acoustic to electrical energy operates on the principle of electromagnetic induction. A representative microphone in a body-style aid of three transistors measures 0.67″ by 1.05″ by 0.32″. Figure 14.1 shows a schematic diagram of the magnetic microphone.

The mechanism of a magnetic microphone consists of a permanent magnet attached to an iron armature, and a movable iron piece. The lines of force of the permanent magnet pass through the iron armature, on through the air gap between the armature and the movable iron piece, and then back to the magnet again, forming a complete circuit. As the air gap offers a high resistance to the flow of the magnetic force, it follows that the width of the air gap will determine the energy of the magnetic lines of force that will flow through the circuit (110).

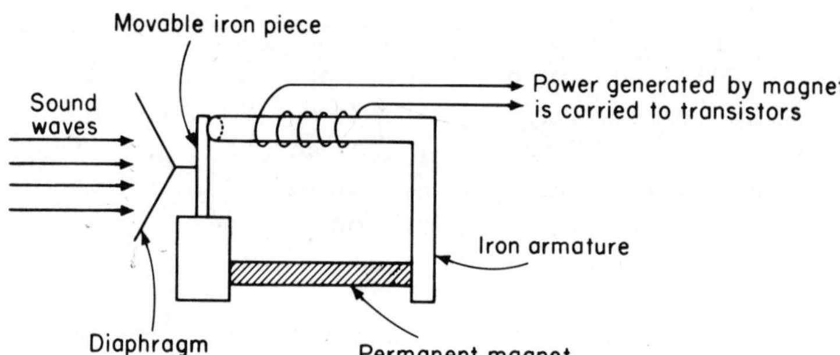

FIGURE 14.1 Magnetic microphone shown diagramatically. (After Sedacca.)

The movable iron piece is connected to the diaphragm by a pin, and will vibrate with the diaphragm, thereby varying the width of the air gap and, hence, the strength of the magnetic field in the circuit. Although sound energy cannot be directly amplified, the electrical voltage from the microphone may be amplified relatively easily.

The microphone in the older body-type hearing aids was usually at the front of the aid and was concealed by a design in the case. Many contemporary body aids have the microphone at the top of the aid, which reduces much of the sound of rubbing clothing which in the past was so annoying to the listener. The top-mounted microphone not only reduces clothing noise, because of the smaller surface of the top, but clothing is less likely to rub across the top of the aid than the front. Clothing noise is further lessened if the case of the aid is highly polished, and the individual can wear the aid in unstarched, soft-textured clothing. The body aid can also be worn in a harness with a cotton pocket. This is of advantage to the young hearing aid wearer since the parent or the teacher can easily check to see if the aid is turned on and is set to the best level for the child.

Depending upon the brand, various ear-level aids have the microphone mounted either at the front, back, or side of the aid. At present there are no good data to show a substantial advantage for any of these three placements.

TRANSISTOR

The invention of the transistor has led to revolutionary changes in amplifiers. Because transistors are ideally suited for miniaturization, their first extensive commercial use was in hearing aid circuits.

Early transistors, also called semiconductors, were made from germanium crystals, to which a tiny amount of another element, such as arsenic, was added to give them special amplifying capabilities. The transistor behaves in a manner analogous to a vacuum-tube triode, in that it allows electrical transmission in one direction only. Among the advantages of the transistor relative to the vacuum tube are: (1) smaller size, (2) no high current consuming filament, (3) more damage resistance, (4) longer life expectancy,

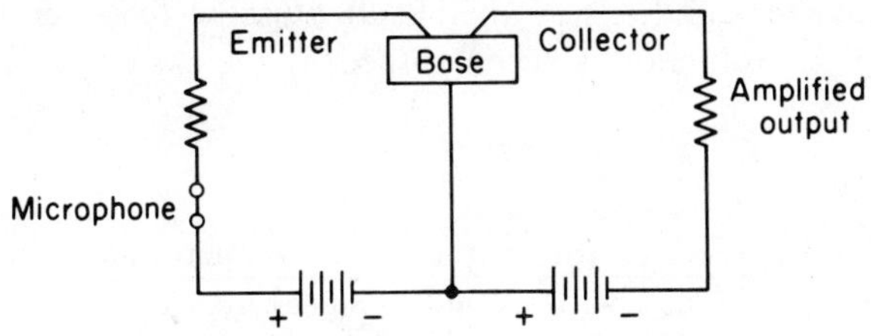

FIGURE 14.2 Diagram of a transistor placed in a very simplified circuit. (After Sedacca.)

and (5) much greater efficiency, i.e., they are less expensive to operate, and only one low-voltage cell is required.

The transistor, developed at Bell Telephone Laboratories, is related to the crystal detector, known since the beginnings of radio. Figure 14.2 shows a diagram of a transistor placed in a very basic system. The transistor is a rectifier in that it allows current to flow in one direction, but in addition it (like the vacuum tube) has a third element by which current flow can be controlled. The transistor has three elements which are usually designated as follows:

1. An emitter, which is analogous to the cathode of a triode vacuum tube;
2. A collector, which has a function similar to the plate of a triode vacuum tube;
3. A base, which usually controls the flow of collector current and is analogous to the grid of a triode vacuum tube.

It is the property of a transistor that small changes in current in the circuit between the emitter and the base produce large, corresponding changes in the current between the collector and the base. The production of this large collector current relative to base current (input) is amplification.

The principle function of the transistor as used in hearing aids is to amplify the alternating electrical signal coming from the microphone. The energy increase is usually on the order of 50 to 300 times. To achieve this, the transistor is adjusted when "no signal" is present by supplying the base with a small D.C. negative voltage (bias) through a base resistor. This subsequently results in a small continuous base current. A negative impulse will increase the negative bias and thus increase the base current. Since the collector current is dependent upon the base current, it can be seen that the large current flow in the collector circuit will constitute an amplified replica of the fluctuating signal with which the base is supplied.

To be useful in a hearing aid, a larger energy increase is needed than is provided by a single transistor stage. Typically three or more transistor amplifiers are coupled to one another in successive stages. Figure 14.3 shows a diagram of a four-transistor hearing aid in simplified form (110).

Once the signal reaches the output stage of the hearing aid, it is still an electrical current and is not audible. It must be reconverted to sound pressure. This transduction is accomplished by the earphone or receiver.

RECEIVER

In principle, a receiver (or earphone) is a microphone in reverse, in which the coil is supplied with an audio signal current. This current flow induces in the coil a varying magnetic field which acts upon the receiver diaphragm.

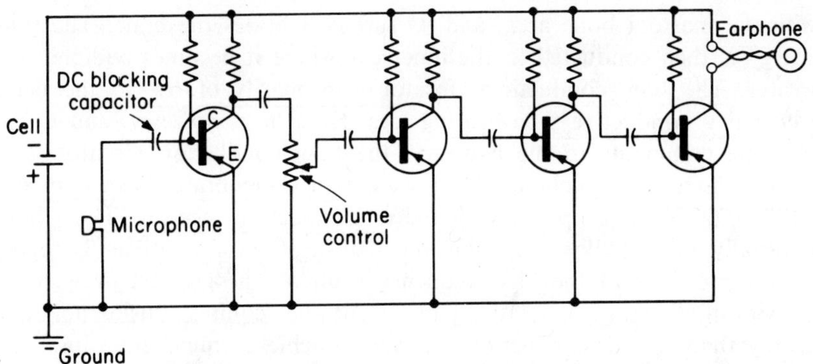

FIGURE 14.3 Simplified diagram of a four-transistor hearing aid. (After Sedacca.)

For practical reasons the receiver is not constructed exactly like a microphone. The gap between the diaphragm and the permanent ring magnet and iron bar (or pole shoe) assembly is kept as small as possible without allowing contact. This fine air gap is accomplished by adjusting the permanent ring magnet and thus securing the best diaphragm response.

The motion of the diaphragm occurs because a current flow in one direction increases the magnetic pull on the diaphragm, while a flow in the opposite direction decreases the pull. The change of current direction in the tiny electromagnetic coil produces a resultant change in polarity which assists or opposes the permanent magnet. In this manner the pattern of the audio output signal is transformed into mechanical vibrations of the diaphragm, which in turn produces corresponding audible air-pressure variations.

There are two fundamental types of receivers used with hearing aids, the air-conduction type as illustrated in Figure 14.4, and the bone-conduction type. The bone-conduction vibrator is also a magnetic device, the armature of which is connected directly to the housing enclosure. Thus, in the bone-conduction vibrator, the entire housing vibrates with the amplified sound rather than simply generating airborne sounds.

The bone-conduction vibrator is placed behind the ear, making contact

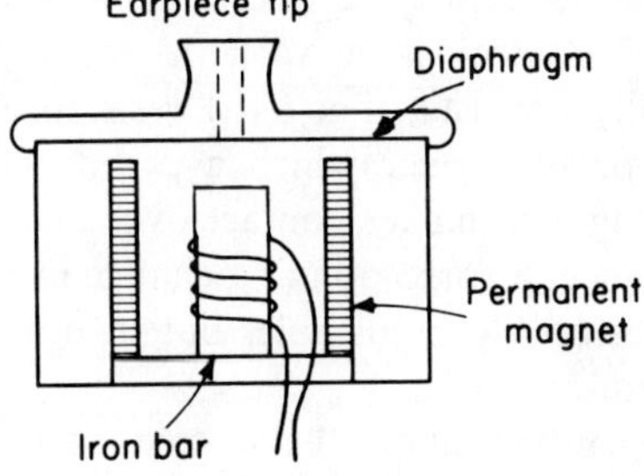

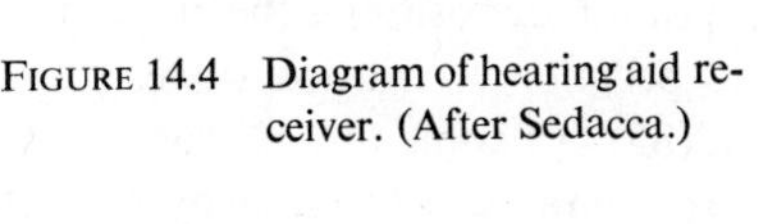
FIGURE 14.4 Diagram of hearing aid receiver. (After Sedacca.)

with the mastoid bone area, and its surface vibrates the bone. The sound energy is then conducted to the inner ear where it becomes audible to the wearer. The bone-conduction vibrator is primarily of use to the person who has a conductive type hearing loss. Even here, however, and in spite of some comments to the contrary, the bone-conduction vibrator is not usually the receiver of choice. The bone-conduction vibrator has a number of disadvantages as compared with the air-conduction receiver. The vibrator is usually more bulky and, from an acoustical standpoint, tends to be a poor reproducer of the high-frequency sounds. The greatest drawback to the vibrator is that it is relatively inefficient and requires considerably more energy than the air-conduction receiver to achieve equivalent stimulation. Part of this inefficiency is due to the thickness of the skull, the skin, and perhaps hair in the area where the vibrator rests in normal use. It should be noted, on the other hand, that if an individual has about a 35-dB air-bone gap, the bone-conduction vibrator is at least as efficient as the air-conduction receiver. The bone-conduction vibrator is of value in hearing-aid use mostly in those cases where the external ear canal is absent or deformed, where there is a large air-bone gap but the person cannot or chooses not to have surgery, or where there is a chronic drainage problem which precludes the closure of the ear canal by the earmold of the air-conduction arrangement.

Some ear-level hearing instruments have internal receivers, that is, the amplified sound is converted to mechanical energy within the physical enclosure of the aid and then conducted to the earmold by means of a small plastic tube. We know of no good data which favor the internal over the external receiver with these aids.

Differences in electromechanical characteristics of receivers can have a pronounced effect on the response of the hearing aid. They can be deliberately altered, and they serve as one means whereby hearing aid responses may be changed to help a particular hearing impairment. Figure 14.5 shows two response curves with the same hearing aid and the same input, but with different receivers.

VOLUME CONTROL

Most hearing aids have a volume control or gain control that allows the user to adjust the output level from minimum to maximum gain. The volume control is a variable resistor known as a potentiometer. This generally consists of a fixed resistance strip, usually a circular section of paper or fiber over which a carbon compound deposit has been painted. A sliding arm makes contact over this and permits a variation of resistance and, hence, a corresponding change in gain (85). In some models the control is continuously adjustable, but in others the gain is adjustable by discrete steps only.

Depending upon the degree of hearing loss, an instrument of mild, moderate, or large maximum gain may be recommended. Most audiologists feel that an aid with less than a 30-dB gain is seldom of value and should not be recommended.

AUTOMATIC VOLUME CONTROL

The terms automatic volume control, automatic gain control, and compression amplification are considered to be interchangeable. Automatic volume control offers the user four principal advantages where some limitation in output is necessary: (1) the maximum output of the aid can be limited to a level below the user's threshold of discomfort without reducing the gain for weak sounds, (2) the waveform distortion produced by "peak clipping" is avoided, thus maintaining better fidelity, (3) the signal-to-noise ratio of the incoming sound is maintained, and (4) the ratio of weak to loud components of speech is improved in favor of the listener in many instances. Let us briefly review each of these features individually.

The maximum output for various settings of the automatic volume control (AVC) are listed in the specification sheets for most hearing aids that employ compression circuitry. Once the threshold of discomfort for a patient has been established by speech audiometry, a setting may be chosen which assures that output will not reach or exceed this level. It must not be forgotten, however, that hearing-aid specifications are stated in sound pressure level (SPL) and not in terms of speech audiometric zero. (Thus, usually about 20-dB must be subtracted from the values given on the specification sheet for the values to coincide with the Threshold of Discomfort as established by speech audiometry.) The gain function of a compression

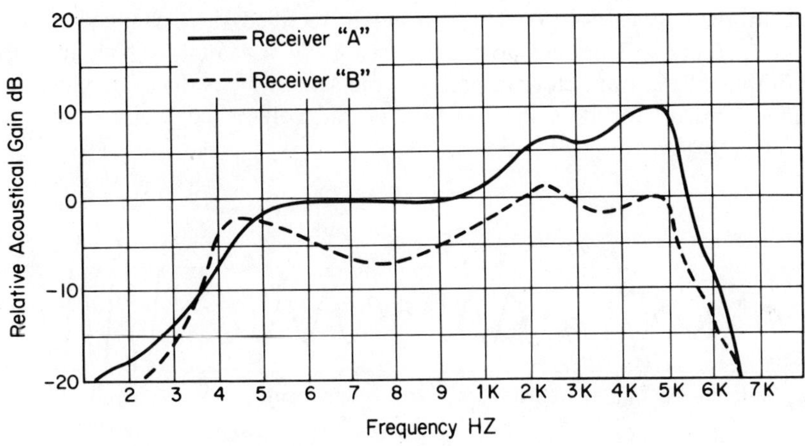

FIGURE 14.5 Hearing aid response curves which vary with the receiver used.

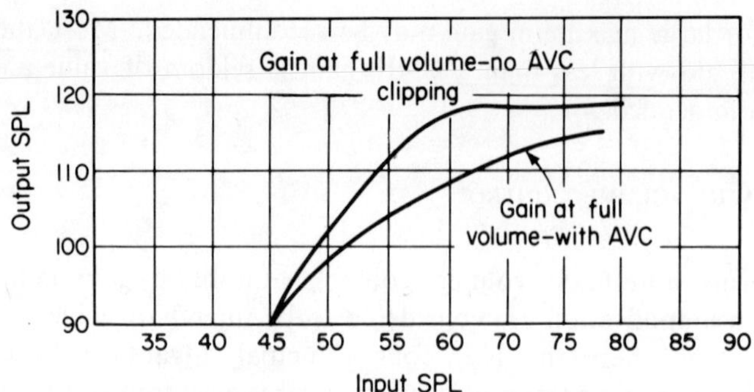

FIGURE 14.6 Gain function of hearing aids with and without automatic volume control.

circuit will be altered from non-AVC circuits in much the same way as shown in Figure 14.6.

When the input signal to a hearing aid reaches a sufficiently high level, saturation output occurs. This simply means that the amplifier has reached its maximum current-carrying capacity. Further increases in the input intensity will not result in further increases in output. This is illustrated in Figure 14.7.

As shown in Figure 14.7, the peaks of each cycle are clipped, thus distorting sound quality. Surprisingly, discrimination for speech is not seriously affected by this clipping unless it is rather severe.

Automatic volume control operates to prevent "clipping" by feeding back a bias to the transistors which do the basic amplifying. This is done by providing a secondary output circuit which is not activated until the output reaches a predetermined value. When this value is exceeded, the secondary circuit "bleeds" off a small amount of the current and feeds it back to the transistors (9). This current is rectified (i.e., changed into a direct current) and applied to the transistors in a manner which reduces the output of the transistors in precisely the same way as does changing the volume control, for it is the function of the volume control to regulate

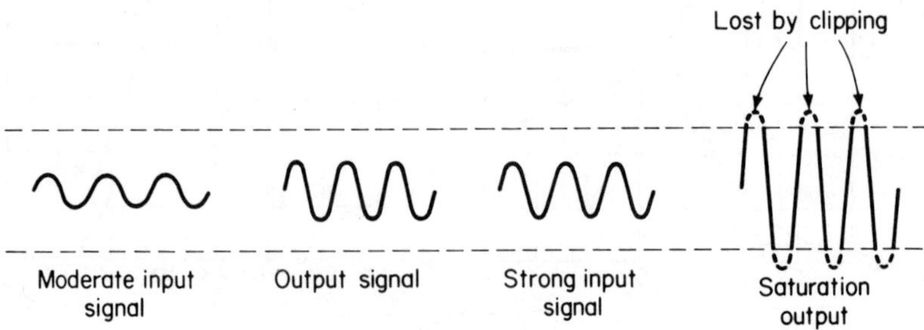

FIGURE 14.7 Comparison of input and output for moderate and strong signals without AVC.

the amount of bias applied to the transistors. This reduction in gain prevents the instrument from reaching the saturation output, and thus the peaks are never clipped and the signal waveform retains its essential shape. Figure 14.8 compares a waveform as a clipped and as an AVC signal.

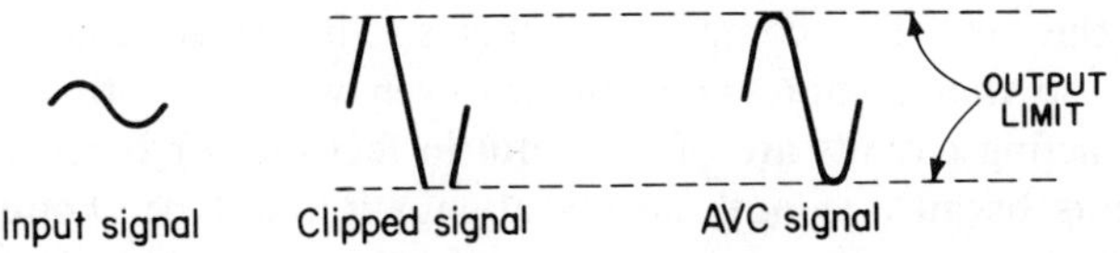

FIGURE 14.8 Comparison of clipped and AVC signals with strong input.

A hearing aid without AVC can drastically reduce intelligibility by reducing a desirable signal-to-noise ratio. Consider a hearing aid with a saturation output of 120-dB SPL, a gain set at 50 dB, and placed in an environment with a steady noise level of 70-dB SPL and a person talking at 90-dB SPL (i.e., the talking is 20 dB higher than the background noise). The amplifier will increase the noise to 120-dB SPL (70 dB plus 50 dB gain equals 120 dB). But the hearing aid, because of its maximum output limitation, can increase the speech level by only 30 dB to a total of 120-dB SPL. The speech and the noise levels are now equal, which in effect means that the noise has been amplified more than the speech.

In the case of AVC, however, the high speech input will "bias" the transistors in such a manner as to reduce the gain level, thus attenuating both speech and noise, rather than clipping the speech alone. The 20-dB difference between speech and noise, in the example above, will therefore be maintained. This particular action is often useful to all hearing-aid users, not just those with a tolerance problem.

If the response of the compression circuit is rapid enough, it can be seen that it can be made to act as a "selective amplifier" or "automatic tone control." Consider the word *so*, which contains the high-frequency voiceless fricative *s*, which is relatively weak in energy, followed by the low-frequency voiced vowel *o* of relatively great energy. The weaker *s* sound will not activate the AVC circuit and thus will be maximally amplified. The stronger *o*, on the other hand, can activate the compression circuit and thus be attenuated. The patient with a high-frequency hearing loss will thereby be protected against excessive low-frequency outputs, but will receive relatively greater high-frequency emphasis.

The features we have been discussing under AVC have been assumed to be advantages when, in fact, they can occasionally be detrimental to hearing function. For example, in the nonrecruiting ear, the compression of loud sounds and low frequencies will produce an unpleasant, monotonous sound, particularly if the amount of compression is excessive. Furthermore, if the patient's loss is flat, the compression of low-frequency components of speech may over emphasize the high-frequency sibilants. This effect is similar to what most of us notice when a radio or TV announcer speaks too close to the microphone and produces an annoying lisping sound.

In addition, compression circuits rarely work with the neat precision described above. Some circuits react slowly, permitting some high energy to pass to the ear before compression begins. The circuits may also be slow to recover, so that compression remains even when the stimulus is weak. Such slow-acting circuits are often useful in factories or other steady noise environments because smooth steady attenuation will be produced, which in these particular environments is preferable to rapid fluctuations of volume. Slow-acting compression circuits often have a switch that enables the wearer to turn off the AVC when in quieter environments. Considerable research on the effect of various attack and release times has been described in audiological literature. The findings, in general, suggest we should caution the reader that AVC is a general term applying to numerous individual circuit designs which are frequently very different. Thus, the type of AVC, type of hearing loss, and the environment in which the hearing aid will be used are important considerations in deciding when and how AVC might affect the listening performance of a particular patient (3, 6, 83).

TONE CONTROL

The tone control is sometimes positioned so that it can be manipulated externally, or it may be inside the case and accessible only to the hearing aid dealer. Occasionally both internal and external controls are built into a hearing aid model. The tone control is a filter network designed to alter the relative strength of high-frequency and low-frequency energy passing through it. A tone control setting for high-frequency emphasis consists of circuitry designed to efficiently transmit high frequencies and to block or inefficiently pass low frequencies. It is more accurate to think of tone control as a suppression of the range of frequencies least in need of amplification, rather than as emphasizing those needing amplification (9).

In addition to the internal and external tone control, the receiver, earmold, and tubing (if any) may, because of their resonant properties, provide the audiologist or hearing aid dealer with means of suppressing or emphasizing certain frequency areas as desired. Most hearing aid specification sheets describe and illustrate the effect of the various tone control settings on overall frequency response.

HAIC STANDARDS

It has long been the practice of hearing aid manufacturers to include specifications with their various models, but in the past there was no uniform way of reporting gain, frequency response, and other important acoustic parameters. In January, 1961, the Hearing Aid Industry Conference, Inc., adopted a standard method of expressing some of the important hearing aid performance factors (82). The HAIC Standard Method is based on the use of USASI Standard S3.3–1960, which describes the method whereby the measurements are to be made. In 1967 the HAIC Standard Method became USASI Standard S3.8–1967, with minor changes. The HAIC Standard concerns itself with expressing gain, output, and frequency range. Several related matters are also included. Although the HAIC Standard Method will undoubtedly be altered and expanded in the future, we so strongly believe that it is a good step in the right direction that we suggest the audiologist not recommend any hearing aid unless the specification sheet for that hearing aid includes data that are expressed using that standard.

BATTERY

Perhaps the most commonly used hearing aid battery is the mercury cell, originally known as the *Ruben* or *RM* cell. Technically, the term battery applies to two or more cells, but we shall follow custom by using cell and battery as synonyms in discussing their use in hearing aids. Most hearing aids today require a single mercury cell, or the newer silver-oxide cell (introduced in 1961); but more recent types, such as the manganese cell and gold cell, are becoming increasingly popular. A few hearing aids, though, still use the older dry cell (12, 46, 137).

Hearing aid manufacturers estimate that 80 per cent of all hearing aid failures are related to the battery circuit. These failures include: incorrect batteries, batteries in backwards, dead batteries, and the failure to periodically remove the corrosion that develops in the instrument battery compartment.

The basic chemical combination determines the voltage of the single cell. All higher voltages are obtained by adding one or more single cells in series, that is, the negative terminal of one cell to the positive terminal of the next cell. A fresh dry cell (zinc-carbon) provides 1.5 volts; fresh mercury cells provide about 1.24 volts; and silver-oxide cells about 1.5 volts.

Single cells connected in series produce a voltage equal to the sum of the separate cells. Thus the No. 152 mercury battery employs two No. 450 cells within a single pasteooard wrapper to produce a total of 2.6 volts. Cells connected in parallel (positive terminal to positive terminal and negative terminal to negative terminal) do not add voltages, so the total voltage is only equal to a single cell, but two cells connected in parallel double the total battery size and thus double its life.

Relationships between battery life, size, and voltage can be demonstrated by discussing the performance of various combinations if placed in a circuit with fixed resistance. For a given type of mercury cell, the operating life is directly related to size, so that if mercury cell X is twice as large as mercury cell Y, cell X will last twice as long as cell Y. However, if the effective voltage is doubled by connecting two cells in series, the current drain is also doubled, thus reducing battery life to what it would be if a single cell were used.

Figure 14.9A compares the power versus the life of the dry cell and the mercury cell. Dry cells gradually diminish in voltage to zero as the chemicals within them are consumed. Mercury cells diminish only slightly throughout their life and then drop very suddenly to a substandard voltage somewhere between 0 and 0.6 volts. When this drop in voltage occurs, the battery is useless, although inexperienced users will often continue to use it. At this reduced level, most hearing aids will tend to amplify only a narrow band of frequencies as shown in Figure 14.9B. Because some sound gets through, the user may assume that the battery is good. This is a frequent user error and the alert audiologist will discover exhausted batteries in patient's aids time and again.

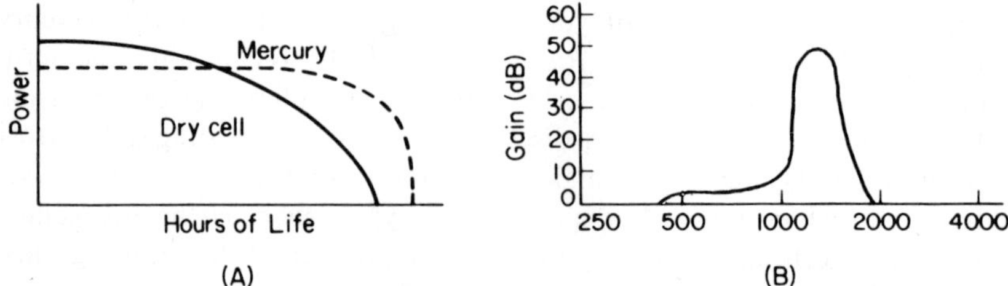

FIGURE 14.9 Hearing aid battery performance. (A) Comparison of discharge rate between dry cell and mercury cell. (B) Distortion caused by exhausted battery which causes a single frequency area to peak.

Advantages of the mercury cell over the older dry cell include: (1) a higher power-output-to-weight ratio, (2) an almost flat discharge-voltage curve, and (3) relatively long shelf life even under conditions of high temperature and humidity. The newer silver-oxide cell promises even further advantages.

Mercury cells have a tendency to develop a carbonate or salt formation on their surfaces. This coating is such an effective insulator that the current flow may stop completely. The coating does not affect battery operation or reduce its life, provided it is removed; brushing the battery with ammonia-soaked Q-tips is a handy way of doing this. If the coating is very light it is often sufficient to wipe it off, or to rub it off with a pencil eraser. This coating will frequently transfer to the contacts in the battery compartment, and, if not removed, will prevent hearing aid function even when fresh batteries are inserted. Periodic cleaning of battery compartments is important, both because the salts tend to corrode the contacts and because the coating will often reduce the power without cutting off the instrument completely.

It is often recommended that dry cells be rotated during their useful life because some energy is recovered if they are given a "rest." This is not true of mercury cells, and they should be used until exhausted. Also dry cells benefit from refrigeration, which slows down their natural degeneration; mercury cells degenerate so slowly that refrigeration is pointless. Stored in a reasonably cool, dry place, mercury cells have been known to provide normal life after several years of storage. Some manufacturers guarantee twelve months of storage life.

The voltage of hearing aid batteries may be checked by battery meters. Because of the current release inherent in the various types of cells and because of current requirements in particular battery meters, the obtained voltage readings are only approximate. Furthermore, meters designed to test dry cells tend to exhaust mercury cells rapidly. Thus, the battery tester should be used sparingly. As soon as the needle stabilizes on the tester a quick reading should be taken and the battery should be promptly removed from the tester. The hearing aid user should also be cautioned never to put batteries with coins, keys, or any metal. Even a momentary "short" can reduce the total operating battery life by many hours.

TELEPHONE PICKUP

Many hearing aids have a telephone pickup, which can be activated by a switch marked on the case as TEL, or T (for telephone) and M (for microphone). This is an audiomagnetic or inductive pickup coil that is mounted inside the case. The switch allows the user to substitute the telephone pickup for the microphone as the input to the hearing aid. With the microphone out of the circuit, noise from the local environment is excluded, and only the telephone signal is amplified. With some hearing aids, particularly those used by deaf children in a schoolroom with a loop system, the instrument is provided with a microphone, a telephone, and a combined microphone-telephone input. To use the telephone with the hearing aid, the telephone is positioned against the hearing aid, near the telephone pickup. With a little practice the user can find the most efficient placement of the telephone receiver.

The telephones that are now gradually being installed in homes do not provide for the use of a hearing aid with a telephone pickup. It is anticipated that within a decade or two few telephones will be in use with which the telephone pickup can be employed. To date no substitute circuit has been developed to help thc hearing impaired individual in using the telephone (9).

EARMOLD

The earmold, which couples the hearing aid receiver to the listener's ear, is an important part of the hearing aid. It is surprising that relatively performance while aided. Thus, an aid which, on the basis of the initial little interest in the earmold has been displayed by the audiologist, at least if one uses published research as the yardstick of interest (89). The pamphlet by Lybarger (81) is an excellent exception to the scarcity of research on the earmold, and this publication also discusses the acoustic effect of tubing length as well as receiver alterations. (*See also* 24, 39, 40, 48.)

Earmolds are available in many styles, and unfortunately the names for these designs vary from one manufacturer or laboratory to the next. The earmold may have on its outer or flat surface a round hole with a retainer ring to receive either the nubbin of the receiver or the nubbin of a plastic tube which, in turn, is connected to the receiver. Or, the tubing may go directly to the earmold and be attached to it by a plastic glue.

The so-called "regular" earmold is made of rigid plastic and fills the bowl of the external ear and the outer part of the external auditory canal. The regular earmold is used for body aid and for many ear-level aids. Less bulky molds are available, made in such a way that a thin ring of material fits just inside the bowl of the external ear and extends into the external auditory canal. This style is often called the "invisible" or "shell" or "phantom" earmold. If there is no ring to hold the mold in the external bowl of the ear but merely an insert portion in the external auditory canal, the mold is usually called by some superlative form of "invisible." In general, the more completely the earmold fills the concha, the less likelihood of acoustic feedback; so when high power is required, the regular earmold is usually preferred.

The making of an ear impression from which the earmold will be cast is somewhat of an art, and in most cases it is made by the hearing aid dealer. Some audiologists prefer to make their own earmold impressions, particularly if a trial period of auditory training is recommended before the aid is purchased. In those cases where the audiologist needs to make an earmold impression, he will find adequate directions accompanying the impression materials available from the various earmold laboratories. A nonallergic material is available for earmolds in those few cases where allergy is a problem.

Making the impression for earmolds in infants and young children presents some unique problems, particularly because of the child's inability to tell how satisfactory the fitting is. An explanation of the steps used in making the earmold impression should be given to the parents, and they should be informed of matters concerning the care of the completed earmold (27). We know of no good data which show how often the child "outgrows" an earmold. Clinically, we have found considerable variation at the preschool age, but the need for larger molds is much less frequent once the child is school age.

History and Philosophies of Hearing Aid Evaluation

At present most audiologic clinics in the United States are involved in some way with hearing aids and in advising persons with hearing losses who may need amplification. The service offered by the audiologist or the clinics goes by an assortment of names, including hearing aid evaluation, hearing aid selection, and hearing aid consultation. There is no generally agreed-upon meaning for any of these terms, but the following descriptions seem to be reasonably appropriate. It should be recognized that regardless of the name of the process, the ultimate goal is to make an amplification recommendation to the patient.

HEARING AID EVALUATION

After it has been determined on the basis of standard audiometric evaluation that the patient might benefit from amplification, various hearing aids are actually tried on the individual. With these instruments various gain and frequency settings may be tried and comparisons are made not only between settings for a specific brand and model but also among other brands and models. A comparison of aided SRT, speech discrimination, TD, and perhaps discrimination in noise scores with various hearing aid models and settings, as well as the comparison of these aided scores with those obtained unaided, is at the heart of the traditional hearing aid evaluation. These comparisons often also include a subjective evaluation by the patient.

The hearing aid evaluation will suggest either that no hearing aid is likely to be satisfactory, or that the person should purchase model X of brand Y. Sometimes the recommendation is not only for a specific model and brand, but for the precise receiver, gain setting, output, frequency response, or other acoustic property. Or, instead of a specific brand and model, the patient may be given a general recommendation for instrument performance characteristics (such as gain, frequency response, etc.) and told of one or more nearby hearing aid dealers whose aids can meet the recommendations. As can be seen, this procedure emphasizes comparing or *evaluating hearing aids* in terms of how they influence patient performance.

MODIFIED HEARING-AID EVALUATION

After it has been determined that the patient might benefit from amplification, he is tested while wearing a hearing aid in free field. Here the audiologist is not so much concerned with specifying a particular instrument or setting as he is with determining the patient's general speech audiometric performance while aided. Thus, an aid which, on the basis of the initial hearing evaluation, would appear to meet the approximate needs of the patient is tested on the patient to determine the effect of amplification in general. If amplification is found to be worthwhile, the patient is directed to one or more hearing aid dealers who will be responsible for selecting the specific hearing aid.

In this procedure the emphasis is actually on *selecting the patient* who might profit from amplification and getting him to a qualified hearing aid dealer for fitting. Instead of, or in addition to, the short trial under speech audiometry with an aid, the audiologist may want to test the patient with the so-called "master hearing aid" to determine approximate hearing aid gain and frequency response requirements (44, 125). The master hearing aid is usually a desk-mounted amplifier with controls that permit the examiner to select a variety of acoustic characteristics. In this manner he can "construct" an aid of low gain, moderate high frequency emphasis, and modest maximum output, for instance. Thus he can, to some extent, duplicate the performance of various hearing aid models.

HEARING-AID CONSULTATION

In this procedure, often little more than routine speech audiometry is employed in determining whether the patient will derive benefit from amplification. The accent is on *counseling the patient* about his hearing loss, and what difficulties he is likely to encounter in social and vocational environments. Referral is then made to one or more qualified hearing aid dealers with little or no specific recommendation for instrument performance.

During the hearing aid consultation, a great deal of time is spent, as the term implies, in consulting with and counseling the patient. It should be stressed that much counseling is also included in either form of the hearing aid evaluation. Thus, the traditional hearing aid evaluation is usually the most time-consuming of the evaluative procedures.

The patient needs to know what the hearing aid will do and what it will not do. He needs to be directed to a qualified hearing aid dealer. He needs advice on the sizes and styles of aids available to him, and how each differs from the other. He needs counseling so that he will be willing to accept the hearing aid just as he would eyeglasses if he had a vision problem. He needs advice about adjusting to amplification, about the general price range of hearing instruments, about trials, about guarantees, about earmolds, about repair service, about upkeep, and other matters. He needs to have possible misconceptions corrected, if he believes the hearing aid might "cure" the hearing loss, or, on the other hand, make it worse. He needs to be informed that hearing aids cannot be fitted (or hearing measured) with the precision that eyeglasses are fitted, and when speaking of hearing aids, that "fitted" means only a general "application" of the capabilities of the hearing aid to his particular hearing loss, rather than a so-called "prescription." All these, and many more questions can best be answered by the audiologist.

Amplification may do no more for the person with a severe hearing loss than to enable him to hear some noises and to determine the presence and absence of speech. Even this little help, however, may well make the purchase of an aid worthwhile. An aid may enable the deaf individual to differentiate the number of syllables in a word or perhaps even to discriminate vowels but not consonants. The individual may not be able to obtain adequate speech perception with an aid unless it is complemented by speech-reading therapy, but here again the aid is very important since numerous studies have shown that the amount of information received by audition together with vision is greater than by either singly.

We should expect any properly selected and fitted aid to enable the wearer to hear fainter sounds than by unaided listening. We also hope to maintain or even improve speech discrimination. The person with a hearing aid should be able to function better in a social or vocational situation than he would without amplification.

Because of some misleading advertising by manufacturers and misunderstandings on the part of the lay public, it is wise to counsel the new hearing aid user on the limitations of amplification. A hearing aid cannot restore hearing to normal, nor can the best electronic device in the world make an impaired ear hear perfectly. In sensori-neural hearing losses there are many cases where no *amount* of amplification will help the auditory nerve or its ending to function adequately. In the process of amplification all hearing instruments introduce some distortion—some of which is introduced purposefully—but the better aids introduce the least amount of undesirable distortion. A hearing aid will not of itself enable a deaf child to understand what he hears; much auditory habilitation is necessary to develop this skill. Even the adult with a long-standing hearing loss may have to relearn to recognize many sounds.

Most individuals need a period of adjustment to amplified sound. They need time to determine the best volume and tone control settings for themselves under a variety of circumstances. They must learn to tolerate the earmold. Hearing-aid users must realize that the aid will amplify unwanted and undesired sounds just as it amplifies speech, and a period of adaptation to amplified noises must be endured.

In spite of its many drawbacks, the hearing aid is a blessing to countless hearing-impaired individuals for whom no medical or surgical treatment has yet been developed to overcome their impairment. The embarrassing fact is that the otologist, the audiologist, and the hearing aid dealer are still not reaching numerous individuals who could profit from amplification.[2]

[2] The ratio of sales to population for hearing aids sold in the United States in 1968 was estimated at 2.05 per 1,000 persons. The ratio of sales to population was substantially lower in western Europe, and was as low as 0.02 to 0.04 in other parts of the world (119).

It is the experience of the authors that few persons with a hearing loss between a marginal and a profound degree cannot profit from amplification once the psychological block to wearing a hearing aid has been overcome.

Regardless of which of the evaluative procedures broadly described above, or combinations or variations of them, are followed by the audiologist, it is almost always the hearing aid dealer who makes the actual hearing aid fitting. By "fitting" we mean the precise instrument as well as the precise frequency response, maximum output, earmold type, tubing length and diameter, and all the detailed parameters which constitute the final amplifier and its associated components. It is the hearing aid dealer who takes the audiometric results of the audiologist and such suggestions or recommendations as the audiologist thinks proper, and decides what the specific fitting should be. Seldom is the audiologist involved with the detailed fitting of the aid, and by present ASHA requirements, members of that organization are prohibited from involvement in the actual sale of an aid.

A report published by the National Bureau of Standards (26) dealt with hearing-aid characteristics. Hearing aid selection matters are discussed in a booklet published by this same agency (25) which includes a listing of hearing clinics in the United States.[3] An early effort to evaluate hearing aid selection procedures was made by Hughson and Thompson (67). They sent questionnaires to individuals who had their hearing aids selected for them at a hospital clinic and found that 90 per cent of those fitted were satisfied with their hearing aids.

In Illinois, those persons who had received hearing aid services through the Division of Vocational Rehabilitation were surveyed (106). Of the respondents, 86 per cent felt their aids were performing acceptably. Of this 86 per cent the data were broken down according to whether the aid was selected at a hearing clinic or not; 90 per cent of the clinic-selected aids were considered to be acceptable. In considering only the "difficult" cases, 94 per cent acceptability was found in the clinic-selected instrument cases and 70 per cent acceptibility was found for those not selected at a clinic; 96 per cent felt the hearing clinic service was worthwhile. The results of this survey suggest that for the "average" hearing aid case the clinic and the nonclinic service will produce similar results, but for difficult cases the clinic's services are superior. Since we don't know in advance which cases will be easy and which will not, it might well be argued that all persons needing amplification should be seen by a clinic for some sort of hearing aid evaluation.

The selection and fitting of hearing aids to children and infants produces

[3] A complete list of audiologic clinics in the United States and Canada appears annually in the *American Annals of the Deaf*. A similar list has appeared periodically in the *Archives of Otolaryngology*, and this information may be obtained from the American Speech and Hearing Association or the National Association of Hearing and Speech Agencies.

special problems (34, 112). There is really no great problem in putting the aid on the infant or child, but there is considerable difficulty in determining if an aid is indeed needed, and also if the hearing aid is helping once it has been fit. The child's adjustment to the aid requires the interest and the cooperation of his parents. One of the first procedural suggestions for evaluating aids with children was by Bangs and Bangs (3), who worked with children as young as eighteen months of age. They suggest selecting an aid which appears logically to fit the child's needs, then teaching the child to recognize gross sounds or pictured words, while observing the speech and hearing behavior for several days; another aid is then tried under the same observational conditions in an effort to find the best fit under the circumstances. In determining the benefits of amplification with young children, the audiologist is likely to find that working with a teacher of the deaf or a hearing therapist will produce more meaningful information than merely one or two efforts at formal test comparisons.

Recent studies in language development and in the education of the deaf have revived emphasis on the importance of early systematic and concentrated auditory stimulation of children with severe hearing losses. The present authors have observed that many teachers of the deaf seem to greatly emphasize lip-reading and to look upon auditory stimulation as a supplementary, less fruitful sensory avenue for teaching. Thus, teaching materials are sometimes chosen more because they differ visually on the lips than for their acoustic contrasts. As Fry (43) and Hirsh (64) have pointed out, there is growing evidence that even cases with minimal residual hearing seem to be able to make much greater use of their auditory capability than has hitherto been supposed possible. If intensive auditory stimulation is an important as these authors say, and we are inclined to agree that it often is, then the audiologist's responsibility in fitting hearing aids on children takes on new importance. Failure to provide effective amplification for such cases as early as possible could result in a delay in speech and language development, or perhaps more likely, a tragic failure even to approach ultimate language capability.

HEARING AID COMPARISONS

Probably the greatest disagreement among audiologists, and between audiologists and hearing aid dealers, is the matter of hearing aid comparisons. Comparisons between two or more hearing aids, or between several settings of the same hearing aid, are the essence of the traditional hearing aid evaluation procedure. Intertwined with this disagreement is the matter of clinic versus nonclinic "fitting" of hearing aids. Some would argue that no differences between hearing aids can be shown in a typical free field clinical audiometric testing. This may be so, but that does not mean that significant differences do not exist. At the opposite extreme is the belief that performance will be influenced by small changes in hearing aid response, a belief that appears to us to be equally indefensible.

Obviously there may be quite different responses between several hearing aids, and persons needing or using a hearing aid will produce different scores by speech audiometry when wearing these aids. It is likely, however, that differences in hearing aids of similar characteristics from brand to brand are no longer great enough to be reflected by the relatively insensitive tests we employ to evaluate them. The matter that evolves from the question of hearing aid comparisons thus becomes a consideration of whether minor changes in hearing aid response characteristics can routinely be found from clinic patient to clinic patient. And, if this is true, is the time required to make tests after each adjustment in gain or frequency response worthwhile?

An early report on procedures used to compare listener responses when wearing carbon and vacuum-tube aids is outlined by Wiener and Miller (131). Their suggested steps are as follows:

A. Monaural tests without the aid.
   1. Pure-tone thresholds.
   2. Thresholds for speech.
   3. Tolerance for pure-tones.
   4. Tolerance for speech.
   5. Discrimination tests.

B. Free field tests without the hearing aid.
   1–5. Same tests as listed under A.

C. Free field tests with the hearing aid.
   1. Pure-tone threshold(s).
   2. Threshold for speech.
   3. Tolerance for loud speech.
   4. Discrimination test(s).
   5. Judgments of quality.
   6. The effect on speech thresholds or discrimination when annoying sounds and various background noises are present.

With some modifications, hearing aid evaluation (i.e., comparison) procedures today follow much the same outline as proposed by Wiener and Miller. The arguments for and against comparison scores have, however, been numerous. In particular, the matter of testing or comparing aided performance in a sound room has been questioned, even when a competing noise has been added to compare scores in the presence of noise. Nor is the typical use of white noise considered meaningful by many, but the problems of controlling most other types of noise in a test comparison situation have not been solved. It is quite possible that comparing aids in a "typical room" would be more meaningful than in a sound room, but the concept of a typical room is not rigorously tenable, and one can imagine the problems inherent in trying to precisely specify the characteristics of such a room.

At about the time Wiener and Miller were developing procedures for their hearing aid comparisons, a twelve-step procedure was developed at one of the army rehabilitation centers at the close of World War II (18). One step of this fairly lengthy and involved procedure was the "hearing aid evaluation," and this is further discussed (19), with the suggestion that the selection of an appropriate instrument be based on the following aided test comparisons: (1) differences of SRT, (2) tolerance, (3) efficiency in background noise, and (4) speech discrimination. A procedure was outlined whereby several trial aids could be compared; this requires the patient to adjust the gain of each aid under test to a comfort level while listening to connected discourse at 40 dB (re speech audiometer zero). An SRT was then determined and discrimination testing was done at 25 dB above aided SRT.

At the Harvard Psycho Acoustic Laboratory (PAL) both hearing-aid fitting and hearing-aid evaluation procedures were examined (28, 29). The resulting well-known "Harvard Report" stressed, among other things, that the effectiveness of the principle of selective amplification is fallacious. Selective amplification is an attempt to restore amounts of energy equal to the patient's hearing loss at various frequencies. It was also concluded that elaborate fitting procedures were unnecessary for most patients, but might have some value for difficult cases. The report was critical of Carhart's gain control setting method as having too much variability from patient to patient, and tests of TD were criticised since tolerance seems often to increase with each presentation. The PAL group suggested a three-step testing program. First, the patient would be tested to determine if he could accurately identify spondees at 60 or 70 dB (re speech audiometer zero); and next, the same determination was made at 20 or 40 dB. Finally, tolerance was examined at 100 dB. If the patient could tolerate speech at 100 dB and could understand simple speech materials at the 40-dB level, he would have an acceptable operating range of 60 dB. The Harvard investigators suggested these rules, designed to allow a 90 per cent successful hearing-aid fitting.

1. Try a high-pass pattern with a smooth rise of 6 dB per octave from 100 to 7,000 Hz for everyone. Use this pattern unless the quality of the flat pattern is preferred by the patient.
2. Use a flat pattern (within ± 1 dB from 100 to 7,000 Hz) for all patients with flat or rising threshold audiograms.
3. If neither of the above two patterns is satisfactory, use an intermediate slope.

Early studies and discussions of selective fitting versus the use of flat amplification, and efforts to differentiate the responses among hearing aids have been reported by Hedgecock (59), Anderson and Black (2), Edgardh (36), Fry and Denes (42), Glorig (45), Groen and Tappin (47), and Herdt (61), among others. These studies and discussions were concerned with vacuum-tube aids or very early models of the transistor aid. Whether selective amplification is more or less valid with transistor aids than with vacuum-tube instruments remains to be satisfactorily determined. Reddell and Calvert (102) suggested that selective amplification matters regarding the older hearing aids are not appropriate to today's aids, and that the older research may be obsolete. We also recall patients who made the change from vacuum-tube aids to transistor aids and had considerable difficulty in adjusting to the "new" sound.

Since the publication of these early reports on hearing-aid evaluations and on the users' impressions of this service, there have been numerous conflicts of opinion between audiologists and hearing aid dealers, and among audiologists, over the value of hearing aid evaluations in general, or over the value of some of the evaluative procedures. The hearing aid dealers appear to be more apt to accept subjective impressions of the aid's value to individuals, while the audiologist may be too insistent upon wanting objective test data to support the value or lack of value of an aid for a particular individual. Since the science of hearing aid fitting is still inexact, few positive conclusions can be made. More recently the entire question of the clinical evaluation of specific hearing aids, based on comparisons of listener performance with various instruments, has again become a controversial issue.

As early as 1946, Davis and his associates suggested that hearing-aid evaluations be limited to problem cases. Although Carhart developed the procedures which are in most common use today (usually in modified form), he essentially concurred with Davis et al. when he stated, "... the time should come when otology is exerting positive guidance by referring problem cases to hearing clinics" while other cases could be sent directly to reputable hearing aid dealers.

In 1960, Shore, Bilger, and Hirsh (116) reported an experiment which concluded that comparative measures of SRT and speech discrimination in quiet and in noise, obtained from listeners wearing several hearing aids which differed acoustically, were not reliable. In short, the relative effectiveness of hearing aids, as reflected by these measures, was sometimes shown to change on repeated testing. The authors asserted that "one does not find substantial or striking differences among the results of hearing tests obtained from patients using different hearing aids or different tone settings of hearing aids." They concluded, therefore, "... that the reliability of these measures is not good enough to warrant the investment of a large amount of clinical time with them in selecting hearing aids." Although the authors of this experiment challenged the reliability of the Carhart procedures, they did not use his recommended method of hearing aid gain adjustment. Since Carhart considered his method (called "functional equivalence") to be an important control in the use of his procedures, any conclusions drawn by the authors would seem, therefore, to apply more to their own procedures than to those of Carhart.

Millin (92), in a reply to the Shore et al. study, suggested that the gain adjustment method used by them may require the use of levels well above those which the user might choose for himself. As Yantis et al. (134) pointed out, excessive gain could result in intensity levels which drive the ear into nonlinear response. This could result, among other things, in an amount of variability greater than that produced by Carhart's method.

Two studies, one by McConnell et al. (88) and the other by Jeffers (70), both of which were published soon after the study of Shore and his associates, reasserted the value of the traditional evaluative methods. Nonetheless Shore and Kramer (115) described a change in hearing services at the Central Institute for the Deaf in which "the testing of a series of hearing aids was eliminated and a specific aid was not recommended." Resnick and Becker (105) also announced the discontinuation of hearing aid evaluations at the Washington D.C. Hospital Center, an action based, at least in part, upon the findings of the study by Shore et al. The abandoning of comparison procedures aroused strong reactions from those who felt that such procedures were of value, despite the Shore, Bilger, and Hirsh study (71). Among the effects of transferring the responsibility of hearing aid selection from disinterested professionals to the hearing aid dealer is the possibility that further research on hearing aid selection will be discouraged.

Resnick and Becker (105) also presented three assumptions which they assert to be the basis of conventional hearing aid evaluation procedures: (1) that there are significant differences among hearing aids in how they enable the user to understand everyday speech; (2) that these differences change from one user to the next, that is, that there is an interaction between people and hearing aids; and (3) that these differences can be demonstrated by PB word intelligibility scores. It is reasoned by Resnick and Becker that if the effect of differences among hearing aids is consistent from user to user, the audiologist need only determine which hearing aid is "best" and recommend it to every potential user. Since, as Shore et al. (116) state, "... there is no good evidence concerning a relation between the performance of an aid as measured through listening tests and the physical performance of an aid as measured through acoustical tests," it is a curious paradox that a determination of which is the best aid would presumably have to be made by comparative tests of hearing aids placed on the heads of listeners, a procedure which the authors claim to be unreliable.

They also express doubt about the assumption that there is an interaction between people and hearing aids and state that they see no reason why such interaction should exist. Yet, there is little doubt that interaction will exist, certainly with certain combinations of extreme hearing loss patterns and hearing aid frequency responses. For example, patients with abrupt high-frequency losses ("waterfall" drops) and no hearing whatever for high frequencies could hardly be expected to benefit from an amplifier which provides energy only at those frequencies to which the patient's auditory system is completely unresponsive. The same instrument might be of use to other listeners, however. The issue would appear to be, therefore, not whether interaction could exist, but rather whether hearing aids currently available on the market differ sufficiently to yield such interactions. Some clinicians, not to mention hearing aid users, insist that they do. Resnick and Becker apparently suspect that they do not.

The acceptance of the Shore et al. (116) position does not settle the issue, nor do Shore et al. make any such claim. They do not say that differences among hearing aids do not influence listener performance, but only that traditional listening tests do not reflect these differences.

Judging from the emphasis of subsequent research, investigators seem to assume that differences in amplifiers are important and have sought either to develop more sensitive tests or to isolate acoustic variables that can be demonstrated to influence performance. For instance, Jerger and his coworkers (73) used a modification of PAL No. 8 sentences, which were reported to be effective in revealing instrument differences; and they later demonstrated that monosyllabic word intelligibility scores were not successful in revealing such differences (74). In the concluding remarks of the second report, the authors note that their "purpose was merely to determine whether monosyllabic word lists, *as they are used in conventional hearing aid selection procedures*, are capable of reflecting the performance differences that can be demonstrated by a suitable behavioral measure" (italics in the original). Yet, the procedure used in this study are, in many respects, atypical of conventional hearing aid selection methods; and the reader is left to guess at other important procedures. Nonetheless, both these reports and one by Harris et al. (55) succeeded in demonstrating a consistent inverse relationship between discrimination scores and the percentage of harmonic distortion present in various hearing aids.

It should be noted that both of these groups of experimenters deliberately, by electronic and mechanical manipulation, exaggerated differences in instrument distortion far beyond that which would be found among aids typically available for clinical trial, and this was acknowledged. In fact, they so greatly increased the degree of harmonic distortion in some aids that the finding of a significant effect was almost inevitable. In clinical practice, the process of preselection tends to reduce, rather than increase, electrophysical differences among aids. While these experiments demonstrated that the effect of instrument differences on performance can be measured, the deliberate overemphasis of distortion casts considerable doubt on the relevance of these experiments to practical problems of hearing aid selection.

One cannot question the desirability of objective measures which will predict the degree of benefit a potential hearing aid user may expect from amplification. The problems involved, however, in developing such measurement procedures are immense. In addition to the problems of reliability of speech audiometry, as discussed in a previous chapter, the following issues are among those which need to be resolved before we can, with greater confidence, predict how amplification will affect the listener's communicative behavior.

1. Validity. Even if more reliable measures of hearing aid performance are developed for sound room use, we have no assurance that they will accurately predict performance outside the test room in the problem environments of everyday life.

2. Short duration tests cannot reflect the adjustments to amplification that many hearing aid users seem to make with experience.

3. Tests in noise suffer from the lack of resemblance between the test noises and noises encountered in everyday life. The development of valid noise stimuli is urgently needed. As a related issue, the influence of competing speech is not yet quantifiable in any practical manner.

4. Speech stimuli presented in largely nonreverberant sound rooms differ significantly from speech as heard in hard-walled rooms such as offices, kitchens, schoolrooms, and living rooms (95).

5. Hearing aids used for clinical testing may differ in acoustical performance from the instrument of the same model which is ultimately delivered to the hearing aid buyer.

6. The dynamics of psychological adjustment to amplifications have not been well delineated or tested experimentally.

Attempts to clarify some of these problems are discussed elsewhere in this chapter. They are far from being resolved at present and offer numerous opportunities for the interested researcher. Until these and other vital questions are answered, the use of clinical hearing aid comparison procedures will doubtless remain a matter of individual conviction. It might also be added that while most audiologists are critical of the evaluative shortcomings, at worst they seem to be better than most suggested alternatives. Whether one is for or against selective amplification, or clinical evaluations, the inescapable point remains that sometime and somewhere a choice of which is likely to be the best aid for that person must be made and in some manner evaluated. Some audiologists and most hearing aid dealers apparently feel that this choice should be made by the dealer; obviously we do not. Thus, the usefulness, reliability, and validity of selective amplification as well as the related matter of clinic versus nonclinic hearing aid "fitting" await solution. As research data slowly but gradually accumulate, we are finding many parameters which will require still further study.

Undoubtedly there are many variables and interactions involved which have not been defined or controlled.

To several questions regarding the clinical "fitting" of hearing aids, preliminary answers can be given. Aided speech audiometric test-retest results, during the same day or separated by about a month, are fairly good, but hopefully can be improved further (88). Possible performance differences which might exist between a specific hearing aid on loan to a clinic and an aid of the same model which is later purchased have also been examined (57). Good test-retest results were obtained for SRT and speech discrimination. Furthermore, the clinic can now readily compare hearing aid responses, either from the loaned aid in the clinic to the purchased aid, or of either aid to the manufacturer's specification, by means of a hearing-aid test unit.[4]

An example of renewed interest in the application of selective amplification is the low-frequency hearing aid. In this case, however, the objective is not to amplify most the frequency range which has the greater loss, but rather, in the case of persons with profound hearing loss, to emphasize amplification of the frequency range in which the patient has the most residual hearing (80, 16). Many manufacturers now have models designed specifically to amplify the low-frequency range of sounds.

The Traditional Hearing Aid Evaluation

Prior to hearing aid evaluation (or consultation) there should be a thorough hearing evaluation which includes as a minimum: pure-tone air- and bone-conduction thresholds, monaural and free field SRT and speech discrimination testing, and such other suprathreshold tests as may be deemed useful. The tympanic membrane should be examined during this initial appointment; this is particularly vital when an earmold for testing purposes is required since, obviously, if there is impacted cerumen or any other deviation in the normal route of sound to the eardrum, the test scores may be invalid.

Obviously it is not possible, or even desirable, to try every model of hearing aid in the clinic on the patient. Some kind of *preselection* of aids to be evaluated must be made. Such preselection should be made on some logical basis. If we knew, however, precisely what kind of acoustic performance would best serve the user, there would be no need for comparative testing; we would simply recommend the most suitable instrument.

In the preselection of aids for evaluation purposes, there are certain acoustic and nonacoustic factors which are well-enough understood to permit us to reduce to a minimum the number of trial aids to be evaluated.

[4] Hearing aid test units are available from: B & K Instruments, Inc.; Kamplex (distributed in the U.S. by Dahlberg Electronics, Inc.); and Vicon Instrument Co.

We know, for example, that severe to profound hearing losses cannot achieve maximum correction with instruments of low gain. Persons with such losses will usually be limited to body-style aids which provide more gain and power than ear-level models. Milder loss cases may have to exclude eyeglass temple aids because they do not need glasses or they do not wear glasses regularly.

Of major concern in the preselection of hearing aids is the matter of hearing aid gain. Millin (93) found that sensori-neural loss patients tended rather consistently to choose a gain setting amounting to approximately two-thirds of their hearing loss for speech. If some additional reserve is provided for the influence of such factors as temporary head colds or a gradually worsening of hearing over the useful life of the aid, one can settle for a maximum gain capability which is approximately equal to two-thirds of the patient's SRT plus about 10 dB in the ear to be fitted. In other words, a patient with an SRT of 60 dB would tend to use about a 40-dB gain; if an additional reserve is added, an appropriate instrument will have a gain of about 50 dB. There are many other formulas for predicting gain needs, based on similar reasoning (87).

The principle of preselection according to frequency response generates great disagreement among audiologists. Perhaps the preselection should include at least one aid of appropriate gain which has a flat frequency response and one in which the gain increases with frequency. Should the latter work poorly, the audiologist can try an aid of low-frequency emphasis.

Evidence of tolerance difficulty suggests the need for a reduced upper power limit. In extreme tolerance cases or projected use in noisy environments, AVC should be considered. Preselection is an area in which the use of a master hearing aid may help to isolate rather quickly the general type of instrument response which is most appropriate.

How many hearing aids should be preselected for evaluation? We feel that three models is a minimum and probably six is a maximum. If it is obvious during the evaluation process that the aid under evaluation is not producing scores comparable to those obtained with previously evaluated aids, there is little point in carrying out the complete evaluation procedure for that aid. Certainly not only the audiologist's time, but also the patient's time and how much concentrated listening he can endure should be considered.

HEARING-AID EVALUATION PROCEDURES

After the preselection of aids has been made, the audiologist proceeds to what is sometimes called the "traditional" hearing aid evaluation (or comparison) procedures. Usually a hearing aid evaluation form is employed so that differences among the tested aids may be readily compared. Figure 14.10 shows a typical hearing aid evaluation test form. We give now, step by

KENT STATE UNIVERSITY
HEARING AID EVALUATION FORM

Date________________ Name________________ Audiologist________________

MAKE OF AID									
MODEL									
RECEIVER									
TONE									
VOLUME									
BATTERY VOLTAGE									
EAR									
dB COMFORT LEVEL SETTING (40 dB unless specified)	SRT	R	L	FF					
	TOLERANCE IN dB								
	DISCRIMINATION IN QUIET	%	%	%	%	%	%	%	%
	DISCRIMINATION IN NOISE	%	%	%	%	%	%	%	%
	dB SPEECH INPUT								
	dB NOISE INPUT								
SETTING FULL VOLUME	SRT								
	TOLERANCE IN dB								
	REMARKS								
	RATING OF AID								

RECOMMENDATION: Make__________ Model__________ Tone__________

Receiver__________ Ear__________ Battery__________

FIGURE 14.10 Kent State University hearing aid evaluation form.

step, a typical traditional procedure for the evaluation of aids based primarily on patient performance.

1. With the speech audiometer at 40 dB (i.e., 62-dB SPL) a recording of cold running speech is played, or the audiologist reads informative but nonemotional speech materials. With the aid in place the patient experiments

with the volume control, and perhaps the tone control, until he feels he can most clearly and easily understand the speech. The patient is then cautioned not to touch the controls of the aid until the conclusion of this particular testing procedure.

2. With recordings or by monitored live voice, the aided free field SRT is obtained.

3. At SRT plus 40 dB (or SRT plus 25 dB, or MCL, or any other level used at that clinic, such as a constant 62-dB SPL) discrimination testing is done with a recording or by monitored live voice.

While the traditional level is SRT plus a given number of decibels, we feel that aided discrimination testing is more realistic and useful when done at a level approximating normal conversation. To test a person with an aided SRT of, for instance, 30 dB, at SRT plus 40 dB (i.e., 70 dB according to speech audiometer zero) is merely to determine how well the patient hears shouted speech. Our real interest should be how well he performs at conversation level when wearing a hearing aid, and 40 dB (according to speech audiometer zero) approximates the lower range of average conversation level.

4. Speech-in-Noise Tests. There are two common methods. In the first, an SRT is obtained in the presence of noise (usually white noise) coming from a loudspeaker separate from the speech. Noise is added to determine the amount needed to alter the SRT. The second method, and one more commonly used, is to set the audiometer for a predetermined signal-to-noise ratio (commonly +10, +5, or 0) and to obtain a discrimination score in noise.

5. Next the audiologist determines tolerance for loud sound. For this he usually uses a recording of cold running speech. As was mentioned in the chapter on speech audiometry, the patient must be cautioned to signal only when the speech is really uncomfortable.

6. With the completion of the speech audiometric tests, the aid is removed from the patient and the volume and tone control settings which were made by the patient are noted. If the volume control is numbered or lettered, this is written on the evaluation sheet. If the volume control is continuously variable, the audiologist estimates the setting, such as one-fourth, two-thirds, or full. This step is important since the patient should not have an aid that requires a full gain setting; and if the hearing loss is progressive, no more than half gain should be required at the initial fitting.

7. Some clinics add or substitute a step for steps four and five. This is to turn the aid to full volume setting and to obtain discrimination and tolerance scores.

Before putting this particular aid aside, the audiologist should also complete the hearing aid evaluation form, noting the ear on which the aid was evaluated, the brand and model number of the instrument and receiver, and the battery voltage. Only when all aids have been evaluated should the patient be asked to informally rate them, and the relative costs of the aids should be discussed only at this time. If the patient was referred by an agency which has a maximum price it will pay for an aid, the preselection of aids should include only those within the allowable price limits.

Succeeding hearing aids will be evaluated by going through steps one through seven above in the same manner. After all aids and settings which might be expected to help this particular patient have been evaluated, the audiologist should examine the various test scores and the rating by the patient. At some clinics the next step is to advise the patient which aid (if any), in the estimation of the audiologist, should be purchased. Other clinics prefer to rank the aids 1, 2, 3, etc., and perhaps let the patient go out and try them at the hearing aid dealer's office. Psychologically there seems to be value in advising the patient to purchase a specific aid rather than sending him to try several aids or visit several dealers. The fear is that he will probably purchase the aid on the basis of sales persuasiveness rather than on the basis of hearing aid performance. There is far from unanimous agreement among audiologists, however, on this point.

Of course the audiologist cannot ethically recommend a specific aid unless his battery of tests or other considerations suggest that this aid is significantly better than the other aids on one or more factors. Improvement in SRT and lack of deterioration (or, hopefully improvement) of speech discrimination are usually major determinants in this recommendation. The aided SRT as a measure of improvement in sensitivity is useful in hearing aid comparisons. But, it does not necessarily follow that a hearing aid which provides great improvement in SRT will also provide good discrimination at ordinary speech levels. Of the two parameters, improved understanding seems to be the more important consideration. It is conceivable that a hearing aid might provide good improvement in the SRT but inferior discrimination. It is difficult, however, to support the view that a listener can demonstrate good aided discrimination with inferior sensitivity. Thus, it might be asserted that good discrimination is, of itself, direct evidence of adequate aided sensitivity.

In making hearing aid recommendations some nonaudiologic factors bear consideration also, such as nearness of dealer to patient for service problems, and the cost of the aid as well as the required batteries. It is assumed that there will be no aids from unethical dealers in the clinic for evaluation purposes.

Most clinics have some sort of follow-up program to insure that the correct aid has been purchased and the patient understands its operation. The better dealers will adequately counsel the new user about the aid, but this should not be left to chance. Ideally the purchaser will return to the clinic within a few weeks of the purchase, at which time the audiologist can again perform some of the aided speech audiometric tests and also counsel the user further about any problems. The purchased aid may also be evaluated to determine whether the gain, frequency range, etc., are within reasonable agreement with the specifications for that aid. If direct follow-up is not possible, it is well for the clinic to keep in contact with the user by mail to make sure the aid is functioning properly and the user is giving the aid a fair chance to prove its value by usage.

The Hearing Aid Candidate

Although the audiologist should probably perform a hearing aid evaluation (or consultation) for any individual who so desires it, there are some general rules which suggest that a person may or may not be a good hearing aid candidate. In addition to some as yet uncorroborated psychological factors (37, 90), the individuals's likelihood of benefiting from an aid depends to some extent upon the degree of hearing loss, the pure-tone threshold configuration, the discrimination for speech, the tolerance for loud sounds, and undoubtedly other measurable factors. The chart in Figure 14.11 gives a general outline of the help an individual might achieve from amplification, based solely on the *degree* of loss. The various levels shown in Figure 14.11 are, of course, arbitrary.

Certainly as important as the degree of hearing loss in predicting success in hearing aid use is the pure-tone threshold contour. In general these patterns might be summarized as follows:

1. Most favorable: flat, gradually rising, or gradually falling.
2. Less favorable: steep falling, deep saucer-shape, or irregular dips and peaks.
3. Least favorable: sharp drop at any lower frequency, islands of hearing only, or a remnant of hearing at lowest frequencies only.

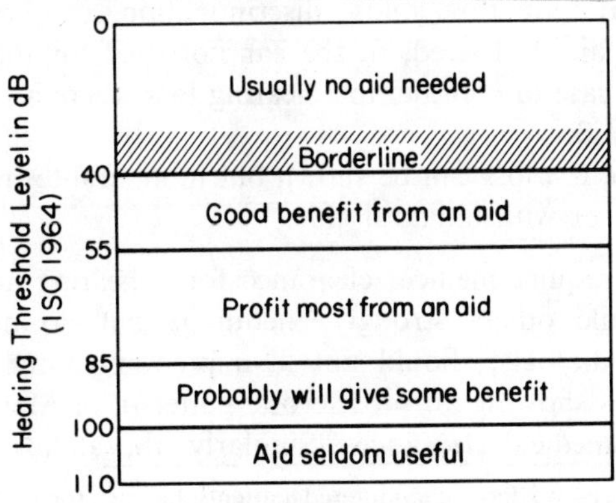

FIGURE 14.11 Expected benefits from amplification.

Unaided discrimination scores provide one of the better indicators of the probable success with an aid, and also of the choice of the ear to be fitted. An unaided discrimination score of 90 per cent or higher with the W–22 records or lists suggests probable good results with amplification; 70 to 90 per cent indicates mild difficulty; 50 to 70 per cent indicates substantial difficulty; and scores lower than 50 per cent should alert us to the probability that amplification will not be entirely successful. On the other hand, it should be stressed that an aided score of, for instance, 40 per cent may be very important and "successful" if the user has a severe hearing loss and can hear nothing without a hearing aid. The discrimination scores, like the other predictive criteria, should not be taken as a definite rule, since frequent exceptions are found. Nor is experimental data available to support most of the statements above; we present only clinical observation.

The question of which ear should be fitted with the hearing aid seems simple to answer, but the fitting of an aid in the incorrect ear is probably the greatest error found in cases of nonclinic fitting. The wrong ear is chosen mostly because of improper masking during initial testing and consequent failure to detect a dead or essentially nonfunctioning ear. The following rules (based in part on the suggestions by Watson and Tolan [126]), although often overlapping, will apply to most cases:

1. Fit the ear with the best speech discrimination.
2. Fit the ear with the greatest conductive component to the loss.
3. Fit the ear with the best tolerance for loud speech.
4. If the better ear has a loss of less than 55 to 60 dB (ISO, 1964) in the speech frequencies, fit the worst ear. Or, if the better ear has a loss greater than 70 to 80 dB, fit the better ear.
5. Don't fit the ear having recruitment; or, if there is bilateral recruitment, fit the ear with the least amount.
6. If one ear has chronic drainage, fit the opposite ear where bone-conduction fitting is not chosen.
7. If the pure-tone thresholds, discrimination, etc., are about equal and a monaural aid is desired, fit the ear not used for the telephone, but vice versa in the case of considerable hearing loss where a telephone pickup is built into the aid.
8. In children, if a loss can be shown but monaural testing is impossible, fit with a Y-cord or with binaural aids.

Some clinics require medical clearance for a hearing aid evaluation or consultation, while others strongly encourage but do not require this. Ethically, the audiologist should not fit a predominantly conductive loss (particularly cases showing an otosclerotic pattern), or Meniere's syndrome without specific medical clearance.[5] Similarly, the audiologist should not

[5] In some instances we have encountered patients having, for instance, a pattern of hearing that strongly suggests otosclerosis; even with the knowledge that surgery might

recommend a hearing aid under any circumstances for persons: (1) suspected of having a retrocochlear loss, (2) having a predominantly nonorganic loss, (3) whose problem is primarily that of phonemic regression, and (4) not showing an improvement of aided over unaided speech in one or more kinds of measurement (e.g., discrimination, SRT, etc.).

Other Hearing Aid Fittings

The directing of the amplified sound to a single ear is referred to as monaural amplification. The division of the amplified sound to the two ears is called pseudobinaural, or a Y-cord fitting. When the sound, by separate microphone, amplifier, and receiver, is directed to each ear, this is referred to as a binaural hearing aid.

The concept of binaural fitting is hardly new, but the past decade has seen a flurry of reports and experiments concerned with this matter. Evidence for and against binaural fitting has been almost evenly split. The opinions of hearing aid dealers (and to some extent hearing aid users) have been quite positive in favor of binaural aids. The expected advantages, under ideal circumstances, in binaural over monaural fitting would include: (1) improved SRT, (2) improved discrimination, particularly in noise, (3) improved threshold of discomfort, and (4) better localization of sound. These expected improvements, particularly discrimination, however, have been elusive when submitted to experimental testing. Even the wearer's beliefs in the superiority of binaural over monaural hearing aids have been difficult if not impossible to quantify to date (33).

The arguments continue. The audiologist apparently suspects that the hearing aid dealer is often merely trying to sell binaural aids to double his profit, and the hearing aid dealer, in turn, wonders why the audiologist can't appreciate the value of binaural aids when the user often reports greater satisfaction with them. The difficulties in demonstrating significant differences between monaural and binaural hearing aids in the clinic may revolve around our relative lack of precision in speech audiometry (as was discussed in Chapter 7), or we may simply have failed to find the tests or test parameters that might reveal these differences. The rich—if confusing—research in this matter will not be reviewed here; the bibliography at the end of this chapter contains important items on the subject which the interested reader will want to study. For a more complete review of binaural hearing and hearing aids, see the article by Berger (8).

---

in their case correct the hearing loss, they refuse to have such surgery and are, in fact, adamant in their unwillingness to seek medical opinion. With a clear explanation of the alternatives in these cases, we have gone ahead with the hearing aid evaluation. Nor should we refuse help to those whose religious beliefs forbid medical consultation, but who do not consider a hearing aid in this category.

Since the audiologist has difficulty in objectively showing an improvement in speech audiometric test scores in favor of binaural aids, and since he is loathe to recommend binaural aids unless he can show such evidence, a few suggested guidelines may be helpful. The audiologist will need to consider each patient from the standpoint of his own needs and impairment when considering a binaural hearing aid. Thus, if a person's vocation requires localization or communication from both sides, a binaural aid may be recommended. Perhaps it should not be a primary consideration, but often the fact that a person does not wear eyeglasses tends to rule out the binaural aid, since the glasses afford a handy method of binaural fitting. Two behind-the-ear aids, of course, can just as easily be fitted. In cases of more severe hearing losses, the binaural fitting can be done by means of two body-style hearing aids, although there have been few binaural body aids manufactured. Another consideration that suggests the likelihood of better hearing through binaural amplification occurs when the patient's work requires him to be in intermittent noise that is not too high in intensity. The price of binaural aids is, of course, a factor that cannot be dismissed, which is probably one of the main reasons why the audiologist is rather conservative in his approach to this matter.

As a general rule we have found that the more different the two ears are in the threshold pure-tone audiogram, or the more different the two ears are in the speech discrimination score, the less likely a binaural aid will be useful.

Undoubtedly the most common hearing aid fitting provides for a microphone on one side of the head, connected via the amplifier unit to a receiver in the ear on the same side of the head. Thus, usually the entire hearing aid is situated on or near the right ear, or left ear (which are monaural fittings), or there are aids at both ears (binaural fitting). Figure 14.12 shows this in diagrammatic form. There are quite a number of other variations for particular hearing problems which have lately interested the audiologist. Referring to Figure 14.12, we can see these more common fittings as well as a number of other possibilities:

1. Monaural fitting. The aid is at the right ear or left ear.
2. Binaural fitting. Aids are at both the right and left ears.
3. Across-head fitting. The microphone at the right ear leads to a receiver at the left ear (usually via a headband or through eyeglass frames), or a microphone at the left ear leads to the receiver at the right ear. This is sometimes referred to as CROS fitting.
4. Criss-cross fitting. A microphone at the right ear leads to a receiver at the left ear, *and* a microphone at the left ear leads to a receiver at the right ear.
5. Monaural and Across-head fitting. A microphone at the right ear leads to receivers in *both* ears, or a microphone at the left ear leads to

receivers in both ears. This is an ear-level version of the Y-cord fitting.

6. Binaural and Across-head fitting. A microphone at the right ear leads to receivers in each ear and a microphone at the left ear leads to receivers in each ear.

The usefulness of each of these variations in fitting is far from clear, but they do make it possible to help some individuals with particular hearing impairments and particular amplification needs. For instance, they enable us to avoid a chronic draining ear and to still receive sound from that side; or they allow the person with a unilateral hearing loss to gain some binaural hearing. Initial research and reports on these various fittings to appear include the articles by Fowler (41), Harford and Barry (51), Harford and Musket (53), Malles (84), and Miller (91).

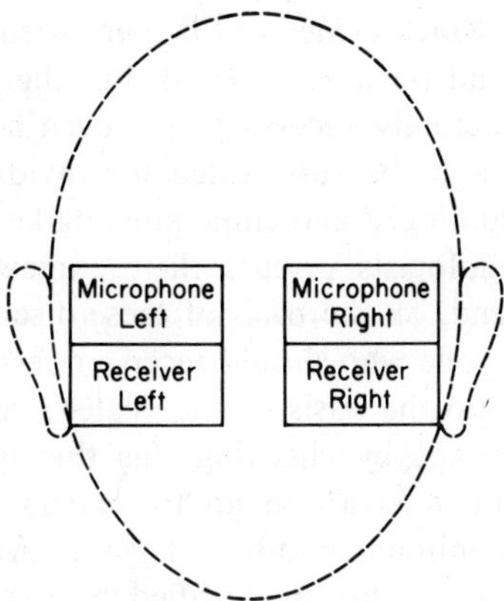

FIGURE 14.12 Typical location of microphone(s) and receiver(s) for hearing aid fitting.

Related to the renewed attention to various types of across-the-head hearing aid fittings, modifications of the earmold has also been of great help for special hearing aid needs. An example of this is the so-called open earmold. This usually consists of a plasting ring which fits around the bowl of the external ear and to which is attached the tubing leading from the hearing aid; the canal portion found in most earmolds is absent or else so open that it forms only a thin cylinder around the outer opening of the external auditory canal.

With the open earmold the ear can receive unamplified sound, for instance from the telephone, but amplified sound (from either the same side or the other side of the head) is also directed to the ear. Because of feedback problems, the open earmold is not useful in the case of a severe hearing loss.

The Hearing Aid Dealer

Enough has been written and said in meetings and in the journals of the professions of otology, audiology, and hearing aid dealers, as well as in several government reports (e.g., subcommittee on antitrust and monopoly, 120, 122) about the practices of hearing aid dealers, that further discussion here is unwarranted. Needless to say, the dealers and the manufacturer who are just barely within legal limits or who practice and advertise unethically have received considerable comment. It is perhaps unfortunate that much of the discussion and publication regarding dealers has been negative, and while some of this is justified, it does not do justice to the hearing aid dealer who does perform and advertise ethically and who does try to keep up with the latest professional matters in his field.

One of the problems the audiologist and the clinic must face is which dealers to refer to, and which dealer will be permitted to have representative aids in the clinic for trial purposes.[6] In all but the hearing aid evaluation procedure no aids are actually necessary, and even here the use of a master hearing aid test unit might be substituted for invidual instruments.

In some way the audiologist and clinic must make choices among hearing aid dealers. Some audiologists discuss their clinical evaluation programs with the local dealers and, on the basis of these discussions, decide whether the dealer in question is one who should receive referrals. Other audiologists choose referral dealers on the basis of the dealer's reputation and standing in the community, perhaps by checking this through the Better Business Bureau, or by requiring referrals to go to dealers who have been in the community for some minimum number of years. Another possibility is to refer to hearing aid dealers who are certified by the National Hearing Aid Society. Certification by N.H.A.S. requires the dealer to pass a written examination covering a twenty-lesson home study course and to subscribe to that organization's code of ethics. Since the audiologist's main concern in referring to dealers is that they have reasonable training and abide by ethical practices, this solution seems practical. On the other hand, some audiologists criticize the training requirements of N.H.A.S. as being too little; but it is our personal feeling that although the requirements are not high, they are far better than anything to date in the hearing aid industry. For those clinics making occasional referrals to distant points, it is handy to have the national list of members certified by N.H.A.S.[7]

The clinic that has representative models of several brands of hearing

[6] That referrals to hearing aid dealers by clinics is a small but still substantial part of their sales is revealed by H.A.I.C. data for July 1, 1965 through July 1, 1966, which shows that 18 per cent of hearing aid sales had been referred by clinics and 11 per cent by physicians (*National Hearing Aid Journal*, **20**: No. 1, 1966).

[7] Available from the National Hearing Aid Society, 24261 Grand River Ave., Detroit, Michigan 48219.

aids on loan from the local dealers or from manufacturers also has certain obligations to those dealers and manufacturers. First, the clinic should not request more models of hearing aids than can routinely be evaluated in the course of a typical schedule for that clinic. A huge number of loan aids in the clinic is not desirable from any standpoint; representative aids, insofar as frequency and gain response are concerned, are sufficient for most clinical evaluation procedures. Some clinics find it useful to use a "master hearing aid" and keep on hand only one or two models of each style of aid, or even simple "dummy" models of the various styles. The local hearing aid dealer or the manufacturer's representative should have ready access to his own aids, so that he may check their condition and replace them with newer models periodically, and he should be expected to make such checks. Finally, the dealer or manufacturer and the clinic should have a clear agreement that either may request the removal of any or all aids upon proper notice to the other party. Precautions to avoid damage to the aids on loan to the clinic are, of course, the responsibility of the audiologist, and he should not loan an aid to an individual without permission from the dealer or the manufacturer originally loaning the instrument.

HEARING AID LEGISLATION

The first state to enact a law regulating the sale and fitting of hearing aids was Oregon (6, 13, 14). Now, after a decade under that law, the hearing-aid dealers in Oregon are evidently performing their work in a more ethical manner than before; and the majority seem to feel that the law has not hampered them. Since the Oregon law went into effect, a number of other states have had similar legislation introduced.

In 1966 Michigan passed a hearing aid licensing act, somewhat more strict than that of Oregon. It requires that all hearing aid dealers be licensed, which in turn requires them to pass a test of competency. Also, like the Oregon law, the Michigan law forbids unethical advertising, but the specifics are not entirely clear. In addition, the Michigan law forbids soliciting from door-to-door and requires that children (defined as sixteen years old and younger) have certain otological and audiological examinations prior to fitting.

Following the enactment of the Michigan law, the Hearing Aid Industry Conference (H.A.I.C.) went on record against all such licensing, but amended their stand to support decisions of state associations of dealers regarding licensing. The National Hearing Aid Society supported licensing in those states where the state association favored a specific bill, and opposed legislation in those states where that association was against the specific bill.[8] Not all dealers or manufacturers are in agreement with the stands of H.A.I.C. or N.H.A.S.

[8] In 1966, the Federal Trade Commission recommended that legislation regarding sales and fitting of hearing aids be introduced in each state. The Council of State Governments, in turn, published a suggested bill.

At the present time there are a total of nineteen states with legislation on the fitting and selling of hearing aids. Most of these laws require the licensed dealer to pass some sort of written and practical state-administered examination covering basic audiometric testing and hearing aid fitting, and most laws outline, in broad form, some restriction of so-called "bait" advertising and door-to-door canvassing. The laws generally set up a board of hearing aid dealers (or dealers and otologists and audiologists) to handle the testing of candidates and sometimes to actually administer the law.

The various laws and acts are generally restrictive in that they forbid the dealer from doing certain specific things. The earliest bills were usually introduced into state legislatures as a result of complaints about excesses in hearing aid sales. The audiologist could, but usually does not and should not, add numerous confirmed reports of grossly misfit hearing aids. How shall the audiologist react to such hearing aid dealer licensing?

There are good and bad features to the various hearing aid licensing laws and bills. Most of them do provide penalties for gross misrepresentation and gross unethical conduct. Thus, the laws are likely to hurt the unethical dealer most—and many hearing aid dealers who are in favor of licensing recognize this. There is some dissatisfaction on the part of the audiologist inasmuch as licensing gives the dealer an aura of professionalism as an audiologist, without requiring formal training on his part. In other words, weak bills give the hearing aid dealer a legal santion to do what he is now doing and may not be doing well. For this reason, the audiologist is often opposed to such licensing unless the bill requires that the individual purchasing the aid receive audiological and otological evaluation first. In particular, the audiologist feels children must be protected by having professional audiologic evaluation before being fit with a hearing aid; and such evaluation for the geriatric patient is probably just as necessary.

Ideally the audiologist would like all persons, regardless of age, who have a hearing loss to be examined by an otolaryngologist, then evaluated by an audiologist, and if a hearing aid is likely to be of value, to be referred to the hearing aid dealer. The hearing aid dealer is quick to state that he does not believe a person should be sold a hearing aid if he does not need one or cannot use one; if the procedures just mentioned were followed, it is difficult to see how the dealer would sell any fewer hearing aids. And, certainly, the hearing-impaired patient would have the best of professional advice from three groups which are interested in his welfare.

The authors are mindful of how tentative many of their statements have been and must be. What we have tried to discuss and review herein may soon be dated. We only need recall that Mandl's book (85) on hearing aid repair contained little more than a paragraph about the transistor, yet in a few years the vacuum tube disappeared from hearing aid design and the transistor became the basic component of all electronic aids.

It is quite possible that many questions and problems of today will be clear in a few years; they may be answered by the rather impressive growth in research in audiology clinics and manufacturer's laboratories around the world. The future, then affords great promise for the public in need of hearing aids. The by-products of military and space research may be expected to provide amplification in a smaller package but also with better control of acoustic performance. A surgically implanted hearing aid with a long-life battery has been reported, but the practicality of this procedure still seems somewhere in the hazy future. Meanwhile, we can expect greater knowledge of genetic, prenatal, and natal influences to lessen the number of congenital hearing losses, while our longer life expectancy will undoubtedly increase hearing aid needs in the geriatric population. The future, too, will be challenging to the otolaryngologist, the audiologist, and the hearing aid dealer, in that they must keep abreast of what promises to be rapid changes in the use of hearing aid amplification.

Bibliography

1. Adams, E. L. "Adjustment of the hard-of-hearing after leaving the service." *U.S. Naval Medical Bulletin*, Supplement: 249–52, March 1946.
2. Anderson, T. B. and J. W. Black. "An experimental study of the evaluation of hearing aids." *Southern Speech Journal*, **16**: 278–80, 1951.
3. Bangs, J. L. and T. E. Bangs. "Hearing aids for young children." *Archives of Otolaryngology*, **55**: 528–35, 1952.
4. Barton, R. T. "Relationships between private practitioners in medicine, speech pathology, and audiology." *EENT Monthly*, **40**: 492–93, 1961.
5. Belzile, M. and D. M. Markle. "A clinical comparison of monaural and binaural hearing aids worn by patients with conductive or perceptive deafness." *Laryngoscope*, **69**: 1317–23, 1959.
6. Bennett, F. C. "Licensing in Oregon." *Audecibel*, **11:5**: 10, 16, 18, 20, 1962.
7. Bentzen, O. "Audiology and hearing-aid therapy." *Acta Oto-Laryngologica*, Supplement **140**: 24–32, 61–62, 1958.
8. Berger, K. W. "Binaural hearing—A review." *Audecibel*, **13:1**: 14–17, 32–34, 1964.
9. Berger, K. W. *The Hearing Aid: Its Operation and Development*. Detroit: National Hearing Aid Society, 1970.
10. Bergman, M. "Binaural hearing." *Archives of Otolaryngology*, **66**: 572–78, 1957.
11. Berkey, M. A. "The role of the hearing-aid audiologist." *Hearing Dealer*, **12:1**: 16–17, 1962.
12. Bishop, O. E. "Packaged power from tubes to transistors." *National Hearing Aid Journal*, **17:9**: 8, 25, 1964.
13. Blakely, R. W., D. H. Holden, and G. J. Leshin. "A preliminary report of the implementation of the Oregon hearing-aid law." *ASHA*, **2**: 171–74, 1960.

14. Blakely, R. W. and G. J. Leshin. "One year of implementation of the Oregon hearing aid law." *ASHA*, **4**: 7–14, 1962.
15. Borrild, K., E. Christiansen, H. H. Ohrt, and C. Rojskjaer. "Some results of hearing aid treatment at a boarding school for profoundly deaf children." *Acta Oto-Laryngologica*, Supplement **140**: 111–14, 1958.
16. Briskey, R. J. "The importance of low frequency amplification in deaf children." *Audecibel*, **15:1**: 7–10, 12–20, 1966.
17. Carhart, R. "Hearing aid selection by university clinics." *Journal of Speech and Hearing Disorders*, **15**: 106–13, 1950.
18. Carhart, R. "A practical approach to the selection of hearing aids." *Transactions of the American Academy of Ophthalmology and Otolaryngology*, **50**: 123–31, 1946.
19. Carhart, R. "Selection of hearing aids." *Archives of Otolaryngology*, **44**: 1–18, 1946.
20. Carhart, R. "Tests for selection of hearing aids." *Laryngoscope*, **56**: 680–794, 1946.
21. Carhart, R. "Volume control adjustment in hearing aid selection." *Laryngoscope*, **56**: 510–26, 1946.
22. Carhart, R. "The usefulness of the binaural hearing aid." *Journal of Speech and Hearing Disorders*, **23**: 42–51, 1958.
23. Carhart, R. and E. Thompson. "The fitting of hearing aids." *Transactions of the American Academy of Ophthalmology and Otolaryngology*, **51**: 354–61, 1947.
24. Coogle, K. L. "Acoustics of the earmold." *National Hearing Aid Journal*, **16:3**: 10–11, 1963.
25. Corliss, E. L. *Selection of Hearing Aids*. Washington, D.C.: National Bureau of Standards, Circular 516, 1951.
26. Corliss, E. L. and G. S. Cook. "Cavity pressure method for measuring the gain of hearing aids." *Journal of Research of the National Bureau of Standards*, **40**: 85–91, 1948.
27. Daniel, E. and J. Delk. "Taking impressions for earmolds for infants and children." *Audecibel*, **10**: 8, 11, 1961.
28. Davis, H., S. S. Stevens, and R. H. Nichols, Jr. *Hearing Aids*. Cambridge, Mass.: Harvard University Press, 1947. (*See* also next item.)
29. Davis, H., C. V. Hudgins, R. J. Marquis, R. H. Nichols, Jr., G. E. Peterson, D. A. Ross, and S. S. Stevens. "The selection of hearing aids." *Laryngoscope*, **56**: 85–115, 135–63, 1946.
30. Davis, H. and S. R. Silverman, eds. *Hearing and Deafness*. New York: Holt, Rinehart, & Winston, Inc., 1947 (1962). See particularly Chapter 10, "Hearing Aids" by Silverman, Taylor, and Davis; Chapter 11, "The choice and use of hearing aids" by Silverman and Taylor.
31. Day, K. M. "Aids to hearing." *Laryngoscope*, **64**: 1–9, 1954.
32. DiCarlo, L. M. and W. J. Brown. "The effectiveness of binaural hearing for adults with hearing impairment." *Journal of Auditory Research*, **1**: 35–76, 1960.
33. Dirks, D. and R. Carhart. "A survey of reactions from users of binaural and monaural hearing aids." *Journal of Speech and Hearing Disorders*, **27**: 311–22, 1962.

34. Downs, M. P. "Hearing aids and the young child." *Audecibel*, **13**: 56–59, 76–77, 1964.
35. Downs, M. P. "Children are different." *National Hearing Aid Journal*, **19:7**: 10, 34, 1966.
36. Edgardh, B. H. "The use of extreme limitation for the dynamic equalization of vowels and consonants in hearing aids." *Acta Oto-Laryngologica*, **40**: 376–82, 1951–52.
37. Elkin, V. B. "The relationship between personality characteristics and efficiency in the use of aural sensory aids by a group of acoustically handicapped patients." Ph.D. dissertation. New York: New York University, 1952.
38. Ewertsen, H. W. "Hearing-aid evaluation." *Archives of Otolaryngology*, **64**: 520–25, 1956.
39. Ewertsen, H. W., J. B. Ipsen, and S. S. Nielsen. "On acoustical characteristics of earmolds." *Acta Oto-Laryngologica*, **47**: 312–17, 1957.
40. Ewertsen, H. W. and M. Nielsen. "Soft earmold." *Acta Oto-Laryngologica*, **47**: 231–32, 1957.
41. Fowler, E. P. "Bilateral hearing aids for monaural total deafness." *Archives of Otolaryngology*, **72**: 41–42, 1960.
42. Fry, D. and P. Denes. *The Testing of Hearing Aids*. (Booklet 490). London: National Institute for the Deaf, 1951.
43. Fry, D. B. "The development of the phonological system in the normal and the deaf child." In F. Smith and G. A. Miller, eds., *The Genesis of Language*. Cambridge, Mass.: M. I. T. Press, 1966.
44. Gillespie, M. E., M. R. Gillespie, and J. E. Creston. "Clinical evaluation of a 'master hearing aid.'" *Archives of Otolaryngology*, **82**: 515–17, 1965.
45. Glorig, A. "Principles involved in selecting a hearing aid." *Acta Oto-Laryngologica*, **41**: 49–57, 1952.
46. Greenbaum, W. H. "Why choose the silver oxide battery?" *National Hearing Aid Journal*, **16**: 4–5, 19, 30, 1963.
47. Groen, J. J. and J. W. Tappin. "A comparison of the physical characteristics of five well-known hearing aids with the theoretical and apparent subjective needs of the patient." *Journal of Laryngology and Otology*, **56**: 604–13, 1952.
48. Grossman, F. M. "Acoustic sound filtration and hearing aids." *Archives of Otolaryngology*, **38**: 101–12, 1943.
49. Guilford, F. R. and C. O. Haug. "The otologist and the hearing aid." *Archives of Otolaryngology*, **61**: 9–15, 1955.
50. Güttner, W. "History of the hearing aid." Reprint from *SRW Nachrichten*, n.d., No. 21, 23, 24.
51. Harford, E. and J. Barry. "A rehabilitation approach to the problem of unilateral hearing impairment with contralateral routing of signals (CROS)." *Journal of Speech and Hearing Disorders*, **30**: 121–38, 1965. (Also see correction on p. 268).
52. Harford, E. R. and D. M. Markle. "The typical effect of a hearing aid on one patient with congenital deafness." *Laryngoscope*, **65**: 970–72, 1955.
53. Harford, E. R. and C. H. Musket. "Binaural hearing with one aid." *Journal of Speech and Hearing Disorders*, **29**: 133–46, 1964.
54. Harford, E. R. and C. H. Musket. "Some considerations in the organization

and administration of a clinical hearing aid selection program." *ASHA*, **6**: 35–40, 1964.

55. Harris, J. D., H. L. Haines, P. A. Keisey, and T. D. Clack. "The relation between speech intelligibility and the electroacoustic characteristics of low fidelity circuitry." *Journal of Audiological Research*, **1**: 357–81, 1961.
56. Haskins, H. L. and W. G. Hardy. "Clinical studies in stereophonic hearing." *Laryngoscope*, **70**: 1427–32, 1960.
57. Haug, O., F. R. Guilford, R. R. Sattin, and P. A. Baccaro. "A comparison of hearing aid evaluation test instruments and aids purchased from dealers." *Volta Review*, **65**: 26–29, 1963.
58. Hedgecock, L. D. and B. V. Sheets. "A comparison of monaural and ninaural hearing aids for listening to speech." *Archives of Otolaryngology*, **68**: 624–29, 1958.
59. Hedgecock, L. D. "Prediction of the efficiency of hearing aids from the audiogram." Doctoral dissertation. Madison: University of Wisconsin, 1949.
60. Hedgecock, L. D. "A university hearing aid clinic." *Journal of Speech Disorders*, **12**: 323–30, 1947.
61. Herdt, M. P. "A comparison of the performance of five pairs of transistor and vacuum tube hearing aids." Masters thesis. College Park: University of Maryland, 1954.
62. Hilger, J. A., A. Glorig, and W. Mueller. "The facts about hearing aid fitting." *Transactions of the American Academy of Ophthalmology and Otolaryngology*, **59**: 617–29, 1955.
63. Hirsh, I. J. "Binaural hearing aids: A review of some experiments." *Journal of Speech and Hearing Disorders*, **15**: 114–23, 1950.
64. Hirsh, I. J. "Teaching the deaf to speak." In F. Smith and G. A. Miller, eds., *The Genesis of Language*. Cambridge, Mass.: M. I. T. Press, 1966.
65. Holcomb, A. L. "Adjusting the patient to the hearing aid." *Archives of Otolaryngology*, **68**: 367–71, 1958.
66. Hughson, W. and E. Thompson. "The hearing aid from the patient's point of view." *Archives of Otolaryngology*, **38**: 252–60, 1943.
67. Hughson, W. and E. Thompson. "Hearing aids." *Archives of Otolaryngology*, **39**: 245–49, 1944.
68. Huitzing, H. C. and M. Taselaar. "Experiments on binaural hearing." *Acta Oto-Laryngologica*, **53**: 151–54, 1961.
69. Ingall, B. I. "Discussion on the use of hearing aid equipment in schools for the deaf." *Teacher of the Deaf*, **58**: 239–43, 1960.
70. Jeffers, J. "Quality judgement in hearing aid selection." *Journal of Speech and Hearing Disorders*, **25**: 259–66, 1960.
71. Jeffers, J. and C. Smith. "On hearing aid selection, in part a reply to Resnick and Becker." *ASHA*, **6**: 504–06, 1964.
72. Jerger, J. and D. Dirks. "Binaural hearing aids—an enigma." *Journal of the Acoustical Society of America*, **33**: 537–38, 1961.
73. Jerger, J., C. Speaks, and C. Malmquist. "Hearing aid performance and hearing aid selection." *Journal of Speech and Hearing Research*, **9**: 136–49, 1966.
74. Jerger, J., C. Malmquist, and C. Speaks. "Comparison of some speech intelligibility tests in the evaluation of hearing aid performance." *Journal of Speech and Hearing Research*, **9**: 253–58, 1966.

75. Keys, J. W. "Binaural versus monaural hearing." *Journal of the Acoustical Society of America*, **19**: 629–31, 1947.
76. Kinney, C. E. "The further destruction of partially deafened children's hearing by the use of powerful hearing aids." *Annals of Otology, Rhinology and Laryngology*, **70**: 828–35 1961. Also see *Transactions of the American Otological Society*, 230–44, 1961, which includes discussion.
77. Kodicek, J. and J. Garrard. "The hearing aid in use." *Journal of Laryngology and Otology*, **68**: 406–09, 1954.
78. Kodman, F., Jr. "Some attitudes of unsuccessful hearing aid users." *Eye, Ear, Nose, and Throat Monthly*, **40**: 405–7, 1961.
79. Kodman, F., Jr. "Successful binaural hearing aid users." *Archives of Otolaryngology*, **74**: 302–04, 1961.
80. Ling, D. "Implications of hearing aid amplification below 300 cps." *Volta Review*, **66**: 723–29, 1964.
81. Lybarger, S. F. *The Earmold as a Part of the Receiver Acoustic System.* Canonsburg, Pa.: Radioear Corp., n.d.
82. Lybarger, S. F. "A new standard for measuring hearing-aid performance." *ASHA*, **3**: 121–22, 1961. Also see *Audecibel*, **10**: 2, 8–10, 24–25, 1961.
83. Lynn, G. and R. Carhart. "Influence of attack and release in compression amplification on understanding of speech by hypoacusics." *Journal of Speech and Hearing Disorders*, **28**: 124–39, 1963.
84. Malles, I. "Hearing aid effect in unilateral conductive deafness." *Archives of Otolaryngology*, **77**: 406–8, 1963.
85. Mandl, M. *Hearing Aids.* New York: The Macmillan Company, 1953.
86. Markle, D. M. and W. Aber. "A clinical evaluation of monaural and binaural hearing aids." *Archives of Otolaryngology*, **67**: 606–08, 1958.
87. Markle, D. M. and A. Zaner. "The determination of 'gain requirements' of hearing aids: A new method." *Journal of Auditory Research*, **6**: 371–77, 1966.
88. McConnell, F., E. F. Silver, and D. McDonald. "Test-retest consistency of clinical hearing aid tests." *Journal of Speech and Hearing Disorders*, **25**: 273–80, 1960.
89. Menzel, O. J. "The earmold: Orphan of the hearing aid industry." *EENT Monthly*, **43**: 104–5, 1964.
90. Miller, A. A., J. M. McCauley, C. Fraser, and C. Cubert. "Psychological factors in adaptation to hearing aids." *American Journal of Orthopsychiatry*, **29**: 121–29, 1959.
91. Miller, A. L. "A case of severe unilateral hearing loss helped by a hearing aid." *Journal of Speech and Hearing Disorders*, **30**: 186–87, 1965.
92. Millin, J. P. "Conventional hearing aid selection." *ASHA*, **5**: 880–81, 1963.
93. Millin, J. P. "Speech discrimination as a function of hearing-aid gain: Implications in hearing-aid evaluation." Masters thesis. Cleveland, Ohio: Western Reserve University, 1965.
94. Millin, J. P. "Counseling the adventitiously hearing impaired adults." *Ohio Journal of Speech and Hearing*, **2**: 46–54, 1966.
95. Millin, J. P. "The effect of small room reverberation on discrimination tests." Doctoral dissertation. Cleveland, Ohio: Case-Western Reserve University, 1968.

96. Mueller, W. "The fitting of hearing aids as an office procedure." *Laryngoscope*, **63**: 581–92, 1953.
97. Naunton, R. F. "The effect of hearing aid use upon the user's residual hearing." *Laryngoscope*, **67**: 569–76, 1957.
98. Nichols, R. H., Jr., R. J. Marquis, W. J. Wiklund, A. S. Filler, C. V. Hudgins, and G. E. Peterson. "The influence of body-effects on the performance of hearing aids." *Journal of the Acoustical Society of America*, **19**: 943–51, 1947.
99. Oyer, H. J. *Auditory Communication for the Hard of Hearing*. Englewood Cliffs, N.J.: Prentice-Hall, Inc., 1966.
100. Pattee, G. L. and L. A. Cary. "The use and abuse of hearing aids." *Archives of Otolaryngology*, **65**: 269–74, 1957.
101. Raymond, T. H. and G. P. Proud. "Audiofrequency conversion." *Archives of Otolaryngology*, **76**: 436–46, 1962.
102. Reddell, R. C. and D. R. Calvert. "Selecting a hearing aid by interpreting audiologic data." *Journal of Auditory Research*, **6**: 445–52, 1966.
103. Reeves, J. K. "The use of hearing aids by children with defective hearing." *Teacher of the Deaf*, **59**: 181–90, 1961.
104. Reeves, J. K. "Listen to this—some parental attitudes and social attitudes toward children using hearing aids." *Volta Review*, **64**: 314–16, 1962.
105. Resnick, D. M. and M. Becker. "Hearing aid evaluation—a new approach." *ASHA*, **5**: 695–99, 1963.
106. Roach, R. E. "A study of the comparative value of the hearing clinic program and commercial service for the difficult hearing aid case." Illinois Division of Vocational Rehabilitation, n.d.
107. Romanow, F. F. "Methods for measuring the performance of hearing aids." *Bell Technical Monograph*, B-1314, 1940. Also see *Journal of the Acoustical Society of America*, **13**: 294–304, 1942.
108. Rushford, G. and E. L. Lowell. "Use of hearing aids by young children." *Journal of Speech and Hearing Research*, **3**: 354–60, 1960.
109. Schachtel, I. I. *Know Your Hearing Aid.* Elmsford, N.Y.: Sonotone Corp., n.d. Seven articles reprinted from *Hearing News*, 1948.
110. Sedacca, Y. C. *Basic Audio Information for Hearing Aid Consultants.* New York: Hal-Hen Widex, Inc., n.d. Also appeared in *National Hearing Aid Journal*, **15:4**: 10–11, 1962 and **15**: 5, 10, 12, 38, 1962.
111. Segard, J. J., E. C. Hinnant, and R. L. McCroskey. "Georgia takes a critical look at aural rehabilitation." *Journal of Rehabilitation*, **27**: 6, 24–25, 1961.
112. Seligman, D. "Hearing aid orientation for young hard of hearing children." *Exceptional Children*, **28**: 268–70, 1962.
113. Senturia, E., S. R. Silverman, and C. E. Harrison. "A hearing aid clinic." *Journal of Speech and Hearing Disorders*, **8**: 215–26, 1943.
114. Sheets, B. V. and L. D. Hedgecock. "Hearing aid amplification for optimum speech reproduction." *Journal of Speech and Hearing Disorders*, **14**: 373–79, 1949.
115. Shore, I. and J. C. Kramer. "A comparison of two procedures for hearing-aid evaluation." *Journal of Speech and Hearing Disorders*, **28**: 159–70, 1963.
116. Shore, I., R. C. Bilger, and I. J. Hirsh. "Hearing aid evaluation: Reliability of repeated measurements." *Journal of Speech and Hearing Disorders*, **25**: 152–70, 1960.

117. Siegenthaler, B. M. "The use of hearing aids by public school children." *Archives of Otolaryngology*, **68**: 367–71, 1958.
118. Silverman, S. R. "A clinical comparison of air and bone conduction hearing aids in cases of conductive impairment of hearing." *Journal of the Acoustical Society of America*, **16**: 108–12, 1944.
119. Simonsen, B. "The world situation in hearing aids—1969." *National Hearing Aid Journal*, **22:6**: 10–11, 1969.
120. Stein, L. "Special report on the Senate antitrust subcommittee hearing on the prices of hearing aids." *ASHA*, **4**: 206–16, 1962.
121. Strommen, E. "Statistical trends among hearing aid users." *Journal of the Acoustical Society of America*, **15**: 211–22, 1944.
122. Subcommittee on antitrust and monopoly. *Prices of Hearing Aids*. 87th Congress, 2nd Session. Washington, D.C.: U.S. Government Printing office, 1962, 533 pp. Supplementary report, 123 pp.
123. Victoreen, J. A. "The audiologist and the hearing instrument dispenser." *Volta Review*, **65**: 76–78, 87, 1963.
124. Wansdronk, C. "On the influence of the diffraction of sound waves around the human head on the characteristics of hearing aids." *Journal of the Acoustical Society of America*, **31**: 1609–12, 1959.
125. Wasson, H. W. "A multifilter circuit simulating representative hearing aids suggested for hearing aid selection." *Journal of Auditory Research*, **3**: 185–88, 1963.
126. Watson, L. and T. Tolan. *Hearing Tests and Hearing Instruments*. Baltimore: The Williams and Wilkins Co., 1949.
127. Watson, H. Z. and V. O. Knudsen. "Selective amplification in hearing aids." *Journal of the Acoustical Society of America*, **11**: 406–19, 1940.
128. Watson, T. J. "The use of hearing aids for severely deaf children." *Archives of Otolaryngology*, **64**: 151–56, 1956.
129. Watson, T. J. "The use of residual hearing in the education of deaf children. Part III: Hearing aids." *Volta Review*, **63**: 435–40, 1961.
130. Whetnall, E. "The Medresco aid: Running a deafness clinic." *Acta Oto-Laryngologica*, Supplement **90**: 73–84, 1950.
131. Wiener, F. M. and G. A. Miller. "Hearing aids." In *Combat Instrumentation II*. Washington, D.C.: NDRC Report **117**: 216–32, 1946.
132. Wright, H. N. "Binaural hearing and the hearing-impaired." *Archives of Otolaryngology*, **70**: 485–94, 1959.
133. Wright, H. N. and R. Carhart. "The efficiency of binaural listening among the hearing impaired." *Archives of Otolaryngology*, **72**: 789–97, 1960.
134. Yantis, P. A., J. P. Millin, and I. Shapiro. "Speech discrimination in sensori-neural hearing loss: Two experiments on the role of intensity." *Journal of Speech and Hearing Research*, **9**: 178–93, 1966.
135. Zerlin, S. "A new approach to hearing-aid selection." *Journal of Speech and Hearing Research*, **5**: 370–76, 1962.
136. Zerlin, S. and E. D. Burnett. "Effects of harmonic and intermodulation distortion on speech intelligibility." *Journal of the Acoustical Society of America*, **32**: 1501–02, 1960.
137. Zymkowitz, E. C. "A new era of energy sources." *Audecibel*, **12:4**: 20–22, 24, 1963.

Index

B

C

D

G

H

I

J

K

L

M

P

Q

R

S

T